Immune System and Immunology

Immune System and Immunology

Edited by Dallas Ford

STATES
ACADEMIC PRESS
www.statesacademicpress.com

States Academic Press,
109 South 5th Street,
Brooklyn, NY 11249, USA

Visit us on the World Wide Web at:
www.statesacademicpress.com

ISBN: 978-1-63989-282-2

Cataloging-in-Publication Data

Immune system and immunology / edited by Dallas Ford.
p. cm.
Includes bibliographical references and index.
ISBN 978-1-63989-282-2
1. Immune system. 2. immunology. I. Ford, Dallas.
QR181 .I46 2022
616.079--dc23

Table of Contents

Preface

Immune system refers to the network of all the biological processes that protect an organism from diseases and foreign micro-organisms. It detects a wide range of pathogens, cancer cells and other objects, distinguishes them from the healthy tissues of the organism and responds to them. There are two major subsystems of the immune system, namely, innate immune system and adaptive immune system. Innate immune system relies on the body's ability to recognize the pathogens while adaptive immune response is based on specialized, systemic cells and processes that prevent the growth of pathogens and eliminate them. Immunology is the branch of science that deals with the study of immune systems in all organisms. It has applications in several disciplines of medicine such as oncology, virology, organ transplantation, etc. This book unravels the recent studies in the field of immunology. It presents researches and studies performed by experts across the globe. This book will serve as a reference to a broad spectrum of readers.

Various studies have approached the subject by analyzing it with a single perspective, but the present book provides diverse methodologies and techniques to address this field. This book contains theories and applications needed for understanding the subject from different perspectives. The aim is to keep the readers informed about the progresses in the field; therefore, the contributions were carefully examined to compile novel researches by specialists from across the globe.

Indeed, the job of the editor is the most crucial and challenging in compiling all chapters into a single book. In the end, I would extend my sincere thanks to the chapter authors for their profound work. I am also thankful for the support provided by my family and colleagues during the compilation of this book.

Editor

Preface

1

Stressful presentations: mild cold stress in laboratory mice influences phenotype of dendritic cells in naïve and tumor-bearing mice

Kathleen M. Kokolus, Haley M. Spangler, Benjamin J. Povinelli, Matthew R. Farren, Kelvin P. Lee and Elizabeth A. Repasky*

Department of Immunology, Roswell Park Cancer Institute, Buffalo, NY, USA

Edited by:
Lisa Helene Butterfield, University of Pittsburgh, USA

Reviewed by:
Gregory B. Lesinski, The Ohio State University Comprehensive Cancer Center, USA
Masoud H. Manjili, Virginia Commonwealth University, USA
Shari Pilon-Thomas, Moffitt Cancer Center, USA

****Correspondence:***
Elizabeth A. Repasky, Department of Immunology, Roswell Park Cancer Institute, Elm and Carlton Streets, Buffalo, NY 14263, USA
e-mail: elizabeth.repasky@roswellpark.org

The ability of dendritic cells (DCs) to stimulate and regulate T cells is critical to effective anti-tumor immunity. Therefore, it is important to fully recognize any inherent factors which may influence DC function under experimental conditions, especially in laboratory mice since they are used so heavily to model immune responses. The goals of this report are to 1) briefly summarize previous work revealing how DCs respond to various forms of physiological stress and 2) to present new data highlighting the potential for chronic mild cold stress inherent to mice housed at the required standard ambient temperatures to influence baseline DCs properties in naïve and tumor-bearing mice. As recent data from our group shows that $CD8^{+}$ T cell function is significantly altered by chronic mild cold stress and since DC function is crucial for $CD8^{+}$ T cell activation, we wondered whether housing temperature may also be influencing DC function. Here we report that there are several significant phenotypical and functional differences among DC subsets in naïve and tumor-bearing mice housed at either standard housing temperature or at a thermoneutral ambient temperature, which significantly reduces the extent of cold stress. The new data presented here strongly suggests that, by itself, the housing temperature of mice can affect fundamental properties and functions of DCs. Therefore differences in basal levels of stress due to housing should be taken into consideration when interpreting experiments designed to evaluate the impact of additional variables, including other stressors on DC function.

Keywords: cold stress, thermoregulation, norepinephrine, mouse models of cancer, anti-tumor immunity

INTRODUCTION

Dendritic cells (DCs) play a vital role in the generation of effective and long-term immune protection from cancer and other diseases. DCs are antigen presenting cells, which educate tumor-specific T cells and provide signals for T cell proliferation and expansion (1, 2). Importantly, DCs bridge the innate and adaptive immune responses so their presence and functional capacity affect both arms of anti-tumor immunity (3, 4). Properties of DCs that are investigated to determine their stage of development include surface expression of major histocompatibility complex (MHC) class II molecules and co-stimulatory CD86 as well as cytokine production. Additionally, DCs are also being used clinically in cancer vaccines (5, 6) and this approach has rendered promising results; however, considerable room for improvement remains (7–9).

In addition to anti-tumor immunity and immune surveillance, DCs also participate in tolerizing the immune system to tumor antigens, which can render the anti-tumor immune response ineffective (10). Cross-presentation, a process that DCs undergo in order to activate $CD8^{+}$ T cells, plays a major role in generating anti-tumor immunity (11), however; when DCs of tumor-bearing hosts undergo this vital process, T cell tolerance often results (5). Recently, it has been reported that DCs able to up-regulate MHC II (signal 1) in the absence of CD86 (signal 2) become tolerogenic DCs (12, 13). Although considerable progress has been made toward understanding how DCs become tolerogenic (10, 14, 15), the precise mechanisms by which tumors modulate cross-priming to suppress the $CD8^{+}$ T cell response remain largely unknown. This incomplete understanding of the role DCs play in immune evasion remains a vital question as DCs are being actively investigated in mouse models to help reveal their role in the anti-tumor immune response. Therefore, it is important to fully recognize the impact of any inherent physiological factors in mice, which can alter DC function and to understand the impact these factors could have on experimental models of antigen presentation and immunotherapy.

We have been interested in the effects of various types of biologically relevant stress on the functional properties of immune cells (16) and have previously reported on the impact of mild (fever-range) heat stress on DC function (17, 18). It is important to note that there are a wide variety of stressors including physical, environmental, and emotional forms of stress that can alter homeostasis in cells or in the whole organism (19). Two major hormonally driven mechanisms are believed to mediate the influence of stress on the immune response. Glucocorticoids are released following stress leading to increased glucose metabolism necessary to provide extra energy to combat that stressor. Additionally, catecholamines, such as norepinephrine (NE), are released from sympathetic nerves and bind receptors on immune cells thereby impacting the immune response. Both of these hormonal mediators can influence immune processes including cell proliferation, migration, and cytokine production (20). Here, we first briefly summarize some of the previous work done to investigate the more specific effects of stress on DC function. While some studies show that acute, short term, stress may enhance DC function *in vitro*, resulting in a better ability to prime naïve T cells, other studies, particularly those which utilize the addition of exogenous stress hormones, reveal that stress impedes DC function *in vivo*. We outline reports suggesting a vital role of the stress hormone NE on DC function *in vivo* but not *in vitro*. We also summarize literature showing beneficial effects of a mild thermal stress on DC function both *in vitro* and *in vivo*. Finally, we report that when mice used to investigate DC function are housed at standard ambient temperatures they experience an underappreciated form of chronic physiological cold stress that alters the baseline used to understand the impact of experimental stressors or other treatments on DC function. We suggest that chronic mild cold stress, similar to other forms of stress inherent to mouse caging conditions including stress caused by lack of exercise and overeating (21), should be taken into consideration when assessing baseline properties of DCs in naïve or tumor-bearing mice.

STRESS CAN TARGET DC FUNCTION

Dendritic cells have already been the subject of many studies investigating the impact of stress on immune function. Acute stressors, lasting minutes to hours, have been shown to augment DC function as seen by enhanced maturation and increased trafficking from skin to lymph nodes (22, 23). Prior to immunization, specific kinds of acute stress, such as psychological stress induced by placing mice in restraints or on a slow moving shaker works as an adjuvant leading to increased DC migration from the skin to the lymph nodes and also improves antigen-specific T cell priming (24, 25). The impact of such acute psychological stress on DCs has also been investigated in humans. Social stress in human participants (induced by public speaking) generates a decrease in skin DCs, which the authors suggest indicates that these cells have trafficked to the lymph node (26) where they are available to interact with T cells and initiate immune activation. However, while some stressors may elicit beneficial effects on DC function and general immunity, chronic or excessive exposure to stress is generally thought to negatively influence immune function (27). Many studies, particularly those using exogenous administration of glucocorticoids, stress hormones which signal to turn down immune activity, suggest inhibitory effects of stress on DC function (28, 29). Both oral (30) and topical (31) application of glucocorticoids leads to a marked reduction in DC numbers. Many studies specifically investigate the impact of dexamethasone (DEX), a commonly prescribed glucocorticoid, on DC development and function. It has been shown that DEX greatly reduces epidermal DC numbers in mice (32, 33) as well as in the spleen, lymph node, and liver (34, 35). DEX treatment also limits DC migration to the draining lymph node (36). Additionally, DEX is correlated with reduced expression of surface maturation markers on DCs including CD86 and MHC class II (35, 37, 38). *In vitro*, DEX treatment reduces the ability of bone marrow (39, 40) and skin derived DCs (32, 41) as well as a murine epidermal DC line (42) to stimulate T cells. DEX also impairs antigen presentation by DCs reducing T cell activation *in vivo* (35). It has also been shown that following DEX treatment, DCs are unable to fully mature and these immature DCs induced a subpopulation of immunosuppressive regulatory T (T_{reg}) cells (39). Additionally a reduction of interleukin (IL)-1β and IL-12p70 secretion from DCs has been shown following DEX treatment (37). Compared to control cells, glucocorticoid-treated DCs produce less granulocyte macrophage colony-stimulating factor (GM-CSF), tumor necrosis factor-alpha (TNF-α) and IL-1α, all cytokines required for survival and maturation, and are less apt to initiate antigen presentation and migration (43). Further, treatment with other glucocorticoids (hydrocortisone or clobetasol) led to DC apoptosis identified by DNA damage, caspase-3 activity, and CD95 up-regulation (43).

Catecholamines, such as NE and epinephrine, also play an important role in mediating the relationship between stress and DCs. Manipulating the function of stress induced catecholamines has been linked to altered DC function (44). For example, when healthy patients were administered a β-adrenergic agonist (oral salbutamol), which mimics NE signaling, IL-12 production by DCs was decreased, inhibiting Th1 development (45). Another study found that NE similarly suppressed IL-12 production in a dose-dependent manner and that this was reversible with a glucocorticoid agonist, RU 486 (46). As Th1 and Th2 responses are mutually inhibitory, this leads to an increasingly prominent Th2 environment, which is defined by various immunosuppressive properties including inhibition of macrophage activation, T cell proliferation, and pro-inflammatory cytokine production (47). The effects of catecholamines may be most important to DCs in the early stages of antigen processing (44). Short term exposure of bone marrow-derived DCs to NE or epinephrine at the early stage of stimulation inhibits IL-12 and favors IL-10 production as well as a reduced ability to stimulate T cells (48). Skin DCs are also sensitive to catecholamine signaling. *In vitro*, treatment with NE, epinephrine, or β-adrenergic agonist (isoproterenol) hindered skin DCs from presenting antigen and this effect was reversed by treatment with ICI 118,551, a β_2-adrenergic antagonist (49). DC migration is NE dependent as demonstrated by decreased DC migration *in vivo* following NE depletion with 6-hydroxydopamine treatment (25). Additionally, NE has been shown to enhance phosphatidylinositol 3-kinase mediated antigen uptake by DCs (50). Taken together, these reports suggest that although some types of stress may benefit DCs under certain circumstances, it is generally accepted that chronic stress dampens many aspects of DC function.

EFFECTS OF MILD HYPERTHERMIA ON DCs

Environmental conditions have long been manipulated to create physiologically relevant stress. Thermal stress, induced when environmental conditions are either too hot or too cold to allow basal metabolism to maintain normal body temperature, is a classically studied stress in mice and humans (51). While conditions of severe heat or cold can be quite damaging to immunity, mild heat stress has been studied for its positive effects since ancient times because of its potential relationship to fever (52–55). In response to infection, body temperature increases to varying extents among different animals, but in all cases, homeostatic functions shift toward producing and conserving heat (52).

Generally, temperature elevation during fever ranges between 1 and 5°C above normal body temperatures (56–58). The physiological effects of fever have been mimicked experimentally by using mild hyperthermia treatments in mice, where body temperature is temporarily raised to fever-range (16). Many studies, including those from our own group, have examined how mild hyperthermia affects DCs and their function (17, 59–64).

Dendritic cell maturation is determined by the up-regulation of surface markers including MHC class II and CD86 (65, 66). Mild thermal stress increases levels of both of these markers on DCs (59). *In vitro* heating accelerates DC maturation as demonstrated by up-regulation of both CD86 and MHC class II (60, 61, 67). *In vivo* studies have also shown that up-regulation of both MHC class II and CD86 molecules on the surface of DCs from mice treated with whole body hyperthermia (61, 68). Additionally, hyperthermia in combination with other treatments including ionizing radiation (69), magnetic nanoparticles (70, 71), radiofrequency ablation (72) and vaccination (73, 74) results in enhanced DC function.

Dendritic cell migration to the lymph node is an important function required for efficient antigen presentation and our group and others have shown that mild heat stress can promote migratory activity of DCs. DCs in ear skin subjected to thermal stress in culture show increased migration compared to control samples (75), while increased DC migration into the lymph nodes of thermally stressed mice has also been demonstrated (61).

Heat treatment results in improved stimulatory function of DCs (59, 63, 67). Heated OVA-loaded DCs induce greater interferon-gamma (IFN-γ) responses from SINFEKL-specific T cells (64). Heat-treated SINFEKL pulsed DCs elicit greater antigen-specific $CD8^+$ T cell proliferation than unheated DCs (67). Heat also enhances the ability of DCs to cross-present to $CD8^+$ T (76) and activates $CD4^+$ T cells leading to antigen dependent memory (77). Additionally, mild hyperthermia alters the production of cytokines and chemokines from DCs, which are important for ensuring effective T cell priming. Mild heating increases DC production of inflammatory cytokines including IFN-γ, IL-17, IL-10, IL-12, and TNF-α (60, 61, 63). Taken together, the growing body of literature describing the effects of mild heat stress on DCs indicates that mild heat stress enhances DC function by promoting maturation and migration and increasing inflammatory cytokine production to assist with mediation of T cell priming to elicit T cell proliferation.

EFFECTS OF COLD STRESS ON DCs

We have summarized some of the previously reported complex effects of stress on DCs, including the general beneficial effects of temporary mild hyperthermia. We wondered whether the baseline function of DCs in these types of studies is influenced by ambient temperature used to house mice in research facilities. Laboratory mice are under a mild, yet constant cold stress as they are group housed at a cool (sub-thermoneutral) temperature (78–80). Additionally, since laboratory mice are provided with unlimited access to food and housed in small cages, which do not allow adequate room to exercise, they also experience additional metabolic stresses (21). Although these stressors have been identified as being important in other fields of research, such as obesity (81), they are not generally accounted for in the field of cancer immunology.

The fact that mice are mildly, yet chronically, cold stressed is not determined simply by body temperature measurements. In fact, while body temperature appears normal (~37°C) for mice housed at standard ambient temperatures required for research facilities (55), thermal preference studies over many decades have shown that mice prefer a warmer housing temperature near thermoneutrality (57, 78, 82, 83) indicating the degree of cold stress prompted by such housing. The degree to which underlying chronic cold stress has impacted the interpretation of the effects of other types of stress on immune function remains to be determined. Importantly, NE is released in response to stressors, including cold stress and, as detailed above, has a very significant influence on DC function.

Recent literature has detailed the impact of chronic cold stress in mice. The relationship between cold stress and metabolism has been investigated and alterations in insulin production (84), NE secretion (85), function of uncoupling proteins (81), and energy expenditure (86, 87) have been identified. Developmental and behavioral effects including differences in limb and tail length (88), cardiac tone and heart rate (89), and sleep (90) have also been observed when comparing cold stressed to non-stressed mice. Most recently, our group has shown that mild cold stress associated with standard housing conditions negatively impacts $CD8^+$ T cell dependent anti-tumor immune responses (55). To test whether DC function is influenced by chronic cold stress, we studied the impact of sub-thermoneutral housing temperatures on DC phenotype and function comparing the results to that seen from mice housed at thermoneutrality. Importantly, core body temperature in both groups of mice is the same, as shown previously (55).

We examined splenocytes from tumor-free and 4T1 tumor-bearing mice housed at standard (ST; 22°C) and thermoneutral (TT; 30°C) temperature. Because at 30°C the metabolic cold stress is greatly reduced, these mice represent un-cold stressed animals whereas their counterparts at 22°C are under chronic cold stress. We found that the number of splenocytes is similar in naïve (tumor-free) mice at ST and TT (**Figure 1A**). However, inoculation of mice with tumors induces an increase in splenocyte number at both ambient temperatures, however, this increase is larger at ST than at TT (**Figure 1A**). Confirming previous data (55), tumors grew slower in mice at TT compared to ST; tumor weight (**Figure 1B**) and volume (**Figure 1C**) were reduced in TT mice compared to ST mice. We also examined body weight for mice housed at each ambient temperature and found that prior to tumor inoculation mice at ST gained weight faster than mice at TT (**Figure 1D**). As tumors began to grow, mice at ST continued to gain even more weight than mice at TT (**Figure 1D**). These data show that animals housed at TT are physically smaller than those mice used as standard control models, while 4T1 tumor growth is accelerated in ST control mice.

We previously reported that spleens from mice at TT have fewer $CD11b^+GR\text{-}1^+$ myeloid derived suppressor cells (MDSCs) (55), so we wondered whether pan myeloid cells ($CD11b^+$) were similarly impacted by temperature (**Figure 2A**). We first determined that tumor-bearing mice at ST have significantly more $CD11b^+$ myeloid cells as well as a higher percentage of $CD11b^+$ cells

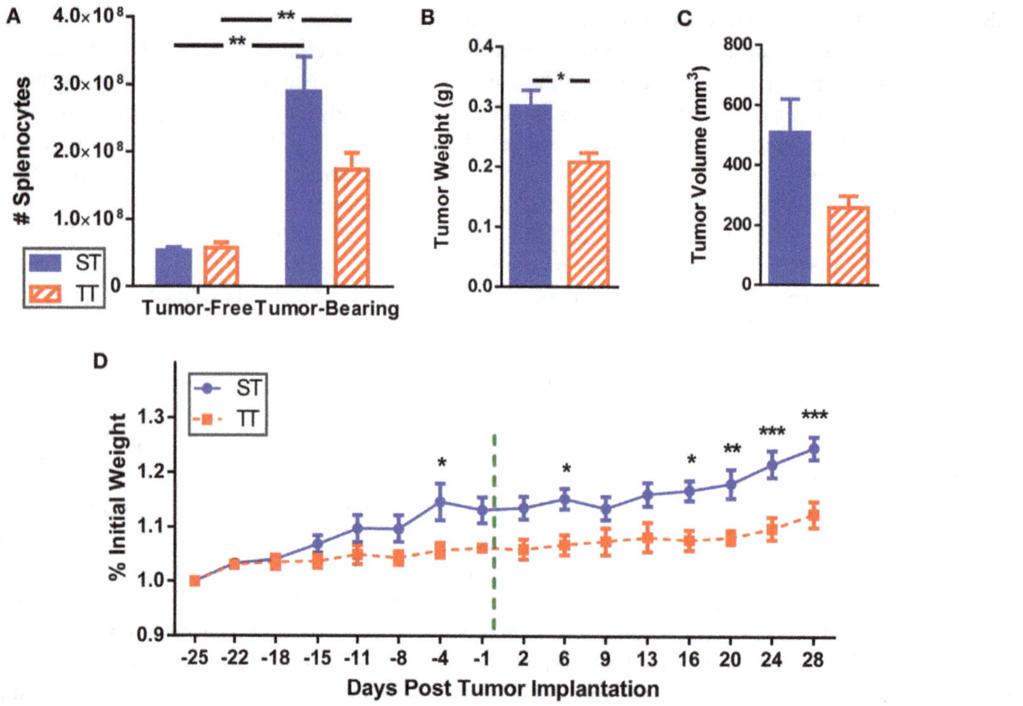

FIGURE 1 | Splenocytes, tumor size, and body weight are increased when mice are maintained at ST compared to TT. 4T1 tumor-bearing BALB/c mice and age-matched controls were maintained at ST or TT. **(A)** Splenocytes obtained from control and tumor-bearing mice were counted and **(B)** tumor weight and **(C)** volume were measured. Data presented as mean ± SEM; $n = 5$/group; Student's t-test; $^{*}p < 0.05$, $^{**}p < 0.01$. **(D)** Change in weight from the start of the experiment was measured. ---- indicates day of tumor inoculation. Data presented as mean ± SEM; $n = 5$/group; two-way ANOVA with Bonferroni post-tests; $^{*}p < 0.05$, $^{**}p < 0.01$, $^{***}p < 0.001$.

compared to tumor-bearing mice at TT (**Figure 2B**). The number and proportion of splenic myeloid cells in tumor-free animals was unchanged (**Figure 2C**). These results suggest that the effects of 4T1 tumor growth on the accumulation of myeloid cells in the spleen may be overestimated in mice housed under standard conditions since the cellular increase is also dependent on ambient temperature.

It has been reported that DC numbers in cancer patients are reduced compared to healthy controls (91); thus, we next investigated numbers of splenic DCs in tumor-free and tumor-bearing mice maintained at ST and TT based on CD11c expression. Total DCs were identified as $CD11c^{+}$ cells. We found that absolute numbers of splenic DCs (**Figure 3A**) increased following tumor implantation in mice at ST but not at TT (**Figure 3B**). However, the proportion of DCs decreased at both ST and TT following tumor inoculation (**Figure 3C**). We next examined plasmacytoid DCs ($B220^{+}CD11c^{+}$) (**Figure 3D**) which, following stimulation, are major interferon producers (92). We discovered that absolute numbers of plasmacytoid DCs increase following tumor inoculation in mice at ST but not at TT (**Figure 3E**), whereas percentages significantly decrease following tumor inoculation in mice at TT but not at ST (**Figure 3F**). When we investigated non-plasmacytoid DCs ($B220^{-}CD11c^{+}$) (**Figure 3D**) (93–95), we again found that absolute numbers increase following tumor inoculation in mice at ST but not at TT (**Figure 3G**) but that percentages of these cells significantly decrease following tumor inoculation in mice at TT only (**Figure 3H**). These data demonstrate that the number of DCs found in the spleens of laboratory mice do not show the expected increase in numbers after tumor inoculation when mice are maintained at thermoneutrality. Thus, ambient temperature should be considered when interpreting data regarding immune cell subsets in the spleens from mice used for cancer immunology studies.

We further dissected the non-plasmacytoid cell population by quantifying a subset of immature ($MHCII^{-}CD86^{-}$) and two subsets of mature ($CD11c^{+}MHCII^{+}CD86$, $CD11c^{+}MHCII^{+}CD86^{-}$) cells among $CD8\alpha^{+}$ and $CD4^{+}$ non-plasmacytoid DCs (**Figure 4A**). $CD8\alpha^{+}$ DCs are major producers of IL-12, able to initiate a robust inflammatory response as well as efficiently presenting antigen to $CD8^{+}$ T cells (96–99). We found that both absolute numbers (**Figure 4B**) and percentages (**Figure 4C**) of immature $CD8\alpha^{+}$ non-plasmacytoid DCs are increased to a greater extent following tumor inoculation in mice at ST compared to TT. Absolute numbers of $CD86^{-}$ mature $CD8\alpha^{+}$ non-plasmacytoid DCs increased following tumor inoculation in mice at ST but not TT (**Figure 4D**). The percentage of $CD86^{-}$ mature $CD8\alpha^{+}$ non-plasmacytoid DCs decreased at ST but not TT following tumor inoculation (**Figure 4E**). $CD86^{+}$ mature $CD8\alpha^{+}$ non-plasmacytoid DCs were unchanged in absolute number (**Figure 4F**) but their proportion in the spleen was modestly, yet significantly decreased at both ST and TT following tumor inoculation (**Figure 4G**). The increased numbers of immature and $CD86^{-}$ mature $CD8\alpha$ non-plasmacytoid DCs present in mice at

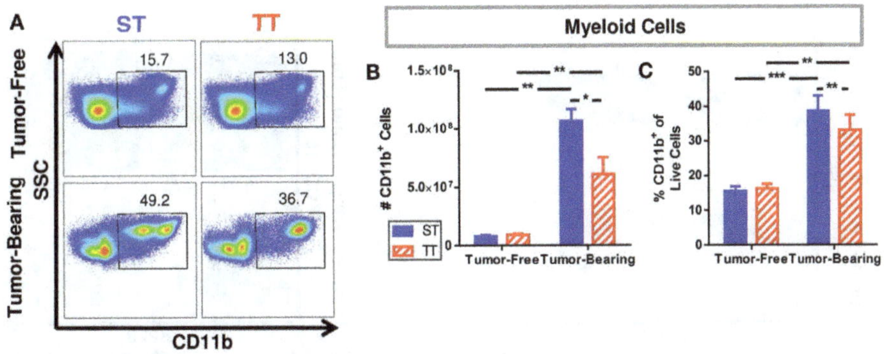

FIGURE 2 | Splenic myeloid cells are increased in tumor-bearing mice maintained at ST compared to TT. Single cell suspensions of splenocytes from 4T1 tumor-bearing mice and age-matched controls were stained for CD11b and analyzed by flow cytometry. **(A)** Representative dot plots from each group show the gating strategy used to select CD11b+ cells. Percentage of cells are shown above their respective gate. **(B)** The absolute number of CD11b+ cells calculated from the total number of splenocytes counted in each individual mouse. **(C)** The percentage of CD11b+ cells of the total population of live cells as determined by DAPI staining. Data presented as mean ± SEM; $n = 5$/group; Student's *t*-test; $^{*}p < 0.05$, $^{**}p < 0.01$, $^{***}p < 0.001$.

ST suggests that many of the DCs from these mice may not be able to become activated.

Further, we investigated the same subsets of immature and mature CD4+ non-plasmacytoid DCs (**Figure 4A**). We also found a major increase in absolute numbers (**Figure 4H**) and percentage (**Figure 4I**) of immature CD4+ non-plasmacytoid DCs in mice at ST but not TT following tumor inoculation. At ST, there was an increase in absolute number (**Figure 4J**) and a decrease in the percentage (**Figure 4K**) of CD86− mature CD4+ non-plasmacytoid DCs in response to tumor, but no significant changes were observed at TT. Again we saw no changes in absolute numbers of CD86+ mature CD4+ non-plasmacytoid DCs at either temperature (**Figure 4L**). We did see a reduced percentage of CD86+ mature CD4+ non-plasmacytoid DCs at ST but not at TT following tumor inoculation (**Figure 4M**). Interestingly, despite the increased number of non-plasmacytoid DCs in mice at ST (**Figure 3G**), there are no differences in the number of mature DCs (**Figures 4F,L**) suggesting that although DC numbers appear to be increased in cold stressed mice, many of these cells are unable to become activated in the presence of a 4T1 tumor.

Due to the increased overall numbers but relatively low number of mature splenic DCs seen in mice at ST, we asked whether DCs from mice at ST were impaired at antigen presentation and their ability to activate naïve T cells. To answer this question, we performed mixed lymphocyte reactions using irradiated splenocytes from ST and TT tumor-free and tumor-bearing mice as stimulator cells and T cells from naïve ST mice as the responders. Responder and stimulator cells were co-cultured at a 2:1 ratio for 72 h and then T cell proliferation was measured by ^{3}H-thymidine incorporation. As expected, we found that stimulator cells from tumor-free mice at both ST and TT were able to induce significant T cell proliferation (**Figure 5**; tumor-free). However, stimulator cells from tumor-free mice at ST elicited significantly more T cell proliferation than those from mice at TT (**Figure 5**; tumor-free, + T cells). Interestingly, when we looked at tumor-bearing mice, we found that stimulator cells from mice at TT were able to initiate T cell proliferation while those from mice at ST were not (**Figure 5**; tumor-bearing). These results suggest that the activated DCs found in 4T1 tumor-bearing mice at TT are more efficient antigen presenting cells than DCs from tumor-bearing ST mice as demonstrated by the superior ability of TT splenocytes to elicit T cell proliferation. As the *in vitro* portion of this work was all done at 37°C, these findings also suggest that cold stress can alter DC function over a prolonged period of time after DCs are removed from the mouse.

DISCUSSION

The relationships between stress and DC function are complex and depend upon the type and duration of stress, and whether the stressor is applied *in vivo* or *in vitro*. The type of DC (i.e., isolated from the bone marrow or skin) or stage of DC maturation when a stressor is encountered may also influence the impact of a particular stress (39). Additionally, DC function is dependent on the timing of antigen exposure and/or the type of antigen used, so these factors may also affect the observed relationship between stress and DC function (44).

In addition to summarizing some of the existing data on the effects of various stressors and stress hormones on DC function, we show here that the numbers and percentages of different subsets of DCs can be dependent upon housing temperature. Since sub-thermoneutral housing temperature is the standard condition under which mice are housed throughout the world, our data suggests that only using mice which are mildly cold stressed could be limiting our full understanding of the role of DCs in immune responses, including their role in anti-tumor immunity. Specifically, we have shown that tumor-bearing mice at ST have significantly more DCs compared to tumor-bearing mice at TT. However, the increased DCs seen at ST primarily display an immature phenotype (MHC II−CD86−) or they up-regulate MHC II but not CD86 rendering them unable to activate CD8+ T cells. The induction of signal 1 in the absence of signal 2 has been shown to lead to immune tolerance (12, 13). Thus, our studies suggest the potential for greater tolerance in mice at ST versus TT as splenocytes from ST mice were unable to activate T cell proliferation likely contributing to faster tumor growth. We observed

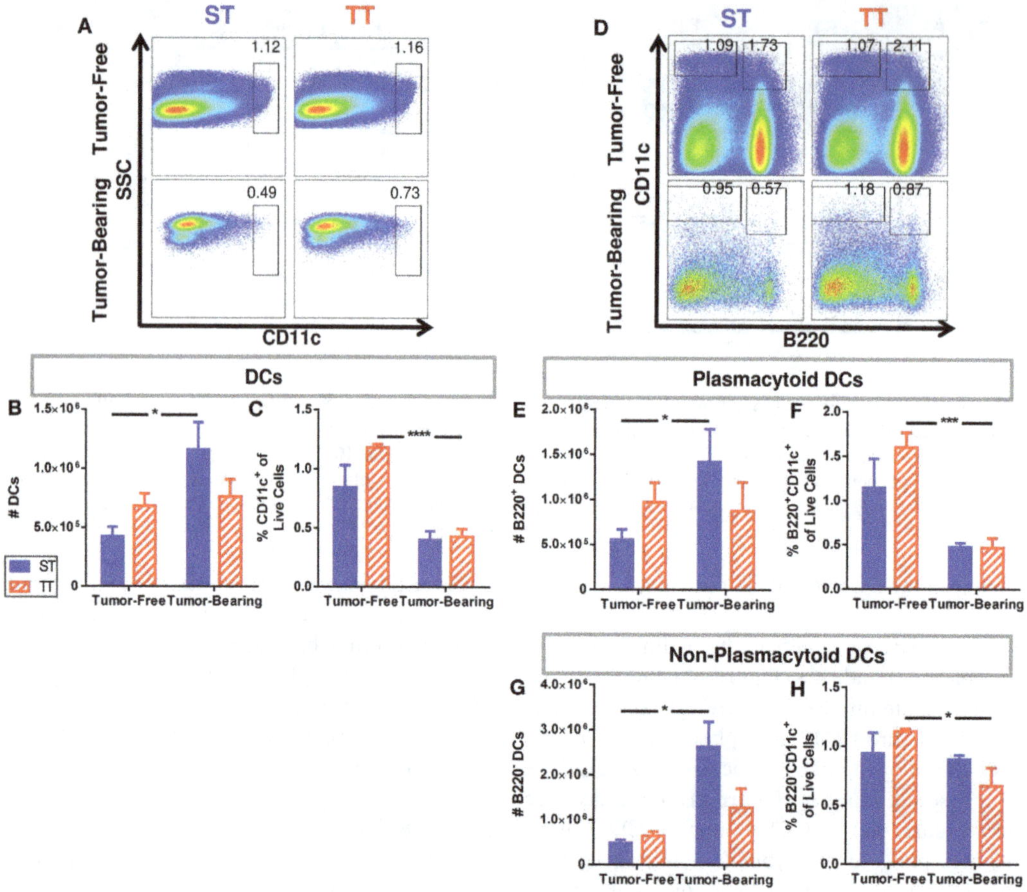

FIGURE 3 | Tumor-bearing mice maintained at ST have an increased frequency of DCs compared to those at TT. Single cell suspensions of splenocytes from 4T1 tumor-bearing mice and age-matched controls were stained for CD11c and **(D–H)** B220 and analyzed by flow cytometry. **(A)** Representative dot plots from each group show the gating strategy used to select CD11c$^+$ cells. Percentage of cells are shown above their respective gate. **(B)** The absolute number of CD11c$^+$ cells calculated from the total number of splenocytes counted in each individual mouse. **(C)** The percentage of CD11c$^+$ cells of the total population of live cells as determined by DAPI staining. **(D)** Representative dot plots from each group show the gating strategy used to select B220$^+$CD11c$^+$ and B220$^-$CD11c$^+$ cells. Percentage of cells are shown above their respective gate. **(E)** The absolute number of B220$^+$CD11c$^+$ cells calculated from the total number of splenocytes counted in each individual mouse. **(F)** The percentage of B220$^+$CD11c$^+$ cells of the total population of live cells as determined by DAPI staining. **(G)** The absolute number of B220$^-$CD11c$^+$ cells calculated from the total number of splenocytes counted in each individual mouse. **(H)** The percentage of B220$^-$CD11c$^+$ cells of the total population of live cells as determined by DAPI staining. Data presented as mean ± SEM; $n = 5$/group; Student's t-test; $^*p < 0.05$, $^{***}p < 0.001$, $^{****}p < 0.0001$.

enhanced T cell stimulatory ability by splenocytes from tumor-free mice at ST versus TT; however, when tumors were present the ability of ST splenocytes to activate T cells was diminished. While these data presented here is limited by the fact that we used whole splenocytes instead of isolated DCs to quantify the ability of cells from mice at ST and TT to activate T cells, the results presented strongly suggest that DCs from mice under mild cold stress are less able to undergo maturation prime T cells and elicit efficient T cell responses than mice maintained under thermoneutral conditions.

One possible explanation for the differences in tumor growth in mice from ST and TT is that DCs from mice at ST are more suppressive than those from mice at TT. It has been shown that a subset of murine DCs become particularly suppressive throughout tumor growth (100–103). Our previous observations suggest that when a tumor is present, the impact of cold stress is greatly exacerbated (55). This idea is further supported by these findings showing that T cell stimulation is greatly suppressed by splenocytes from mice at ST, but not TT.

The data presented here, along with other recent publications (81, 84–90) strongly suggest that the effects of chronic mild cold stress are important to consider when working with mouse models. Moreover, when studying the impact of experimentally induced stress, such as social or psychological stress, on DCs and other immune cells, it may be important to recognize that baseline data could be significantly influenced by inherent cold stress induced by standard housing conditions for laboratory mice.

FUTURE RESEARCH QUESTIONS

New questions emerge from the data presented here with regard to the effects of stress on DCs. Most importantly, what is the mechanism by which mild cold stress influences DC function? NE is involved in activation of thermogenesis in order to increase heat

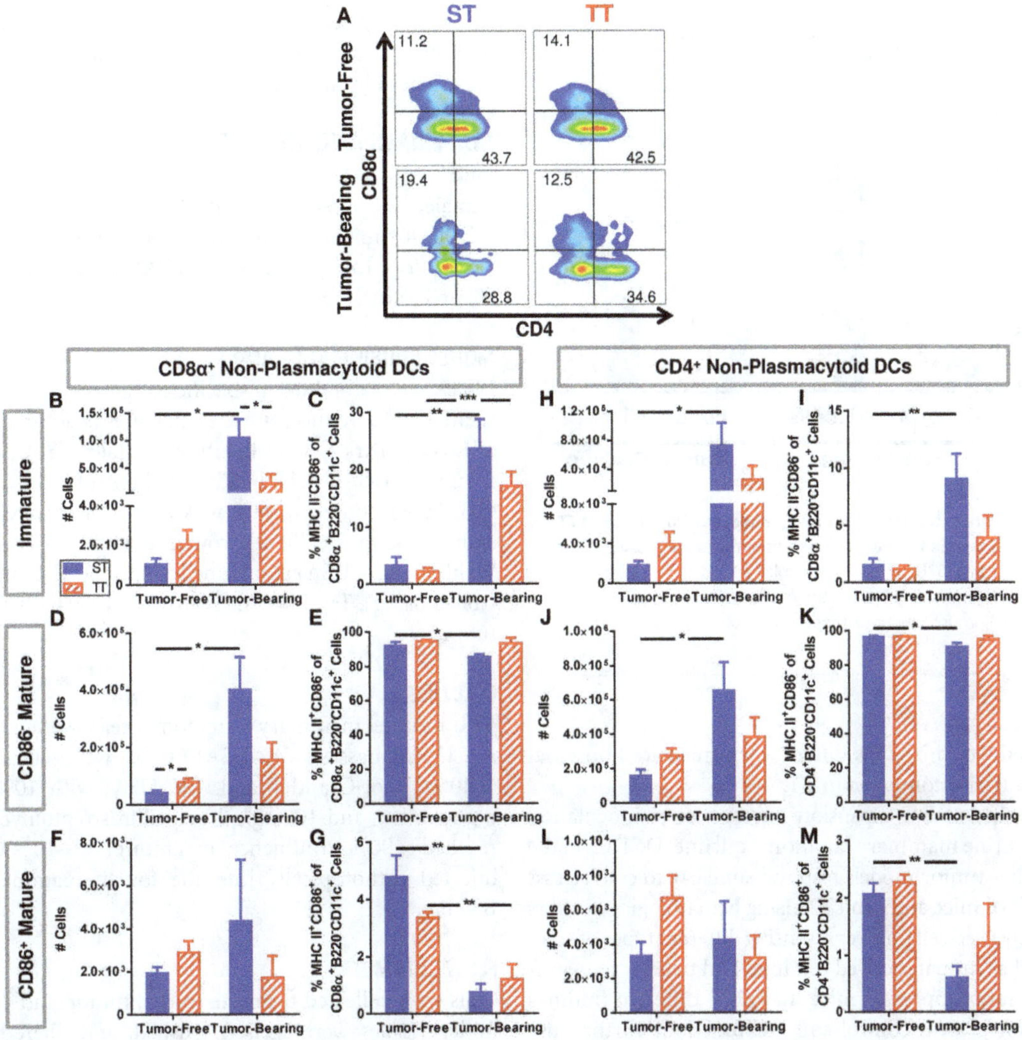

FIGURE 4 | Tumor-bearing mice maintained at ST have proportionally more non-plasmacytoid DCs than those at TT, but these DCs primarily display an immature phenotype. Single cell suspensions of splenocytes from 4T1 tumor-bearing mice and age-matched controls were stained for CD8α, CD4, CD11c, MHCII, CD86 and analyzed by flow cytometry. **(B–G)** Quantification of data describing CD8α+ non-plasmacytoid DCs. **(A)** Representative dot plots from each group show the gating strategy used to select CD4 and CD8α cells from the non-plasmacytoid parent population shown in **Figure 3D**. Percentage of cells are shown above their respective gate. **(B)** The absolute number of CD8α+MHC II−CD86−B220−CD11c+ cells calculated from the total number of non-plasmacytoid cells. **(C)** The percentage of MHC II−CD86− cells of the total population of CD8α+ non-plasmacytoid cells. **(D)** The absolute number of CD8α+MHC II+CD86−B220−CD11c+ cells calculated from the total number of non-plasmacytoid cells. **(E)** The percentage of MHC II+CD86− cells of the total population of CD8α+ non-plasmacytoid cells. **(F)** The absolute number of CD8α+MHC II+CD86+B220−CD11c+ cells calculated from the total number of non-plasmacytoid cells. **(G)** The percentage of MHC II+CD86+ cells of the total population of CD8α+ non-plasmacytoid cells. **(H–M)** Quantification of data describing CD4+ non-plasmacytoid DCs. **(H)** The absolute number of CD4+MHC II−CD86−B220−CD11c+ cells calculated from the total number of non-plasmacytoid cells. **(I)** The percentage of MHC II−CD86− cells of the total population of CD4+ non-plasmacytoid cells. **(J)** The absolute number of CD4+MHC II+CD86−B220−CD11c+ cells calculated from the total number of non-plasmacytoid cells. **(K)** The percentage of MHC II+CD86− cells of the total population of CD4+ non-plasmacytoid cells. **(L)** The absolute number of CD4+MHC II+CD86+B220−CD11c+ cells calculated from the total number of non-plasmacytoid cells. **(M)** The percentage of MHC II+CD86+ cells of the total population of CD4+ non-plasmacytoid cells. Data presented as mean ± SEM; $n = 5$/group; Student's t-test; $*p < 0.05$, $**p < 0.01$, $***p < 0.001$.

production to maintain normal body temperature (51, 85) and has already been strongly implicated for its roles in immunosuppression (20) and in regulating the polarization of macrophages (85). These observations strongly point to NE being a key player in the underlying relationship between cold stress and impaired DC function (55).

As mentioned earlier, cytokines affected by glucocorticoid treatment (43) or mild heating (60, 61, 63) include TNF-α, IFN-γ, IL-1α, IL-17, IL-10, and IL-12. How is the expression of these cytokines impacted by pre-existing mild cold stress in mice? In order to fully understand the impact of other types of stress in mouse models, it will be imperative to understand

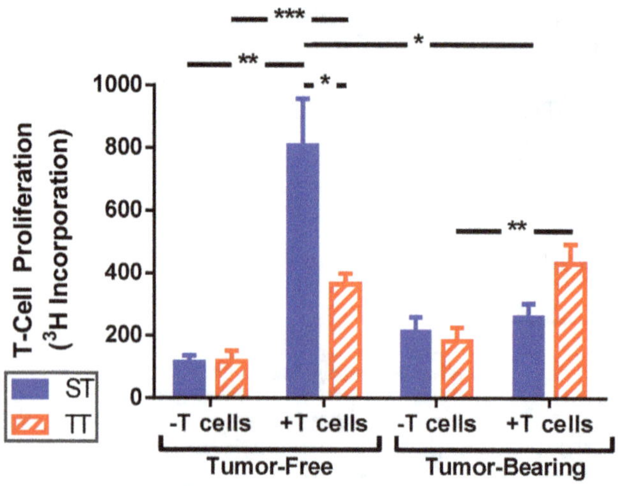

FIGURE 5 | T cells are activated better by splenocytes from mice at TT than ST. Total splenocytes from tumor-free and tumor-bearing BALB/c mice and lymphocytes from C57BL/6 mice were cultured 1:2. T cell proliferation was measured by ^{3}H-thymidine incorporation. Data presented as mean ± SEM; $n = 5$/group; Student's t-test; $*p < 0.05$, $**p < 0.01$, $***p < 0.001$.

if cytokine production by DCs differs when mice are housed at sub-thermoneutrality compared to TT.

Here, we looked at DC expansion in response to inoculation with the 4T1 murine mammary carcinoma cell line. Do DCs in the presence of other tumor models respond similarly to cold stress? Similar analysis of mice at ST and TT using hematological tumors and other widely used cell lines representing different types of solid tumors, as well as human derived cell lines and patient xenograft models in immunosuppressed mice may elicit different findings regarding tumor growth control and DC function. Further, use of carcinogen-induced or transgenic mouse tumor models will all be important to establish the overall impact of cold stress on DC function.

We have shown that eliminating cold stress influences baseline properties of DCs in tumor-free and tumor-bearing mice. Therefore, a major question which should be addressed is how this may be influencing data interpretation of experiments in which additional stressors (such as social isolation) are imposed on pre-existing cold stress. It is also possible that previously demonstrated beneficial effects of mild hyperthermia on DC function could be related to the fact that control (non-heated) mice are actually cold stressed. In other words, applications of mild heat could have a similar effect on DCs as thermoneutural housing in which body temperature is not elevated. It is clear that the study of stress responses in mice should be done at more than one ambient temperature in order to understand the impact of this variable on data interpretation. Conducting experiments under thermoneutral conditions as well as sub-thermoneutral housing would help to eliminate the impact of pre-existent cold stress while studying the effects of other stressors on DC function.

In summary, since a complete understanding of DCs is critical for development of effective immunotherapies for cancer patients, it is essential to recognize that the function of these critical cells may be dependent upon ambient housing temperature and other factors which influence physiologic or metabolic stress experienced by laboratory mice used in preclinical studies.

MATERIALS AND METHODS

MICE

Female, 8–10-week-old BALB/cAnNcr (BALB/c) and C57BL/6NCr (C57BL/6) mice were purchased from the NCI (Bethesda, MD, USA). Prior to experimentation, BALB/c mice were acclimated to ST or TT for 2 weeks.

MOUSE HOUSING AT ST AND TT

Mice were maintained in specific pathogen-free facilities and were treated in accordance with the guidelines established by the IACUC at Roswell Park Cancer Institute (Buffalo, NY, USA). Cages containing Enrich-o'Cobs bedding (The Andersons, Inc., Maumee, OH, USA) housed mice 5 to a cage. Cages were held in Precision® Refrigerated Plant-Growth Incubators (Thermo Scientific; Waltham, MA, USA) maintained at 22 or 30°C. Humidity was controlled using a Top Fin® Air Pump AIR 1000 with Top Fin® airline tubing.

CELL LINE

4T1 murine mammary carcinoma cells were purchased from ATCC (Manassas, VA, USA). Cells were cultured in RPMI 1640 (Gibco, Grand Island, NY, USA) with 10% FBS, 10 mM L-glutamine, and 100 μg/ml penicillin/streptomycin. When cells reached ~90% confluence in culture, 1×10^4 4T1 cells were injected orthotopically into the fourth mammary fat pad of BALB/c, mice.

FLOW CYTOMETRY

Cells were collected from the spleen, tumor, and draining lymph node. Tissues were excised, washed, and filtered into a single cell suspension. Cells were counted with a hemocytometer and Trypan Blue solution. Cells were stained with Brilliant Violet 711™ anti-mouse CD4 (clone RM4-5; BioLegend; San Diego, CA, USA), Brilliant Violet 650™ anti-mouse CD3 (clone 17A2; BioLegend), Pacific Blue™ anti-mouse CDllb (clone M1/70; BioLegend), APC anti-mouse CD11c (clone N418; BioLegend), FITC anti-mouse CD86 (clone GL1; BD Pharmingen; San Jose, CA, USA), PerCp/Cy5.5 anti-mouse MHC (clone M5/114.15.2; BioLegend). Live cells were determined by staining cells with 4′,6-diamidino-2-phenylindole (DAPI; Life Technologies; Grand Island, NY, USA) and defined as DAPI-negative. Samples were analyzed on an LSRII flow cytometer (BD Pharmingen) and analyzed using FlowJo (Ashland, OR, USA) version 10.0.6.

MIXED LYMPHOCYTE REACTIONS

Spleens were excised from tumor-free and tumor-bearing BALB/c mice, and lymph nodes were excised from C57BL/6 mice. BALB/c splenocytes were irradiated at 30 Gy. BALB/c splenocytes (stimulator cells) and C57BL/6 lymphocytes (responder cells) were filtered, washed, and cultured at a ratio of one stimulator cell to two responder cells in 200 μl RPMI (10% FBS, 100 mM L-Glutamate, and 100 U/ml Penicillin–Streptomycin). After 72 h

1 μCi ^{3}H-thymidine was added for 14–18 h. T cell proliferation was determined by ^{3}H-thymidine incorporation.

DATA ANALYSIS AND STATISTICS

All data are presented as mean ± SEM All p values were determined using Student's t-tests or two-way ANOVA with Bonferroni post-tests. All statistical analysis was completed using Prism software.

ACKNOWLEDGMENTS

The authors thank Louise Carlson, Bonnie Hylander, Michael Nemeth, Adam Utley, Jason Eng, Michelle Messmer, and Jeanne Prendergast for technical or editorial assistance. This work was supported by National Institute of Health Grants R01 CA135368 and T32 CA085183 and Peter T. Rowley Breast Cancer Research Grant. Work in this manuscript used shared resources supported by the Roswell Park Cancer Institute's Comprehensive Cancer Center Support Grant CA016056.

REFERENCES

1. Lipscomb MF, Masten BJ. Dendritic cells: immune regulators in health and disease. *Physiol Rev* (2002) **82**(1):97–130. doi:10.1152/physrev.00023.2001
2. Steinman RM. Lasker basic medical research award. Dendritic cells: versatile controllers of the immune system. *Nat Med* (2007) **13**(10):1155–9. doi:10.1038/nm1643
3. Lewis KL, Reizis B. Dendritic cells: arbiters of immunity and immunological tolerance. *Cold Spring Harb Perspect Biol* (2012) **4**(8):a007401. doi:10.1101/cshperspect.a007401
4. Reis e Sousa C. Activation of dendritic cells: translating innate into adaptive immunity. *Curr Opin Immunol* (2004) **16**:21–5. doi:10.1016/j.coi.2003.11.007
5. Melief CJ. Cancer immunotherapy by dendritic cells. *Immunity* (2008) **29**(3):372–83. doi:10.1016/j.immuni.2008.08.004
6. Steinman RM, Banchereau J. Taking dendritic cells into medicine. *Nature* (2007) **449**(7161):419–26. doi:10.1038/nature06175
7. Kalinski P, Edington H, Zeh HJ, Okada H, Butterfield LH, Kirkwood JM, et al. Dendritic cells in cancer immunotherapy: vaccines or autologous transplants? *Immunol Res* (2011) **50**(2–3):235–47. doi:10.1007/s12026-011-8224-z
8. Palucka K, Banchereau J. Cancer immunotherapy via dendritic cells. *Nat Rev Cancer* (2012) **12**(4):265–77. doi:10.1038/nrc3258
9. Palucka K, Banchereau J. Dendritic-cell-based therapeutic cancer vaccines. *Immunity* (2013) **39**(1):38–48. doi:10.1016/j.immuni.2013.07.004
10. Lin A, Schildknecht A, Nguyen LT, Ohashi PS. Dendritic cells integrate signals from the tumor microenvironment to modulate immunity and tumor growth. *Immunol Lett* (2010) **127**(2):77–84. doi:10.1016/j.imlet.2009.09.003
11. Bevan MJ. Minor H antigens introduced on H-2 different stimulating cells cross-react at the cytotoxic T cell level during in vivo priming. *J Immunol* (1976) **117**(6):2233–8.
12. Granucci F, Lutz MB, Zanoni I. The nature of activatory and tolerogenic dendritic cell-derived signal 2. *Front Immunol* (2013) **4**:198. doi:10.3389/fimmu.2013.00198
13. Bakdash G, Sittig SP, van Dijk T, Figdor CG, de Vries IJ. The nature of activatory and tolerogenic dendritic cell-derived signal II. *Front Immunol* (2013) **4**:53. doi:10.3389/fimmu.2013.00053
14. Gabrilovich DI, Ostrand-Rosenberg S, Bronte V. Coordinated regulation of myeloid cells by tumours. *Nat Rev Immunol* (2012) **12**(4):253–68. doi:10.1038/nri3175
15. Apetoh L, Locher C, Ghiringhelli F, Kroemer G, Zitvogel L. Harnessing dendritic cells in cancer. *Semin Immunol* (2011) **23**(1):42–9. doi:10.1016/j.smim.2011.01.003
16. Repasky EA, Evans SS, Dewhirst MW. Temperature matters! And why it should matter to tumor immunologists. *Cancer Immunol Res* (2013) **1**(4):1–7. doi:10.1158/2326-6066.CIR-13-0118
17. Ostberg JR, Repasky EA. Emerging evidence indicates that physiologically relevant thermal stress regulates dendritic cell function. *Cancer Immunol Immunother* (2006) **55**(3):292–8. doi:10.1007/s00262-005-0689-y
18. Ostberg JR, Gellin C, Patel R, Repasky EA. Regulatory potential of fever-range whole body hyperthermia on Langerhans cells and lymphocytes in an antigen-dependent cellular immune response. *J Immunol* (2001) **167**(5):2666–70.
19. Chrousos GP. Stress and disorders of the stress system. *Nat Rev Endocrinol* (2009) **5**(7):374–81. doi:10.1038/nrendo.2009.106
20. Padgett DA, Glaser R. How stress influences the immune response. *Trends Immunol* (2003) **24**(8):444–8. doi:10.1016/S1471-4906(03)00173-X
21. Martin B, Ji S, Maudsley S, Mattson MP. Control laboratory rodents are metabolically morbid: why it matters. *Proc Natl Acad Sci U S A* (2010) **107**(14):6127–33. doi:10.1073/pnas.0912955107
22. Dhabhar FS. Psychological stress and immunoprotection versus immunopathology in the skin. *Clin Dermatol* (2013) **31**(1):18–30. doi:10.1016/j.clindermatol.2011.11.003
23. Dhabhar FS. Enhancing versus suppressive effects of stress on immune function: implications for immunoprotection versus immunopathology. *Allergy Asthma Clin Immunol* (2008) **4**(1):2–11. doi:10.1186/1710-1492-4-1-2
24. Viswanathan K, Daugherty C, Dhabhar FS. Stress as an endogenous adjuvant: augmentation of the immunization phase of cell-mediated immunity. *Int Immunol* (2005) **17**(8):1059–69. doi:10.1093/intimm/dxh286
25. Saint-Mezard P, Chavagnac C, Bosset S, Ionescu M, Peyron E, Kaiserlian D, et al. Psychological stress exerts an adjuvant effect on skin dendritic cell functions in vivo. *J Immunol* (2003) **171**(8):4073–80.
26. Kleyn CE, Schneider L, Saraceno R, Mantovani C, Richards HL, Fortune DG, et al. The effects of acute social stress on epidermal Langerhans' cell frequency and expression of cutaneous neuropeptides. *J Invest Dermatol* (2008) **128**(5):1273–9. doi:10.1038/sj.jid.5701144
27. Hall JM, Cruser D, Podawiltz A, Mummert DI, Jones H, Mummert ME. Psychological stress and the cutaneous immune response: roles of the HPA axis and the sympathetic nervous system in atopic dermatitis and psoriasis. *Dermatol Res Pract* (2012) **2012**:403908. doi:10.1155/2012/403908
28. Abe M, Thomson AW. Influence of immunosuppressive drugs on dendritic cells. *Transpl Immunol* (2003) **11**(3–4):357–65. doi:10.1016/S0966-3274(03)00050-9
29. Elenkov IJ, Chrousos GP. Stress system – organization, physiology and immunoregulation. *Neuroimmunomodulation* (2006) **13**(5–6):257–67. doi:10.1159/000104853
30. Shodell M, Siegal FP. Corticosteroids depress IFN-alpha-producing plasmacytoid dendritic cells in human blood. *J Allergy Clin Immunol* (2001) **108**(3):446–8. doi:10.1067/mai.2001.117928
31. Ashworth J, Booker J, Breathnach SM. Effects of topical corticosteroid therapy on Langerhans cell antigen presenting function in human skin. *Br J Dermatol* (1988) **118**(4):457–69. doi:10.1111/j.1365-2133.1988.tb02453.x
32. Furue M, Katz SI. Direct effects of glucocorticosteroids on epidermal Langerhans cells. *J Invest Dermatol* (1989) **92**(3):342–7. doi:10.1111/1523-1747.ep12277165
33. Halliday GM, Knight BA, Muller HK. Reduction in murine Langerhans cell ATPase staining following topical but not systemic treatment with steroid and non-steroid immunosuppressants. *Br J Dermatol* (1986) **114**(1):83–9. doi:10.1111/j.1365-2133.1986.tb02782.x
34. Abe M, Thomson AW. Dexamethasone preferentially suppresses plasmacytoid dendritic cell differentiation and enhances their apoptotic death. *Clin Immunol* (2006) **118**(2–3):300–6. doi:10.1016/j.clim.2005.09.019
35. Moser M, De Smedt T, Sornasse T, Tielemans F, Chentoufi AA, Muraille E, et al. Glucocorticoids down-regulate dendritic cell function in vitro and in vivo. *Eur J Immunol* (1995) **25**(10):2818–24. doi:10.1002/eji.1830251016
36. Cumberbatch M, Dearman RJ, Kimber I. Inhibition by dexamethasone of Langerhans cell migration: influence of epidermal cytokine signals. *Immunopharmacology* (1999) **41**(3):235–43. doi:10.1016/S0162-3109(99)00037-5
37. Pan J, Ju D, Wang Q, Zhang M, Xia D, Zhang L, et al. Dexamethasone inhibits the antigen presentation of dendritic cells in MHC class II pathway. *Immunol Lett* (2001) **76**(3):153–61. doi:10.1016/S0165-2478(01)00183-3
38. Matasic R, Dietz AB, Vuk-Pavlovic S. Dexamethasone inhibits dendritic cell maturation by redirecting differentiation of a subset of cells. *J Leukoc Biol* (1999) **66**(6):909–14.
39. Matyszak MK, Citterio S, Rescigno M, Ricciardi-Castagnoli P. Differential effects of corticosteroids during different stages of dendritic cell maturation.

Eur J Immunol (2000) **30**(4):1233–42. doi:10.1002/(SICI)1521-4141(200004)30:43.0.CO;2-F
40. Matsue H, Yang C, Matsue K, Edelbaum D, Mummert M, Takashima A. Contrasting impacts of immunosuppressive agents (rapamycin, FK506, cyclosporin A, and dexamethasone) on bidirectional dendritic cell-T cell interaction during antigen presentation. *J Immunol* (2002) **169**(7):3555–64.
41. Salgado CG, Nakamura K, Sugaya M, Tada Y, Asahina A, Fukuda S, et al. Differential effects of cytokines and immunosuppressive drugs on CD40, B7-1, and B7-2 expression on purified epidermal Langerhans cells1. *J Invest Dermatol* (1999) **113**(6):1021–7. doi:10.1046/j.1523-1747.1999.00785.x
42. Kitajima T, Ariizumi K, Bergstresser PR, Takashima A. A novel mechanism of glucocorticoid-induced immune suppression: the inhibition of T cell-mediated terminal maturation of a murine dendritic cell line. *J Clin Invest* (1996) **98**(1):142–7. doi:10.1172/JCI118759
43. Hoetzenecker W, Meingassner JG, Ecker R, Stingl G, Stuetz A, Elbe-Burger A. Corticosteroids but not pimecrolimus affect viability, maturation and immune function of murine epidermal Langerhans cells. *J Invest Dermatol* (2004) **122**(3):673–84. doi:10.1111/j.0022-202X.2004.22324.x
44. Seiffert K, Granstein RD. Neuroendocrine regulation of skin dendritic cells. *Ann N Y Acad Sci* (2006) **1088**:195–206. doi:10.1196/annals.1366.011
45. Panina-Bordignon P, Mazzeo D, Lucia PD, D'Ambrosio D, Lang R, Fabbri L, et al. Beta2-agonists prevent Th1 development by selective inhibition of interleukin 12. *J Clin Invest* (1997) **100**(6):1513–9. doi:10.1172/JCI119674
46. Elenkov IJ, Papanicolaou DA, Wilder RL, Chrousos GP. Modulatory effects of glucocorticoids and catecholamines on human interleukin-12 and interleukin-10 production: clinical implications. *Proc Assoc Am Physicians* (1996) **108**(5):374–81.
47. Elenkov IJ, Chrousos GP, Wilder RL. Neuroendocrine regulation of IL-12 and TNF-alpha/IL-10 balance. Clinical implications. *Ann N Y Acad Sci* (2000) **917**:94–105. doi:10.1111/j.1749-6632.2000.tb05374.x
48. Maestroni GJ. Short exposure of maturing, bone marrow-derived dendritic cells to norepinephrine: impact on kinetics of cytokine production and the development. *J Neuroimmunol* (2002) **129**(1–2):106–14. doi:10.1016/S0165-5728(02)00188-1
49. Seiffert K, Hosoi J, Torii H, Ozawa H, Ding W, Campton K, et al. Catecholamines inhibit the antigen-presenting capability of epidermal Langerhans cells. *J Immunol* (2002) **168**(12):6128–35.
50. Yanagawa Y, Matsumoto M, Togashi H. Enhanced dendritic cell antigen uptake via alpha2 adrenoceptor-mediated PI3K activation following brief exposure to noradrenaline. *J Immunol* (2010) **185**(10):5762–8. doi:10.4049/jimmunol.1001899
51. Cannon B, Nedergaard J. Brown adipose tissue: function and physiological significance. *Physiol Rev* (2004) **84**(1):277–359. doi:10.1152/physrev.00015.2003
52. Kluger MJ, Kozak W, Conn CA, Leon LR, Soszynski D. The adaptive value of fever. *Infect Dis Clin North Am* (1996) **10**(1):1–20. doi:10.1016/S0891-5520(05)70282-8
53. Kluger MJ, Ringler DH, Anver MR. Fever and survival. *Science* (1975) **188**(4184):166–8. doi:10.1126/science.1114347
54. Hasday JD, Fairchild KD, Shanholtz C. The role of fever in the infected host. *Microbes Infect* (2000) **2**(15):1891–904. doi:10.1016/S1286-4579(00)01337-X
55. Kokolus KM, Capitano ML, Lee CT, Eng JW, Waight JD, Hylander BL, et al. Baseline tumor growth and immune control in laboratory mice are significantly influenced by subthermoneutral housing temperature. *Proc Natl Acad Sci U S A* (2013) **110**(50)20176–81. doi:10.1073/pnas.1304291110
56. Singh IS, Hasday JD. Fever, hyperthermia and the heat shock response. *Int J Hyperthermia* (2013) **29**(5):423–35. doi:10.3109/02656736.2013.808766
57. Gordon CJ. *Temperature Regulation in Laboratory Rodents.* Cambridge: Cambridge University Press (1993).
58. Dinarello CA. Review: infection, fever, and exogenous and endogenous pyrogens: some concepts have changed. *J Endotoxin Res* (2004) **10**(4):201–22. doi:10.1177/09680519040100040301
59. Ostberg JR, Kabingu E, Repasky EA. Thermal regulation of dendritic cell activation and migration from skin explants. *Int J Hyperthermia* (2003) **19**(5):520–33. doi:10.1080/02656730310001607986
60. Knippertz I, Stein MF, Dorrie J, Schaft N, Muller I, Deinzer A, et al. Mild hyperthermia enhances human monocyte-derived dendritic cell functions and offers potential for applications in vaccination strategies. *Int J Hyperthermia* (2011) **27**(6):591–603. doi:10.3109/02656736.2011.589234
61. Joshi N, Duhan V, Lingwal N, Bhaskar S, Upadhyay P. Adjuvant properties of thermal component of hyperthermia enhanced transdermal immunization: effect on dendritic cells. *PLoS One* (2012) **7**(2):e32067. doi:10.1371/journal.pone.0032067
62. Zhang HG, Mehta K, Cohen P, Guha C. Hyperthermia on immune regulation: a temperature's story. *Cancer Lett* (2008) **271**(2):191–204. doi:10.1016/j.canlet.2008.05.026
63. Tournier JN, Hellmann AQ, Lesca G, Jouan A, Drouet E, Mathieu J. Fever-like thermal conditions regulate the activation of maturing dendritic cells. *J Leukoc Biol* (2003) **73**(4):493–501. doi:10.1189/jlb.1002506
64. Basu S, Srivastava PK. Fever-like temperature induces maturation of dendritic cells through induction of hsp90. *Int Immunol* (2003) **15**(9):1053–61. doi:10.1093/intimm/dxg104
65. Banchereau J, Briere F, Caux C, Davoust J, Lebecque S, Liu YJ, et al. Immunobiology of dendritic cells. *Annu Rev Immunol* (2000) **18**:767–811. doi:10.1146/annurev.immunol.18.1.767
66. Ohashi PS, DeFranco AL. Making and breaking tolerance. *Curr Opin Immunol* (2002) **14**(6):744–59. doi:10.1016/S0952-7915(02)00406-5
67. Zheng H, Benjamin IJ, Basu S, Li Z. Heat shock factor 1-independent activation of dendritic cells by heat shock: implication for the uncoupling of heat-mediated immunoregulation from the heat shock response. *Eur J Immunol* (2003) **33**(6):1754–62. doi:10.1002/eji.200323687
68. Matsumoto K, Yamamoto N, Hagiwara S, Saito M, Furue H, Shigetomi T, et al. Optimization of hyperthermia and dendritic cell immunotherapy for squamous cell carcinoma. *Oncol Rep* (2011) **25**(6):1525–32. doi:10.3892/or.2011.1232
69. Schildkopf P, Frey B, Ott OJ, Rubner Y, Multhoff G, Sauer R, et al. Radiation combined with hyperthermia induces HSP70-dependent maturation of dendritic cells and release of pro-inflammatory cytokines by dendritic cells and macrophages. *Radiother Oncol* (2011) **101**(1):109–15. doi:10.1016/j.radonc.2011.05.056
70. Tanaka K, Ito A, Kobayashi T, Kawamura T, Shimada S, Matsumoto K, et al. Intratumoral injection of immature dendritic cells enhances antitumor effect of hyperthermia using magnetic nanoparticles. *Int J Cancer* (2005) **116**(4):624–33. doi:10.1002/ijc.21061
71. Tanaka K, Ito A, Kobayashi T, Kawamura T, Shimada S, Matsumoto K, et al. Heat immunotherapy using magnetic nanoparticles and dendritic cells for T-lymphoma. *J Biosci Bioeng* (2005) **100**(1):112–5. doi:10.1263/jbb.100.112
72. Liu Q, Zhai B, Yang W, Yu LX, Dong W, He YQ, et al. Abrogation of local cancer recurrence after radiofrequency ablation by dendritic cell-based hyperthermic tumor vaccine. *Mol Ther* (2009) **17**(12):2049–57. doi:10.1038/mt.2009.221
73. Schueller G, Stift A, Friedl J, Dubsky P, Bachleitner-Hofmann T, Benkoe T, et al. Hyperthermia improves cellular immune response to human hepatocellular carcinoma subsequent to co-culture with tumor lysate pulsed dendritic cells. *Int J Oncol* (2003) **22**(6):1397–402.
74. Mukhopadhaya A, Mendecki J, Dong X, Liu L, Kalnicki S, Garg M, et al. Localized hyperthermia combined with intratumoral dendritic cells induces systemic antitumor immunity. *Cancer Res* (2007) **67**(16):7798–806. doi:10.1158/0008-5472.CAN-07-0203
75. Ostberg JR, Taylor SL, Baumann H, Repasky EA. Regulatory effects of fever-range whole-body hyperthermia on the LPS-induced acute inflammatory response. *J Leukoc Biol* (2000) **68**(6):815–20.
76. Shi H, Cao T, Connolly JE, Monnet L, Bennett L, Chapel S, et al. Hyperthermia enhances CTL cross-priming. *J Immunol* (2006) **176**(4):2134–41.
77. Wang Y, Seidl T, Whittall T, Babaahmady K, Lehner T. Stress-activated dendritic cells interact with CD4+ T cells to elicit homeostatic memory. *Eur J Immunol* (2010) **40**(6):1628–38. doi:10.1002/eji.200940251
78. Gordon CJ. Thermal physiology of laboratory mice: defining thermoneutrality. *J Therm Biol* (2012) **37**:654–85. doi:10.1016/j.jtherbio.2012.08.004
79. Karp CL. Unstressing intemperate models: how cold stress undermines mouse modeling. *J Exp Med* (2012) **209**(6):1069–74. doi:10.1084/jem.20120988
80. Overton JM. Phenotyping small animals as models for the human metabolic syndrome: thermoneutrality matters. *Int J Obes* (2010) **34**(Suppl 2):S53–8. doi:10.1038/ijo.2010.240

81. Feldmann HM, Golozoubova V, Cannon B, Nedergaard J. UCP1 ablation induces obesity and abolishes diet-induced thermogenesis in mice exempt from thermal stress by living at thermoneutrality. *Cell Metab* (2009) **9**(2):203–9. doi:10.1016/j.cmet.2008.12.014
82. Shimizu I, Iida T, Guan Y, Zhao C, Raja SN, Jarvis MF, et al. Enhanced thermal avoidance in mice lacking the ATP receptor P2X3. *Pain* (2005) **116**(1–2):96–108. doi:10.1016/j.pain.2005.03.030
83. Gordon CJ, Becker P, Ali J. Behavioral thermoregulatory responses of single- and group-housed mice. *Physiol Behav* (1998) **65**(2):255–62. doi:10.1016/S0031-9384(98)00148-6
84. Uchida K, Shiuchi T, Inada H, Minokoshi Y, Tominaga M. Metabolic adaptation of mice in a cool environment. *Pflugers Arch* (2010) **459**(5):765–74. doi:10.1007/s00424-010-0795-3
85. Nguyen KD, Qiu Y, Cui X, Goh YP, Mwangi J, David T, et al. Alternatively activated macrophages produce catecholamines to sustain adaptive thermogenesis. *Nature* (2011) **480**(7375):104–8. doi:10.1038/nature10653
86. Virtue S, Even P, Vidal-Puig A. Below thermoneutrality, changes in activity do not drive changes in total daily energy expenditure between groups of mice. *Cell Metab* (2012) **16**(5):665–71. doi:10.1016/j.cmet.2012.10.008
87. Ravussin Y, LeDuc CA, Watanabe K, Leibel RL. Effects of ambient temperature on adaptive thermogenesis during maintenance of reduced body weight in mice. *Am J Physiol Regul Integr Comp Physiol* (2012) **303**(4):R438–48. doi:10.1152/ajpregu.00092.2012
88. Serrat MA, King D, Lovejoy CO. Temperature regulates limb length in homeotherms by directly modulating cartilage growth. *Proc Natl Acad Sci U S A* (2008) **105**(49):19348–53. doi:10.1073/pnas.0803319105
89. Swoap SJ, Li C, Wess J, Parsons AD, Williams TD, Overton JM. Vagal tone dominates autonomic control of mouse heart rate at thermoneutrality. *Am J Physiol Heart Circ Physiol* (2008) **294**(4):H1581–8. doi:10.1152/ajpheart.01000.2007
90. Lo Martire V, Silvani A, Bastianini S, Berteotti C, Zoccoli G. Effects of ambient temperature on sleep and cardiovascular regulation in mice: the role of hypocretin/orexin neurons. *PLoS One* (2012) **7**(10):e47032. doi:10.1371/journal.pone.0047032
91. Almand B, Resser JR, Lindman B, Nadaf S, Clark JI, Kwon ED, et al. Clinical significance of defective dendritic cell differentiation in cancer. *Clin Cancer Res* (2000) **6**(5):1755–66.
92. Gill MA, Bajwa G, George TA, Dong CC, Dougherty II, Jiang N, et al. Counterregulation between the FcepsilonRI pathway and antiviral responses in human plasmacytoid dendritic cells. *J Immunol* (2010) **184**(11):5999–6006. doi:10.4049/jimmunol.0901194
93. Diebold SS, Montoya M, Unger H, Alexopoulou L, Roy P, Haswell LE, et al. Viral infection switches non-plasmacytoid dendritic cells into high interferon producers. *Nature* (2003) **424**(6946):324–8. doi:10.1038/nature01783
94. O'Keeffe M, Fancke B, Suter M, Ramm G, Clark J, Wu L, et al. Nonplasmacytoid, high IFN-alpha-producing, bone marrow dendritic cells. *J Immunol* (2012) **188**(8):3774–83. doi:10.4049/jimmunol.1101365
95. Voisine C, Mastelic B, Sponaas AM, Langhorne J. Classical CD11c+ dendritic cells, not plasmacytoid dendritic cells, induce T cell responses to *Plasmodium chabaudi* malaria. *Int J Parasitol* (2010) **40**(6):711–9. doi:10.1016/j.ijpara.2009.11.005
96. Lin ML, Zhan Y, Proietto AI, Prato S, Wu L, Heath WR, et al. Selective suicide of cross-presenting CD8+ dendritic cells by cytochrome *c* injection shows functional heterogeneity within this subset. *Proc Natl Acad Sci U S A* (2008) **105**(8):3029–34. doi:10.1073/pnas.0712394105
97. Edelson BT, Bradstreet TR, Hildner K, Carrero JA, Frederick KE, KC W, et al. CD8alpha(+) dendritic cells are an obligate cellular entry point for productive infection by *Listeria monocytogenes*. *Immunity* (2011) **35**(2):236–48. doi:10.1016/j.immuni.2011.06.012
98. Vremec D, Pooley J, Hochrein H, Wu L, Shortman K. CD4 and CD8 expression by dendritic cell subtypes in mouse thymus and spleen. *J Immunol* (2000) **164**(6):2978–86.
99. Hildner K, Edelson BT, Purtha WE, Diamond M, Matsushita H, Kohyama M, et al. Batf3 deficiency reveals a critical role for CD8alpha+ dendritic cells in cytotoxic T cell immunity. *Science* (2008) **322**(5904):1097–100. doi:10.1126/science.1164206
100. Hurwitz AA, Watkins SK. Immune suppression in the tumor microenvironment: a role for dendritic cell-mediated tolerization of T cells. *Cancer Immunol Immunother* (2012) **61**(2):289–93. doi:10.1007/s00262-011-1181-5
101. Watkins SK, Hurwitz AA. FOXO3: a master switch for regulating tolerance and immunity in dendritic cells. *Oncoimmunology* (2012) **1**(2):252–4. doi:10.4161/onci.1.2.18241
102. Watkins SK, Zhu Z, Riboldi E, Shafer-Weaver KA, Stagliano KE, Sklavos MM, et al. FOXO3 programs tumor-associated DCs to become tolerogenic in human and murine prostate cancer. *J Clin Invest* (2011) **121**(4):1361–72. doi:10.1172/JCI44325
103. Shafer-Weaver KA, Watkins SK, Anderson MJ, Draper LJ, Malyguine A, Alvord WG, et al. Immunity to murine prostatic tumors: continuous provision of T-cell help prevents CD8 T-cell tolerance and activates tumor-infiltrating dendritic cells. *Cancer Res* (2009) **69**(15):6256–64. doi:10.1158/0008-5472.CAN-08-4516

2

Immunoglobulin gene repertoire diversification and selection in the stomach – from gastritis to gastric lymphomas

Miri Michaeli[1†], Hilla Tabibian-Keissar[1,2†], Ginette Schiby[2†], Gitit Shahaf[1], Yishai Pickman[1], Lena Hazanov[1], Kinneret Rosenblatt[2], Deborah K. Dunn-Walters[3], Iris Barshack[2,4‡] and Ramit Mehr[1*‡]

[1] The Mina and Everard Goodman Faculty of Life Sciences, Bar-Ilan University, Ramat Gan, Israel
[2] Department of Pathology, Sheba Medical Center, Ramat Gan, Israel
[3] Division of Immunology, Infection, and Inflammatory Diseases, King's College London School of Medicine, London, UK
[4] Sackler Faculty of Medicine, Tel Aviv University, Tel Aviv, Israel

Edited by:
Michal Or-Guil, Humboldt University Berlin, Germany

Reviewed by:
Jose Faro, Universidade de Vigo, Spain
Andrew M. Collins, University of New South Wales, Australia

***Correspondence:**
Ramit Mehr, The Mina and Everard Goodman Faculty of Life Sciences, Bar-Ilan University, Ramat Gan 52900, Israel
e-mail: ramit.mehr@biu.ac.il

† Miri Michaeli, Hilla Tabibian-Keissar and Ginette Schiby have contributed equally to this work.

‡ Iris Barshack and Ramit Mehr have equally supervised this study.

Chronic gastritis is characterized by gastric mucosal inflammation due to autoimmune responses or infection, frequently with *Helicobacter pylori*. Gastritis with *H. pylori* background can cause gastric mucosa-associated lymphoid tissue lymphoma (MALT-L), which sometimes further transforms into diffuse large B-cell lymphoma (DLBCL). However, gastric DLBCL can also be initiated *de novo*. The mechanisms underlying transformation into DLBCL are not completely understood. We analyzed immunoglobulin repertoires and clonal trees to investigate whether and how immunoglobulin gene repertoires, clonal diversification, and selection in gastritis, gastric MALT-L, and DLBCL differ from each other and from normal responses. The two gastritis types (positive or negative for *H. pylori*) had similarly diverse repertoires. MALT-L dominant clones (defined as the largest clones in each sample) presented higher diversification and longer mutational histories compared with all other conditions. DLBCL dominant clones displayed lower clonal diversification, suggesting the transforming events are triggered by similar responses in different patients. These results are surprising, as we expected to find similarities between the dominant clones of gastritis and MALT-L and between those of MALT-L and DLBCL.

Keywords: B-cells, gastritis, *H. pylori*, MALT lymphoma, DLBCL, Ig gene, repertoire, somatic hypermutation

INTRODUCTION

Chronic gastritis is a common disorder characterized by chronic inflammation of gastric mucosa. In acute gastritis, patients suffer from dyspeptic symptoms including epigastric burning, distention or bloating, belching, episodic nausea, flatulence, and halitosis. In contrast, most patients with chronic gastritis are asymptomatic (1). One of the major causes of gastritis is bacterial infection, most frequently with *Helicobacter pylori* (*H. pylori*). *H. pylori* are Gram-negative bacteria that are present in the gastric mucosa of more than 50% of people and may persist lifelong unless treated (2). *H. pylori* are resistant to elimination by the immune response so the immune system fails to remove the infection effectively (3). Previous studies have shown a strong association between gastritis and *H. pylori* infection, at least in the early stages of gastritis (3, 4). Although rare, organisms other than *H. pylori* (e.g., *Mycobacterium avium*-intracellulare, Herpes simplex, Cytomegalovirus, and Epstein–Barr virus) can invade the gastric mucosa and cause inflammation (5, 6). Gastritis can also be initiated *de novo*, as an autoimmune disease (7). In either case, prolonged antigenic stimulation causing chronic inflammation might further contribute to the development of some malignancies (8), such as gastric mucosa-associated lymphoid tissue (MALT) lymphoma (9–16).

Mucosa-associated lymphoid tissue lymphoma (MALT-L) is a low-grade B-cell lymphoma. It grows slowly and remains confined to one organ for a relatively long time. Stomach MALT-L exemplifies the close link between chronic inflammation and lymphomagenesis. B-cells of MALT-L are related to normal marginal zone cells. Their IgH variable region gene sequences exhibit features of post germinal center B-cells, such as somatic hypermutation (SHM), implying that the clone has expanded in the presence of an antigen (17). MALT-L is often associated with bacterial infection, most commonly by *H. pylori* bacterium (7–9, 15–17).

A possible outcome of low-grade B-cell lymphomas such as MALT-L is the transformation into a more aggressive lymphoma such as diffuse large B-cell lymphoma (DLBCL) (18, 19). Gastric DLBCL is a fast-growing, aggressive B-cell malignancy characterized by diffuse proliferation of large neoplastic lymphoid B-cells (20, 21). DLBCL is known to represent a heterogeneous group of malignancies, comprising either germinal center-like cells exhibiting intra-clonal diversity or "activated B-cell-like" cells, which do not (22, 23).

Abbreviations: AML, acute myeloid leukemia; B-CLL, chronic lymphocytic leukemia; BCR, B-cell receptor; CDR, complementary determining region; CI, confidence intervals; CLN, control lymph node; DLBCL, diffuse large B-cell lymphoma; FL, follicular lymphoma; GHP, gastritis with *H. pylori* background; GNHP, gastritis without *H. pylori* background; *H. pylori*, *Helicobacter pylori*; HTS, high-throughput sequencing; Indels, insertions and/or deletions; MALT, mucosa-associated lymphoid tissue; MALT-L, MALT lymphoma; MID, molecular identification; MM, multiple myeloma; SHM, somatic hypermutation.

During the clonal expansion of B-cells in response to an antigen, Ig gene sequences from clonally related B-cells (i.e., B-cells that are derivatives of the same B-cell ancestor) accumulate mutations via SHM and thus diversify. Clonally related cells are identified by identical V(D)J segments and by highly homologous sequences of the complementary determining region (CDR) 3 of their Ig genes. An easy way to track and analyze the relationships between clonally related Ig gene sequences is by using lineage trees. The tree root is the ancestor sequence, usually the rearranged, pre-mutation sequence. Each tree node represents a single mutation (point mutation, insertion, or deletion). Lineage trees have been used in order to quantify the differences between the dynamics of SHM and antigen-driven selection in different lymphoid tissues, species, and disease situations. Our lineage trees-based mutation analysis has demonstrated its usefulness in previous studies of aging (24), autoimmunity (25–28), and chronic inflammation (29). Recent work on B-cell malignancies done in our lab (30–32) showed differences in tree properties between lymphomas and controls. Lymphoma trees were more branched and had longer trunks compared to controls, indicating a higher intra-clonal diversification and a longer mutational history. Intra-clonal diversification was also shown in chronic lymphocytic leukemia cases (33–35), in marginal zone lymphoma cases (36, 37) and in intestinal DLBCL cases (21). In addition, lymphoma and controls exhibited similar mutation rates and same SHM motifs. Follicular lymphoma (FL), which is considered a less aggressive lymphoma, displayed higher diversity than DLBCL and highest recent diversification events, suggesting that the more aggressive lymphoma diversifies the least (38–40).

In the present study, we used repertoire, lineage tree, and mutation analyses to investigate whether and how B-cell repertoires, clonal diversification, and selection mechanisms in gastritis, gastric MALT-L, and DLBCL differ from each other and from normal responses. The two types of gastritis (positive or negative for *H. pylori*) were found to have similar repertoires and diversification. MALT-L clones were found to be more diversified and had longer mutational histories compared with all other conditions, but the dominant clones of MALT-L (defined as the largest clones in each sample) were different from those of all other conditions. DLBCL dominant clones, however, displayed lower diversification. These results are surprising, as we expected to find similarities between the dominant clones of gastritis and MALT-L and between those of MALT-L and DLBCL, according to the hypothesis that these are often sequential steps of inflammation and transformation.

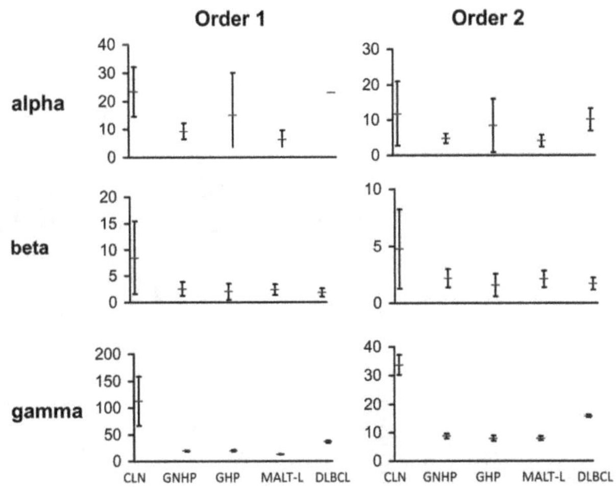

FIGURE 1 | Graphic presentation of alpha, beta, and gamma diversity indices of order 1 and 2. Diversity measures were calculated, as described in the Section "Materials and Methods," based on the Shannon entropy and the Simpson concentration diversity indices. The alpha diversity measure represents the average sample diversity in each condition/population. The gamma diversity measure represents the "global" repertoire diversity across all samples studied in each condition/population. The beta diversity measure represents the diversity component resulting from the variability between samples. In our Ig gene repertoire studies, the abundance data (numbers of unique sequences) of antibody clones in each sample was used to estimate the mean, standard error, and 95% confidence intervals (CI) of the total number of unique sequences in clones within each sample. The CI allows us to compare between diversity indices of different conditions. The error bars show the standard errors.

RESULTS

REPERTOIRES IN GASTRITIS WITH *H. PYLORI* BACKGROUND WERE AS DIVERSE AS THOSE IN GASTRITIS NEGATIVE FOR *H. PYLORI*, AND CONTAINED SIMILAR V(D)J COMBINATIONS

We compared the repertoires in both types of gastritis, with *H. pylori* background (GHP) or without *H. pylori* background (GNHP), and examined the differences between them. We expected the repertoire in GHP to be less diverse due to the response to the bacterium, as previous studies showed that monoclonality is frequently found in GHP samples [(41–43) and others]. In contrast to our expectation, the confidence intervals (CI) of alpha, beta, and gamma diversity indices of both orders were overlapping (**Figure 1**), implying the average individual biopsy diversities, the variability of diversities between individual biopsies, and the overall pool diversities in GHP and GNHP were not statistically different. Indeed, most V(D)J combinations observed were expressed in both gastritis types (**Figures 2A,B**).

Gastritis with *H. pylori* background and GNHP were the most similar conditions (similarity index of 0.543, **Table 1**), although one GHP sample (the second GHP sample in Table S1 in Supplementary Material) had an extremely high alpha diversity index compared to the other two samples (data not shown). This contradicts our expectation of narrower repertoires in GHP samples due to the presence of *H. pylori*. However, if the one highly diverse GHP sample is excluded from the analysis, the confidence interval of alpha of GHP becomes narrower (3.9–11.25), and lower than that of GNHP. It is possible that the highly diverse sample reflected additional ongoing responses.

VH1-3/JH4 was a common combination in both GNHP and GHP VH–JH repertoires, but not so prominent in repertoires of other conditions (**Figures 2A,B**). These combinations contained several DH genes in both GNHP and GHP. However, identification of D genes should be taken with caution, as SoDA always finds a D gene, even when this is based on too-few nucleotides to be reliable. **Table 2** summarizes all common combinations and genes found in our study and their relationships with other clinical conditions as implicated in the literature.

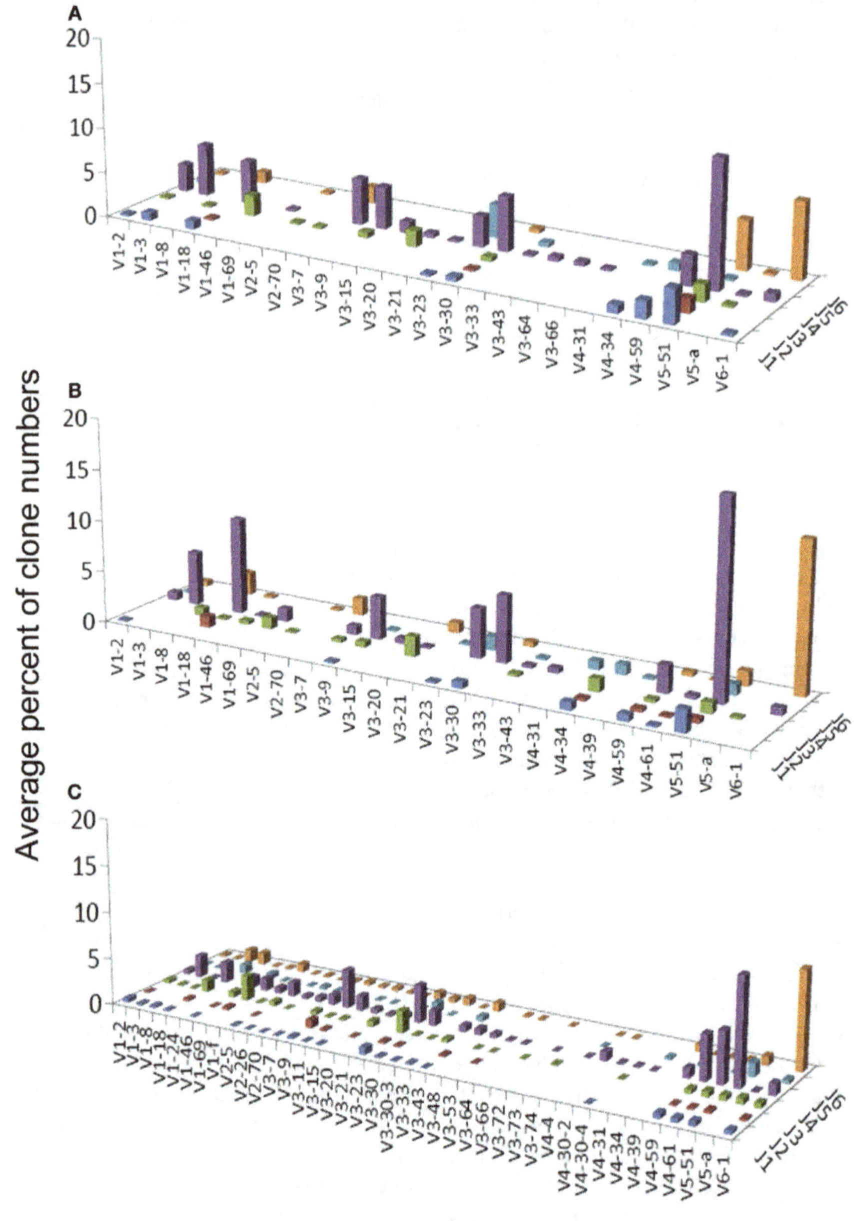

FIGURE 2 | Average percentages of clones in each VH–JH combination, in (A) GHP, (B) GNHP, and (C) CLN samples.

Table 1 | The average similarity between each pair of conditions.

	CLN	GNHP	GHP
CLN	0.211	0.295	0.343
GNHP		0.408	0.543
GHP			0.478

Similarity measures were calculated between all clones in all samples in the compared conditions. In lymphomas, only the dominant clone(s) are relevant, as the rest of the clones in each sample represent other B-cells present in the tissue, which are not related to the malignancy. Thus, MALT-L and DLBCL are not included in the calculation of similarity measures because the dominant clones in these conditions cannot be compared to the full repertoire samples from other conditions.

In the case of GNHP, the DH3 and DH6 families were found to be preferred, as combinations of V6D3J6 and V6D6J6 were used significantly more than expected (**Table 3; Figure 2B**). Other over-expressed DH genes were used in less prominent combinations in the observed repertoire. Other combinations used in GNHP and GHP, such as VH3-7, VH3-23, and VH3-30 – all with JH4 – used several DH genes from different DH families.

Gastritis without *H. pylori* background and GHP presented almost identical gene usage patterns, having VH5-51/JH4 and VH6-1/JH6 as the two most frequent combinations (**Figures 2A,B**). VH5-51 and VH6-1 have been shown to often participate in earlier stages of repertoire development via positive selection by auto-antigens (**Table 2**). These two combinations also appeared in our control lymph node (CLN) samples (**Figure 2C**),

Table 2 | A summary of frequent combinations and genes in conditions from our study and from other studies.

Gene or combination	Common in our study in	Appeared in the literature in relation to
VH1-2	MALT-L[a]	Self-reactive antibodies, Bahler et al. (44) Chronic lymphocytic leukemia (B-CLL), primary central nervous system lymphomas, and splenic marginal zone lymphomas, Walsh and Rosenquist (45)
VH1-3	GNHP, GHP	B-CLL, Fais et al. (46)
VH1-18	GNHP, GHP, DLBCL	B-CLL, Fais et al. (46) Autoreactive gene, Yamashita et al. (47) BM-DLBCL, gastric MALT-Ls, Bende et al. (48)
VH1-8	DLBCL	B-CLL, Pimentel et al. (49)
VH1-69	MALT-L[a], DLBCL	Rheumatoid factor, Bende et al. (48), Matsuda et al. (50) Gastric MALT-Ls, Bende et al. (48) B-CLL, Fais et al. (46), Pimentel et al. (49), Johnson et al. (51)
VH2-26/JH5	MALT-L[a]	FL, Bayerl et al. (52)
VH2-26	MALT-L[a]	B-CLL, Pimentel et al. (49) Hairy cell leukemia, Hashimoto et al. (53)
VH3-7	MALT-L Dominant, DLBCL	Rheumatoid factor, Bende et al. (48), Matsuda et al. (50) Rheumatoid arthritis, Nakamura-Kikuoka et al. (54) Sjögren syndrome, Bahler and Swerdlow (55) B-CLL, Fais et al. (46) BM-DLBCL, Yamashita et al. (47) Gastric MALT-Ls, Bende et al. (48)
VH3-23	DLBCL	IgM+ B-cells, Brezinschek et al. (56) Naïve B-cells, Wu et al. (57) Anti-DNA auto-antibodies, Matsuda et al. (50) Hepatitis C virus-related mixed cryoglobulinemia, Perotti et al. (58) Unmutated VH3-23 in transformation from B-CLL into DLBCL, Mao et al. (59) Gastric MALT lymphomagenesis, Sakuma et al. (60), Lenze et al. (61), Alpen et al. (62), Siakantaris et al. (63) BM-DLBCL, Yamashita et al. (47) B-CLL, Pimentel et al. (49)
VH3-30	DLBCL	Rheumatoid factor, Bende et al. (48), Matsuda et al. (50) Gastric MALT lymphomagenesis, Sakuma et al. (60), Lenze et al. (61), Alpen et al. (62), Siakantaris et al. (63) B-CLL, Pimentel et al. (49)
VH3-30/JH4	DLBCL	FL, Bayerl et al. (52)
VH5-51 and VH6-1	CLN, GNHP, GHP, and DLBCL Dominant	Auto-antigens, Matsuda et al. (50)

The dominant segments are marked with "Dominant" indication. The dominant segments/combinations are those that appeared in the largest clone in each sample.
[a]Represents frequent genes or combinations in the repertoire of unique sequences.

so they probably have no specific connection to gastritis or *H. pylori* response. However, the VH1-18/JH4 combination was more frequently used in GNHP than in GHP, and was not prominently observed in other conditions. As VH1-18 is an autoreactive gene and was found in several gastric MALT-Ls (**Table 2**), VH1-18 may be involved in the development of gastritis regardless of the presence of *H. pylori*.

One combination was over-expressed in both types of gastritis (V3D0J5), and two combinations (V6D3J6 and V6D6J6, **Table 3**) were over-expressed in GNHP (as dominant clones) and in DLBCL samples (not the dominant clones). As can be seen in **Figures 2B,C** and **3A**, many sequences used the V6–J6 combination in GNHP and DLBCL, but also in the controls. Thus, this combination is very frequent in immune responses, and cannot be ascribed to a

Table 3 | VDJ combinations that were over-expressed in each condition[a].

Condition	Combination	*p*-Value	Mean difference[b]
GNHP	V2D1J6	0.009	3.57
	V3D5J4	0.002	4.38
	V3D0J5	0.001	7.84
	V6D6J6	0.035	3.84
	V6D3J6	0.042	3.60
GHP	V3D0J5	0.035	10.44
	V5D3J2	0.015	3.26
DLBCL	V1D1J6 Dominant[c]	0.011	1.30
	V1D4J3	0.000	4.94
	V4D6J4	0.046	2.70
	V5D1J4 Dominant[d]	0.001	1.80
	V5D7J4	0.036	2.20
	V6D6J6	0.000	3.47
	V6D3J6	0.003	3.50

[a]*There were no VDJ combinations that where over-expressed in MALT-L samples, thus MALT-L does not appear in the table.*

[b]*Represents the value of $\log_2$(observed/expected).*

[c]*This combination was found in DLBCL samples number 1, 2, 3 (sample numbers according to Table S1 in Supplementary Material). The dominant combinations are those that appeared in the largest clone in each sample.*

[d]*This combination was found in DLBCL sample number 5.*

specific condition. However, the combination V3D0J5 may represent an antibody that is effective in the gastric environment, related to inflammatory processes, or participates in both.

To conclude, both types of gastritis presented similar repertoires and diversity properties, in contrast to our expectation.

GASTRIC MALT-L EXHIBITED UNIQUE V(D)J COMBINATIONS

Several studies have demonstrated that gastric MALT-L is often associated with a bacterial infection, most commonly by *H. pylori*; another association has been revealed between gastritis and gastric MALT-L (11–13). Therefore, we expected to find similar V(D)J combinations when comparing the two conditions. Surprisingly, the dominant MALT-L V(D)J combinations were very different from those in GHP. While GHP showed an extensive use of JH4 family genes and several common combinations, of which the most frequent was VH5-51/JH4, in MALT-L dominant clones were VH3-7/JH4, VH1-69/JH6, and VH1-2/JH1. VH3-7 is frequently found in rheumatoid factors and was selectively expressed by patients with rheumatoid arthritis and Sjögren syndrome. Preferential use of these genes and combinations has been reported in several types of lymphomas and leukemias (**Table 2**).

Table S2 in Supplementary Material presents the combinations that were over-expressed in one condition while under-represented in the other. It can be seen (from the "Mean deviation" column) that over-expressed combinations were almost absolutely from either MALT-L or DLBCL samples (dominant clones only). As DLBCL contained dominant combinations that also appeared in other conditions, this supports the observation of different dominant combinations in MALT-L compared to those observed in other conditions. These combinations may relate to the malignancy, but this remains to be explored.

We also compared the dominant clones in DLBCL and MALT-L samples, as in some cases DLBCL appears in association with MALT-L (18, 19). DLBCL is considered in these cases to result from clonal transformation of large cells within the low-grade lymphoma (64, 65). Hence, we expected to identify similar segment combinations on the dominant clones from the two conditions. However, the dominant clones of MALT-L samples were different from those of DLBCL (**Figures 3A,B**). As mentioned above, the dominant clones in MALT-Ls were VH3-7/JH4, VH1-69/JH6, and VH1-2/JH1, while in DLBCLs these combinations were found, but were not the dominant clones. VH5-51/JH4 and VH6-1/JH6 were frequent combinations in all conditions, except in MALT-L, suggesting they may have some advantage in binding common antigens. In terms of unique sequences, MALT-Ls presented completely different dominant combinations from DLBCL (VH1-2/JH1, VH1-69/JH6, VH2-26/JH5, and VH3-7/JH4, data not shown). Preferential use of these genes and combinations has been reported in several types of lymphomas and leukemias (**Table 2**). In addition, VH3-7/JH4, which was the most frequent combination in MALT-L dominant clones, appeared in all other conditions but with dramatically lower numbers. As mentioned above, VH3-7 participates in the formation of auto-antibodies and was found in several gastric MALT-Ls. Some MALT-Ls were found to use VH genes previously associated with auto-reactivity. This suggests that B-cells in MALT-L react with self-antigens (66), different from those that arouse in GHP and DLBCL responses.

MALT-L DOMINANT CLONES HAD LONGER DIVERSIFICATION HISTORY, IN CONTRAST TO DLBCL CLONES

Lineage trees of the MALT-L dominant clones had significantly longer trunks (T) and path lengths (PLmin), which are tree length measures, than all other conditions (**Figure 4**; Figure S1 in Supplementary Material). In addition, according to the correlation of tree properties with the dynamic parameters of the secondary B-cell response (67), longer trunks correlate with a lower initial affinity, and longer paths also correlate with a lower selection threshold. This suggests that diversification history in MALT-L dominant clones was longer than that of other conditions.

On the contrary, DLBCL dominant clones had significantly shorter trunks and path lengths than those of GHP (and MALT-L), and in general, the lowest tree length measures. Dominant clones of DLBCL presented similar tree length measures to those of CLN (**Figure 4**; Figure S1 in Supplementary Material). This is in line with the above-described observation of similarity between DLBCL and CLN. The shorter lengths observed in DLBCL, which correlate with high initial affinity and selection threshold, may indicate a shorter diversification process compared to MALT-L and GHP (21). A possible explanation for this is that, because MALT-L

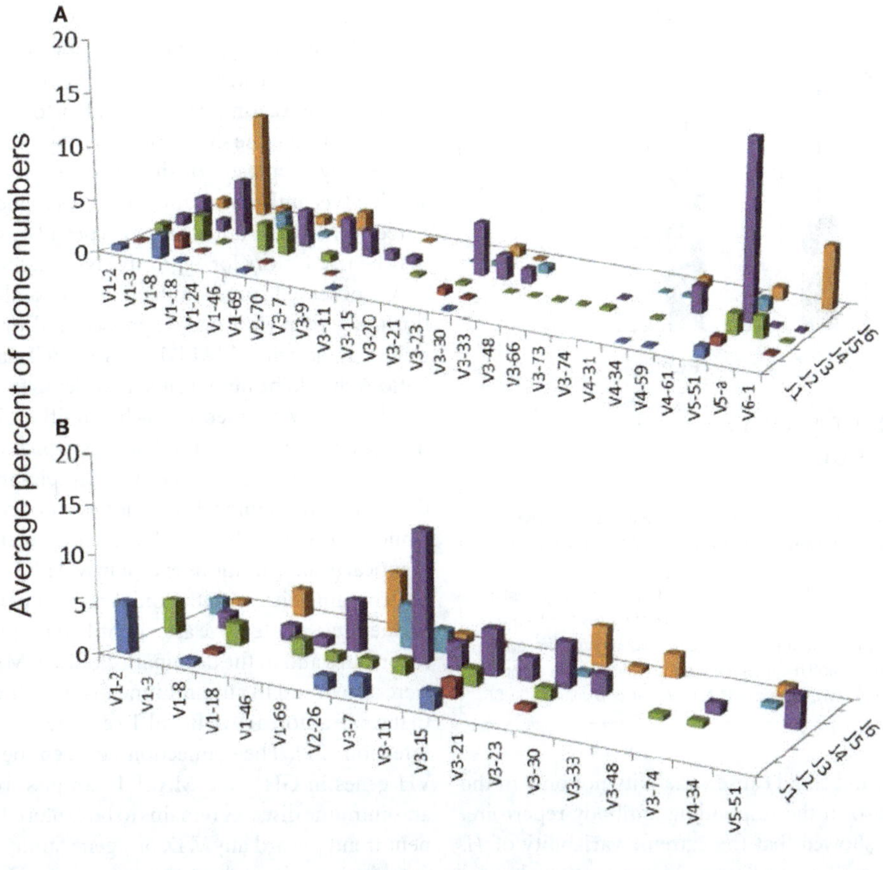

FIGURE 3 | Average percentages of clones in each VH–JH combination, in (A) DLBCL and (B) MALT-L samples.

is an indolent lymphoma and DLBCL is an aggressive lymphoma, the latter usually has less time to diversify until it is discovered and treated. Figures S2 and S3 in Supplementary Material show representative examples for MALT-L and DLBCL dominant trees, respectively.

The fact that MALT-L dominant clones had larger trunks, path lengths, and distance from the root to any split node, thus probably lower initial affinity than DLBCL dominant clones, suggests that DLBCL dominant clones started as responses to specific (yet-unknown) antigens, with probably higher initial affinity than the responses that initiated MALT-Ls. That is, high affinity and vigorous response may be risk factors for aggressive lymphoma development. In terms of selection, these results show that selection thresholds in MALT-L dominant clones were the lowest among all other conditions. Low selection pressure may simply be the result of abundance of antigen, and this may indeed be the case in gastric MALT-Ls.

Dominant clones from the two types of gastritis presented similar tree length measures, which correlate with the observed similar repertoires.

DISCUSSION

In this study, we investigated the relationships between four related conditions of the stomach: gastritis positive or negative for *H. pylori*, gastric MALT-L, and gastric DLBCL. As previous studies showed, these conditions sometimes appear successively, as prolonged stimulation during chronic gastritis may result in the development of gastric MALT-L, which in some cases further transforms into DLBCL. We examined the clonal repertoires of the IgH variable region genes (or in the case of lymphomas, the dominant clones, which are defined as the largest clone in each sample) and the lineage tree characteristics in each condition, in order to find similarities or differences between these conditions.

Both types of gastritis presented similar IgH variable region gene repertoires and lineage tree characteristics, in contrast to our pre-study assumptions. However, although the GNHP biopsies were negative for *H. pylori*, it could be present in the tissue in undetectable amounts, and thus affect the repertoire of the B-cells in its surroundings. Moreover, both types of gastritis used the VH1-18 gene, which may be involved in the development of gastritis regardless of the presence of *H. pylori*; this remains to be elucidated, as this was not the dominant combination in both type of gastritis. We expected the repertoire in GHP to be less diverse than that of GNHP due to the response to the bacterium, which is expected to elicit only specific clones. In contrast to our expectations, GHP samples showed at least as diverse repertoires as GNHP (**Figures 1** and **2A,B**). An explanation for a high diversity in GHP might be the phase variation of *H. pylori*, which is the generation of intra-strain diversity that is important for bacterial

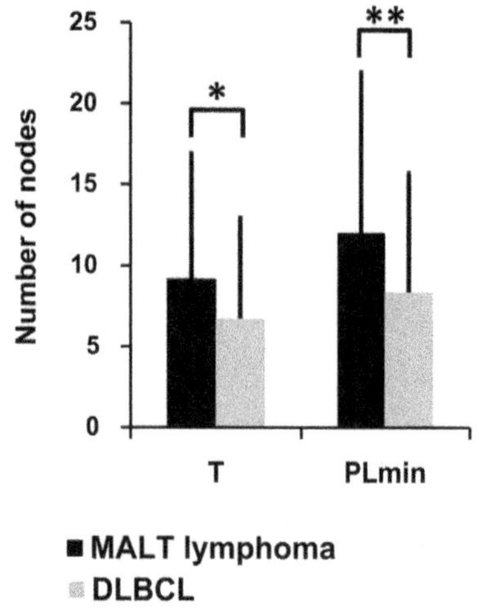

FIGURE 4 | Lineage tree analysis – comparison between dominant clones from the three MALT-L samples (24 trees) and the five DLBCL samples (47 trees). There was more than one tree per sample, as we included all clones with the same VH and JH genes (but different alleles) in the dominant clone in each sample, because they might be related to the dominant clone and falsely attributed to other alleles. Significant differences were found in trunk length (T) and minimal path length (PLmin). An asterisk (*) represents p-value <0.01; two asterisks (**) represents p-value <0.005.

niche adaptation (68), and could cause variability not only in the bacterial strains but also in the responding antibody repertoire. Hussell et al. (69, 70) showed that the extreme variability of *H. pylori* strains led to diverse T cell responses. Moreover, they showed that B-cells did not respond to *H. pylori* themselves, but required contact-dependent help from *H. pylori*-specific T cells, and their Ig genes responded to auto-antigens, similar to our observations. Alternatively, the repertoires in the biopsies – even GHP biopsies – may reflect immune responses to a variety of pathogens, including but not limited to *H. pylori.*

Although in many cases DLBCL is associated with MALT-L, the two types of lymphomas presented different dominant clone combinations and lineage tree characteristics. DLBCL may develop after prolonged stimulation during gastritis, derive from a low-grade malignant clone, or it can initiate *de novo*, depending on the mutations in each clone. In this study, as MALT-L and DLBCL presented different dominant clone combinations, in contrast to our expectations; we speculate that in these cases DLBCL may have initiated *de novo*. MALT-L samples presented different lineage tree characteristics from those of all other conditions, although we expected MALT-L to resemble GHP. In fact, we identified preferential use of the autoreactive gene VH3-7 in MALT-L samples. VH3-7 was one of the common VH genes in GHP (but not the dominant clone). These findings suggest that gastric MALT-L is derived from highly restricted B-cell subsets probably resulting from specific antigenic stimulation, such as with *H. pylori* (15). It is possible that B-cells in MALT-L react with self-antigens (66), however, the role of self-antigens in the development of the malignancy has yet to be examined. Moreover, lineage tree drawings demonstrated longer trunks and path lengths in MALT-L dominant clones, compared with all other conditions. These differences in tree characteristics correlate with lower initial affinity and lower selection threshold, respectively. Low selection pressure may simply be the result of abundance of antigen, and this may indeed be the case in gastric MALT-L. The above may indicate that MALT-L has undergone a longer mutational history than other conditions. On the contrary, the shorter lengths observed in DLBCL dominant clones may be a result of shorter diversification and responses to specific (yet-unknown) antigens, with higher initial affinity compared to MALT-L and the two types of gastritis (21). The latter may be risk factors for aggressive lymphoma development.

We observed some similar VH–JH combinations in all conditions, together with over-expressed and preferred combinations unique to gastritis, MALT-L, and DLBCL samples. These combinations should be investigated in order to further understand their role in the development of each condition. For example, the relatively extensive use of combinations, which were previously found in other malignancies, in DLBCL samples in this study reinforces the notion that some DLBCL clones had developed from MALT-L clones. Moreover, the fact that the dominant combinations were identical in all conditions except in MALT-L (and that MALT-L did not contain this combination at all) is interesting and should be further investigated. We also identified frequent VH genes in GHP repertoires and in the dominant clones in MALT-L samples, which were also found in autoimmune diseases. It was previously shown that some autoreactive B and T cells are activated during *H. pylori* infection (71). The connection between the appearances of these VH genes in GHP and MALT-L samples from our study and in autoimmune diseases remains to be explored. There was no prominent trend toward any V, D, or J gene family in the over-expressed combinations in each of the conditions. However, combinations that were over-expressed in lymphoma dominant clones compared to other conditions had a clear preference toward the use of VH2, JH1 in MALT-L and VH1, JH2 in DLBCL. The role of these combinations and gene families in lymphomas is still unknown.

It should be noted that, because we studied formalin-fixed paraffin-embedded archival biopsies, we had access to only a limited number of biopsies, and limited amounts of DNA, as DNA in the preserved biopsies is often denatured (72). More samples in more conditions will have to be studied in order to give a clearer picture of the roles of specific V(D)J genes and combinations in inflammation and malignancies. Moreover, the similarity between conditions is also affected by the limited number of samples in each condition. This may cause the similarity calculations to be biased toward random features of the samples that may characterize a certain condition, and thus affect the interpretations. However, the similarity between samples within each condition was not very large, so it is unlikely that some random feature is common to all samples of the same condition. Coincident with obtaining more samples, we intend to use the Illumina high-throughput sequencing (HTS) in future studies, in order to avoid the 454 sequencing artifacts, which resulted in discarding many sequences (73). A possible argument could be raised regarding the exclusion of duplicate sequences from our analysis. As mentioned in the Section "Materials and Methods," duplicate sequences may stem from the PCR amplification, and may cause misidentification of dominant clones. Although we stringently defined duplicate sequences as those that had the exact nucleotide composition and equal lengths, most of the sequences differed not only by their lengths, but also in the mutations they include. Table S5 in Supplementary Material summarizes the distributions of the number of sequences in the tree-nodes in the dominant and second dominant clones in lymphoma samples. As can be seen from Table S5 in Supplementary Material, most of the nodes contained only one sequence, implying that most of the sequences differed not only in their lengths, but also in the mutations they include. There were, however, several nodes that contained more than one sequence. This does not necessarily indicate that those sequences are duplicates, as the clone-tree is built according to the aligned sub-sequences that are shared between all sequences in the clone. This means that sequences included in a specific node could differ in their ends, and not necessarily be duplicates.

All conditions in this study presented similar mutation rates and the same SHM targeting motifs. Replacement and silent mutation analysis revealed a strong selection against replacement mutations in the CDR regions of all conditions. This may indicate that most of the examined IgH variable region gene sequences represented B-cell receptors (BCRs) that were already highly specific to their antigens and thus selection operated against replacement mutations in their CDR regions, which are responsible for antigen binding. These results are also consistent with previous work on lymphomas from our lab (30).

In this study, we used the Morisita similarity index in order to measure similarity between conditions (as mentioned in the Section "Materials and Methods"). Similarity measures were calculated between all clones in all samples in the compared conditions. In lymphomas, only the dominant clone(s) are relevant, as the rest of the clones in each sample represent other B-cells that are also present in the tissue, but are not related to the malignancy. Thus, the MALT-L and DLBCL conditions were not included in calculation of similarity measures exactly because the dominant clones in these conditions cannot be compared to the whole other samples in other conditions. In addition, Morisita similarity index is of order 2, which emphasizes large clones. This affects the similarity results. However, we are interested in the larger clones in each condition as they probably represent the dominant responses.

In summary, we showed that gastritis positive or negative for *H. pylori* presented very similar IgH variable region gene repertoires. This suggests that the diverse stomach repertories do not change much due to the presence of the bacteria, and moreover, GHP does not become oligoclonal (or at least with narrower repertoire) due to *H. pylori*. MALT-L, however, presented different and unique dominant clone gene combinations, which can result from specific antigenic stimulation. As was mentioned in the Section "Introduction," several studies showed that *H. pylori* causes gastritis, and suggested that prolonged gastritis can lead to MALT-L, and that prolonged MALT-L can develop into DLBCL. This flow and graduation of diseases led us to the assumption that the repertoires (VDJ combinations) in these conditions would be similar, because these conditions were initiated by the bacteria, and several clones got out of control to progress into lymphoma. Moreover, the diversity in these conditions was expected to be narrower than that in CLN, and to be progressively lower as the conditions proceed toward the aggressive lymphoma. However, the results differed from what we expected. In addition, some combinations did appear in several conditions, but not in MALT-L, and the DLBCL dominant clones also appear in other conditions (so they were not unique to the cancer). We speculate that the transformation into MALT-L, after the prolonged stimulation by the chronic GHP, amplified specific combination(s) that were also found in GHP but in a lower frequency (such as VH3-7). The two types of lymphomas differed in their dominant clone gene combinations and lineage tree characteristics, suggesting differences in the abundance of antigens, if not in their nature, which remain to be explored.

MATERIALS AND METHODS

HISTOPATHOLOGICAL SPECIMENS

Five gastric DLBCL biopsies, 3 gastric MALT-L biopsies, 10 chronic gastritis biopsies (3 with *H. pylori* background and 7 that were negative for *H. pylori*), and 19 reactive lymph node biopsies (which served as controls), each from a different patient, were selected from the pathology department archives in the Sheba Medical Center (Table S1 in Supplementary Material). Tissue biopsies were taken during resection procedures and were used in this study in accordance with institutional Helsinki committee guidelines and approval. Histochemical stains, by Hematoxylin-Eosin (H&E) and Giemsa, were performed for histological evaluation and *H. pylori* identification. For diagnosis of lymphoproliferative disease and characterization of lymphocyte populations, immunohistochemical stains (e.g., CD20, CD3, CD23, CD21, cyclin-D1, Ki67, and IgD) were also performed. All cases were revised by two independent pathologists to confirm the diagnosis.

DNA EXTRACTION

Paraffin-embedded blocks were cut using a microtome to get extremely thin slices of tissues (sections). Each of the biopsies was consecutively cut to yield 10–20 sections of 4 μ each, depending on tissue size. All sections from each biopsy were inserted into an eppendorf tube with 200 μl water (Sigma) and were heated in 90°C until the paraffin was melted. After the tubes were centrifuged at full speed (14000 rpm) for 1 min, a paraffin ring was created and could easily be removed from each of the tubes. Water was drawn from the tubes while tissues remained in the tubes. Extraction of DNA was then performed using the QIAamp DNA Mini Kit (or the QIAamp DNA Micro Kit for very small samples) according to the QIAGEN protocol.

In some cases, a micro-dissection was needed. First, H&E stained thin sections were reviewed by a pathologist, and areas of interest were outlined. The tissues were cut from 5 to 10 sections that were placed onto five slides per tissue. The slides were heated in 90°C for 15 min. Next, the slides were hydrated (5 min soaking in Xylene, brief immersion in Ethanol 100, 96, and 70% in this order). The slides were then placed to dry. According to the outlined stained slides of each tissue, the hydrated slides were scratched with buffer ATL (QIAamp DNA Mini Kit, QIAGEN) and sample scrapings were picked up into eppendorf tubes. Extraction of DNA was then performed using the QIAamp DNA Mini Kit (or the QIAamp DNA Micro Kit for very small samples) according to the QIAGEN protocol.

PCR AMPLIFICATION AND HIGH-THROUGHPUT SEQUENCING

For each sample taken from each biopsy, semi-nested PCR was performed using the same forward primers for the two PCR rounds and two different reverse primers as described below.

Forward primers from FR2 region:

VH1: 5′-TGCGMCAGGCCCCYGGACAAR-3′,
VH2: 5′-ARGRAAGGCCCTGGAGTGG-3′,
VH3: 5′-CCAGGCTCCAGGSAAG-3′,
VH4: 5′-MGGGAAGGGRCTGGAGTGG-3′,
VH5: 5′-GAAAGGCCTGGAGTGGATGGG-3′,
VH6: 5′-TTGAGTGGCTGGGRAGGAC-3′.

Reverse primers:

First round – JH1R: 5′-TGAGGAGACGGTGACCAGGGT-3′,
Second round – JH2R: 5′-TGACCRKGGTHCCYTGGCCC-3′.

There is no specific primer for VH7 gene family in the FR2 region, as the VH7 primer in this region is very similar to that of VH1, thus, it amplifies the VH1 family and creates a very strong VH1 bias.

The primers were augmented for HTS experiments by the addition of 5′ sequencing adapter elements and 10-nucleotide unique sample molecular identification (MID) tags according to the 454 FLX Titanium chemistry protocol (Roche) (74). Proofreading Taq DNA polymerase (ABgene) was used in PCR reactions according to the manufacturer's protocol. PCR reaction was performed on a sample of 50 ng DNA from each sample, with slight changes according to calibration (because DNA was taken from different tissues, and each tissue can differ in the percentages of lymphocytes). PCR products were separated on a 2% agarose gel stained by ethidium bromide. Clear bands were cut from the gel and DNA was extracted using the MinElute Gel Extraction kit (QIAGEN), according to the manufacturer's protocol. Sequencing of small samples of the PCR products by the classic Sanger method (after cloning to pGEM – T-easy vector) was performed in order to make sure they are Ig gene amplifications and the sequences of the primers and the tags are intact. DNA concentration of PCR products from each sample were determined by PicoGreen dye and fluorospectrometer (Nanodrop). According to these results, a mixture containing 10^9 molecules of PCR products from each sample was prepared and sent to sequencing. HTS was performed using the 454 GS FLX Titanium platform by DYN Diagnostics Ltd., the sole representative in Israel of Roche Diagnostics. Raw data files containing a total of ~120,000 reads were received when the HTS was completed. Raw data files can be downloaded from the SRA database, accession number PRJNA206548 (Runs: SRR873440, SRR873441, SRR873442).

HTS RAW DATA PRE-PROCESSING

To process the 454 raw data, we used our program Ig-HTS-cleaner (73). Ig-HTS-cleaner discards artifact sequences, assigns the sequences to samples according to their MID tags, identifies primers, and discards sequences much shorter or longer than the expected length of an Ig variable region gene, or sequences with average quality scores below a defined threshold. Parameters used in the Ig-HTS-Cleaner run were as follows. Average quality score threshold of 20, a maximum of 2 allowed mismatches in the primer search, 75% of the primer's length to search, and a range of 25 bases at the ends of the read for the MID and primers search (Table S3 in Supplementary Material).

Next, we discarded duplicate sequences, which are completely identical sequences, from each sample. We cannot exclude the possibility that duplicate sequences are a result of the PCR amplification; hence the existence of many identical sequences in a sample does not necessarily indicate that the sequence is found in the original biopsy in the same frequency.

Afterward, we used our program Ig-Indel-Identifier (Ig Insertion – Deletion Identifier) (73), in order to identify legitimate and artifact insertions and/or deletions (indels) in the sequences. Parameters used in the Ig-Indel-Identifier run were as follows. HPT length was set to 2, quality score threshold (for suspected point mutations) of 25, and the number of sequences in the same clone containing the same indel was set to 1 (Table S4 in Supplementary Material). **Table 4** presents the numbers of unique sequences from each condition after discarding sequences with suspected indels. These were the final numbers of sequences that were analyzed.

GERMLINE VDJ SEGMENT IDENTIFICATION AND ASSIGNMENT INTO CLONES

Clonally related sequences were identified by identical V(D)J segments and by highly homologous sequences of the CDR3 of their Ig genes. For gene segment identification, we used SoDA (75). We computationally grouped the sequences into clones based only on their V, D, and J segments. We aligned clonally related sequences using ClustalW2 (76), in order to confirm that the CDR3 in the clonally related sequences were highly homologous. If not, we separated the sequences into clonally related groups according to the different CDR3 sequences.

REPERTOIRE ANALYSIS

We enumerated the clones based on V(D)J combinations. Results are presented as the average sample percentages of clones of each VH–JH combination, across all samples within the same group. Using the percentages normalizes for different numbers of sequences and/or clones, due to sampling of different numbers of B-cells or obtaining different DNA quantities in each case.

In order to examine the relationships between the VDJ combinations used in each repertoire, we needed to compare the observed repertoires to repertoires predicted under some model, for example, under the assumption that the expression of each gene in each VDJ combination (e.g., V1D1J1) is independent of that of other genes. Immunologists call this assumption "the product rule" (77). Deviations from this assumption can thus point at interdependencies between the V, D, and J genes. We decided to look only at the gene family level, as higher resolution (genes, alleles) would give extremely large numbers of possible combinations, far from the number of combinations observed and therefore the frequencies of each expected combination at the gene or allele level would be close to zero. Thus, each observed gene combination would be significantly different from the expected. Using only families of the VDJ segments would solve this problem. For each sample, we counted the number of unique sequences that used each V, D, or J family. We then calculated the frequency of each V/D/J family as the number of unique sequences using this family divided by the total number of unique sequences in the sample. We then created all possible

Table 4 | Number of unique sequences[a], without suspected indels[b], from each condition.

	CLN	GNHP	GHP	MALT-L	DLBCL	Total
Number of patients (samples)	19	7	3	3	5	37
Number of unique sequences	23,308	4,676	3,373	3,851	4,389	39,597
Range of sequences[c]	384–3,353	75–1,105	513–1,406	838–1,854	267–1,601	
Dominant clone sizes[d]				360 (249)	162 (49)	
				461 (399)	325 (257)	
				408 (321)	58 (42)	
					78 (47)	
					418 (193)	

[a] *Unique sequence: a sequence that differs from all other sequences due to one or more insertion(s), deletion(s), or point mutation(s).*

[b] *After sequences with suspected indels were discarded.*

[c] *The lowest-to-highest numbers of unique sequences without suspected indels in each sample from each condition.*

[d] *The number of unique sequences in the dominant clone, and the number of the second dominant clone (in parentheses), in the lymphoma samples. Each couple of numbers represents one-sample.*

combinations that can be made using the observed VDJ families, and defined their expected frequencies as the product of the V/D/J family frequencies calculated in the previous step. Next, we calculated the actual frequencies of the observed combinations (number of unique sequences in each observed combination divided by the total number of unique sequences). There was no point in creating combinations with families that did not appear in the sample, as there was no meaning of calculating frequencies of non-existing combinations.

In order to know whether a combination was expressed more or less than expected, we calculated the expression: $\log_2$(observed/expected). If a specific combination was over-expressed compared to the expected frequency, the ratio inside the logarithm would be larger than 1, as the observed frequency would be larger than the expected, and thus the logarithm would be positive. On the other hand, if a specific combination was under-expressed compared to the expected frequency, the ratio inside the logarithm would be smaller than 1, and thus the logarithm will be negative. Combinations that were not observed at all received the value ($-\infty$), because the expression inside the logarithm was zero. This step was repeated for each sample. It is important to note that most of the combinations (>80%) were observed in a significantly different frequency than expected. Out of these combinations, 99% were under-represented (because the number of combinations observed is smaller than the potential number), and only 1% of the combinations were over-expressed compared to the expected frequency, and any such case of over-expression was thus particularly noticeable.

The final step was to unite all combinations from all samples as follows: we created a matrix, where rows represented samples and columns represented VDJ combinations. For each combination and for each sample, we inserted the logarithm that was calculated as above. If a sample did not have a specific combination, the cell would be left unfilled. The full matrix was used to carry out the statistical tests. In order to examine whether some combinations tend to appear more or less than expected, we carried out a one-sample t-test on each of the conditions. In order to examine differences in combination usage between conditions, we carried out a two-sample ANOVA test.

In order to graphically present repertoires, we only plotted V–J repertoires, not showing the DH segments used in each VH–JH combination. There are several ways of presenting also the DH genes used in the repertoires (78, 79). However, as mentioned above, DH segments are sometimes misidentified, so we preferred to focus on V and J segments.

DIVERSITY ANALYSIS

Clones in samples can be regarded as species in habitats

In the case of lymphocyte clonal repertoire samples (e.g., those obtained from tissue biopsies), we treat each sample as a sample from a habitat, in which the "species" are the BCR or TCR clones found in the sample. Each of the clones may be composed of a number of different sequences. In TCR clones, all sequences are identical, but in BCR clones sequences from the same clone may be different due to SHM, and one may choose to use only unique sequences found, or all sequences including multiplicate ones. The latter choice depends on whether identical sequences coming from different cells can be identified as such, or cannot be distinguished from sequence duplications caused by PCR amplification. If the former is true (as when using random barcoding in the PCR primers), then the number of sequences that come from different cells is known, and can be used to estimate diversity. If not, then TCR diversity cannot be estimated, and BCR diversity can only be estimated based on the numbers of unique sequences and thus would usually only gives a minimum estimate of the total diversity, as we have done in this study.

Diversity indices

In order to quantify the diversity of clonal repertoires (such as antibody/BCR or TCR gene repertoires) in each experimental or clinical condition, and later to be able to compare between two or more conditions, we used diversity indices (such as the Species Richness, the Shannon entropy, or the Simpson concentration, which are indices of order 0, 1, and 2, respectively) (80). These indices take into account the number of species and (in indices of order >0) the frequency of members of a species (in our case, sequences) of each species (in our case, clone) in each habitat sample. In indices of order 0, diversity is defined simply as number of species (in our case, lymphocyte clones) in a sample. In order 1 indices, clone size (or frequency) is taken into account, as in the Shannon entropy when diversity is the sum of $\left[-p_i^{*}\ln\left(p_i\right)\right]$, where i represents a species or clone and p_i represents its size (the number of members/sequences, see below). Order 2 indices attribute more weight to large clones, as in the Simpson concentration, which is the sum of p_i^2. In our studies, we used both order 1 and 2 diversity indices, i.e., the Shannon entropy and the Simpson concentration.

Diversity measures

From the sample diversity indices, we have calculated the alpha, beta, and gamma diversity measures for each condition (80). The alpha diversity measure represents the average sample diversity in each condition/population. In order to calculate alpha, we calculate the alpha diversity of each sample, and then average over all samples from the same condition. The gamma diversity measure represents the "global" repertoire diversity across all samples studied in each condition/population. It is calculated as the diversity of the pool containing all the sequences from all the samples from the same condition/population.

Finally, the beta diversity measure, which represents the diversity component resulting from the variability between samples, is derived from the alpha and gamma measures using the method of Jost et al. (80). The beta diversity measure is calculated as the gamma diversity of each condition/population divided by the alpha diversity (average of the diversities of individual samples). In order to allow an intuitive comparison between the diversities of each of the groups, all the diversity measures can be expressed as their number equivalents (80), which reflect the number of equally sized clones needed to produce the given value of the diversity index.

Estimating the full repertoire from the sample

Considering the large number of sequences that were observed only once in each sample, it is likely that many rare clones in an individual's original full repertoire were not detected. To account for the presence of unobserved "species" (clones), all diversity measures can be estimated for whole repertoires (rather than calculated for the sample) using the method described by Chao and Shen (81), which is based on a non-parametric estimation of diversity indices where there are undetected species. Chao and Shen's approach utilizes the concept of sample coverage to adjust the diversity indices for clones that escaped sampling. The sample coverage is estimated from the proportion of species/sequences that are observed only once within a sample.

In our Ig gene repertoire studies, the abundance data (numbers of unique sequences) of antibody clones in each sample were used to estimate the mean, standard error, and 95% CI of the total number of unique sequences in clones within each sample. This was done using SPADE©, a program designed for diversity calculations (81). The alpha diversity for each sample, and the gamma diversities for combined samples in each condition, were then calculated from the order 1 or 2 diversity indices of the estimated total repertoires, also using SPADE©(81). In principle, beta is calculated as the average alpha of all samples in the condition divided by the gamma of the condition, as explained above. In order to compare between conditions, however, we needed to calculate CI for beta. This was done by calculating beta index per sample (alpha of the sample divided by the gamma of the condition) and then calculating the CI for each condition (**Figure 5**).

SIMILARITY ANALYSIS

Another method we used to compare between conditions is the Morisita similarity index (82). SPADE©(81) was used to calculate a similarity matrix, in which we measured each individual repertoire's similarity to all other individual repertoires. The average of similarity indices of individuals in a given group to those in another group represents the similarity index for the comparison between the two groups. A value close to 1 represents high similarity between two groups, and a value close to 0 represents low similarity.

The highest values of the Morisita similarity indices representing the highest similarity were rather low and relatively far from 1, indicating the sensitivity of this method. However, they were consistent with observed repertoire diversities.

Ig LINEAGE TREE ANALYSES

Clonally related Ig gene sequences from each sample were used to create mutational lineage trees using our program IgTree©(83), as described in previous work (29, 30). All trees were measured using our program MTree©, quantifying the graphical properties of the trees (84, 85). A thorough statistical analysis has concluded that seven specific tree characteristics possess the highest correlation values with the biological parameters and are hence most informative (67). As described there, these properties are the minimum root to leaf path length, the average distance from a leaf to the first split node/fork, the average outgoing degree, that is the average number of branches coming out of any node, the root's outgoing

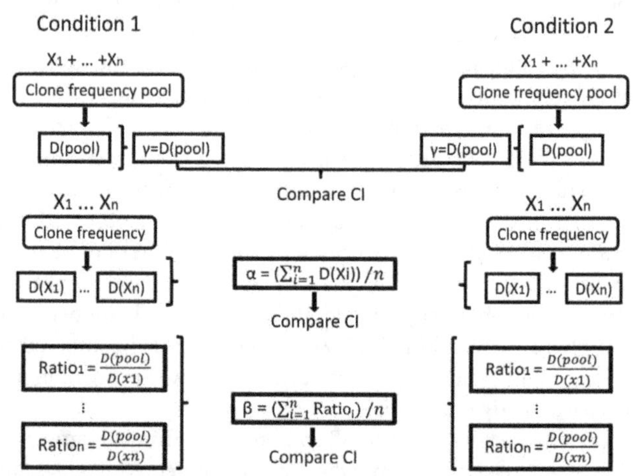

FIGURE 5 | Illustration of the calculation of repertoire diversity. First, the diversity indices (Shannon entropy, Simpson concentration index, etc.) are calculated for the pool of samples in each condition and also for each sample separately (samples are denoted by $X_1, \ldots, X_n$. Diversity indices are denoted by D (sample) or D (pool)). Next, the distribution measures (α, β, γ) are calculated for each condition using the samples. γ is the pool diversity, α is the mean sample diversity, and β for each sample is γ divided by D (sample). Finally, the CIs of the distribution measures are compared between the populations/conditions.

degree, minimum distance between adjacent split nodes/forks, the length of the tree's trunk and minimum distance from the root to any split node/fork. The analysis in this study has thus focused on these properties. Comparison between lineage tree characteristics of different conditions was done using the non-parametric Mann–Whitney U-test, as normal distributions (required by tests such as Student's t-test) could not be assumed. We used the FDR correction (86) for multiple comparisons.

Replacement (R) and silent (S) mutation analysis methods attempt to measure the extent of selection operating on the diversifying clones. These methods compare the frequencies of replacement mutations found in the frame-work and CDR regions of mutated Ig gene sequences to their expected frequency, based on codon usage of the germline sequence. We used the updated focused binomial test by Hershberg et al. (87, 88). The numbers of observed mutations were pooled for each data group by IgTree©, and the new focused binomial formula (88) was calculated using Microsoft Excel©. This measure was also performed for each sample separately, yielding the same results; however, when comparing conditions, we chose to show the pooled analysis for simplicity. Additional mutational analyses were carried out as described in previous studies (27, 28, 30), however, no significant differences between the conditions were found.

AUTHOR CONTRIBUTIONS

Miri Michaeli performed all steps from DNA extraction from samples to bioinformatical analysis of the sequences, and wrote the manuscript. Hilla Tabibian-Keissar supervised the molecular process. Ginette Schiby revised the samples to confirm the diagnosis. Gitit Shahaf and Yishai Pickman developed the diversity analysis. Lena Hazanov developed the bioinformatical analyses. Kinneret Rosenblatt was in charge of the laboratory in which the molecular work was performed. Deborah K. Dunn-Walters advised the author throughout the study. Ramit Mehr and Iris Barshack supervised the molecular work and the analyses performed, and finalized the manuscript. All authors read and approved the final manuscript.

ACKNOWLEDGMENTS

This work was supported in parts by an Israel Science Foundation (grant number 270/09, to Ramit Mehr); and a Human Frontiers Science Program Research Grant (to Ramit Mehr and Deborah K. Dunn-Walters). The work was part of Miri Michaeli's studies toward a combined M.Sc/Ph.D. degree in Bar-Ilan University, and she was supported by a Combined Technologies M.Sc Scholarship from the Israeli Council for Higher Education.

REFERENCES

1. Schubert TT, Schubert AB, MA CK. Symptoms, gastritis, and *Helicobacter pylori* in patients referred for endoscopy. *Gastrointest Endosc* (1992) **38**:357–60. doi:10.1016/S0016-5107(92)70432-5
2. Kusters JG, van Vliet AHM, Kuipers EJ. Pathogenesis of *Helicobacter pylori* infection. *Clin Microbiol Rev* (2006) **19**:449–90. doi:10.1128/CMR.00054-05
3. Sipponen P, Hyuarinen H. Role of *Helicobacter pylori* in the pathogenesis of gastritis, peptic ulcer and gastric cancer. *Scand J Gastroenterol* (1993) **28**:3–6. doi:10.3109/00365529309098333
4. Veldhuyzen van Zanten SJ, Sherman PM. *Helicobacter pylori* infection as a cause of gastritis, duodenal ulcer, gastric cancer and nonulcer dyspepsia: a systematic overview. *Can Med Assoc J* (1994) **150**:177–85.
5. Nordenstedt H, Graham DY, Kramer JR, Rugge M, Verstovsek G, Fitzgerald S, et al. *Helicobacter pylori*-negative gastritis: prevalence and risk factors. *Am J Gastroenterol* (2013) **108**:65–71. doi:10.1038/ajg.2012.372
6. Ryan JL, Shen Y-J, Morgan DR, Thorne LB, Kenney SC, Dominguez RL, et al. Epstein-Barr virus infection is common in inflamed gastrointestinal mucosa. *Dig Dis Sci* (2012) **57**:1887–98. doi:10.1007/s10620-012-2116-5
7. Karlsson FA, Burman P, Loof L, Mardh S. Major parietal cell antigen in autoimmune gastritis with pernicious anemia is the acid-producing H+,K+-adenosine triphosphatase of the stomach. *J Clin Invest* (1988) **81**:475–9. doi:10.1172/JCI113344
8. Sipponen P, Kosunen TU, Valle J, Riihelä M, Seppälä K. *Helicobacter pylori* infection and chronic gastritis in gastric cancer. *J Clin Pathol* (1992) **45**:319–23. doi:10.1136/jcp.45.4.319
9. Segal ED, Cha J, Lo J, Falkow S, Tompkins LS. Altered states: involvement of phosphorylated CagA in the induction of host cellular growth changes by *Helicobacter pylori*. *Proc Natl Acad Sci U S A* (1999) **96**:14559–64. doi:10.1073/pnas.96.25.14559
10. Lin W-C, Tsai H-F, Kuo S-H, Wu M-S, Lin C-W, Hsu P-I, et al. Translocation of *Helicobacter pylori* CagA into human B lymphocytes, the origin of mucosa-associated lymphoid tissue lymphoma. *Cancer Res* (2010) **70**:5740–8. doi:10.1158/0008-5472.CAN-09-4690
11. Fujimori K, Shimodaira S, Akamatsu T, Furihata K, Katsuyama T, Hosaka S. Effect of *Helicobacter pylori* eradication on ongoing mutation of immunoglobulin genes in gastric MALT lymphoma. *Br J Cancer* (2005) **92**:312–9. doi:10.1038/sj.bjc.6602262
12. Suzuki H, Saito Y, Hibi T. *Helicobacter pylori* and gastric mucosa-associated lymphoid tissue (MALT) lymphoma: updated review of clinical outcomes and the molecular pathogenesis. *Gut Liver* (2009) **3**:81–7. doi:10.5009/gnl.2009.3.2.81
13. Lochhead P, El-Omar E. *Helicobacter pylori* infection and gastric cancer. *Best Pract Res Clin Gastroenterol* (2007) **21**:281–97. doi:10.1016/j.bpg.2007.02.002
14. Wotherspoon AC, Ortiz Hidalgo C, Falzon MR, Isaacson PG. *Helicobacter pylori*-associated gastritis and primary B-cell gastric lymphoma. *Lancet* (1991) **338**:1175–6. doi:10.1016/0140-6736(91)92035-Z
15. Zucca E, Bertoni F, Roggero E, Bosshard G, Cazzaniga G, Pedrinis E, et al. Molecular analysis of the progression from *Helicobacter pylori*-associated chronic gastritis to mucosa-associated lymphoid-tissue lymphoma of the stomach. *N Engl J Med* (1998) **338**:804–10. doi:10.1056/NEJM199803193381205
16. Isaacson PG. Lymphomas of mucosa associated lymphoid tissue (MALT). *Am J Surg Pathol* (1992) **16**:201–5. doi:10.1097/00000478-199202000-00023
17. Cavalli F, Isaacson PG, Gascoyne RD, Zucca E. MALT lymphomas. *Hematology Am Soc Hematol Educ Program* (2001) **2001**:241–58. doi:10.1182/asheducation-2001.1.241
18. Chan JKC, Ng CS, Isaacson PG. Relationship between high-grade lymphoma and low-grade B-cell mucosa-associated lymphoid tissue lymphoma (MALToma) of the stomach. *Am J Pathol* (1990) **136**:1153–64.
19. Peng H, Du M, Diss TC, Isaacson PG, Pan L. Genetic evidence for a clonal link between low and high-grade components in gastric MALT B-cell lymphoma. *Histopathology* (1997) **30**:425–9. doi:10.1046/j.1365-2559.1997.5450786.x
20. Freeman C, Berg JW, Cutler SJ. Occurrence and prognosis of extranodal lymphomas. *Cancer* (1972) **29**:252–60. doi:10.1002/1097-0142(197201)29:1<252::AID-CNCR2820290138>3.0.CO;2-\#
21. Go JH, Kim DS, Kim TJ, Ko YH, Ra HK, Rhee JC, et al. Comparative studies of somatic and ongoing mutations in immunoglobulin heavy-chain variable region genes in diffuse large B-cell lymphomas of the stomach and the small intestine. *Arch Pathol Lab Med* (2003) **127**:1443–50. doi:10.1043/1543-2165(2003)127<1443:CSOSAO>2.0.CO;2
22. Alizadeh AA, Eisen MB, Davis RE, Ma C, Lossos IS, Rosenwald A, et al. Distinct types of diffuse large B-cell lymphoma identified by gene expression profiling. *Nature* (2000) **403**:503–11. doi:10.1038/35000501
23. De Paepe P, De Wolf-Peeters C. Diffuse large B-cell lymphoma: a heterogeneous group of non-Hodgkin lymphomas comprising several distinct clinicopathological entities. *Leukemia* (2007) **21**:37–43. doi:10.1038/sj.leu.2404449

24. Banerjee M, Mehr R, Belelovsky A, Spencer J, Dunn-Walters DK. Age- and tissue-specific differences in human germinal center B cell selection revealed by analysis of IgVH gene hypermutation and lineage trees. *Eur J Immunol* (2002) **32**:1947–57. doi:10.1002/1521-4141(200207)32:7<1947::AID-IMMU1947>3.0.CO;2-1
25. Steiman-Shimony A, Edelman H, Barak M, Shahaf G, Dunn-Walters DK, Stott DI, et al. Immunoglobulin variable-region gene mutational lineage tree analysis: application to autoimmune diseases. *Autoimmun Rev* (2006) **5**:242–51. doi:10.1016/j.autrev.2005.07.008
26. Steiman-Shimony A, Edelman H, Hutzler A, Barak M, Zuckerman NS, Shahaf G, et al. Lineage tree analysis of immunoglobulin variable-region gene mutations in autoimmune diseases: chronic activation, normal selection. *Cell Immunol* (2006) **244**:130–6. doi:10.1016/j.cellimm.2007.01.009
27. Zuckerman NS, Hazanov H, Barak M, Edelman H, Hess S, Shcolnik H, et al. Somatic hypermutation and antigen-driven selection of B cells are altered in autoimmune diseases. *J Autoimmun* (2010) **35**:325–35. doi:10.1016/j.jaut.2010.07.004
28. Zuckerman NS, Howard WA, Bismuth J, Gibson KL, Edelman H, Berrih-Aknin S, et al. Ectopic GC in the thymus of myasthenia gravis patients show characteristics of normal GC. *Eur J Immunol* (2010) **40**:1150–61. doi:10.1002/eji.200939914
29. Tabibian-Keissar H, Zuckerman NS, Barak M, Dunn-Walters DK, Steiman-Shimony A, Chowers Y, et al. B-cell clonal diversification and gut-lymph node trafficking in ulcerative colitis revealed using lineage tree analysis. *Eur J Immunol* (2008) **38**:2600–9. doi:10.1002/eji.200838333
30. Zuckerman NS, McCann KJ, Ottensmeier CH, Barak M, Shahaf G, Edelman H, et al. Ig gene diversification and selection in follicular lymphoma, diffuse large B cell lymphoma and primary central nervous system lymphoma revealed by lineage tree and mutation analyses. *Int Immunol* (2010) **22**:875–87. doi:10.1093/intimm/dxq441
31. Manske MK, Zuckerman NS, Timm MM, Maiden S, Edelman H, Shahaf G, et al. Quantitative analysis of clonal bone marrow CD19+ B cells: use of B cell lineage trees to delineate their role in the pathogenesis of light chain amyloidosis. *Clin Immunol* (2006) **120**:106–20. doi:10.1016/j.clim.2006.01.008
32. Abraham RS, Manske MK, Zuckerman NS, Sohni A, Edelman H, Shahaf G, et al. Novel analysis of clonal diversification in blood B cell and bone marrow plasma cell clones in immunoglobulin light chain amyloidosis. *J Clin Immunol* (2007) **27**:69–87. doi:10.1007/s10875-006-9056-9
33. Gurrieri C, McGuire P, Zan H, Yan X-J, Cerutti A, Albesiano E, et al. Chronic lymphocytic leukemia B cells can undergo somatic hypermutation and intraclonal immunoglobulin V(H)DJ(H) gene diversification. *J Exp Med* (2002) **196**:629–39. doi:10.1084/jem.20011693
34. Kostareli E, Sutton L, Hadzidimitriou A, Darzentas N, Kouvatsi A, Tsaftaris A, et al. Intraclonal diversification of immunoglobulin light chains in a subset of chronic lymphocytic leukemia alludes to antigen-driven clonal evolution. *Leukemia* (2010) **24**:1317–24. doi:10.1038/leu.2010.90
35. Bashford-Rogers RJM, Palser AL, Huntly BJ, Rance R, Vassiliou GS, Follows GA, et al. Network properties derived from deep sequencing of human B-cell receptor repertoires delineate B-cell populations. *Genome Res* (2013) **23**(11):1874–84. doi:10.1101/gr.154815.113
36. Zhu D, Orchard J, Oscier DG, Wright DH, Stevenson FK. V(H) gene analysis of splenic marginal zone lymphomas reveals diversity in mutational status and initiation of somatic mutation in vivo. *Blood* (2002) **100**:2659–61. doi:10.1182/blood-2002-01-0169
37. Traverse-Glehen A, Davi F, Ben Simon E, Callet-Bauchu E, Felman P, Baseggio L, et al. Analysis of VH genes in marginal zone lymphoma reveals marked heterogeneity between splenic and nodal tumors and suggests the existence of clonal selection. *Haematologica* (2005) **90**:470–8.
38. Matolcsy A, Schattner EJ, Knowles DM, Casali P. Clonal evolution of B cells in transformation from low- to high-grade lymphoma. *Eur J Immunol* (1999) **29**:1253–64. doi:10.1002/(SICI)1521-4141(199904)29:04<1253::AID-IMMU1253>3.0.CO;2-8
39. Carlotti E, Wrench D, Matthews J, Iqbal S, Davies A, Norton A, et al. Transformation of follicular lymphoma to diffuse large B-cell lymphoma may occur by divergent evolution from a common progenitor cell or by direct evolution from the follicular lymphoma clone. *Blood* (2009) **113**:3553–7. doi:10.1182/blood-2008-08-174839
40. Green MR, Gentles AJ, Nair RV, Irish JM, Kihira S, Liu CL, et al. Hierarchy in somatic mutations arising during genomic evolution and progression of follicular lymphoma. *Blood* (2013) **121**:1604–11. doi:10.1182/blood-2012-09-457283
41. Wündisch T, Thiede C, Alpen B, Stolte M, Neubauer A. Are lymphocytic monoclonality and immunoglobulin heavy chain (IgH) rearrangement premalignant conditions in chronic gastritis? *Microsc Res Tech* (2001) **53**:414–8. doi:10.1002/jemt.1110
42. Miyamoto M, Haruma K, Hiyama T, Kamada T, Masuda H, Shimamoto F, et al. High incidence of B-cell monoclonality in follicular gastritis: a possible association between follicular gastritis and MALT lymphoma. *Virchows Arch* (2002) **440**:376–80. doi:10.1007/s00428-001-0575-8
43. Georgopoulos SD, Triantafyllou K, Fameli M, Kitsanta P, Spiliadi C, Anagnostou D, et al. Molecular analysis of B-cell clonality in *Helicobacter pylori* gastritis. *Dig Dis Sci* (2005) **50**:1616–20. doi:10.1007/s10620-005-2905-1
44. Bahler DW, Szankasi P, Kulkarni S, Tubbs RR, Cook JR, Swerdlow SH. Use of similar immunoglobulin VH gene segments by MALT lymphomas of the ocular adnexa. *Mod Pathol* (2009) **22**:833–8. doi:10.1038/modpathol.2009.42
45. Walsh SH, Rosenquist R. Immunoglobulin gene analysis of mature B-cell malignancies: reconsideration of cellular origin and potential antigen involvement in pathogenesis. *Med Oncol* (2005) **22**:327–41. doi:10.1385/MO:22:4:327
46. Fais F, Ghiotto F, Hashimoto S, Sellars B, Valetto A, Allen SL, et al. Chronic lymphocytic leukemia B cells express restricted sets of mutated and unmutated antigen receptors. *J Clin Invest* (1998) **102**:1515–25. doi:10.1172/JCI3009
47. Yamashita Y, Kajiura D, Tang L, Hasegawa Y, Kinoshita T, Nakamura S, et al. XCR1 expression and biased VH gene usage are distinct features of diffuse large B-cell lymphoma initially manifesting in the bone marrow. *Am J Clin Pathol* (2011) **135**:556–64. doi:10.1309/AJCPCTDC5PY3LXBP
48. Bende RJ, Aarts WM, Riedl RG, de Jong D, Pals ST, van Noesel CJM. Among B cell non-Hodgkin's lymphomas, MALT lymphomas express a unique antibody repertoire with frequent rheumatoid factor reactivity. *J Exp Med* (2005) **201**:1229–41. doi:10.1084/jem.20050068
49. Pimentel BJ, Stefanoff CG, Moreira AS, Seuánez HN, Zalcberg IR. Use of V H, D and J H immunoglobulin gene segments in Brazilian patients with chronic lymphocytic leukaemia (CLL). *Genet Mol Biol* (2008) **31**:643–8. doi:10.1590/S1415-47572008000400007
50. Matsuda F, Shin EK, Nagaoka H, Matsumura R, Haino M, Fukita Y, et al. Structure and physical map of 64 variable segments in the 3'0.8-megabase region of the human immunoglobulin heavy-chain locus. *Nat Genet* (1993) **3**:88–94. doi:10.1038/ng0193-88
51. Johnson TA, Rassenti LZ, Kipps TJ. Ig VH1 genes expressed in B cell chronic lymphocytic leukemia exhibit distinctive molecular features. *J Immunol* (1997) **158**:235–46.
52. Bayerl MG, Bentley G, Bellan C, Leoncini L, Ehmann WC, Palutke M. Lacunar and Reed-Sternberg – like cells in follicular lymphomas are clonally related to the centrocytic and centroblastic cells as demonstrated by laser capture microdissection. *Am J Clin Pathol* (2004) **122**:858–64. doi:10.1309/PMR86PHKK4J3RUH3
53. Hashimoto Y, Tsukamoto N, Nakahashi H, Yokohama A, Saitoh T, Handa H, et al. Hairy cell leukemia-related disorders consistently show low CD27 expression. *Pathol Oncol Res* (2009) **15**:615–21. doi:10.1007/s12253-009-9161-1
54. Nakamura-Kikuoka S, Takahi K, Tsuboi H, Toyosaki-Maeda T, Maeda-Tanimura M, Wakasa C, et al. Limited VH gene usage in B-cell clones established with nurse-like cells from patients with rheumatoid arthritis. *Rheumatology* (2006) **45**:549–57. doi:10.1093/rheumatology/kei170
55. Bahler DW, Swerdlow SH. Clonal salivary gland infiltrates associated with myoepithelial sialadenitis (Sjögren's syndrome) begin as nonmalignant antigen-selected expansions. *Blood* (1998) **91**:1864–72.
56. Brezinschek HP, Foster SJ, Brezinschek RI, Dörner T, Domiati-Saad R, Lipsky PE. Analysis of the human VH gene repertoire. Differential effects of selection and somatic hypermutation on human peripheral CD5(+)/IgM+ and CD5(-)/IgM+ B cells. *J Clin Invest* (1997) **99**:2488–501. doi:10.1172/JCI119433
57. Wu Y-C, Kipling D, Leong HS, Martin V, Ademokun A, Dunn-Walters DK. High-throughput immunoglobulin repertoire analysis distinguishes between human IgM memory and switched memory B-cell populations. *Blood* (2010) **116**:1070–8. doi:10.1182/blood-2010-03-275859
58. Perotti M, Ghidoli N, Altara R, Diotti RA, Clementi N, De Marco D, et al. Hepatitis C virus (HCV)-driven stimulation of subfamily-restricted natural IgM antibodies in mixed cryoglobulinemia. *Autoimmun Rev* (2008) **7**:468–72. doi:10.1016/j.autrev.2008.03.008

59. Mao Z, Quintanilla-Martinez L, Raffeld M, Richter M, Krugmann J, Burek C, et al. IgVH mutational status and clonality analysis of Richter's transformation: diffuse large B-cell lymphoma and Hodgkin lymphoma in association with B-cell chronic lymphocytic leukemia (B-CLL) represent 2 different pathways of disease evolution. *Am J Surg Pathol* (2007) **31**:1605–14. doi:10.1097/PAS.0b013e31804bdaf8
60. Sakuma H, Nakamura T, Uemura N, Chiba T, Sugiyama T, Asaka M, et al. Immunoglobulin VH gene analysis in gastric MALT lymphomas. *Mod Pathol* (2007) **20**:460–6. doi:10.1038/modpathol.3800758
61. Lenze D, Greiner A, Knörr C, Anagnostopoulos I, Stein H, Hummel M. Receptor revision of immunoglobulin heavy chain genes in human MALT lymphomas. *Mol Pathol* (2003) **56**:249–55. doi:10.1136/mp.56.5.249
62. Alpen B, Wündisch T, Dierlamm J, Börsch G, Stolte M, Neubauer A. Clonal relationship in multifocal non-Hodgkin's lymphoma of mucosa-associated lymphoid tissue (MALT). *Ann Hematol* (2004) **83**:124–6. doi:10.1007/s00277-003-0763-5
63. Siakantaris MP, Pangalis GA, Dimitriadou E, Kontopidou FN, Vassilakopoulos TP, Kalpadakis C, et al. Early-stage gastric MALT lymphoma: is it a truly localized disease? *Oncologist* (2009) **14**:148–54. doi:10.1634/theoncologist.2008-0178
64. De Wolf-Peeters C, Achten R. The histogenesis of large-cell gastric lymphomas. *Histopathology* (1999) **34**:71–5. doi:10.1046/j.1365-2559.1999.00602.x
65. Friedberg JW. Diffuse large B-cell lymphoma. *J Hematol Oncol* (2008) **22**:941–52. doi:10.1016/j.hoc.2008.07.002
66. Lenze D, Berg E, Volkmer-Engert R, Weiser A, Greiner A, Knörr-Wittmann C, et al. Influence of antigen on the development of MALT lymphoma. *Blood* (2006) **107**:1141–8. doi:10.1182/blood-2005-04-1722
67. Shahaf G, Barak M, Zuckerman NS, Swerdlin N, Gorfine M, Mehr R. Antigen-driven selection in germinal centers as reflected by the shape characteristics of immunoglobulin gene lineage trees: a large-scale simulation study. *J Theor Biol* (2008) **255**:210–22. doi:10.1016/j.jtbi.2008.08.005
68. Salau L, Linz B, Suerbaum S, Saunders NJ, Saunders N. The diversity within an expanded and redefined repertoire of phase-variable genes in *Helicobacter pylori*. *Microbiology* (2004) **150**:817–30. doi:10.1099/mic.0.26993-0
69. Hussell T, Isaacson PG, Crabtree JE, Spencer J. The response of cells from low-grade B-cell gastric lymphomas of mucosa-associated lymphoid tissue to *Helicobacter pylori*. *Lancet* (1993) **342**:571–4. doi:10.1016/0140-6736(93)91408-E
70. Hussell T, Isaacson PG, Crabtree JE, Spencer J. *Helicobacter pylori*-specific tumour-infiltrating T cells provide contact dependent help for the growth of malignant B cells in low-grade gastric lymphoma of mucosa-associated lymphoid tissue. *J Pathol* (1996) **178**:122–7. doi:10.1002/(SICI)1096-9896(199602)178:2<122::AID-PATH486>3.0.CO;2-D
71. Ernst PB, Gold BD. The disease spectrum of *Helicobacter pylori*: the immunopathogenesis of gastroduodenal ulcer and gastric cancer. *Annu Rev Microbiol* (2000) **54**:615–40. doi:10.1146/annurev.micro.54.1.615
72. Tabibian-Keissar H, Schibby G, Michaeli M, Rakovsky-Shapira A, Azogui-Rosenthal N, Dunn-Walters DK, et al. PCR amplification and high throughput sequencing of immunoglobulin heavy chain genes from formalin-fixed paraffin-embedded human biopsies. *Exp Mol Pathol* (2012) **94**:182–7. doi:10.1016/j.yexmp.2012.08.002
73. Michaeli M, Noga H, Tabibian-Keissar H, Barshack I, Mehr R. Automated cleaning and pre-processing of immunoglobulin gene sequences from high-throughput sequencing. *Front Immunol* (2012) **3**:386. doi:10.3389/fimmu.2012.00386
74. Ansorge WJ. Next-generation DNA sequencing techniques. *N Biotechnol* (2009) **25**:195–203. doi:10.1016/j.nbt.2008.12.009
75. Volpe JM, Cowell LG, Kepler TB. SoDA: implementation of a 3D alignment algorithm for inference of antigen receptor recombinations. *Bioinformatics* (2006) **22**:438–44. doi:10.1093/bioinformatics/btk004
76. Larkin MA, Blackshields G, Brown NP, Chenna R, McGettigan PA, McWilliam H, et al. Clustal W and Clustal X version 2.0. *Bioinformatics* (2007) **23**:2947–8. doi:10.1093/bioinformatics/btm404
77. Mehr R, Sternberg-Simon M, Michaeli M, Pickman Y. Models and methods for analysis of lymphocyte repertoire generation, development, selection and evolution. *Immunol Lett* (2012) **148**:11–22. doi:10.1016/j.imlet.2012.08.002
78. Weinstein JA, Jiang N, White RA, Fisher DS, Quake SR. High-throughput sequencing of the zebrafish antibody repertoire. *Science* (2009) **324**:807–10. doi:10.1126/science.1170020
79. Briney BS, Willis JR, McKinney BA, Crowe JE. High-throughput antibody sequencing reveals genetic evidence of global regulation of the naïve and memory repertoires that extends across individuals. *Genes Immun* (2012) **13**:469–73. doi:10.1038/gene.2012.20
80. Jost L. Partitioning diversity into independent alpha and beta components. *Ecology* (2007) **88**:2427–39. doi:10.1890/06-1736.1
81. Chao A, Shen TJ. *Program SPADE (Species Prediction and Diversity Estimation): Program and User's Guide.* (2003). Available from: http://chao.stat.nthu.edu.tw
82. Chao A, Jost L, Chiang SC, Jiang Y-H, Chazdon RL. A two-stage probabilistic approach to multiple-community similarity indices. *Biometrics* (2008) **64**:1178–86. doi:10.1111/j.1541-0420.2008.01010.x
83. Barak M, Zuckerman NS, Edelman H, Unger R, Mehr R. IgTree: creating immunoglobulin variable region gene lineage trees. *J Immunol Methods* (2008) **338**:67–74. doi:10.1016/j.jim.2008.06.006
84. Dunn-Walters DK, Belelovsky A, Edelman H, Banerjee M, Mehr R. The dynamics of germinal centre selection as measured by graph-theoretical analysis of mutational lineage trees. *Dev Immunol* (2002) **9**:233–43. doi:10.1080/10446670310001593541
85. Dunn-Walters DK, Edelman H, Mehr R. Immune system learning and memory quantified by graphical analysis of B-lymphocyte phylogenetic trees. *Biosystems* (2004) **76**:141–55. doi:10.1016/j.biosystems.2004.05.011
86. Benjamini Y, Hochberg Y. Controlling the false discovery rate: a practical and powerful approach to multiple testing. *J R Stat Soc Ser B* (1995) **57**:289–300.
87. Hershberg U, Uduman M, Shlomchik MJ, Kleinstein SH. Improved methods for detecting selection by mutation analysis of Ig V region sequences. *Int Immunol* (2008) **20**:683–94. doi:10.1093/intimm/dxn026
88. Uduman M, Yaari G, Hershberg U, Stern JA, Shlomchik MJ, Kleinstein SH. Detecting selection in immunoglobulin sequences. *Nucleic Acids Res* (2011) **39**:W499–504. doi:10.1093/nar/gkr413

3

Significance of interleukin-33 and its related cytokines in patients with breast cancers

Jing Liu[1†], Jia-Xin Shen[1,2†], Jia-Lin Hu[1,2†], Wen-He Huang[2] and Guo-Jun Zhang[2*]

[1] *Cancer Research Center, Shantou University Medical College, Shantou, China*
[2] *Breast Center, Cancer Hospital of Shantou University Medical College, Shantou, China*

Edited by:
Fang-Ping Huang, Imperial College London, UK

Reviewed by:
Federica Cavallo, University of Turin, Italy
Carlos Alfaro, Clínica Universidad de Navarra, Spain

***Correspondence:**
Guo-Jun Zhang, Breast Center, Cancer Hospital of Shantou University Medical College, 7 Raoping Road, Shantou 515031, China
e-mail: guoj_zhang@yahoo.com

[†] *Jing Liu, Jia-Xin Shen and Jia-Lin Hu have contributed equally to this work.*

Interleukin-33 (IL-33) is a recently identified cytokine, an important member of the interleukin-1 family. IL-33 binds to its receptor ST2 to induce type 2 cytokines and exert both pro-inflammatory and protective functions in host defense and disease. Murine breast carcinoma models suggest disruption of ST2 signaling may enhance the anti-tumor immune response, suggesting IL-33 impedes anti-tumor immunity. However, the role of IL-33 in patients with breast cancers (BC) is not elucidated. We detected the expression of IL-33 in tumor tissue, and IL-33 and its related cytokines in serum from BC patients. Using Luminex and immunohistochemistry methods, we found that serum levels of IL-33 were nearly twofold higher in patients with BC, compared to patients with benign breast diseases. In cancer tissues, expression of IL-33 was higher than matched normal breast tissues from the same patients, and was also associated with a well-differentiated phenotype, HER2 overexpression, more lymph nodes involvement, and a family history of malignant carcinoma. These results suggest that IL-33 may play an important role in the progress of BC and may be a useful biomarker for predicting the progress and metastasis of BC.

Keywords: interleukin-33, ST2/ST2L, breast cancer, cytokines, immunosuppression

INTRODUCTION

Breast cancer (BC) is the second leading cause of cancer-related deaths amongst women in the United States, and morbidity and mortality of this disease increases each year (1). Although standard multi-modality treatment has improved the overall outcome and quality of life for patients with BC, identification of new prognostic markers, therapeutic targets, and new therapeutic approaches are needed. Recent insights into the cancer development mechanisms have revealed that immune system functionally regulates development and progression of epithelial malignancies and tumor-infiltrating leukocytes may be causal players in cancer development (2).

The interleukin-1 (IL-1) family is a growing group of cytokines, consisting of at least 11 members, and the balance between pro- and anti-inflammatory cytokines is crucial in the pathogenesis of many human diseases (3). Interleukin-33 (IL-33) is an important member of the IL-1 family, and in humans is expressed predominantly in skin, lung, adipocytes, and synovial fibroblasts (4). IL-33 is an endogenous ligand for the ST2/T1 receptor, and depending on the cellular and cytokine context, participates in many immune diseases with dual, pro-inflammatory, or protective roles. IL-33 induces T cells to produce IL-4, IL-5, and IL-13, and potently induces pro-inflammatory cytokines and chemokines through a Th2-dependent pathway, and also promotes Th1-type responses (5). IL-33 is involved in the pathogenesis of immune diseases, such as rheumatoid arthritis and atopic dermatitis, and may reflect the degree of inflammation in patients with immune diseases (6, 7). Deletion of IL-33/ST2 function enhances cytotoxicity of NK cells and increases levels of TNF-α, IFN-γ, and IL-17, and systemic pro-inflammatory cytokines, leading to attenuated tumor growth (8).

Recent studies demonstrated that high serum levels of soluble ST2 (sST2) are a worse prognostic factor in hepatocellular carcinoma (9), and that serum IL-33 is a diagnostic and prognostic marker in non-small cell lung cancer, independent of the therapeutic intervention (10). In studies on mouse mammary carcinoma, the IL-33/ST2 pathway promotes BC progression and metastasis through increased intratumoral accumulation of immunosuppressive cells and by diminishing innate anti-tumor immunity (11). Conversely, Gao et al. reported that transgenic expression of IL-33 may activate CD8(+) T cells and NK cells, and inhibit tumor growth and metastasis in B16 melanoma and Lewis lung carcinoma metastatic models (12). Thus, the data on the role of IL-33 in cancer progression was limited, and in particular, the function mediated by IL-33 in human BC is under-investigated. In this study, we aim to determine the serum level and to detect the expression of IL-33 in human tissues in patients with breast carcinoma, using Luminex-based measurements and immunohistochemistry, to further explore the role of IL-33 in anti-tumor immunity in BC.

MATERIALS AND METHODS

PATIENTS

This study was approved by the Ethics Committee of Shantou University Medical College and conducted according to the principles in the Declaration of Helsinki (13).

Blood samples were drawn from 64 patients with BC and 10 patients with benign breast diseases (BBD) as controls, who visited the Shantou University Medical College Cancer Hospital Breast Center between April 2013 and July 2013. The mean age was 52 ± 11 years (25–80 years old) for patients with BC, and 41 ± 11 years (28–68 years old) for patients with BBD. All patients were pathologically diagnosed using specimens obtained either by core-needle biopsy or by surgery. The clinicopathological characters of the BC patients are summarized in **Table 1**.

The central regions of tumors were collected from 29 BC patients, as well as microscopic normal tissues from either tumor-adjacent normal tissue (<1 cm) or normal tissue ≥5 cm away from the tumor margins, for which paraffin-embedded samples were available. The mean age was 53 ± 13 years (25–80 years old) for all enrolled patient. The clinicopathological characteristics of the 29 BC patients are summarized in **Table 3**.

ASSESSMENT OF SERUM CYTOKINES

The levels of IL-33, IL-12, IL-13, IL-17, IFN-γ, and TNF-α in serum were measured based on a Luminex assay, using Milliplex™ MAP (Millipore, MA, USA) multiplex magnetic bead-based antibody detection kits according to the manufacturer's protocols (14).

Blood from patients was collected and centrifuged for 10 min at room temperature. Serum was removed carefully and stored at −80°C until use. Twenty-five microliters of neat samples were added into each well of 96-well plate, and then 25 μl mixed beads were added to the samples. The plate was incubated with agitation on a plate shaker overnight at 4°C. Twenty-five microliters of anti-cytokine antibody was then added and incubated for 1 h at room temperature. Lastly, 25 μl streptavidin–phycoerythrin was added into each well containing the detection antibodies for 30 min at room temperature. Cytokines were quantified using a BioPlex 200 platform (BioRad, CA, USA).

IMMUNOHISTOCHEMISTRY

Surgical specimens of cancer tissues, adjacent tissues to tumors, and normal tissues collected from patients with BC were formalin-fixed, paraffin-embedded, and cut into four-micron-thick sections. Sections were deparaffinized by immersion in xylene, and rehydrated in a series of graded alcohols. Epitope retrieval and inactivation of endogenous peroxidase activity was achieved as described (15). Samples were incubated overnight at 4°C with anti-IL-33 (R&D Systems, Minneapolis, MN, USA), then visualized using 3,3′-diaminobenzidine tetrahydrochloride (DAB). Sections without primary antibody were used as negative controls. Counterstaining was carried out with hematoxylin, and sections were visualized and photographed under a bright-field microscope (Olympus, Tokyo, Japan). Immunohistochemical staining was mainly cytoplasmic, and the percentage of positive cells for IL-33 was calculated for analysis by counting at least 200 cells in five or more high power fields.

Estrogen receptor (ER) and progesterone receptor (PR) were interpreted as negative or positive, if equal to and less than 1% or more than 1% of tumor showed nuclear positivity, respectively. HER2 was interpreted as negative or over-expressed, if there was 0–1+ or 3+ membranous staining, respectively. If there was 2+ membranous staining, FISH was conducted to determine whether HER2 was over-expressed (16). A Ki-67 cut-off point of 15% was defined according to the experience of different pathologists as well as national and international recommendations at present (17).

Table 1 | Relationship of serum IL-33 levels with clinicopathological parameters of breast cancer patients.

Variables	IL-33 level (pg/ml)			
	N	Mean	SD	P value
Age				
≤50 years	30	35.87	11.00	0.481
>50 years	34	38.21	14.78	
Menopausal status[a]				
No	33	36.19	11.33	0.992
Yes	30	36.52	12.26	
Size				
≤2 cm	26	36.50	11.52	0.760
>2 cm	38	37.53	14.21	
AJCC stage				
I + II	44	37.93	12.11	0.465
III	20	35.32	15.23	
Histological grade[b]				
1 + 2	30	36.51	13.58	0.915
3	23	36.14	10.64	
ER expression[c]				
Negative	26	32.79	10.84	0.033
Positive	37	39.92	13.97	
PR expression[c]				
Negative	32	36.76	16.28	0.896
Positive	31	37.20	9.17	
HER2 expression[c]				
No	46	37.82	14.28	0.409
Yes	17	34.71	9.48	
Ki-67 expression[c]				
Low	15	43.74	19.40	0.021
High	48	34.86	9.86	
Lymph node metastasis				
≤3	56	37.59	13.52	0.445
>3	8	33.78	9.67	
Family history				
No	58	36.00	11.69	0.034
Yes	6	47.81	21.29	

[a] *One case missing this information because the patient was male.*

[b] *Two cases with invasive lobular carcinomas, one case with an intraductal papillary carcinoma, and in eight cases, only biopsy samples were available without information on histological grade.*

[c] *One case was discharged after biopsy, without information on ER, PR, HER2, and Ki-67 expression.*

STATISTICAL ANALYSIS

Serum levels and tissue expression are expressed as the mean ± standard deviation (SD). Differences between groups were analyzed using the Student t-test or the non-parametric Mann–Whitney test. All statistical differences were considered significant at the level of $p < 0.05$. All data were analyzed with SPSS 19.0 software for Windows.

RESULTS

SERUM LEVELS OF IL-33 AND RELATED CYTOKINES IN BBD AND BC

Among six cytokines, the concentrations of IL-33 were nearly twofold higher in the BC group (34.49 ± 1.65 pg/ml) compared with BBD group (17.71 ± 2.60 pg/ml) (p = 0.0008), with a non-normal distribution (**Figure 1A**). Conversely, serum levels of IL-13, a Th2-associated cytokine, in the BC group (14.79 ± 0.45) were 40% lower than in the BBD group (24.92 ± 8.68 pg/ml) with borderline difference ($p = 0.0608$) (**Figure 1B**), and the concentrations of IL-12, a Th1-type cytokine, were 35% lower in the BC group (6.143 ± 0.25 pg/ml) than in the BBD group (9.39 ± 2.11 pg/ml) with statistical significance (p = 0.0178) (**Figure 1C**). The concentrations of other cytokines, IL-17, TNF-α, and IFN-γ, did not show any significant difference between the BBD and BC groups (p > 0.05, **Figures 1D–F**).

CLINICOPATHOLOGICAL ANALYSIS OF SERUM LEVELS OF IL-33 IN BREAST CARCINOMA PATIENTS

In patients with ER-positive breast tumors, the serum levels of IL-33 were 39.92 ± 13.97 pg/ml, and were significantly higher than in patients with ER-negative tumors, which were 32.79 ± 10.84 pg/ml, p = 0.033 (**Table 1**). In patients who showed lower Ki-67 expression, the serum levels of IL-33 were higher than the high Ki-67-expressing group (43.74 ± 19.40 pg/ml vs. 34.86 ± 9.86 pg/ml, p = 0.021). The serum concentrations of IL-33 were significantly associated with family history of malignant tumors (p = 0.034). No correlation was observed between serum IL-33 levels and patient age, menopausal status, tumor size, AJCC stage, histological grade, lymph node status, PR, and HER2 expression.

We also analyzed the association of clinicopathological parameters with IL-33-related cytokines. The serum levels of INF-γ were associated with tumor size (p = 0.039), with INF-γ being higher in patients with tumors <2 cm in size (22.57 ± 2.63 pg/ml) than patients with tumors >2 cm (15.22 ± 5.13 pg/ml). In pre-menopausal patients, the serum levels of IL-17 were significantly higher (p = 0.048) than that in post-menopausal group (15.51 ± 6.29 vs. 13.13 ± 2.16 pg/ml), and serum levels of IL-17 were also significantly associated with AJCC stage (p = 0.049) and HER2 expression (p = 0.012). No statistical significance was

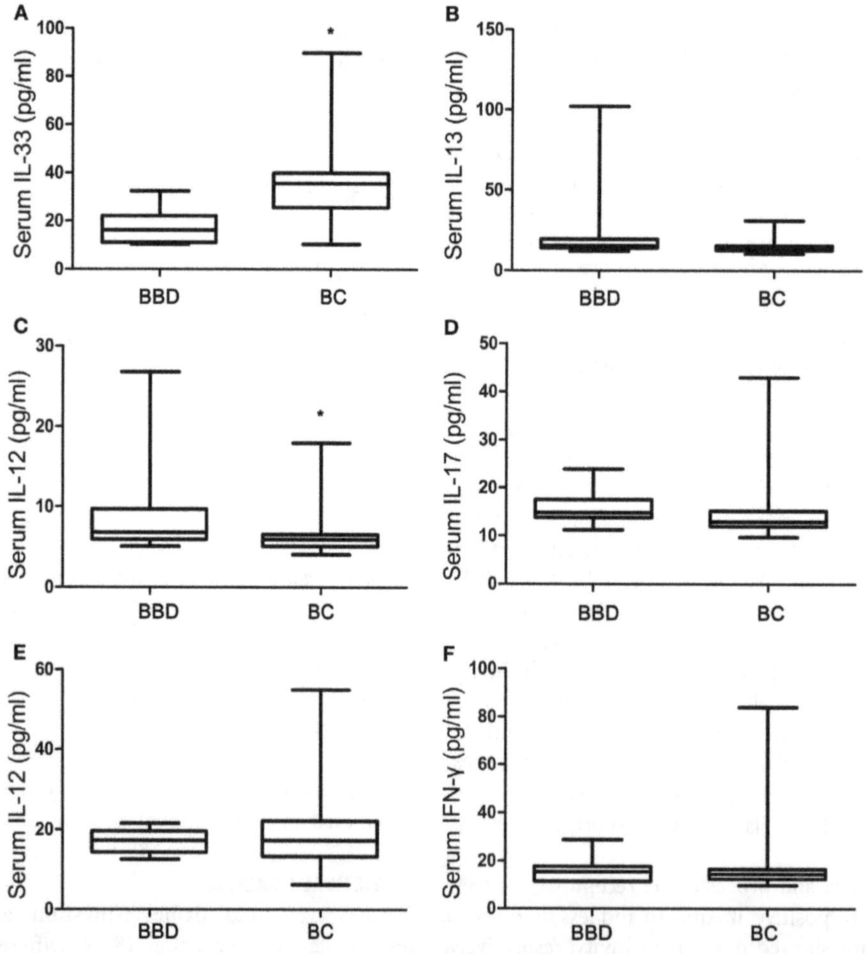

FIGURE 1 | Interleukin-33 and associated cytokine levels in benign breast diseases (BBD) and breast cancers (BC). **(A)** Serum IL-33 expression in BC was significant higher than that in BBD (p = 0.0008); **(B)** no significant difference between serum IL-13 expression in BC and BBD (p = 0.0608); **(C)** serum IL-12 expression in BBD was significant higher than that in BC (p = 0.0178); **(D)** no significant difference between serum IL-17 expression in BC and BBD (p = 0.0526); **(E)** no significant difference between serum TNF-α expression in BC and BBD (p = 0.9748); **(F)** no significant difference between serum IFN-γ expression in BC and BBD (p = 0.7693); *$p < 0.05$ by unpaired two tailed Student's t-test.

found between the serum levels of TNF-α, IL-12, or IL-13 with clinicopathological parameters of BC patients (specific data not shown).

IL-33 IS HIGHER IN CANCER TISSUES, COMPARED WITH ADJACENT AND NORMAL TISSUES

Figure 2 shows a representative immunohistochemical staining of IL-33 in tissues from patients with BC. In 29 patients with BC, mean expression of IL-33 in carcinoma was 72.6% of cells in the tumor, which was significantly higher than in normal breast tissues from the same patients ($p < 0.0001$) as shown in **Table 2.** Interestingly, the mean expression of IL-33 in adjacent tissues to tumor was 64.1%, which was also significantly higher than in normal breast tissues from the same patients ($p = 0.0002$). However, the mean expression level of IL-33 was not statistically different between in cancer and adjacent tissues ($p = 0.3561$).

CLINICOPATHOLOGICAL ANALYSIS OF CYTOPLASMIC IL-33 EXPRESSION IN BREAST CANCER TISSUES

Interleukin-33 was mainly detected in cytoplasm of BC cells as shown in **Figure 2.** With quantitative analysis, mean expressions of IL-33 were not significantly associated with the age at diagnosis, menopausal status, tumor size, AJCC stage, ER, PR, and Ki-67 expression (**Table 3**). In comparison with high grade tumors, low grade tumors showed significant higher IL-33 expression ($p = 0.027$). Interestingly, high IL-33 expression was more frequently observed in tumors with HER2 overexpression ($p = 0.017$). In patients with more than three lymph nodes involved, the expression of IL-33 was significantly higher than the patients with ≤3 metastases ($p = 0.002$). High IL-33 expression was also associated with family history of malignant tumor ($p = 0.002$).

DISCUSSION

Interleukin-33, the newest member of IL-1 family, is a recently identified cytokine with diverse and context-dependent functions, and has been shown to bind to ST2. IL-33 has also been characterized as a potent inducer of T helper (Th) 2 immune responses, and is an important mediator for mucosal healing and epithelial

Table 2 | The percentage of IL-33-positive tissue in breast tumors, tumor-adjacent tissues, and normal tissues from breast cancer patients.

Samples	IL-33 (%)			
	N	Mean	SD	P value[a]
Breast carcinoma tissue	29	72.6	34.5	<0.0001
Adjacent tissues to tumors	29	64.1	34.7	0.0002
Normal breast tissues from BC patients	25[b]	26.8	33.0	

BC, breast cancer.

[a]Statistically significantly different was found between cancer tissues vs. normal breast tissues, and between adjacent tissues vs. normal breast tissues from BC patients, using unpaired Student's t-test. No statistical significance was found between cancer tissues and adjacent tissues.

[b]In four cases, no normal breast tissues were available.

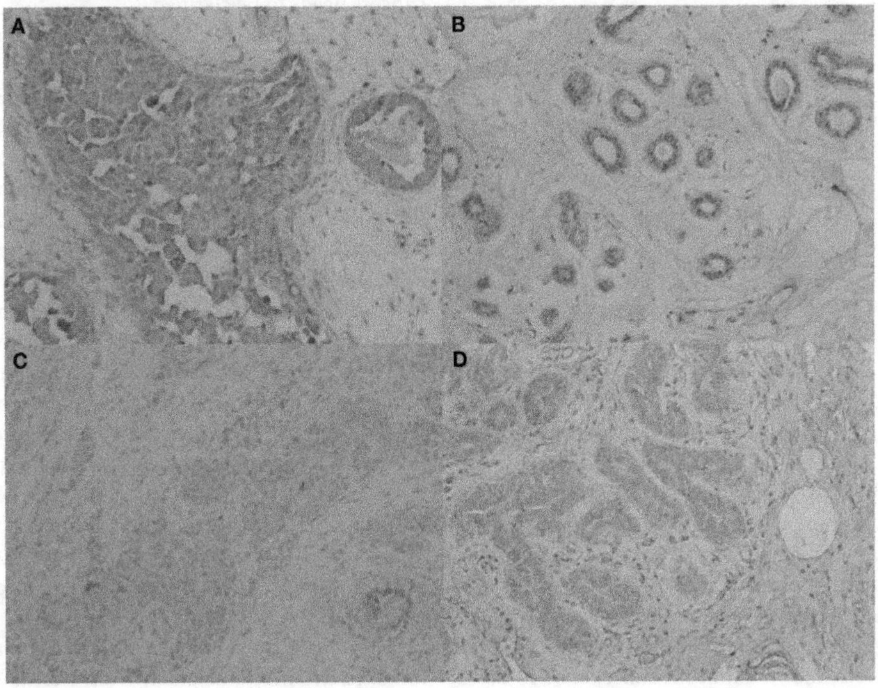

FIGURE 2 | Immunohistochemical staining of IL-33 in patients with breast cancers. Representative images of immunohistochemical staining for IL-33 in breast carcinoma, adjacent tissue to tumor, and normal tissue. **(A)** High IL-33 expression in carcinoma tissues. **(B)** IL-33 expression in tissue adjacent to tumors. **(C)** Low IL-33 expression in carcinoma tissue. **(D)** IL-33 expression in normal breast tissue from BC patients (magnification: ×400).

Table 3 | Clinicopathological analysis of cytoplasmic IL-33 expression in breast carcinoma.

Variables	IL-33 (%)			
	N	Mean	SD	P value
Age				
≤50 years	13	83.85	27.25	0.103
>50 years	16	63.44	37.71	
Menopausal status				
No	13	83.85	27.25	0.114
Yes	16	63.44	37.72	
Size				
≤2 cm	13	68.85	32.28	0.607
>2 cm	16	75.63	36.87	
AJCC stage				
I+II	22	69.09	34.21	0.342
III	7	83.57	35.44	
Histological grade[a]				
1+2	15	87.33	18.70	0.027
3	11	58.64	41.96	
ER expression				
Negative	14	76.8	34.8	0.536
Positive	15	68.7	34.82	
PR expression				
Negative	16	73.44	34.09	0.887
Positive	13	71.54	36.25	
HER2 expression				
No	18	62.50	38.90	0.017
Yes	11	89.09	16.40	
Ki-67 expression				
Low	6	75.00	24.29	0.851
High	23	71.96	37.07	
Lymph node metastasis				
≤3	24	67.71	35.87	0.002
>3	5	96.00	8.94	
Family history				
No	26	69.81	35.34	0.002
Yes	3	96.67	5.77	

[a]*Two cases with invasive lobular carcinomas and one case with an intraductal papillary carcinoma.*

restoration/repair (18). IL-33/ST2 axis can also promote Th1-type responses depending on the presence or absence of IL-12 (5). The influence of the IL-33/ST2 axis may be protective or pathogenic in various disease conditions, as it has a dual role in inflammatory disorders (8, 19). IL-33 plays a crucial role in inflammation and is associated with many diseases, such as giant cell arteritis (20), biliary atresia (21), and chronic obstructive lung disease (22). However, few data have been reported about the role of IL-33/ST2 axis in cancer, and little is known about the function of IL-33 in patients with BC.

In this study, we investigated the serum level and tissue expression of IL-33 in patients with BC. We found significantly higher serum levels of IL-33 in patients with BC, compared with patients with BBD, and higher expression of IL-33 in carcinomas and adjacent tissues to tumors, compared with normal breast tissue from the same patients.

The serum concentration of sST2, the soluble form of the receptor for both IL-33 and IL-1, has been shown to be elevated in patients with metastatic BC, and knockdown of the sST2 decreases ErbB2-induced cell motility in two different cell lines (23). However, there are no previous reports about IL-33 expression in serum or tissues of BC patients. In this study, serum levels of IL-33 are higher in patients with ER-positive tumors, predicting that the IL-33/ST2 axis may be involved in hormone receptor signaling. Moreover, in carcinoma tissues, IL-33 expression is significantly higher in HER2-overexpressing tissues, consistent with the report that its receptor sST2 is over-expressed to promote BC metastases upon ErbB2 activation in BC cell lines (23). In ST knock out mice models, lack of ST2 can suppress BC progression and metastasis, through enhanced cytotoxic activity of NK cells and increased systemic Th1/Th17 cytokines (24). Although we found no association between serum levels of IL-33 and in patients with more than three involved lymph nodes, the higher expression of IL-33 consistent with the IL-33/ST2 axis being involved in progression and metastasis of BC.

Of interest is that serum levels and carcinoma tissue expression of IL-33 are higher in patients with a family history of malignant breast carcinoma. As IL-33 may play an important role in immunosuppression of cancer for subsequent tumor progression and metastasis, and auto-immune diseases are usually hereditary, patients with a family history may be more likely to trigger or promote the process of immunosuppression (11). Whether and how IL-33 expression is linked auto-immune disease and familial cancers needs to be clarified.

Ki-67 is a cancer cell proliferation biomarker (25). IL-33 was higher in the low Ki-67 expression group, suggesting serum levels of IL-33 are negatively associated with BC proliferation. After analyzing cytokines associated with IL-33, only a decrease in IL-12 is observed in patients with BC, suggesting systemic IL-33 may not play an important role in BC immunity. In a murine model, the IL-33/ST2 axis has been demonstrated to facilitate intratumoral accumulation of immunosuppressive and innate lymphoid cells, and then promote BC growth and metastases (11). Similarly, in head and neck squamous cell carcinomas, administration of IL-33 promotes cancer cell migration and invasion through induction of epithelial-to-mesenchymal transition. Moreover, IL-33 has been shown to be a potential prognostic biomarker and target for new therapeutic strategies (26). Recent research suggests that in the breast tumor environment, tumor-infiltrating T lymphocytes (TILs) secrete IL-17A, to activate the MAPK pathway, promoting proliferation and resistance to conventional chemotherapeutic agents (27). The elevations of both IL-33 serum levels and immunohistochemical expression might promote BC progression and metastases through regulation of IL-12 pathway.

The local expression of IL-33 may be an important marker for differentiating malignant from normal/benign tissues. IL-33 expression in adjacent tissues also tends to be higher compared to normal tissues, suggesting that adjacent non-cancerous tissues may be similarly relevant to cancers in terms of anti-tumor immunity. Local IL-33 expression may also increase intratumoral accumulation of immunosuppressive lymphoid cells in patients with BC. However, in high grade tumor tissue, the expression of IL-33 is decreased compared to low grade tumor tissues, indicating that IL-33 may be more important in HER2-over-expressing tumors, and other cytokines may be involved in this crosstalk of regulation. Interestingly, IL-33 expression in serum and cancer tissues was contrary when comparing with ER and HER2 expression, although with statistical significance (**Tables 1** and **3**). Up to now, there were no reports about the relationship between IL-33 and ER or HER2. So we supposed that IL-33 may play different roles in system and in local tissues under different hormone conditions. The IL-33 may be involved in the resistence to endocrine therapy and Herceptin therapy of ER/HER2 positive patients with BC.

It is confirmed that IL-33 could activate, Th1, NK, NKT, and $CD8^+$ T cells under certain pathophysiological conditions (11). On the other hand, IL-33 has a dual role in inflammatory disorders, anti- and pro-inflammatory. The tissue expression of IL-33 is significantly different, indicated that in carcinomas, immune cells may be recruited to anti-inflammatory and subsequent immunosuppression in HER2 overexpression tumors. In summary, this study indicated that serum IL-33 is higher in cancer patients compare to patients with BBD. Immunohistochemical staining demonstrated that IL-33 is higher in both cancerous and adjacent tissues compared to normal tissues, suggesting its role in BC progression and metastases. Thus, IL-33 may be a useful biomarker for prediction of malignant potential and immunosuppression of breast carcinomas.

AUTHOR CONTRIBUTIONS

Jing Liu and Guo-Jun Zhang conceived and designed the experiments; Jing Liu, Jia-Xin Shen, and Jia-Lin Hu performed the experiments; Jing Liu, Wen-He Huang, and Guo-Jun Zhang analyzed the data; Jing Liu, Jia-Xin Shen, Jia-Lin Hu, Wen-He Huang, and Guo-Jun Zhang contributed reagents and materials; Jing Liu, Jia-Xin Shen, and Guo-Jun Zhang wrote the paper.

ACKNOWLEDGMENTS

This study was supported by State Key Development Program for Basic Research of China (No. 2011CB707705), National Natural Science Foundation of China (No. 31271068 and 81320108015), and Seed funding of Guangdong Provincial Key Laboratory for Diagnosis and Treatment of Breast Cancer. We would like to thank Dr. Stanley Lin for his critical and careful reading of the manuscript.

REFERENCES

1. Siegel R, Naishadham D, Jemal A. Cancer statistics, 2013. *CA Cancer J Clin* (2013) **63**(1):11–30. doi:10.3322/caac.21166
2. Jiang X, Shapiro DJ. The immune system and inflammation in breast cancer. *Mol Cell endocrinol* (2014) **382**(1):673–82. doi:10.1016/j.mce.2013.06.003
3. Mattii M, Ayala F, Balato N, Filotico R, Lembo S, Schiattarella M, et al. The balance between pro- and anti-inflammatory cytokines is crucial in human allergic contact dermatitis pathogenesis: the role of IL-1 family members. *Exp Dermatol* (2013) **22**(12):813–9. doi:10.1111/exd.12272
4. Wood IS, Wang B, Trayhurn P. IL-33, a recently identified interleukin-1 gene family member, is expressed in human adipocytes. *Biochem Biophys Res Commun* (2009) **384**(1):105–9. doi:10.1016/j.bbrc.2009.04.081
5. Liew FY, Pitman NI, McInnes IB. Disease-associated functions of IL-33: the new kid in the IL-1 family. *Nat Rev Immunol* (2010) **10**(2):103–10. doi:10.1038/nri2692
6. Hong YS, Moon SJ, Joo YB, Jeon CH, Cho ML, Ju JH, et al. Measurement of interleukin-33 (IL-33) and IL-33 receptors (sST2 and ST2L) in patients with rheumatoid arthritis. *J Korean Med Sci* (2011) **26**(9):1132–9. doi:10.3346/jkms.2011.26.9.1132
7. Salimi M, Barlow JL, Saunders SP, Xue L, Gutowska-Owsiak D, Wang X, et al. A role for IL-25 and IL-33-driven type-2 innate lymphoid cells in atopic dermatitis. *J Exp Med* (2013) **210**(13):2939–50. doi:10.1084/jem.20130351
8. Volarevic V, Mitrovic M, Milovanovic M, Zelen I, Nikolic I, Mitrovic S, et al. Protective role of IL-33/ST2 axis in Con A-induced hepatitis. *J Hepatol* (2012) **56**(1):26–33. doi:10.1016/j.jhep.2011.03.022
9. Bergis D, Kassis V, Ranglack A, Koeberle V, Piiper A, Kronenberger B, et al. High serum levels of the interleukin-33 receptor soluble ST2 as a negative prognostic factor in hepatocellular carcinoma. *Transl Oncol* (2013) **6**(3):311–8.
10. Hu LA, Fu Y, Zhang DN, Zhang J. Serum IL-33 as a diagnostic and prognostic marker in non-small cell lung cancer. *Asian Pac J Cancer Prev* (2013) **14**(4):2563–6. doi:10.7314/APJCP.2013.14.4.2563
11. Jovanovic IP, Pejnovic NN, Radosavljevic GD, Pantic JM, Milovanovic MZ, Arsenijevic NN, et al. Interleukin-33/ST2 axis promotes breast cancer growth and metastases by facilitating intratumoral accumulation of immunosuppressive and innate lymphoid cells. *Int J Cancer* (2013) **134**(7):1669–82. doi:10.1002/ijc.28481
12. Gao K, Li X, Zhang L, Bai L, Dong W, Shi G, et al. Transgenic expression of IL-33 activates CD8(+) T cells and NK cells and inhibits tumor growth and metastasis in mice. *Cancer Lett* (2013) **335**(2):463–71. doi:10.1016/j.canlet.2013.03.002
13. Deutsch E. Medical experimentation: international rules and practice. *Law Rev* (1989) **19**:1–10.
14. Bernhard OK, Mathias RA, Barnes TW, Simpson RJ. A fluorescent microsphere-based method for assay of multiple analytes in plasma. *Methods Mol Biol* (2011) **728**:195–206. doi:10.1007/978-1-61779-068-3_12
15. Liu J, Wei XL, Huang WH, Chen CF, Bai JW, Zhang GJ. Cytoplasmic Skp2 expression is associated with p-Akt1 and predicts poor prognosis in human breast carcinomas. *PLoS One* (2012) **7**(12):e52675. doi:10.1371/journal.pone.0052675
16. Jorns JM, Healy P, Zhao L. Review of estrogen receptor, progesterone receptor, and HER-2/neu immunohistochemistry impacts on treatment for a small subset of breast cancer patients transferring care to another institution. *Arch Pathol Lab Med* (2013) **137**(11):1660–3. doi:10.5858/arpa.2012-0670-OA
17. Inwald EC, Klinkhammer-Schalke M, Hofstädter F, Zeman F, Koller M, Gerstenhauer M, et al. Ki-67 is a prognostic parameter in breast cancer patients: results of a large population-based cohort of a cancerregistry. *Breast Cancer Res Treat* (2013) **139**(2):539–52. doi:10.1007/s10549-013-2560-8
18. Lopetuso LR, Scaldaferri F, Pizarro TT. Emerging role of the interleukin (IL)-33/ST2 axis in gut mucosal wound healing and fibrosis. *Fibrogenesis Tissue Repair* (2012) **5**(1):18. doi:10.1186/1755-1536-5-18
19. Kamijo S, Takeda H, Tokura T, Suzuki M, Inui K, Hara M. IL-33-mediated innate response and adaptive immune cells contribute to maximum responses of protease allergen-induced allergic airway inflammation. *J Immunol* (2013) **190**(9):4489–99. doi:10.4049/jimmunol.1201212
20. Ciccia F, Alessandro R, Rizzo A, Raimondo S, Giardina A, Raiata F, et al. IL-33 is overexpressed in the inflamed arteries of patients with giant cell arteritis. *Ann Rheum Dis* (2013) **72**(2):258–64. doi:10.1136/annrheumdis-2012-201309
21. Dong R, Dong K, Wang X, Chen G, Shen C, Zheng S. Interleukin-33 overexpression is associated with gamma-glutamyl transferase in biliary atresia. *Cytokine* (2013) **61**(2):433–7. doi:10.1016/j.cyto.2012.10.035
22. Byers DE, Alexander-Brett J, Patel AC, Agapov E, Dang-Vu G, Jin X, et al. Long-term IL-33-producing epithelial progenitor cells in chronic obstructive lung disease. *J Clin Invest* (2013) **123**(12):5410. doi:10.1172/JCI65570
23. Gillibert-Duplantier J, Duthey B, Sisirak V, Salaun D, Gargi T, Tredan O, et al. Gene expression profiling identifies sST2 as an effector of ErbB2-driven breast carcinoma cell motility, associated with metastasis. *Oncogene* (2012) **31**(30):3516–24. doi:10.1038/onc.2011.525
24. Jovanovic I, Radosavljevic G, Mitrovic M, Juranic VL, McKenzie AN, Arsenijevic N, et al. ST2 deletion enhances innate and acquired immunity to murine mammary carcinoma. *Eur J Immunol* (2011) **41**(7):1902–12. doi:10.1002/eji.201141417
25. Brown JR, Digiovanna MP, Killelea B, Lannin DR, Rimm DL. Quantitative assessment Ki-67 score for prediction of response to neoadjuvant chemotherapy in breast cancer. *Lab Invest* (2014) **94**(1):98–106. doi:10.1038/labinvest.2013.128

26. Chen SF, Nieh S, Jao SW, Wu MZ, Liu CL, Chang YC, et al. The paracrine effect of cancer-associated fibroblast-induced interleukin-33 regulates the invasiveness of head and neck squamous cell carcinoma. *J Pathol* (2013) **231**(2):180–9. doi:10.1002/path.4226

27. Cochaud S, Giustiniani J, Thomas C, Laprevotte E, Garbar C, Savoye AM, et al. IL-17A is produced by breast cancer TILs and promotes chemoresistance and proliferation through ERK1/2. *Sci Rep* (2013) **3**:3456. doi:10.1038/srep03456

4

The past, present, and future of immune repertoire biology – the rise of next-generation repertoire analysis

Adrien Six[1,2,3,4,5 *†], Maria Encarnita Mariotti-Ferrandiz[1,2,3,5], Wahiba Chaara[1,2,3,4,5], Susana Magadan[6], Hang-Phuong Pham[1,2], Marie-Paule Lefranc[7], Thierry Mora[8], Véronique Thomas-Vaslin[1,2,3,5], Aleksandra M. Walczak[9] and Pierre Boudinot[6†]

[1] UPMC University Paris 06, UMR 7211, Immunology-Immunopathology-Immunotherapy (I3), Paris, France
[2] CNRS, UMR 7211, Immunology-Immunopathology-Immunotherapy (I3), Paris, France
[3] INSERM, UMR_S 959, Immunology-Immunopathology-Immunotherapy (I3), Paris, France
[4] AP-HP, Hôpital Pitié-Salpêtrière, CIC-BTi Biotherapy, Paris, France
[5] AP-HP, Hôpital Pitié-Salpêtrière, Département Hospitalo-Universitaire (DHU), Inflammation-Immunopathology-Biotherapy (i2B), Paris, France
[6] Institut National de la Recherche Agronomique, Unité de Virologie et Immunologie Moléculaires, Jouy-en-Josas, France
[7] IMGT®, The International ImMunoGeneTics Information System®, Institut de Génétique Humaine, UPR CNRS 1142, Université Montpellier 2, Montpellier, France
[8] Laboratoire de Physique Statistique, UMR8550, CNRS and Ecole Normale Supérieure, Paris, France
[9] Laboratoire de Physique Théorique, UMR8549, CNRS and Ecole Normale Supérieure, Paris, France

Edited by:
Miles Davenport, University of New South Wales, Australia

Reviewed by:
Koji Yasutomo, University of Tokushima, Japan
John J. Miles, Queensland Institute of Medical Research, Australia

***Correspondence:**
Adrien Six, CNRS UMR 7211, UPMC, Immunology-Immunopathology-Immunotherapy (I3), BâtimentCervi, 83 bd de l'Hôpital, Paris F-75013, France
e-mail: adrien.six@upmc.fr

†Adrien Six and Pierre Boudinot have contributed equally to this work.

T and B cell repertoires are collections of lymphocytes, each characterized by its antigen-specific receptor. We review here classical technologies and analysis strategies developed to assess immunoglobulin (IG) and T cell receptor (TR) repertoire diversity, and describe recent advances in the field. First, we describe the broad range of available methodological tools developed in the past decades, each of which answering different questions and showing complementarity for progressive identification of the level of repertoire alterations: global overview of the diversity by flow cytometry, IG repertoire descriptions at the protein level for the identification of IG reactivities, IG/TR CDR3 spectratyping strategies, and related molecular quantification or dynamics of T/B cell differentiation. Additionally, we introduce the recent technological advances in molecular biology tools allowing deeper analysis of IG/TR diversity by next-generation sequencing (NGS), offering systematic and comprehensive sequencing of IG/TR transcripts in a short amount of time. NGS provides several angles of analysis such as clonotype frequency, CDR3 diversity, CDR3 sequence analysis, V allele identification with a quantitative dimension, therefore requiring high-throughput analysis tools development. In this line, we discuss the recent efforts made for nomenclature standardization and ontology development. We then present the variety of available statistical analysis and modeling approaches developed with regards to the various levels of diversity analysis, and reveal the increasing sophistication of those modeling approaches. To conclude, we provide some examples of recent mathematical modeling strategies and perspectives that illustrate the active rise of a "next-generation" of repertoire analysis.

Keywords: diversity analysis, immune receptors, next-generation sequencing, modeling, statistics, gene nomenclature, B cell repertoire, T cell repertoire

INTRODUCTION

T and B cell repertoires are collections of lymphocytes, each characterized by its antigen-specific receptor. The resources available to generate the potential repertoires are described by the genomic T cell receptor (TR) and immunoglobulin (IG) loci. TR and IG are produced by random somatic rearrangements of V, D, and J genes during lymphocyte differentiation. The product of the V-(D)-J joining, called the complementarity determining region 3 (CDR3) and corresponding to the signature of the rearrangement, binds the antigen and is responsible for the specificity of the recognition. During their differentiation, lymphocytes are subjected to selective processes, which lead to deletion of most auto-reactive cells, selection, export, and expansion, of mature T and B cells to the periphery. Primary IG and TR repertoires are therefore shaped to generate the available peripheral or mucosal repertoires. In addition, several different functional T and B cells subsets have been identified, with differential dynamics and antigen-specific patterns. These available repertoires are dramatically modified during antigen-driven responses especially in the inflammatory context of pathogen infections, autoimmune syndromes, and cancer to shape actual repertoires. When considering the importance of efficient adaptive immune responses to get rid of infections naturally or to avoid auto-reactive damages, but also for therapeutic purposes such as vaccination or cell therapy, one realizes the relevance of understanding how lymphocyte repertoires are selected during differentiation, from ontogeny to aging, and upon antigenic challenge. However, immune repertoires of expressed antigen receptors are built by an integrated system of genomic recombination and controlled expression, and follow complex time-space developmental patterns. Thus, an efficient repertoire analysis requires both (1) methods that sample and describe the diversity of receptors at different levels for an acceptable cost and from a little amount of material and (2) analysis strategies that reconstitute the best multidimensional picture of the immune diversity from the partial information provided by the repertoire description as reviewed in Ref. (1). In the following sections, we summarize technologies developed over the past decades to describe lymphocyte repertoires and we present the growing number of analysis tools, evolving from basic to sophisticated statistics and modeling strategies with regards to the level of complexity of the data produced.

METHODS DEVELOPED TO DESCRIBE THE IG AND TR REPERTOIRES

B and T lymphocyte repertoires can be studied from different lymphoid tissues and at various biological levels, such as cell membrane or secreted proteins, transcripts or genes, according to the techniques used. Fluorescence microscopy or flow cytometry techniques allow to track and sort particular cell phenotypes and to quantify the expressed repertoire at the single-cell level with V subgroup-specific monoclonal antibodies. Alternatively, the IG or TR diversity may be also analyzed using proteomics methods from either the serum (for IG) or dedicated cell extracts. Finally, molecular biology techniques assess the repertoire at the genomic DNA or transcriptional levels, qualitatively and/or quantitatively.

ANALYSIS OF IG AND TR REPERTOIRES AT THE PROTEIN LEVEL

Flow cytometry single-cell repertoire analysis

The frequency of lymphocytes expressing a given IG or TR can be determined using flow cytometry when specific monoclonal antibodies are available. This technique allows for the combined analysis of the antigen receptor and of other cell surface markers. Currently, using flow cytometry, up to 13 parameters can be routinely studied at once, reaching 20 parameters with the last generation flow cytometers and 70–100 parameters with mass cytometry (2). Seminal studies in mice using specific anti-TRBV antibodies have led to the characterization of the central tolerance selection processes that occur in thymus (3–5). Later on, a comprehensive description of the human TRBV repertoire was setup (6), when monoclonal antibodies became available for most of the TRBV subgroups. Repertoire analysis with flow cytometry provides a qualitative and quantitative analyses of the variable region, often done on heterogeneous cell populations, in order to decipher, for example, selection events related to aging, perturbations, and treatments (7). However, this technology is naturally limited by the availability of specific monoclonal antibodies, and does not address more detailed issues such as junction diversity. Furthermore, polymorphism of the IG or TR genes (8, 9) may constitute a serious limitation for a systematic survey using these approaches.

Proteomic repertoire analysis for serum immunoglobulins

Recent developments of proteomics tools now offer sensitivity levels applicable to IG repertoire analysis. Such a description at the protein level takes into account all post transcriptional and translational modifications.

PANAMA-blot technology. A semi-quantitative immunoblot, called the PANAMA-blot technique (10), allows for the identification of the antibody reactivities present in collection of sera (or cell culture supernatant) against a given source of antigens (10–12). Briefly, a selected source of antigens is subjected to preparative SDS-PAGE, transferred onto nitrocellulose membranes, then incubated with the serum to be tested allowing for the revelation of the bound antibodies using an appropriate secondary antibody coupled to alkaline phosphatase. Computer-assisted analysis of the densitometric profiles allows for the rescaling and the quantitative comparison of patterns of antibody reactivity from individuals in different groups. A large amount of data is generated when testing a range of sera against various sources of antigens. Statistical analyses are included in the PANAMA-Blot approach (as described further). This global analysis helped to reveal that the IgM repertoire in mice is selected by internal ligands and independent of external antigens (13).

This method can also lead to identify IG reactivity patterns specific for a type of pathology or clinical status and has been applied to both fundamental and clinical analysis. In particular, it was used to analyze human self-reactive antibody repertoires and their potential role for down-modulating autoimmune processes (14–16).

Antigen micro-array chips. More recently, antigen micro-array-based technology coupled to a complex two-way clustering bioinformatics analysis was developed to evaluate the serum repertoire antibodies from diabetes-prone individuals and revealed their predictive or diagnostic value. In brief, a range of antigens (proteins, peptides, nucleotides, phospholipids...) were plated onto glass plates and incubated with sera from individuals (human diabetes patients or mice in an experimental model of diabetes). The intensity of reactivity of the serum IG for each peptide was determined and scored against the control reactivity. Clustering analysis was then implemented to determine a potential antigen signature that significantly sorts out diabetes from non-diabetes individuals. In this way, it was found that the patterns of IgG antibodies expressed early in male NOD mice can mark susceptibility or resistance to diabetes induced later and that it is different than the pattern characteristic of healthy or diabetic mice after disease induction (17). Similarly, this clustering approach was applied in humans to successfully separate human subjects that are already diabetic from healthy people (18).

REPERTOIRE ANALYSIS AT THE GENOMIC DNA LEVEL

Other strategies that cover IG or TR repertoire analyses have been developed at the genomic DNA level. Firstly, CDR3 spectratyping studies (detailed in the following section) have been carried out at the DNA level mostly to address issues related to B or T cell development (19, 20). More recently, an original multiplex genomic PCR assay coupled to real-time PCR analysis was developed to provide a comprehensive description of the mouse T cell receptor alpha (TRA) repertoire during development (21). Although these approaches can be applied to all IG isotypes and TR, they have not been used as much as transcript CDR3 spectratyping due to sensitivity and heterozygosity issues.

Immunoglobulin or T cell receptor repertoires can also be assessed by following the diversity of rearrangement deletion circles. Since they are produced by the V-(D)-J recombination machinery when the joint signal is formed and diluted in daughter cells, they give a good representation of recently generated T or B cells. This technique has been particularly useful for describing the restoration of T cell diversity following highly active antiretroviral therapy in HIV-infected patients (22) and has been used to model thymic export (23, 24) as well as to demonstrate continued contribution of the thymus to repertoire diversity, even in older individuals (25). It also reveals that thymic output is genetically determined, and related to the extent of proliferation of T cells at DN4 stage in mice (26). However, their analysis does not provide much insight into the level of diversity since the signal joint does not vary for a given combination of genes. Therefore, the interest of such analyses is reached when combined with CDR3 spectratyping analyses to know whether a repertoire perturbation is rather attributable to newly produced T cells or peripheral T cell proliferation.

V-(D)-J JUNCTION ANALYSIS OF IG AND TR TRANSCRIPT REPERTOIRES

Original molecular-based strategies for analyzing repertoire diversity relied on cloning and hybridization of molecular probes specific for IGHV gene subgroups first by RNA colony blot assay (27). This led to the observation that IGHV gene usage is characteristic of mouse strain and is a process of random genetic combination by equiprobable expression of IGHV genes (28). The study of selection processes revealed that the IGHV region-dependent selection determines clonal persistence of B cells (29) and that selection with age leads to biased IGHV gene expression (30).

In situ hybridization on single-cells revealed that during mouse ontogeny and early development of B cells in bone marrow, there is a non-random position-dependent IGHV gene expression, favoring D-proximal IGHV gene subgroup usage (31). Thereafter, sequencing of PCR-amplified cDNA collections were obtained from samples of interest. Although fastidious, these early studies have been useful in defining the basis of human IG and TR repertoires in terms of overall distribution, CDR3-length distribution, and V-(D)-J use (32–35), sometimes leading to the identification of new IG or TR genes. Later, more practical techniques have been developed for large-scale analysis of lymphocyte repertoires, such as quantitative PCR, micro-array, and junction length spectratyping, as described below.

Quantitative RT-PCR for repertoire analysis

In parallel to qualitative CDR3 spectratyping techniques (see section below), quantitative PCR strategies were developed (36). Coupling the two techniques for all V domain-C region combinations provides a complete qualitative and quantitative picture of the repertoire (37–39) described by up to 2,000 measurements per IG isotype or TR for one sample. With the development of real-time quantitative PCR, this approach opened the possibility for a more precise evaluation of repertoire diversity (39–41). Complementary tools have been also developed in order to allow normalization of spectratype analysis such as studies by Liu et al. (42) and Mugnaini et al. (43).

Matsutani et al. (44) developed another method to quantify the expression of the human TRAV and TRBV repertoires based on hybridization with gene specific primers coated plates. The cDNA from PBMC extracted RNA are ligated to a universal adaptor which allows for a global amplification of all TRAV or TRBV cDNAs. The PCR products are then transferred onto microplates coated with oligonucleotides specific for each TRAV or TRBV regions, and the amount of hybridized material is quantified. This technique was used to analyze the TR repertoire diversity of transplanted patients (45) and adapted to the study of mouse TRAV and TRBV repertoires (46). VanderBorght et al. also developed a semi-quantitative PCR-ELISA-based method for the human TRAV and TRBV repertoire analysis (38). The combined usage of digoxigenin (DIG)-coupled nucleotides and DIG-coupled reverse TRAC or TRBC primers allowed for a quantitative measurement of the amount of amplified DNA by a sandwich ELISA.

Du et al. (47) later setup a megaplex PCR strategy to characterize the antigen-specific TRBV repertoire from sorted IFNγ-producing cells after *Mycobacterium* infection. The clonotypic TRBV PCR products were used for Taqman probes design to quantify the expression of the corresponding clonotypes from ATLAS-amplified SMART cDNAs.

Direct measurement of lymphocyte diversity using micro-arrays

Another technology, similar to the one just discussed, has been developed by the group of Cascalho et al. which allows for a direct measurement of the entire population of lymphocyte-receptors. This is accomplished by hybridization of lymphocyte-receptor specific cRNA of a lymphocyte population of interest to random oligonucleotides on a gene chip; the number of sites undergoing hybridization corresponds to the level of diversity. This method was validated and calibrated using control samples of random oligonucleotides of known diversity (1, 10^3, 10^6, 10^9) (48, 49) and successfully demonstrated that central and peripheral diversification of T lymphocytes is dependent on the diversity of the circulating IG repertoire (49, 50). Similarly, a highly sensitive micro-array-based method has been proposed to monitor TR repertoire at the single-cell level (51).

CDR3 spectratyping techniques

Immunoscope technology. Among various techniques used to analyze the T or B cell repertoires, Immunoscope, also known as CDR3 spectratyping (52, 53) consists in the analysis of the CDR3-length usage so that antigen-specific receptor repertoires can be described by thousands of measurements. In the case of naive murine repertoires, T cell populations are polyclonal and analysis typically yields eight-peak regular bell-shaped CDR3 displays (wrongly assumed to be Gaussian), each peak corresponding to a given CDR3-length. When an immune response occurs, this regular polyclonal display can be perturbed: one can see one or several prominent peaks that correspond to the oligoclonal or clonal expansion of lymphocytes. A complete description of this technique and its applications to clinical studies has been published elsewhere (54).

In the original Immunoscope publication, Cochet et al. (55) analyzed the T cell repertoire after the immunization of mice with the pigeon cytochrome c. They provided the first description of an *ex vivo* follow-up of a primary T cell specific response in a mouse model. Their second paper analyzed the average CDR3-lengths as a function of TRBV-TRBJ combinations. In particular, the authors found a correlation between TRBV CDR1 and major histocompatibility (MH) haplotype (52). This group later published a large amount of original studies in various models such as lymphocyte development (40, 56–63), kinetics of antigen-specific responses (64–67), viral infection (68, 69), autoimmunity (70, 71), tumor-associated disease (72), and analysis of allogeneic T cell response and tolerance after transplantation (73). Notably, the combination of CDR3 spectratyping with flow cytometry-based IG or TR V frequency analysis provides a more comprehensive assessment, such as in Pilch et al. (74). For example, such an approach revealed the constriction of repertoire diversity through age-related clonal CD8 expansion (75). Similarly, a combination of CDR3 spectratyping, flow cytometry, and TR deletion circle analysis has allowed to define age-dependent incidence on thymic renewal in patients (76) or to evaluate the effects of caloric restriction in monkeys to preserve repertoire diversity (77). CDR3-length spectratyping was also used in other models, such as rainbow trout, to analyze TRB repertoire and its modifications induced by viral infection (78–80). While no tool such as monoclonal antibodies to T cell marker(s) was available in this model, this approach demonstrated that fish could mount specific T cell responses against virus, which could be found in all individuals (public clonotypes) or not (private clonotypes). Similar strategies, developed by other groups (81) and following the same approach in parallel, analyzed the IG repertoire in *Xenopus* at different stages of development, describing a more restricted IG junction diversity in the tadpole compared to the adult.

Gorski et al. (82) developed their own CDR3 spectratyping technique to analyze the complexity and stability of circulating αβT cell repertoires in patients following bone marrow transplantation as compared to normal adults. They showed that repertoire complexity of bone marrow recipients correlates with their state of immune function; in particular, individuals suffering from recurrent infections associated with T cell impairment exhibited contractions and gaps in repertoire diversity. The detailed procedure for this technique has been published in Maslanka et al. (83). A variation of this technique has been reported later by Lue et al. (84), relying on a compact glass cassette, a simpler device than the usual automated plate DNA sequencers.

Alternative technologies. Alternative CDR3 spectratyping techniques have been described such as single-strand conformation polymorphism (85–87) and heteroduplex analysis (88–91). These methods differ from the CDR3 spectratyping/Immunoscope technique mostly in the way PCR products are analyzed by performing non-denaturing polyacrylamide electrophoresis. The main advantage of these techniques is a more direct assessment of clonal expansion since PCR products migrate according to their conformation properties; therefore, presence of a predominant peak is strongly indicative of clonality when a smear migration pattern indicates polyclonality. However, these techniques have been less widely used probably because of the difficulty to make clear correlations between the expanded peaks across samples.

Another original alternative technique has been described by Bouffard et al. (92), analyzing products obtained after *in vitro* translation of PCR-amplified TR-specific products by isoelectric focusing. With this technique, clonality can also directly be assessed by looking at the obtained migration profile.

IG/TR REARRANGEMENT SEQUENCING: FROM CLONING-BASED- TO NEXT-GENERATION-SEQUENCING

In order to get a better description of IG/TR diversity at the nucleotide sequence level, thus providing fine-tuned description of the actual diversity, Sanger sequencing approaches relying on bacterial cloning of rearrangements were performed in physiological conditions globally (60, 93–99) or partially to characterize particular expansions identified by other technologies such as CDR3 spectratyping (40, 59, 100–102), flow cytometry (103). They were also used in pathological/infectious conditions (104–107) sometimes leading to antigen-specific T cell TR identification and quantification through the combination of antigen-specific T cell stimulation and cytometry-based cell sorting, anchor-PCR, and bacterial cloning-based sequencing (108).

These studies pioneered the description of the repertoire and provided fruitful information regarding the extent and modification of the diversity. However, besides being time and cost-extensive, such approaches have allowed for the analysis of 10^2–10^3 sequences, far under the estimated diversity reaching 10^6–10^7 unique clonotypes in mice and humans (40, 59, 109).

In the last decade, DNA sequencing technologies have made tremendous progresses (110) with the development of so called next-generation sequencers, already reaching four generations (111). Those instruments are designed to sequence mixtures of up to millions of DNA molecules simultaneously, instead of individual clones separately. Second generation sequencers became affordable in the last 5 years and have been used for immune repertoire analysis, starting with the seminal work of Weinstein et al. (112) where the IG repertoire of Zebrafish has been described by large-scale sequencing. Consequently, exploratory works by other groups provided an overview of the complex sequence landscape of immune repertoires in humans (113–118). More recent work aimed at addressing fundamental questions such as lineage cells commitment (119–122), generation of the diversity processes (123–125), and diversity sharing between individuals (126, 127). Finally, the power of this technology has been validated in the clinic as well (128, 129).

As seen above for other technologies, combinations of approaches have been applied to NGS. Notably, deep sequencing has been used in combination with CDR3-length spectratyping by some groups to study human (130) or rainbow trout IG (131) repertoire modifications after vaccination against bacteria or viruses. In the latter, pyrosequencing performed for relevant VH/Cμ or VH/Cτ junctions identified the clonal structure of responses, and showed, for example, that public responses are made of different clones identified by (1) distinct V-(D)-J junctions encoding the same protein sequence or (2) distinct V-(D)-J sequences differing by one or two conservative amino acid changes (131) as described for public response in mammals (132, 133). These studies showed that NGS and traditional spectratyping techniques lead to remarkably similar CDR3 distributions.

Several NGS have been developed in the past years using different sequencing technologies characterized with different speed, deepness and read length. Metzker thoroughly reviewed their principles and properties (134). Among them, three platforms, all offering benchtop sequencers with reduced cost and setup, fit with immune repertoire analysis in terms of read length and deepness. The 454/Roche platform uses pyrosequencing technology (135), which combines single nucleotide addition (SNA) with chemoluminescent detection on templates that are clonally amplified by emulsion PCR and loaded on a picotiter plate. Pyrosequencing currently has a 500 bp (GS Junior) to 700 bp (GS FLX) sequencing capacity with a respective deepness of 150,000–3,000,000 reads per run (134). The Illumina/Solexa platform technology is based on cyclic reversible termination (CRT) sequencing (an adaptation of Sanger sequencing) performed on templates clonally amplified on solid-phase bridge PCR. Protected fluorescent nucleotides are added, imaged, delabeled, and deprotected cyclically (134), providing a deeper sequencing (from 15 to 6 billion reads per run for the MiSeq to the HiSeq2500/2000) of shorter reads (100–250 bp for the very recent MiSeq) with the possibility to perform pair-end sequencing (two-side sequencing) to increase the read length after aligning the generated complementary sequences. A more recent platform, Ion Torrent/Life Technologies using an imaging free detection system may open a new era in terms of deepness (one billion reads per run) of 200 bp reads (136) in a very short time and on a benchtop sequencer. Importantly, depending on the technology, errors due to the PCR-based sample preparation and the sequencing are of major concern. Bolotin et al. (137) evaluated this issue on TR repertoire analysis of the same donor performed on the three platforms described previously; algorithms for error correction have been developed. Indeed, PCR- and sequencing-related errors represent the major concern for immune repertoire diversity analysis as they may generate artificial diversity. Illumina and 454 appear to be the most robust technologies, with Illumina having the highest throughput and 454 generating the longest reads. The currently available Ion Torrent platform, although very promising, has been shown to display the highest rate of errors in TR (137) and bacterial DNA (138) sequencing. However, such error corrections must be used with caution since they may inadvertently underestimate repertoire diversity by removing rare sequences.

With the power of such approach for genomics and transcriptomics studies in general, constant improvements are achieved to increase the sequencing deepness and read length as well as to reduce the cost, therefore offering multitude of biological explorations (139). NGS now permits a comprehensive and quantitative view of IG and TR diversity by combining and improving the sensitivity of classical approaches with accurate and large-scale sequencing. NGS has the power to identify IG or TR specific for given antigens (in combination with antigen-specific assays) and to define more complex signatures (i.e., TR sets) related to disease and/or treatment from heterogeneous T and B cell populations. Still, most of the deep sequencing efforts have been limited to only one chain of the receptor at the repertoire level (usually the β chain for TR and the heavy chain for IG). Indeed, current high-throughput approaches do not allow one to assign which combination of chains (TRA and TRB, or IGH and IGK or IGL) belong to which cell (140). A recent development by DeKosky et al. proposed a reasonably high-throughput technology to assess massively paired IG VH and VL from bulk population (141). In parallel, Turchaninova et al. (142) have proposed a similar approach for the paired analysis of the TRA and TRB chains. The parallel development of high-throughput microfluidic-based single-cell sorting will certainly push forward new developments in the field (143).

However, despite the technological advance, studies so far have mainly reported CDR3 counting and identification of major expansions. The complexity of immune repertoires is still a matter that such approach cannot completely overcome, due to the paucity of powerful analytical methods. Besides data management tools, studies are now starting to extract most of the benefit from such approach to model the immune repertoire diversity and dynamics (144), an approach that may help in understanding the interplay between cells and repertoire shaping. Accurate and powerful statistical analyses are required to manage such amount of information. Current state will be reviewed in the following sections.

POTENTIAL AND GENOMIC REPERTOIRES: A QUESTION OF ONTOLOGY AND ORTHOLOGY

Immune repertoires *sensu stricto* are expressed by lymphocyte clones, each carrying a single receptor for the antigen. Such receptors comprise IG and TR in jawed vertebrates (8, 9) and VLR in Agnathans (145). The sequences of these receptors are available in databases such as GenBank or EMBL, which are difficult to use for transversal studies due to inconsistent annotation. The IMGT® information system (see below) has largely solved this problem setting standardized gene nomenclatures, ontologies and a universal numbering of the IG/TR V and C domains, thus giving a common access to standardized data from genome, proteome, genetics, two-dimensional, and three-dimensional structures (146). The accuracy and the consistency of the IMGT® data are based on IMGT-ONTOLOGY, the first, and so far, unique ontology for immunogenetics and immunoinformatics (147).

With the development of high-throughput sequencing, large numbers of new sequences of antigen receptor genes have become available, which can be classified into different categories: genomic sequences of IG or TR (in germline configuration in genome assemblies) or fragments of IG/TR transcripts, containing the CDR3 or not. Also, these datasets can be produced from species newly sequenced, as well as from new haplotypes of well-described species.

The annotation of such sequences remains an open question. Manual annotation is not applicable, and no good automated approach has been validated yet. A relevant annotation of these massive datasets will require the integration of genomic and expression data with existing standardized description charts, as offered by IMGT®. A standardized annotation is an important issue since it facilitates the re-utilization of datasets and comparison of analyses. Thus, the description of IG and TR polymorphisms, the integration of repertoire studies with structural features of antigen-specific domains, and even the usage of new genes in genetic engineering rely on a common standard for nomenclature, numbering, and annotation (147).

To take advantage of the current standards that have been established from classical sequencing data during the last 25 years, new, fast, reliable, and human-supervised annotation methods will have to be developed, integrating directly high-throughput sequence information from the increasing number of deep sequencing platforms and technologies, at different genetic levels (genome, transcriptome, clonotype repertoires). Along this line, IMGT/HighV-QUEST offers online tools to the scientific community for the analysis of long IG and TR sequences from NGS (148).

Special attention can be paid to the orthology/paralogy relationships between similar antigen receptor genes from different species. These characteristics are essential to understand the dynamics of IG and TR loci. In fact, with many important lymphocyte subsets characterized by canonical/invariant antigen receptors, such relationships are critical to transfer functional knowledge between models. Importantly, the phylogenetic analyses required to reconstitute the evolution of antigen receptor genes are based on multiple alignments, the quality of which is highly dependent on common numbering and precise annotation of sequences.

As far as immune repertoires are characterized by the diversity of receptors specifically binding antigen/pathogen motifs to initiate a defense response, they might not be limited to lymphocyte diversifying receptors, e.g., IG, TR, and VLR. The particularity of these systems is a somatic diversification combined to a clonal structure of the repertoire, each lymphocyte clone expressing the product of a recombination/hypermutation and/or conversion process. However, many other arrays of diverse receptors binding or sensing pathogens have been discovered in metazoans, in invertebrates as well as in vertebrates.

In some cases, their diversity is really "innate," i.e., encoded in the genome as multiple genes produced by duplications. Fish NLR, finTRIMs, and NITR, primate KIR, chicken CHIR, or TLR in sea urchin, constitute good examples of such situations. While these repertoires may appear as relatively limited, polymorphism within populations, and differential expression of receptors per cell upon stimulation represent complex issues, which fall well into "traditional" repertoire approaches.

In other cases, receptors are subject to diversification processes much faster than gene duplication, which does not comply with a clonal selection pattern. The best examples are probably the DSCAM in arthropods, which hugely diversify by alternative splicing of exons encoding half-IgSF domains (149, 150), and the FREP lectins in mollusks, of which sequences are highly variable at the population level, and even between parents and offspring produced by auto-fecundation (151).

The number of such "innate" repertoires which are not expressed by clonally selected lymphocytes will likely increase with deep sequencing of new genomes/transcriptomes, as illustrated by a recent report from mussel (152). A good example of the importance of a proper structural description of key domains of receptors is provided by the extensive analysis of LRR motifs in studies on TLR evolution (153, 154). Further insights into the functions of such diverse proteins will be provided by the characterization of their expressed (available) repertoire, at different levels such as single-cells, cell populations, and animal populations.

Such analyses will require precise identification of genes and sequences as well as mutations, and a standardized approach of nomenclature and structural description will be as useful as it is for the vertebrate IG and TR sequences. Importantly, these receptors are made of a small number of structural units, such as IgSF domain or LRR domains, which suggests that standardized system(s) for sequence annotation could be developed following IMGT standards (155).

STATISTICAL ANALYSIS AND MODELING OF IMMUNE REPERTOIRE DATA

STATISTICAL REPERTOIRE ANALYSIS

The description of the repertoire modifications using flow cytometry or Immunoscope provided clear-cut and detailed insight into the clonal expansion processes during the responses against a defined antigen (64, 66). However, it is difficult to identify the relevant alterations of the repertoires in more complex situations such as pathogen infections or variable genetic backgrounds. For example, it appeared impossible to identify all significant modifications of TRB Immunoscope profiles during cerebral malaria by direct ocular comparison (107). Different methods were therefore developed to extract from IG and TR repertoire descriptions the relevant information, to encode it as numerical tables and to analyze them with statistical models.

CDR3 spectratype perturbation indices

Since the initial description of the CDR3 spectratyping technique, different scoring indices were developed or derived from the literature: "relative index of stimulation" (RIS) (55), "overall complexity score" (156), Reperturb (157), "complexity scoring system" (158), COPOM (159), Oligoscore (160), TcLandscape (161), "spectratype diversity scoring system" (162), Morisita-Horn index and Jaccard index (95–97), "absolute perturbance value" (163). A comparative review of such scoring strategies was published by Miqueu et al. (164).

In particular, the perturbation index Reperturb was developed by Gorochov et al. to perform TR repertoire analysis in HIV patient during progression to AIDS and under antiretroviral therapy. They could show drastic restrictions in the $CD8^+$ T cell repertoire at all stages of natural progression that persisted during the first 6 months of treatment. In contrast, $CD4^+$ T cell repertoire perturbations correlated with progression to AIDS with a return to a diversified repertoire in good responders to treatment (157).

Soulillou et al. refined this approach by combining the qualitative information obtained with usual CDR3 spectratyping with quantitative information of TRBV usage obtained by real-time quantitative PCR. They devised a four-dimension representation that represents TRBV subgroups, CDR3-length and percentage of TRBV use on three axis chart in addition to a color-coded representation of the CDR3 profile perturbation. Using this original approach, they were able to show that graft rejection is associated with a vigorous polyclonal accumulation of TRBV mRNA among graft-infiltrating T lymphocytes, whereas in tolerated grafts T cell repertoire is strongly altered (161, 165). Their study puts the emphasis on the importance of not only qualitative but also quantitative analysis of lymphocyte repertoires.

Platforms for repertoire data management and statistical analysis

Several platforms have been developed and rely mostly on CDR3 spectratyping and sequencing data, with recent developments to manage and analyze NGS data.

The ISEApeaks strategy and software were developed in order to satisfy the needs for efficient automated electrophoresis data retrieval and management (160, 166). ISEApeaks extracts peak area and length data generated by software used to determine fragment intensity and size. CDR3 spectratype raw data, consisting of peak areas and nucleotide lengths for each V-(D)-J-C combination, is extracted, smoothed, managed, and analyzed. The repertoires of different samples are gathered in a peak database and CDR3 spectratypes can be analyzed by different perturbation indices and multivariate statistical methods implemented in ISEApeaks. We have applied our ISEApeaks strategy in several studies. In an experimental model of cerebral malaria, we established a correlation between the quality of TR repertoire alterations and the clinical status of infected mice, whether they developed cerebral malaria or not (107). We contributed to the characterization of the membrane-associated *Leishmania* antigens (MLA) that stimulates a large fraction of naive CD4 lymphocytes. Repertoire analyses showed that MLA-induced T cell expansions used TR with various TRBV rearrangements and CDR3 lengths, a feature closer to that of polyclonal activators than of a classic antigen (167). We also revealed repertoire age-related perturbations in mice (7). ISEApeaks functions for statistical analysis was successfully applied to analyze the TR repertoire in fish as shown by our detailed analysis of the TRB repertoire of rainbow trout IELs, performed in both naive and virus-infected animals. Rainbow trout IEL TRBV transcripts were highly diverse and polyclonal in adult naive individuals, in sharp contrast with the restricted diversity of IEL oligoclonal repertoires described in birds and mammals (102). More recently, our study of the $CD8^+$ and $CD8^-$ αβ T cell repertoire suggests different regulatory patterns of those T cell patterns in fish and in mammals (168). ISEApeaks was also used to implement a new statistically based strategy for quantification of repertoire diversity (159).

Kepler et al. described another original statistical approach for CDR3 spectratype analysis, using complex procedures for testing hypotheses regarding differences in antigen receptor distribution and variable repertoire diversity in different treatment groups. This approach is based on the derivation of probability distributions directly from spectratype data instead of using *ad hoc* measures of spectratype differences (169). A software (called SpA) implementing this method has been developed and made available online (170). This approach has been used in a longitudinal analysis of TRBV repertoire during acute GvHD after stem cell transplantation (171).

Another group (163) reported the development of a new software platform, REPERTOIRE, which allows handling of CDR3 spectratyping data. This software implements a perturbation index based upon an expected normal Gaussian distribution of CDR3 length profiles.

Owing to the complexity and diversity of the immune system, immunogenetics represents one of the greatest challenges for data interpretation: a large biological expertise, a considerable effort of standardization, and the elaboration of an efficient system for the management of the related knowledge were required. To answer that challenge, IMGT®, the international ImMunoGeneTics information system®(http://www.imgt.org), was created in 1989 by one of the authors (146). Overtime, it developed standards that, since 1995, have been endorsed by the World Health Organization-International Union of Immunological Societies (WHO-IUIS) Nomenclature Committee and by the WHO-International Nonproprietary Names (INN) (172–175). IMGT® comprises seven databases (sequence, gene, and structure databases), 17 online tools and more than 15,000 pages of web resources. Among the databases, IMGT/LIGM-DB, the database for nucleotide sequences (170,685 sequences from 335 species as of July 2013) and IMGT/GENE-DB, the gene database (3,081 genes and 4,687 alleles) are of great interest for repertoire analysis. Freely available since 1997, IMGT/V-QUEST is an integrated system for the standardized analysis of collections of IG and TR rearranged nucleotide sequences (176, 177). A high-throughput version, IMGT/HighV-QUEST (148), has been released in 2010 for the analysis of long IG and TR sequences from NGS using the 454 Life Sciences technology. In the same line, other analysis tools are becoming available showing the renewed interest for repertoire analyses and modeling consecutive to NGS technology developments (178–181).

Altogether, these efforts highlight the relevance of developing more efficient and powerful technologies for the evaluation of repertoire diversity. Notably, two successful French biotech companies (TcLand, Nantes; ImmunID, Grenoble) were created in the field of repertoire analysis, using different technologies. In collaboration with ImmunID, we have proposed a novel strategy for statistical modeling of T lymphocyte repertoire data obtained in humans and humanized mice. With this model, we revealed that half of the human TRB repertoire, in terms of proportion of TRBV-TRBJ combinations, is genetically determined, the other half occurring stochastically (182). In addition, the biotechnology company "Adaptive" and the "Repertoire 10K (R10K) Project" have been recently founded by researchers respectively from the Fred Hutchinson Cancer Research Center (Seattle and Washington) and the HudsonAlpha Institute (Huntsville). Both have developed platforms (immunoSEQ®, iRepertoire®) providing researchers with a global analysis of the T or B cell receptor sequence repertoires (183). However, despite the power of this technology, studies are still limited by the ability to process the complexity of the information provided. Specific software developments for the automatic treatment and annotation of IG and TR sequences and the statistical modeling of repertoire diversity can still be improved.

Multivariate analysis

As mentioned above, the PANAMA-Blot technique also includes statistical analysis of the data. Multi-parametric analysis was introduced to compare the global reactivity of antibodies of different individuals in different groups with a given antigenic extract. This analysis has been successfully implemented to identify reactivity patterns specific for a given pathology or clinical status (10–12, 14, 15, 184). Similarly, multi-parametric analysis was also applied to TRBV spectratype analysis in an experimental cerebral malaria model (107).

Hierarchical clustering or classification algorithms have become very popular with the growing of micro-array-based transcriptome analysis. Although still uncommon for immune repertoire analysis, such approaches have been employed to categorize large sets of repertoire data without *a priori* (17, 102, 107).

Diversity indices

The concept of immune repertoire has been devised to describe the diversity of cells involved in the immune system of an individual (1). As described above, different scoring systems were developed to assess this diversity, some are heuristics but others have been borrowed from theoretical ecology and evolution. As reviewed by Magurran (185), the Shannon entropy, introduced by Claude Shannon in 1948 for the information theory, is the most used because it not only integrates the number of different species but also the relative proportion of each of these species. In 1961, Alfred Rényi generalized this entropy to a family of functions, like Species Richness, Simpson, Quadratic, and Berger–Parker indices, for quantifying the diversity, the uncertainty or randomness of a system. Most of these indices are implemented in the free software application Estimates (http://purl.oclc.org/estimates) (186). Altogether, these diversity indices constitute a collection of tools with their own sensitivity to the variety and the relative abundances of the species that are perfectly suitable for assessing immune repertoire diversity. Indeed, the very famous index of variability proposed by Kabat and Wu (187) corresponds to the ratio of Species Richness and Berger–Parker indices. In 1990, Jores et al. showed that the resolving power of this Wu-Kabat variability coefficient can be enhanced by increasing the weight on the frequency distribution of the amino acids in the formula (188). This approach inspired Stewart et al. (189) to use the Shannon entropy to demonstrate that TR amino acid composition is significantly more diverse than that of IG. In the same way, CDR3 spectratyping data can be analyzed using the relative abundance of each peak within CDR3 length global distribution. By doing so, we adjusted the original Shannon entropy, making it reaching its maximum for a Gaussian distribution, to compare the CDR3 length diversity of splenic IgM, IgD, and IgT in infected Teleost Fish (131). Recently, the Gini index, used in ecology or economics to measure the equality of distributions, was applied to individual TR clones and compared naive and memory repertoires (190). The development of deep sequencing techniques ignited a renewed interest in IG/TR repertoire. Indeed, several studies used high-throughput analysis to describe TR repertoire of key T cell subsets in human peripheral blood (115, 126, 191). This approach assessing the repertoire diversity from the relative abundance of each species in the global distribution can be decomposed hierarchically into components attributable, respectively, to variations in TRBV-TRBJ combinations and in CDR3-length (113, 117). However, most of these studies have been limited to the counting of the observed unique clonotypes. Beside the species richness, ecology-derived indices have also been applied to assess and compare immune repertoire diversity. Föhse et al. (119) used the Morisita-Horn similarity index to compare regulatory T cell repertoires between several lymphoid organs. In addition, Simpson diversity index, associated with Shannon entropy, was used to monitor TR repertoire diversity of HIV-specific CD8 T cells during antiretroviral therapy (192) but also to quantify TR repertoire recovery in the blood after allogeneic hematopoietic stem cell transplantation (128). In the same manner, Koning et al. (193) used Shannon's and Simpson's indices to show the role for the peptide component of the peptide-MH1 complex on the molecular frontline of $CD8^+$ T cell–mediated immune surveillance, by comparing the repertoire diversity of $CD8^+$ T cell populations directed against a variety of epitopes. In parallel, using Simpson's index as a metric allowed Johnson et al. (194) to model mathematically the naïve CD4 T cell repertoire contraction with age leading them to conclude that diversity plummet observed around the age of 70 could be correlated to cell-intrinsic mutations affecting cell division rate or death.

MODELING STRATEGIES

Modeling approaches have a strong tradition in immunology, usually at the boundary with other disciplines such as physics (195). Before deep sequencing data was available, general design principles were proposed as desirable features of immune repertoires, with implications for the observed repertoire diversity and dynamics (196–198). Many efforts have involved the modeling of immune cell dynamics and the effects of antigens on repertoire diversity, using differential equations descriptions of the population dynamics (199–201). Recognition in the immune system is often studied both theoretically and experimentally by probing the dynamics of cells with a specific type of receptor with respect to infections (202). Alternatively one can look at the response of a small set of chosen receptors to a specific pathogenic challenge, or careful biochemical investigation of particular receptor/antigen pairs (203, 204). Much work has been devoted to systems-biology approaches to signal processing in immune cells, as reviewed in Germain et al. (205) and Emonet and Altan-Bonnet (206). Here we focus on approaches inspired by recent advances in sequencing technologies (112, 113, 115, 116, 125, 191, 207, 208) that have opened the way for data-driven modeling of the immune repertoires and interactions between receptors and antigen.

A common modeling approach for describing receptors at the amino acid level is to choose a relevant interaction parameter (e.g., chemical affinity or hydrophobicity) and assign it a simplified digit-string representation (209). These methods are extensions of the string model, which describes both receptor and epitopes as strings of length L, with values chosen from natural numbers, and quantify their interaction by the match between the two strings (197, 210, 211). Such quantitative, physically inspired descriptions of immune receptors, despite the arbitrary choice of interaction coordinates, have proven a valuable first step in statistically describing recognition in T cells (195, 212–215). Recently, lower hydrophilicity of regulatory vs. conventional T cells was suggested from CDR3 sequencing (216).

High-throughput sequencing of immune receptors raises specific challenges compared to traditional genomic sequencing. It is harder to distinguish sequencing errors from new polymorphisms, since no corresponding pre-existing sequence exists. One of the most interesting regions when studying diversity is the CDR3 with its many insertions and deletions added to the germline sequence. These regions are often hard to align to the genomic templates, or with each other (217). Therefore, extra care is needed when generating and analyzing sequence data. Not all sequencing technologies are equally good for all purposes (218): while 454 sequencing gives longer reads than Illumina it is known to have a greater probability of frameshift errors. In addition, primer-dependent PCR amplification biases require that raw sequence counts be normalized using control experiments (112) in order to accurately report clone sizes, as demonstrated by spike-in experiments (219). In TR repertoire studies, this is circumvented by using 5′RACE which provides an unbiased amplification of fully rearranged sequences, as recently demonstrated for TRB V-(D)-J transcripts (191).

Despite sequencing issues, statistical algorithms are often able to extract information from the data. Many studies of diversity focus on the V, D, and J gene usage of each rearranged sequence. Algorithms and tools have been developed to rapidly identify the V, D, and J genes for massive numbers of sequences (148, 178, 181). In many cases however, the assignment of a D gene to each sequence read is unreliable if the D region is too short owing to extensive trimming. Mora et al. (217) learned from data and analyzed statistical models of the D gene flanked by its junctions. These models are based on the principle of maximum entropy and make minimal assumptions about the mechanisms of diversity – they only rely on the observed frequencies of amino acid pairs along the sequence. These models were used to describe global features of the sequence ensemble, such as the probability distribution following Zipf's law (220) – the observation that the probability of sequences is inversely proportional to their frequency-rank, or the observation of peaks of frequency in sequence landscape as possible signatures of past pathogenic challenges. Recently, the estimation of repertoire diversity and clonal size distribution were analyzed by Poisson abundance models (221) and simple bivariate-Poisson-lognormal (BPLN) parametric model for fitting and analyzing TR repertoire data was proposed (222). Similarly, network analysis of IG repertoire from Weinstein et al. study revealed the possibility to identify subgroups of individuals on the basis of IG network similarity (223).

The task of characterizing the CDR3 at the nucleotide level is made difficult by the fact that a deterministic assignment of the V-(D)-J recombination process is impossible, because any given sequence can be generated by many possible recombination processes. A previous study proposed a probabilistic model of nucleotide trimming of rearranged TR genes derived from a benchmark data set of TRA and TRG V-(D)-J junctions obtained by comparison to the germline genes in the IMGT® tools (224). Recently a statistical method based on the expectation-maximization algorithm was proposed to circumvent this issue and to extract the statistical properties of junctional diversity accurately from data (124). Applying it to human non-productive DNA sequences gave insight into a universal generation mechanism, reproducible from individual to individual. It was shown that each sequence could potentially be generated by the equivalent of $\sim$30 equally likely ways by convergent recombination. This method showed that the potential diversity of the recombination machinery was equivalent to $\sim 10^{14}$ *equally likely* sequences (and a practically infinite total number of possible sequences), much more than the estimated 10^{12} T cells that a single human body can hold. The frequencies of the V, D, and J genes is non-uniform, even at the level of recombination, suggesting underlying physical mechanisms at work. Ndifon et al. (125) proposed a polymer model that accounts for the likelihood of connecting given genomic fragments, giving insight into the mechanistic process.

One of the ultimate goals of deep repertoire sequencing is to find signatures of the repertoire's response to its antigenic environment. A combination of clustering methods and tree reconstruction techniques have been developed (225, 226) to identify lineages in B cells and study the response to pathogenic challenges. Statistical methods have been devised to detect and quantify the extent of antigen-driven selection acting on B cells, by analyzing the patterns of hypermutations in a Bayesian framework, with applications to deep sequencing data (227, 228).

A lot remains to be done in terms of both data-driven and small-scale models of repertoire-antigen interactions. Ultimately, a close collaboration and development of experimental techniques and models can shed light on how selection at different stages shapes the repertoire, how affinity maturation changes the diversity and the link between sequence diversity and function.

FUTURE PROSPECTS OF BIOMATHEMATICAL ANALYSIS OF REPERTOIRE DATA

One of the current challenging issues in antigen-specific repertoire analysis is the development of relevant statistical analysis strategies. Biologists are usually keen on parametric tests, such as ANOVA, *t*-test, Fischer's test, among others. However, such statistical methods assume that the inherent probability distribution of the observed variable follows a normal distribution. Rock et al. (229) described that the distribution of the TR diversity is far from following this distribution, thus they proposed the use of non-parametric tests. Nevertheless, different groups are dealing with this issue in order to determine the relevant way to analyze repertoire diversity data and to propose new biostatistics strategies, including principal component analysis, discriminant analysis, hierarchical clustering, specific statistics (164, 169).

In fact, the traditional use of statistics in biology aims at the falsification of a defined hypothesis, i.e., at validating significant differences between defined situations. The recent development of "systems immunology" reverses this point of view and establishes a new usage of multi-parametric statistical approaches to represent the biological data by projections and "landscapes" in the N-dimensional space of considered parameters (230). Thus, the traditional description of separate repertoires for distinct cell subsets defined from a few markers is being replaced by overlapping clouds of data, setting the limits of the different classification groups (tissue of origin, infection contexts, combination of marker expression, repertoire expression...). Moreover, repertoire diversity technologies can now be combined to complementary approaches to decipher the complexity of lymphocyte populations, such as microwell array cell culture and high-resolution imaging (231), mass cytometry (232, 233), cellular barcoding (234), intravital imaging (235, 236), single-cell gene expression (237). In addition, high-throughput repertoire descriptions will enrich mathematical and computer models of lymphocyte repertoire diversity and dynamics such as those proposed by Mehr (238), Ciupe et al. (239), or Stirk et al. (240).

As advocated by others, the concepts developed by systems biology, such as the signatures emerging from clustering and the modularity regulating gene networks, will probably need to be adapted to the constraints of immunology data (241). However, this is probably through this kind of representation that global analysis of immune repertoires will have to be addressed (242).

The upcoming challenge is now to merge data produced through the different technological approaches available to achieve full integration of these data and make them available for interactive meta-analysis. This necessitates more than the simple juxtaposition of annotated raw data but rather requires (1) the codification and standardization of this multi-level data and (2) the integration of complexity science into immunology. Along this line, recent developments of multi-parametric flow cytometry naturally led to systematic clustering and multivariate statistical analysis approaches for searching functional signatures (2, 232, 233, 243–245).

ACKNOWLEDGMENTS

This work was supported by French state funds within the Investissements d'Avenir program (ANR-11-IDEX-0004-02; LabEx Transimmunom), the European Research Council Advanced grant (TRiPoD), the European PCRDT7 (Lifecycle program), the RNSC (ImmunoComplexiT network), CNRS (PEPS BMI), INRA and Université Pierre and Marie Curie.

REFERENCES

1. Boudinot P, Marriotti-Ferrandiz ME, Du Pasquier L, Benmansour A, Cazenave PA, Six A. New perspectives for large-scale repertoire analysis of immune receptors. *Mol Immunol* (2008) **45**:2437–45. doi:10.1016/j.molimm.2007.12.018
2. Bendall SC, Nolan GP, Roederer M, Chattopadhyay PK. A deep profiler's guide to cytometry. *Trends Immunol* (2012) **33**:323–32. doi:10.1016/j.it.2012.02.010
3. MacDonald HR, Pedrazzini T, Schneider R, Louis JA, Zinkernagel RM, Hengartner H. Intrathymic elimination of Mls^a-reactive (Vβ6$^+$) cells during neonatal tolerance induction to Mls^a-encoded antigens. *J Exp Med* (1988) **167**:2005–10. doi:10.1084/jem.167.6.2005
4. MacDonald HR, Schneider R, Lees RK, Howe RC, Acha-Orbea H, Festenstein H, et al. T-cell receptor Vβ use predicts reactivity tolerance to Mls^a-encoded antigens. *Nature* (1988) **332**:40–5. doi:10.1038/332040a0
5. Salaun J, Bandeira A, Khazaal I, Burlen-Defranoux O, Thomas-Vaslin V, Coltey M, et al. Transplantation tolerance is unrelated to superantigen-dependent deletion and anergy. *Proc Natl Acad Sci U S A* (1992) **89**:10420–4. doi:10.1073/pnas.89.21.10420
6. Faint JM, Pilling D, Akbar AN, Kitas GD, Bacon PA, Salmon M. Quantitative flow cytometry for the analysis of T cell receptor Vβ chain expression. *J Immunol Methods* (1999) **225**:53–60. doi:10.1016/S0022-1759(99)00027-7
7. Thomas-Vaslin V, Six A, Pham HP, Dansokho C, Chaara W, Gouritin B, et al. Immunodepression & Immunosuppression during aging. In: Portela MB editor. *Immunosuppression*. Rijeka: InTech open access publisher (2012). p. 125–463.
8. Lefranc MP, Lefranc G. *The Immunoglobulin FactsBook*. London: Academic Press (2001).
9. Lefranc MP, Lefranc G. *The T Cell Receptor FactsBook*. London: Academic Press (2001).
10. Nobrega A, Haury M, Grandien A, Malanchere E, Sundblad A, Coutinho A. Global analysis of antibody repertoires. II. Evidence for specificity, self-selection and the immunological "homunculus" of antibodies in normal serum. *Eur J Immunol* (1993) **23**:2851–9. doi:10.1002/eji.1830231119
11. Haury M, Grandien A, Sundblad A, Coutinho A, Nobrega A. Global analysis of antibody repertoires. 1. An immunoblot method for the quantitative screening of a large number of reactivities. *Scand J Immunol* (1994) **39**:79–87.
12. Fesel C, Coutinho A. Serum IgM repertoire reactions to MBP/CFA immunization reflect the individual status of EAE susceptibility. *J Autoimmun* (2000) **14**:319–24. doi:10.1006/jaut.2000.0373
13. Haury M, Sundblad A, Grandien A, Barreau C, Coutinho A, Nobrega A. The repertoire of serum IgM in normal mice is largely independent of external antigenic contact. *Eur J Immunol* (1997) **27**:1557–63. doi:10.1002/eji.1830270635
14. Stahl D, Lacroix-Desmazes S, Heudes D, Mouthon L, Kaveri SV, Kazatchkine MD. Altered control of self-reactive IgG by autologous IgM in patients with warm autoimmune hemolytic anemia. *Blood* (2000) **95**:328–35.
15. Stahl D, Lacroix-Desmazes S, Mouthon L, Kaveri SV, Kazatchkine MD. Analysis of human self-reactive antibody repertoires by quantitative immunoblotting. *J Immunol Methods* (2000) **240**:1–14. doi:10.1016/S0022-1759(00)00185-X
16. Costa N, Pires AE, Gabriel AM, Goulart LF, Pereira C, Leal B, et al. Broadened T-cell repertoire diversity in ivIg-treated SLE patients is also related to the individual status of regulatory T-cells. *J Clin Immunol* (2013) **33**:349–60. doi:10.1007/s10875-012-9816-7
17. Quintana FJ, Hagedorn PH, Elizur G, Merbl Y, Domany E, Cohen IR. Functional immunomics: microarray analysis of IgG autoantibody repertoires predicts the future response of mice to induced diabetes. *Proc Natl Acad Sci U S A* (2004) **101**:14615–21. doi:10.1073/pnas.0404848101
18. Quintana FJ, Getz G, Hed G, Domany E, Cohen IR. Cluster analysis of human autoantibody reactivities in health and in type 1 diabetes mellitus: a bio-informatic approach to immune complexity. *J Autoimmun* (2003) **21**:65–75. doi:10.1016/S0896-8411(03)00064-7
19. Delassus S, Darche S, Kourilsky P, Cumano A. Ontogeny of the heavy chain immunoglobulin repertoire in fetal liver and bone marrow. *J Immunol* (1998) **160**:3274–80.
20. Yassai M, Gorski J. Thymocyte maturation: selection for in-frame TCRα-chain rearrangement is followed by selection for shorter TCRβ-chain complementarity-determining region 3. *J Immunol* (2000) **165**:3706–12.
21. Pasqual N, Gallagher M, Aude-Garcia C, Loiodice M, Thuderoz F, Demongeot J, et al. Quantitative and qualitative changes in V-Jα rearrangements during mouse thymocytes differentiation: implication for a limited T cell receptor α chain repertoire. *J Exp Med* (2002) **196**:1163–73. doi:10.1084/jem.20021074
22. Douek DC, McFarland RD, Keiser PH, Gage EA, Massey JM, Haynes BF, et al. Changes in thymic function with age and during the treatment of HIV infection. *Nature* (1998) **396**:690–5. doi:10.1038/25374
23. Ribeiro RM, Perelson AS. Determining thymic output quantitatively: using models to interpret experimental T-cell receptor excision circle (TREC) data. *Immunol Rev* (2007) **216**:21–34.
24. Bains I, Thiebaut R, Yates AJ, Callard R. Quantifying thymic export: combining models of naive T cell proliferation and TCR excision circle dynamics gives an explicit measure of thymic output. *J Immunol* (2009) **183**:4329–36. doi:10.4049/jimmunol.0900743
25. Poulin JF, Viswanathan MN, Harris JM, Komanduri KV, Wieder E, Ringuette N, et al. Direct evidence for thymic function in adult humans. *J Exp Med* (1999) **190**:479–86. doi:10.1084/jem.190.4.479
26. Dulude G, Cheynier R, Gauchat D, Abdallah A, Kettaf N, Sékaly RP, et al. The magnitude of thymic output is genetically determined through controlled intrathymic precursor T cell proliferation. *J Immunol* (2008) **181**:7818–24.
27. Wu GE, Paige CJ. VH gene family utilization in colonies derived from B and pre-B cells detected by the RNA colony blot assay. *EMBO J* (1986) **5**:3475–81.
28. Schulze DH, Kelsoe G. Genotypic analysis of B cell colonies by in situ hybridization. Stoichiometric expression of three VH families in adult C57BL/6 and BALB/c mice. *J Exp Med* (1987) **166**:163–72. doi:10.1084/jem.166.1.163
29. Thomas-Vaslin V, Andrade L, Freitas A, Coutinho A. Clonal persistence of B lymphocytes in normal mice is determined by variable region-dependent selection. *Eur J Immunol* (1991) **21**:2239–46. doi:10.1002/eji.1830210935
30. Andrade L, Huetz F, Poncet P, Thomas-Vaslin V, Goodhardt M, Coutinho A. Biased VH gene expression in murine CD5 B cells results from age-dependent cellular selection. *Eur J Immunol* (1991) **21**:2017–23. doi:10.1002/eji.1830210908
31. Freitas AA, Lembezat MP, Coutinho A. Expression of antibody V-regions is genetically and developmentally controlled and modulated by the B lymphocyte environment. *Int Immunol* (1989) **1**:342–54. doi:10.1093/intimm/1.4.342
32. Rosenberg WMC, Moss PAH, Bell JI. Variation in human T cell receptor Vβ and Jβ repertoire: analysis using anchored polymerase reaction. *Eur J Immunol* (1992) **22**:541–9. doi:10.1002/eji.1830220237
33. Moss PAH, Rosenberg WMC, Zintzaras E, Bell JI. Characterization of the human T cell receptor α-chain repertoire and demonstration of α genetic influence on the Vα usage. *Eur J Immunol* (1993) **23**:1155–9. doi:10.1002/eji.1830230526

34. Moss PAH, Bell JI. Sequence analysis of the human αβ T-cell receptor CDR3 region. *Immunogenetics* (1995) **42**:10–8. doi:10.1007/BF00164982
35. Moss PA, Bell JI. Comparative sequence analysis of the human T cell receptor TCRA and TCRB CDR3 regions. *Hum Immunol* (1996) **48**:32–8. doi:10.1016/0198-8859(96)00084-5
36. Pannetier C, Delassus S, Darche S, Saucier C, Kourilsky P. Quantitative titration of nucleic acids by enzymatic amplification reactions run to saturation. *Nucleic Acids Res* (1993) **21**:577–83. doi:10.1093/nar/21.3.577
37. Manfras BJ, Rudert WA, Trucco M, Boehm O. Analysis of the αβ T-cell receptor repertoire by competitive and quantitative family-specific PCR with exogenous standards and high resolution fluorescence based CDR3 size imaging. *J Immunol Methods* (1997) **210**:235–49. doi:10.1016/S0022-1759(97)00197-X
38. VanderBorght A, Van der Aa A, Geusens P, Vandevyver C, Raus J, Stinissen P. Identification of overrepresented T cell receptor genes in blood and tissue biopsies by PCR-ELISA. *J Immunol Methods* (1999) **223**:47–61. doi:10.1016/S0022-1759(98)00201-4
39. Lim A, Baron V, Ferradini L, Bonneville M, Kourilsky P, Pannetier C. Combination of MHC-peptide multimer-based T cell sorting with the Immunoscope permits sensitive ex vivo quantitation and follow-up of human CD8+ T cell immune responses. *J Immunol Methods* (2002) **261**:177–94. doi:10.1016/S0022-1759(02)00004-2
40. Casrouge A, Beaudoing E, Dalle S, Pannetier C, Kanellopoulos J, Kourilsky P. Size estimate of the αβ TCR repertoire of naive mouse splenocytes. *J Immunol* (2000) **164**:5782–7.
41. Gallard A, Foucras G, Coureau C, Guery JC. Tracking T cell clonotypes in complex T lymphocyte populations by real-time quantitative PCR using fluorogenic complementarity-determining region-3-specific probes. *J Immunol Methods* (2002) **270**:269–80. doi:10.1016/S0022-1759(02)00336-8
42. Liu DB, Callahan JP, Dau PC. Intrafamily fragment analysis of the T cell receptor β chain CDR3 region. *J Immunol Methods* (1995) **187**:139–50. doi:10.1016/0022-1759(95)00178-D
43. Mugnaini EN, Egeland T, Syversen AM, Spurkland A, Brinchmann JE. Molecular analysis of the complementarity determining region 3 of the human T cell receptor β chain. Establishment of a reference panel of CDR3 lengths from phytohaemagglutinin activated lymphocytes. *J Immunol Methods* (1999) **223**:207–16. doi:10.1016/S0022-1759(99)00004-6
44. Matsutani T, Yoshioka T, Tsuruta Y, Iwagami S, Suzuki R. Analysis of TCRAV and TCRBV repertoires in healthy individuals by microplate hybridization assay. *Hum Immunol* (1997) **56**:57–69. doi:10.1016/S0198-8859(97)00102-X
45. Matsutani T, Yoshioka T, Tsuruta Y, Iwagami S, Toyosaki-Maeda T, Horiuchi T, et al. Restricted usage of T-cell receptor α-chain variable region (TCRAV) and T-cell receptor β-chain variable region (TCRBV) repertoires after human allogeneic haematopoietic transplantation. *Br J Haematol* (2000) **109**:759–69. doi:10.1046/j.1365-2141.2000.02080.x
46. Yoshida R, Yoshioka T, Yamane S, Matsutani T, Toyosaki-Maeda T, Tsuruta Y, et al. A new method for quantitative analysis of the mouse T-cell receptor V region repertoires: comparison of repertoires among strains. *Immunogenetics* (2000) **52**:35–45. doi:10.1007/s002510000248
47. Du G, Qiu L, Shen L, Sehgal P, Shen Y, Huang D, et al. Combined megaplex TCR isolation and SMART-based real-time quantitation methods for quantitating antigen-specific T cell clones in mycobacterial infection. *J Immunol Methods* (2006) **308**:19–35. doi:10.1016/j.jim.2005.09.009
48. Ogle BM, Cascalho M, Joao C, Taylor W, West LJ, Platt JL. Direct measurement of lymphocyte receptor diversity. *Nucleic Acids Res* (2003) **31**:e139. doi:10.1093/nar/gng139
49. Joao C, Ogle BM, Gay-Rabinstein C, Platt JL, Cascalho M. B cell-dependent TCR diversification. *J Immunol* (2004) **172**:4709–16.
50. Joao C. Immunoglobulin is a highly diverse self-molecule that improves cellular diversity and function during immune reconstitution. *Med Hypotheses* (2007) **68**:158–61. doi:10.1016/j.mehy.2006.05.062
51. Bonarius HP, Baas F, Remmerswaal EB, van Lier RA, ten Berge I, Tak PP, et al. Monitoring the T-cell receptor repertoire at single-clone resolution. *PLoS One* (2006) **1**:e55. doi:10.1371/journal.pone.0000055
52. Pannetier C, Cochet M, Darche S, Casrouge A, Zöller M, Kourilsky P. The size of the CDR3 hypervariable regions of the murine T-cell receptor β chains vary as a function of the recombined germ-line segments. *Proc Natl Acad Sci U S A* (1993) **90**:4319–23. doi:10.1073/pnas.90.9.4319
53. Pannetier C, Even J, Kourilsky P. T-cell repertoire diversity and clonal expansions in normal and clinical samples. *Immunol Today* (1995) **16**:176–81. doi:10.1016/0167-5699(95)80117-0
54. Pannetier C, Levraud JP, Lim A, Even J, Kourilsky P. The immunoscope approach for the analysis of T-cell repertoires. In: Oksenberg J editor. *The Human Antigen T Cell Receptor. Selected Protocols and Applications.* Georgetown, TX: Landes RG (1997). p. 287–325.
55. Cochet M, Pannetier C, Darche S, Leclerc C, Kourilsky P. Molecular detection and *in vivo* analysis of the specific T cell response to a protein antigen. *Eur J Immunol* (1992) **22**:2639–47. doi:10.1002/eji.1830221025
56. Regnault A, Cumano A, Vassalli P, Guy-Grand D, Kourilsky P. Oligoclonal repertoire of the CD8αα and the CD8αβ TCR-α/β murine intestinal intraepithelial T lymphocytes: evidence for the random emergence of T cells. *J Exp Med* (1994) **180**:1345–58. doi:10.1084/jem.180.4.1345
57. Regnault A, Levraud JP, Lim A, Six A, Moreau C, Cumano A, et al. The expansion and selection of T cell receptor αβ intestinal intraepithelial T cell clones. *Eur J Immunol* (1996) **26**:914–21. doi:10.1002/eji.1830260429
58. Ema H, Cumano A, Kourilsky P. TCRβ repertoire development in the mouse embryo. *J Immunol* (1997) **159**:4227–32.
59. Arstila TP, Casrouge A, Baron V, Even J, Kanellopoulos J, Kourilsky P. A direct estimate of the human αβ T cell receptor diversity. *Science* (1999) **286**:958–61. doi:10.1126/science.286.5441.958
60. Bousso P, Lemaître F, Laouini D, Kanellopoulos J, Kourilsky P. The peripheral CD8 T cell repertoire is largely independent of the presence of intestinal flora. *Int Immunol* (2000) **12**:425–30. doi:10.1093/intimm/12.4.425
61. Arstila TP, Even J. Size of the αβ TCR repertoire. *Med Sci (Paris)* (2000) **16**:1257–60. doi:10.4267/10608/1566
62. Cabaniols JP, Fazilleau N, Casrouge A, Kourilsky P, Kanellopoulos JM. Most α/β T cell receptor diversity is due to terminal deoxynucleotidyl transferase. *J Exp Med* (2001) **194**:1385–90. doi:10.1084/jem.194.9.1385
63. Fazilleau N, Cabaniols JP, Lemaitre F, Motta I, Kourilsky P, Kanellopoulos JM. Valpha and Vbeta public repertoires are highly conserved in terminal deoxynucleotidyl transferase-deficient mice. *J Immunol* (2005) **174**:345–55.
64. Cibotti R, Cabaniols JP, Pannetier C, Delarbre C, Vergnon I, Kanellopoulos JM, et al. Public and private Vβ T cell receptor repertoires against hen egg white lysozyme (HEL) in nontransgenic versus HEL transgenic mice. *J Exp Med* (1994) **180**:861–72. doi:10.1084/jem.180.3.861
65. Gapin L, Fukui Y, Kanellopoulos J, Sano T, Casrouge A, Malier V, et al. Quantitative analysis of the T cell repertoire selected by a single peptide-major histocompatibility complex. *J Exp Med* (1998) **187**:1871–83. doi:10.1084/jem.187.11.1871
66. Bouneaud C, Kourilsky P, Bousso P. Impact of negative selection on the T cell repertoire reactive to a self-peptide: a large fraction of T cell clones escapes clonal deletion. *Immunity* (2000) **13**:829–40. doi:10.1016/S1074-7613(00)00080-7
67. Fukui Y, Oono T, Cabaniols JP, Nakao K, Hirokawa K, Inayoshi A, et al. Diversity of T cell repertoire shaped by a single peptide ligand is critically affected by its amino acid residue at a T cell receptor contact. *Proc Natl Acad Sci U S A* (2000) **97**:13760–5. doi:10.1073/pnas.250470797
68. Musette P, Bureau JF, Gachelin G, Kourilsky P, Brahic M. T lymphocyte repertoire in Theiler's virus encephalomyelitis: the nonspecific infiltration of the central nervous system of infected SJL/J mice is associated with a selective local T cell expansion. *Eur J Immunol* (1995) **25**:1589–93. doi:10.1002/eji.1830250618
69. Sourdive DJD, Murali-Krishna K, Altman JD, Zajac AJ, Whitmire JK, Pannetier C, et al. Conserved T cell receptor repertoire in primary and memory CD8 T cell responses to an acute viral infection. *J Exp Med* (1998) **188**:71–82. doi:10.1084/jem.188.1.71
70. Musette P, Bequet D, Delarbre C, Gachelin G, Kourilsky P, Dormont D. Expansion of a recurrent Vβ5.3^{+} T-cell population in newly diagnosed and untreated HLA-DR2 multiple sclerosis patients. *Proc Natl Acad Sci U S A* (1996) **93**:12461–6. doi:10.1073/pnas.93.22.12461
71. Fazilleau N, Delarasse C, Sweenie CH, Anderton SM, Fillatreau S, Lemonnier FA, et al. Persistence of autoreactive myelin oligodendrocyte glycoprotein (MOG)-specific T cell repertoires in MOG-expressing mice. *Eur J Immunol* (2006) **36**:533–43. doi:10.1002/eji.200535021
72. Musette P, Bachelez H, Flageul B, Delarbre C, Kourilsky P, Dubertret L, et al. Immune-mediated destruction of melanocytes in halo nevi is associated with

the local expansion of a limited number of T cell clones. *J Immunol* (1999) **162**:1789–94.

73. Douillard P, Pannetier C, Josien R, Menoret S, Kourilsky P, Soulillou JP, et al. Donor-specific blood transfusion-induced tolerance in adult rats with a dominant TCR-Vβ rearrangement in heart allografts. *J Immunol* (1996) **157**:1250–60.
74. Pilch H, Höhn H, Freitag K, Neukirch C, Necker A, Haddad P, et al. Improved assessment of T-cell receptor (TCR) VB repertoire in clinical specimens: combination of TCR-CDR3 spectratyping with flow cytometry-based TCR VB frequency analysis. *Clin Diagn Lab Immunol* (2002) **9**:257–66.
75. Messaoudi I, LeMaoult J, Guevara-Patino JA, Metzner BM, Nikolich-Zugich J. Age-related CD8 T cell clonal expansions constrict CD8 T cell repertoire and have the potential to impair immune defense. *J Exp Med* (2004) **200**:1347–58. doi:10.1084/jem.20040437
76. Hakim FT, Memon SA, Cepeda R, Jones EC, Chow CK, Kasten-Sportes C, et al. Age-dependent incidence, time course, and consequences of thymic renewal in adults. *J Clin Invest* (2005) **115**:930–9. doi:10.1172/JCI200522492
77. Messaoudi I, Warner J, Fischer M, Park B, Hill B, Mattison J, et al. Delay of T cell senescence by caloric restriction in aged long-lived nonhuman primates. *Proc Natl Acad Sci U S A* (2006) **103**:19448–53. doi:10.1073/pnas.0606661103
78. Boudinot P, Boubekeur S, Benmansour A. Rhabdovirus infection induces public and private T cell responses in teleost fish. *J Immunol* (2001) **167**:6202–9.
79. Boudinot P, Boubekeur S, Benmansour A. Primary structure and complementarity-determining region (CDR) 3 spectratyping of rainbow trout TCRβ transcripts identify ten Vβ families with Vβ6 displaying unusual CDR2 and differently spliced forms. *J Immunol* (2002) **169**:6244–52.
80. Boudinot P, Bernard D, Boubekeur S, Thoulouze MI, Bremont M, Benmansour A. The glycoprotein of a fish rhabdovirus profiles the virus-specific T-cell repertoire in rainbow trout. *J Gen Virol* (2004) **85**:3099–108. doi:10.1099/vir.0.80135-0
81. Desravines S, Hsu E. Measuring CDR3 length variability in individuals during ontogeny. *J Immunol Methods* (1994) **168**:219–25. doi:10.1016/0022-1759(94)90058-2
82. Gorski J, Yassai M, Zhu X, Kissella B, Keever C, Flomenberg N. Circulating T cell repertoire complexity in normal individuals and bone marrow recipients analyzed by CDR3 spectratyping. *J Immunol* (1994) **152**:5109–19.
83. Maslanka K, Piatek T, Gorski J, Yassai M. Molecular analysis of T cell repertoires – Spectratypes generated by multiplex polymerase chain reaction and evaluated by radioactivity or fluorescence. *Hum Immunol* (1995) **44**: 28–34.
84. Lue C, Mitani Y, Crew MD, George JF, Fink LM, Schichman SA. An automated method for the analysis of T-cell receptor repertoires: rapid RT-PCR fragment length analysis of the T-cell receptor β chain complementarity-determining region 3. *Am J Clin Pathol* (1999) **111**:683–90.
85. Yamamoto K, Masuko-Hongo K, Tanaka A, Kurokawa M, Hoeger T, Nishioka K, et al. Establishment and application of a novel T cell clonality analysis using single-strand conformation polymorphism of T cell receptor messenger signals. *Hum Immunol* (1996) **48**:23–31. doi:10.1016/0198-8859(96)00080-8
86. Shiokawa S, Nishimura J, Ohshima K, Uike N, Yamamoto K. Establishment of a novel B cell clonality analysis using single-strand conformation polymorphism of immunoglobulin light chain messenger signals. *Am J Pathol* (1998) **153**:1393–400. doi:10.1016/S0002-9440(10)65726-4
87. Raaphorst FM, Gokmen E, Teale JM. Analysis of clonal diversity in mouse immunoglobulin heavy chain genes selected for size of the antigen combining site. *Immunol Invest* (1998) **27**:355–65. doi:10.3109/08820139809022709
88. Sottini A, Quirós Roldan E, Albertini A, Primi D, Imberti L. Assessment of T-cell receptor beta-chain diversity by heteroduplex analysis. *Hum Immunol* (1996) **48**:12–22. doi:10.1016/0198-8859(96)00087-0
89. Wack A, Montagna D, Dellabona P, Casorati G. An improved PCR-heteroduplex method permits high-sensitivity detection of clonal expansions in complex T cell populations. *J Immunol Methods* (1996) **196**:181–92. doi:10.1016/0022-1759(96)00114-7
90. Shen DF, Doukhan L, Kalam S, Delwart E. High-resolution analysis of T-cell receptor β-chain repertoires using DNA heteroduplex tracking: generally stable, clonal $CD8^+$ expansions in all healthy young adults. *J Immunol Methods* (1998) **215**:113–21. doi:10.1016/S0022-1759(98)00066-0
91. Wedderburn LR, Maini MK, Patel A, Beverley PCL, Woo P. Molecular fingerprinting reveals non-overlapping T cell oligoclonality between an inflamed site and peripheral blood. *Int Immunol* (1999) **11**:535–43. doi:10.1093/intimm/11.4.535
92. Bouffard P, Gagnon C, Cloutier D, MacLean SJ, Souleimani A, Nallainathan D, et al. Analysis of T cell receptor β chain expression by isoelectric focusing following gene amplification and *in vitro* translation. *J Immunol Methods* (1995) **187**:9–21. doi:10.1016/0022-1759(95)00161-3
93. Sant'Angelo DB, Lucas B, Waterbury PG, Cohen B, Brabb T, Goverman J, et al. A molecular map of T cell development. *Immunity* (1998) **9**:179–86. doi:10.1016/S1074-7613(00)80600-7
94. Correia-Neves M, Waltzinger C, Mathis D, Benoist C. The shaping of the T cell repertoire. *Immunity* (2001) **14**:21–32. doi:10.1016/S1074-7613(01)00086-3
95. Hsieh CS, Liang Y, Tyznik AJ, Self SG, Liggitt D, Rudensky AY. Recognition of the peripheral self by naturally arising CD25+ CD4+ T cell receptors. *Immunity* (2004) **21**:267–77. doi:10.1016/j.immuni.2004.07.009
96. Hsieh CS, Zheng Y, Liang Y, Fontenot JD, Rudensky AY. An intersection between the self-reactive regulatory and nonregulatory T cell receptor repertoires. *Nat Immunol* (2006) **7**:401–10. doi:10.1038/ni1318
97. Pacholczyk R, Ignatowicz H, Kraj P, Ignatowicz L. Origin and T cell receptor diversity of $Foxp3^+CD4^+CD25^+$ T cells. *Immunity* (2006) **25**:249–59. doi:10.1016/j.immuni.2006.05.016
98. Pacholczyk R, Kern J, Singh N, Iwashima M, Kraj P, Ignatowicz L. Nonself-antigens are the cognate specificities of $Foxp3^+$ regulatory T cells. *Immunity* (2007) **27**:493–504. doi:10.1016/j.immuni.2007.07.019
99. Wong J, Obst R, Correia-Neves M, Losyev G, Mathis D, Benoist C. Adaptation of TCR repertoires to self-peptides in regulatory and nonregulatory $CD4^+$ T cells. *J Immunol* (2007) **178**:7032–41.
100. Kang JA, Mohindru M, Kang BS, Park SH, Kim BS. Clonal expansion of infiltrating T cells in the spinal cords of SJL/J mice infected with Theiler's virus. *J Immunol* (2000) **165**:583–90.
101. Apostolou I, Cumano A, Gachelin G, Kourilsky P. Evidence for two subgroups of $CD4^-CD8^-$ NKT cells with distinct TCRαβ repertoires and differential distribution in lymphoid tissues. *J Immunol* (2000) **165**:2481–90.
102. Bernard D, Six A, Rigottier-Gois L, Messiaen S, Chilmonczyk S, Quillet E, et al. Phenotypic and functional similarity of gut intraepithelial and systemic T cells in a teleost fish. *J Immunol* (2006) **176**:3942–9.
103. Mancini S, Candéias SM, Fehling HJ, von Boehmer H, Jouvin-Marche E, Marche PN. TCR α-chain repertoire in pTα-deficient mice is diverse and developmentally regulated: implications for pre-TCR functions and TCRA gene rearrangement. *J Immunol* (1999) **163**:6053–9.
104. Halapi E, Werner A, Wahlström J, Österborg A, Jeddi-Tehrani M, Yi Q, et al. T cell repertoire in patients with multiple myeloma and monoclonal gammopathy of undetermined significance: clonal $CD8^+$ T cell expansions are found preferentially in patients with a low tumor burden. *Eur J Immunol* (1997) **27**:2245–52. doi:10.1002/eji.1830270919
105. Brawand P, Cerottini JC, MacDonald HR. Hierarchal utilization of different T-cell receptor Vβ gene segments in the $CD8^+$-T-cell response to an immunodominant Moloney leukemia virus-encoded epitope *in vivo*. *J Virol* (1999) **73**:9161–9.
106. Matsuzaki G, Takada H, Nomoto K. *Escherichia coli* infection induces only fetal thymus-derived γδ T cells at the infected site. *Eur J Immunol* (1999) **29**:3877–86. doi:10.1002/(SICI)1521-4141(199912)29:12<3877::AID-IMMU3877>3.3.CO;2-3
107. Collette A, Bagot S, Ferrandiz ME, Cazenave PA, Six A, Pied S. A profound alteration of blood TCRB repertoire allows prediction of cerebral malaria. *J Immunol* (2004) **173**:4568–75.
108. Douek DC, Betts MR, Brenchley JM, Hill BJ, Ambrozak DR, Ngai KL, et al. A novel approach to the analysis of specificity, clonality, and frequency of HIV-specific T cell responses reveals a potential mechanism for control of viral escape. *J Immunol* (2002) **168**:3099–104.
109. Lim A, Lemercier B, Wertz X, Pottier SL, Huetz F, Kourilsky P. Many human peripheral VH5-expressing IgM+ B cells display a unique heavy-chain rearrangement. *Int Immunol* (2008) **20**:105–16. doi:10.1093/intimm/dxm125
110. Voelkerding KV, Dames SA, Durtschi JD. Next-generation sequencing: from basic research to diagnostics. *Clin Chem* (2009) **55**:641–58. doi:10.1373/clinchem.2008.112789
111. McGinn S, Gut IG. DNA sequencing – spanning the generations. *Nat Biotechnol* (2013) **30**:366–72. doi:10.1016/j.nbt.2012.11.012

112. Weinstein JA, Jiang N, White RA III, Fisher DS, Quake SR. High-throughput sequencing of the zebrafish antibody repertoire. *Science* (2009) **324**:807–10. doi:10.1126/science.1170020
113. Robins HS, Campregher PV, Srivastava SK, Wacher A, Turtle CJ, Kahsai O, et al. Comprehensive assessment of T-cell receptor β-chain diversity in αβ T cells. *Blood* (2009) **114**:4099–107. doi:10.1182/blood-2009-04-217604
114. Freeman JD, Warren RL, Webb JR, Nelson BH, Holt RA. Profiling the T-cell receptor beta-chain repertoire by massively parallel sequencing. *Genome Res* (2009) **19**:1817–24. doi:10.1101/gr.092924.109
115. Wang C, Sanders CM, Yang Q, Schroeder HW, Wang E, Babrzadeh F, et al. High throughput sequencing reveals a complex pattern of dynamic interrelationships among human T cell subsets. *Proc Natl Acad Sci U S A* (2010) **107**:1518–23. doi:10.1073/pnas.0913939107
116. Warren RL, Freeman JD, Zeng T, Choe G, Munro S, Moore R, et al. Exhaustive T-cell repertoire sequencing of human peripheral blood samples reveals signatures of antigen selection and a directly measured repertoire size of at least 1 million clonotypes. *Genome Res* (2011) **21**:790–7. doi:10.1101/gr.115428.110
117. Venturi V, Quigley MF, Greenaway HY, Ng PC, Ende ZS, McIntosh T, et al. A mechanism for TCR sharing between T cell subsets and individuals revealed by pyrosequencing. *J Immunol* (2011) **186**:4285–94. doi:10.4049/jimmunol.1003898
118. Wu D, Sherwood A, Fromm JR, Winter SS, Dunsmore KP, Loh ML, et al. High-throughput sequencing detects minimal residual disease in acute T lymphoblastic leukemia. *Sci Transl Med* (2012) **4**:134ra63. doi:10.1126/scitranslmed.3003656
119. Föhse L, Suffner J, Suhre K, Wahl B, Lindner C, Lee CW, et al. High TCR diversity ensures optimal function and homeostasis of Foxp3$^+$ regulatory T cells. *Eur J Immunol* (2011) **41**:3101–13. doi:10.1002/eji.201141986
120. Sherwood AM, Desmarais C, Livingston RJ, Andriesen J, Haussler M, Carlson CS, et al. Deep sequencing of the human TCRγ and TCRβ repertoires suggests that TCRβ rearranges after αβ and γδ T cell commitment. *Sci Transl Med* (2011) **3**:90ra61. doi:10.1126/scitranslmed.3002536
121. Cebula A, Seweryn M, Rempala GA, Pabla SS, McIndoe RA, Denning TL, et al. Thymus-derived regulatory T cells contribute to tolerance to commensal microbiota. *Nature* (2013) **497**:258–62. doi:10.1038/nature12079
122. Bashford-Rogers RJM, Palser AL, Huntly BJ, Rance R, Vassiliou GS, Follows GA, et al. Network properties derived from deep sequencing of human B-cell receptor repertoires delineate B-cell populations. *Genome Res* (2013) **23**:1874–84. doi:10.1101/gr.154815.113
123. Srivastava SK, Robins HS. Palindromic nucleotide analysis in human T cell receptor rearrangements. *PLoS One* (2012) **7**:e52250. doi:10.1371/journal.pone.0052250
124. Murugan A, Mora T, Walczak AM, Callan CG. Statistical inference of the generation probability of T-cell receptors from sequence repertoires. *Proc Natl Acad Sci U S A* (2012) **109**:16161–6. doi:10.1073/pnas.1212755109
125. Ndifon W, Gal H, Shifrut E, Aharoni R, Yissachar N, Waysbort N, et al. Chromatin conformation governs T-cell receptor Jβ gene segment usage. *Proc Natl Acad Sci U S A* (2012) **109**:15865–70. doi:10.1073/pnas.1203916109
126. Robins HS, Srivastava SK, Campregher PV, Turtle CJ, Andriesen J, Riddell SR, et al. Overlap and effective size of the human CD8$^+$ T cell receptor repertoire. *Sci Transl Med* (2010) **2**:47ra64. doi:10.1126/scitranslmed.3001442
127. Prabakaran P, Chen W, Singarayan MG, Stewart CC, Streaker E, Feng Y, et al. Expressed antibody repertoires in human cord blood cells: 454 sequencing and IMGT/HighV-QUEST analysis of germline gene usage, junctional diversity, and somatic mutations. *Immunogenetics* (2012) **64**:337–50. doi:10.1007/s00251-011-0595-8
128. van Heijst JW, Ceberio I, Lipuma LB, Samilo DW, Wasilewski GD, Gonzales AM, et al. Quantitative assessment of T cell repertoire recovery after hematopoietic stem cell transplantation. *Nat Med* (2013) **19**:372–7. doi:10.1038/nm.3100
129. Meier J, Roberts C, Avent K, Hazlett A, Berrie J, Payne K, et al. Fractal organization of the human T cell repertoire in health and after stem cell transplantation. *Biol Blood Marrow Transplant* (2013) **19**:366–77. doi:10.1016/j.bbmt.2012.12.004
130. Ademokun A, Wu Y-C, Martin V, Mitra R, Sack U, Baxendale H, et al. Vaccination-induced changes in human B-cell repertoire and pneumococcal IgM and IgA antibody at different ages. *Aging Cell* (2011) **10**:922–30. doi:10.1111/j.1474-9726.2011.00732.x
131. Castro R, Jouneau L, Pham HP, Bouchez O, Giudicelli V, Lefranc MP, et al. Teleost fish mount complex clonal IgM and IgT responses in spleen upon systemic viral infection. *PLoS Pathog* (2013) **9**:e1003098. doi:10.1371/journal.ppat.1003098
132. Bousso P, Casrouge A, Altman JD, Haury M, Kanellopoulos J, Abastado JP, et al. Individual variations in the murine T cell response to a specific peptide reflect variability in naive repertoires. *Immunity* (1998) **9**:169–78. doi:10.1016/S1074-7613(00)80599-3
133. Lin MY, Welsh RM. Stability and diversity of T cell receptor repertoire usage during lymphocytic choriomeningitis virus infection of mice. *J Exp Med* (1998) **188**:1993–2005. doi:10.1084/jem.188.11.1993
134. Metzker ML. Sequencing technologies – the next generation. *Nat Rev Genet* (2010) **11**:31–46. doi:10.1038/nrg2626
135. Margulies M, Egholm M, Altman WE, Attiya S, Bader JS, Bemben LA, et al. Genome sequencing in microfabricated high-density picolitre reactors. *Nature* (2005) **437**:376–80.
136. Rothberg JM, Hinz W, Rearick TM, Schultz J, Mileski W, Davey M, et al. An integrated semiconductor device enabling non-optical genome sequencing. *Nature* (2011) **475**:348–52. doi:10.1038/nature10242
137. Bolotin DA, Mamedov IZ, Britanova OV, Zvyagin IV, Shagin D, Ustyugova SV, et al. Next generation sequencing for TCR repertoire profiling: platform-specific features and correction algorithms. *Eur J Immunol* (2012) **42**:3073–83. doi:10.1002/eji.201242517
138. Bragg LM, Stone G, Butler MK, Hugenholtz P, Tyson GW. Shining a light on dark sequencing: characterising errors in Ion Torrent PGM data. *PLoS Comput Biol* (2013) **9**:e1003031. doi:10.1371/journal.pcbi.1003031
139. Shendure J, Aiden EL. The expanding scope of DNA sequencing. *Nat Biotechnol* (2012) **30**:1084–94. doi:10.1038/nbt.2421
140. Dash P, McClaren JL, Oguin TH III, Rothwell W, Todd B, Morris MY, et al. Paired analysis of TCRα and TCRβ chains at the single-cell level in mice. *J Clin Invest* (2011) **121**:288–95. doi:10.1172/JCI44752
141. DeKosky BJ, Ippolito GC, Deschner RP, Lavinder JJ, Wine Y, Rawlings BM, et al. High-throughput sequencing of the paired human immunoglobulin heavy and light chain repertoire. *Nat Biotechnol* (2013) **31**:166–9. doi:10.1038/nbt.2492
142. Turchaninova MA, Britanova OV, Bolotin DA, Shugay M, Putintseva EV, Staroverov DB, et al. Pairing of T-cell receptor chains via emulsion PCR. *Eur J Immunol* (2013) **43**:2507–15. doi:10.1002/eji.201343453
143. Plessy C, Desbois L, Fujii T, Carninci P. Population transcriptomics with single-cell resolution: a new field made possible by microfluidics: a technology for high throughput transcript counting and data-driven definition of cell types. *Bioessays* (2013) **35**:131–40. doi:10.1002/bies.201200093
144. Mehr R, Sternberg-Simon M, Michaeli M, Pickman Y. Models and methods for analysis of lymphocyte repertoire generation, development, selection and evolution. *Immunol Lett* (2012) **148**:11–22. doi:10.1016/j.imlet.2012.08.002
145. Pancer Z, Amemiya CT, Ehrhardt GR, Ceitlin J, Gartland GL, Cooper MD. Somatic diversification of variable lymphocyte receptors in the agnathan sea lamprey. *Nature* (2004) **430**:174–80. doi:10.1038/nature02740
146. Lefranc MP, Giudicelli V, Ginestoux C, Jabado-Michaloud J, Folch G, Bellahcene F, et al. IMGT, the international ImMunoGeneTics information system. *Nucleic Acids Res* (2009) **37**:D1006–12. doi:10.1093/nar/gkn838
147. Giudicelli V, Lefranc MP. IMGT-ONTOLOGY 2012. *Front Genet* (2012) **3**:79. doi:10.3389/fgene.2012.00079
148. Alamyar E, Giudicelli V, Li S, Duroux P, Lefranc MP. IMGT/HighV-QUEST: the IMGT(R) web portal for immunoglobulin (IG) or antibody and T cell receptor (TR) analysis from NGS high throughput and deep sequencing. *Immunome Res* (2012) **8**:26. doi:10.1007/978-1-61779-842-9_32
149. Watson FL, Puttmann-Holgado R, Thomas F, Lamar DL, Hughes M, Kondo M, et al. Extensive diversity of Ig-superfamily proteins in the immune system of insects. *Science* (2005) **309**:1874–8. doi:10.1126/science.1116887
150. Du Pasquier L. Insects diversify one molecule to serve two systems. *Science* (2005) **309**:1826–7. doi:10.1126/science.1118828
151. Zhang SM, Adema CM, Kepler TB, Loker ES. Diversification of Ig superfamily genes in an invertebrate. *Science* (2004) **305**:251–4. doi:10.1126/science.1088069
152. Philipp EER, Kraemer L, Melzner F, Poustka AJ, Thieme S, Findeisen U, et al. Massively parallel RNA sequencing identifies a complex immune gene repertoire in the Lophotrochozoan *Mytilus edulis*. *PLoS One* (2012) **7**:e33091. doi:10.1371/journal.pone.0033091

153. Matsushima N, Tanaka T, Enkhbayar P, Mikami T, Taga M, Yamada K, et al. Comparative sequence analysis of leucine-rich repeats (LRRs) within vertebrate toll-like receptors. *BMC Genomics* (2007) **8**:124. doi:10.1186/1471-2164-8-124
154. Matsushima N, Miyashita H, Mikami T, Kuroki Y. A nested leucine rich repeat (LRR) domain: the precursor of LRRs is a ten or eleven residue motif. *BMC Microbiol* (2010) **10**:235. doi:10.1186/1471-2180-10-235
155. Kaas Q, Ehrenmann F, Lefranc MP. IG, TR and IgSF, MHC and MhcSF: what do we learn from the IMGT Colliers de Perles? *Brief Funct Genomic Proteomic* (2007) **6**:253–64. doi:10.1093/bfgp/elm032
156. Bomberger C, Singh-Jairam M, Rodey G, Guerriero A, Yeager AM, Fleming WH, et al. Lymphoid reconstitution after autologous PBSC transplantation with FACS-sorted CD34+ hematopoietic progenitors. *Blood* (1998) **91**:2588–600.
157. Gorochov G, Neumann AU, Kereveur A, Parizot C, Li TS, Katlama C, et al. Perturbation of $CD4^+$ and $CD8^+$ T-cell repertoires during progression to AIDS and regulation of the $CD4^+$ repertoire during antiviral therapy. *Nat Med* (1998) **4**:215–21. doi:10.1038/nm0298-215
158. Wu CJ, Chillemi A, Alyea EP, Orsini E, Neuberg D, Soiffer RJ, et al. Reconstitution of T-cell receptor repertoire diversity following T-cell depleted allogeneic bone marrow transplantation is related to hematopoietic chimerism. *Blood* (2000) **95**:352–9.
159. Hori S, Collette A, Demengeot J, Stewart J. A new statistical method for quantitative analyses: application to the precise quantification of T cell receptor repertoires. *J Immunol Methods* (2002) **268**:159–70. doi:10.1016/S0022-1759(02)00187-4
160. Collette A, Six A. ISEApeaks: an excel platform for GeneScan and Immunoscope data retrieval, management and analysis. *Bioinformatics* (2002) **18**:329–30. doi:10.1093/bioinformatics/18.2.329
161. Guillet M, Brouard S, Gagne K, Sebille F, Cuturi MC, Delsuc MA, et al. Different qualitative and quantitative regulation of Vβ TCR transcripts during early acute allograft rejection and tolerance induction. *J Immunol* (2002) **168**:5088–95.
162. Peggs KS, Verfuerth S, D'Sa S, Yong K, Mackinnon S. Assessing diversity: immune reconstitution and T-cell receptor BV spectratype analysis following stem cell transplantation. *Br J Haematol* (2003) **120**:154–65. doi:10.1046/j.1365-2141.2003.04036.x
163. Long SA, Khalili J, Ashe J, Berenson R, Ferrand C, Bonyhadi M. Standardized analysis for the quantification of Vbeta CDR3 T-cell receptor diversity. *J Immunol Methods* (2006) **317**:100–13. doi:10.1016/j.jim.2006.09.015
164. Miqueu P, Guillet M, Degauque N, Dore JC, Soulillou JP, Brouard S. Statistical analysis of CDR3 length distributions for the assessment of T and B cell repertoire biases. *Mol Immunol* (2007) **44**:1057–64. doi:10.1016/j.molimm.2006.06.026
165. Guillet M, Sebille F, Soulillou JP. TCR usage in naive and committed alloreactive cells: implications for the understanding of TCR biases in transplantation. *Curr Opin Immunol* (2001) **13**:566–71. doi:10.1016/S0952-7915(00)00260-0
166. Collette A, Cazenave PA, Pied S, Six A. New methods and software tools for high throughput CDR3 spectratyping. Application to T lymphocyte repertoire modifications during experimental malaria. *J Immunol Methods* (2003) **278**:105–16. doi:10.1016/S0022-1759(03)00225-4
167. Sassi A, Largueche-Darwaz B, Collette A, Six A, Laouini D, Cazenave PA, et al. Mechanisms of the natural reactivity of lymphocytes from noninfected individuals to membrane-associated *Leishmania infantum* antigens. *J Immunol* (2005) **174**:3598–607.
168. Castro R, Takizawa F, Chaara W, Lunazzi A, Dang TH, Koellner B, et al. Contrasted TCRβ diversity of $CD8^+$ and $CD8^-$ T cells in rainbow trout. *PLoS One* (2013) **8**:e60175. doi:10.1371/journal.pone.0060175
169. Kepler TB, He M, Tomfohr JK, Devlin BH, Sarzotti M, Markert ML. Statistical analysis of antigen receptor spectratype data. *Bioinformatics* (2005) **21**:3394–400. doi:10.1093/bioinformatics/bti539
170. He M, Tomfohr JK, Devlin BH, Sarzotti M, Markert ML, Kepler TB. SpA: web-accessible spectratype analysis: data management, statistical analysis and visualization. *Bioinformatics* (2005) **21**:3697–9. doi:10.1093/bioinformatics/bti600
171. Liu C, He M, Rooney B, Kepler TB, Chao NJ. Longitudinal analysis of T-cell receptor variable beta chain repertoire in patients with acute graft-versus-host disease after allogeneic stem cell transplantation. *Biol Blood Marrow Transplant* (2006) **12**:335–45. doi:10.1016/j.bbmt.2005.09.019
172. Lefranc MP. From IMGT-ONTOLOGY CLASSIFICATION Axiom to IMGT standardized gene and allele nomenclature: for immunoglobulins (IG) and T cell receptors (TR). *Cold Spring Harb Protoc* (2011) **2011**:627–32. doi:10.1101/pdb.ip84
173. Lefranc MP. From IMGT-ONTOLOGY DESCRIPTION axiom to IMGT standardized labels: for immunoglobulin (IG) and T cell receptor (TR) sequences and structures. *Cold Spring Harb Protoc* (2011) **2011**:614–26. doi:10.1101/pdb.ip84
174. Lefranc MP. From IMGT-ONTOLOGY IDENTIFICATION axiom to IMGT standardized keywords: for immunoglobulins (IG), T cell receptors (TR), and conventional genes. *Cold Spring Harb Protoc* (2011) **2011**:604–13. doi:10.1101/pdb.ip84
175. Lefranc MP. IMGT unique numbering for the variable (V), constant (C), and groove (G) domains of IG, TR, MH, IgSF, and MhSF. *Cold Spring Harb Protoc* (2011) **2011**:633–42. doi:10.1101/pdb.ip85
176. Giudicelli V, Chaume D, Lefranc MP. IMGT/V-QUEST, an integrated software program for immunoglobulin and T cell receptor V-J and V-D-J rearrangement analysis. *Nucleic Acids Res* (2004) **32**:W435–40. doi:10.1093/nar/gkh412
177. Brochet X, Lefranc MP, Giudicelli V. IMGT/V-QUEST: the highly customized and integrated system for IG and TR standardized V-J and V-D-J sequence analysis. *Nucleic Acids Res* (2008) **36**:W503–8. doi:10.1093/nar/gkn316
178. Gaëta BA, Malming HR, Jackson KJL, Bain ME, Wilson P, Collins AM. iHMMune-align: hidden Markov model-based alignment and identification of germline genes in rearranged immunoglobulin gene sequences. *Bioinformatics* (2007) **23**:1580–7. doi:10.1093/bioinformatics/btm147
179. Rogosch T, Kerzel S, Hoi KH, Zhang Z, Maier RF, Ippolito GC, et al. Immunoglobulin analysis tool: a novel tool for the analysis of human and mouse heavy and light chain transcripts. *Front Immunol* (2012) **3**:176. doi:10.3389/fimmu.2012.00176
180. Ye J, Ma N, Madden TL, Ostell JM. IgBLAST: an immunoglobulin variable domain sequence analysis tool. *Nucleic Acids Res* (2013) **41**:W34–40. doi:10.1093/nar/gkt382
181. Thomas N, Heather J, Ndifon W, Shawe-Taylor J, Chain B. Decombinator: a tool for fast, efficient gene assignment in T-cell receptor sequences using a finite state machine. *Bioinformatics* (2013) **29**:542–50. doi:10.1093/bioinformatics/btt004
182. Pham HP, Manuel M, Petit N, Klatzmann D, Cohen-Kaminsky S, Six A, et al. Half of the T-cell repertoire combinatorial diversity is genetically determined in humans and humanized mice. *Eur J Immunol* (2012) **42**:760–70. doi:10.1002/eji.201141798
183. Eisenstein M. Personalized, sequencing-based immune profiling spurs startups. *Nat Biotechnol* (2013) **31**:184–6. doi:10.1038/nbt0313-184b
184. Stahl D, Lacroix-Desmazes S, Barreau C, Sibrowski W, Kazatchkine MD, Kaveri SV. Altered antibody repertoires of plasma IgM and IgG toward nonself antigens in patients with warm autoimmune hemolytic anemia. *Hum Immunol* (2001) **62**:348–61. doi:10.1016/S0198-8859(01)00225-7
185. Magurran AE. *Measuring Biological Diversity*. Oxford: Wiley-Blackwell (2004).
186. Colwell RK. *EstimateS: Statistical Estimation of Species Richness and Shared Species from Samples. [Version 9]. User's Guide and application* (2013). Available from: http://purl.oclc.org/estimates
187. Wu TT, Kabat EA. An analysis of the sequence of the variable regions of Bence Jones proteins and myeloma light chains and their implications for antibody complementarity. *J Exp Med* (1970) **132**:211–50. doi:10.1084/jem.132.2.211
188. Jores R, Alzari PM, Meo T. Resolution of hypervariable regions in T-cell receptor β chains by a modified Wu-Kabat index of amino acid diversity. *Proc Natl Acad Sci U S A* (1990) **87**:9138–42. doi:10.1073/pnas.87.23.9138
189. Stewart JJ, Lee CY, Ibrahim S, Watts P, Shlomchik M, Weigert M, et al. A Shannon entropy analysis of immunoglobulin and T cell receptor. *Mol Immunol* (1997) **34**:1067–82. doi:10.1016/S0161-5890(97)00130-2
190. Thomas PG, Handel A, Doherty PC, La Gruta NL. Ecological analysis of antigen-specific CTL repertoires defines the relationship between naïve and immune T-cell populations. *Proc Natl Acad Sci U S A* (2013) **110**:1839–44. doi:10.1073/pnas.1222149110
191. Li S, Lefranc MP, Miles J, Alamyar E, Giudicelli V, Duroux P, et al. IMGT/HighV-QUEST paradigm for T cell receptor IMGT clonotype diversity and next generation repertoire immunoprofiling. *Nat Commun* (2013) **4**:2333. doi:10.1038/ncomms3333
192. Conrad JA, Ramalingam RK, Duncan CB, Smith RM, Wei J, Barnett L, et al. Antiretroviral therapy reduces the magnitude and T cell receptor repertoire

diversity of HIV-specific T cell responses without changing T cell clonotype dominance. *J Virol* (2012) **86**:4213–21. doi:10.1128/JVI.06000-11
193. Koning D, Costa AI, Hoof I, Miles JJ, Nanlohy NM, Ladell K, et al. CD8+ TCR repertoire formation is guided primarily by the peptide component of the antigenic complex. *J Immunol* (2013) **190**:931–9. doi:10.4049/jimmunol.1202466
194. Johnson PLF, Yates AJ, Goronzy JJ, Antia R. Peripheral selection rather than thymic involution explains sudden contraction in naive CD4 T-cell diversity with age. *Proc Natl Acad Sci U S A* (2012) **109**:21432–7. doi:10.1073/pnas.1209283110
195. Perelson AS, Weisbuch G. Immunology for physicist. *Rev Mod Phys* (1997) **69**:1219–67. doi:10.1103/RevModPhys.69.1219
196. Perelson AS, Oster GF. Theoretical studies of clonal selection: minimal antibody repertoire size and reliability of self-non-self discrimination. *J Theor Biol* (1979) **81**:645–70. doi:10.1016/0022-5193(79)90275-3
197. Percus JK, Percus OE, Perelson AS. Predicting the size of the T-cell receptor and antibody combining region from consideration of efficient self-nonself discrimination. *Proc Natl Acad Sci U S A* (1993) **90**:1691–5. doi:10.1073/pnas.90.5.1691
198. Bergstrom CT, Antia R. How do adaptive immune systems control pathogens while avoiding autoimmunity? *Trends Ecol Evol* (2006) **21**:22–8. doi:10.1016/j.tree.2005.11.008
199. Perelson AS. Modelling viral and immune system dynamics. *Nat Rev Immunol* (2002) **2**:28–36. doi:10.1038/nri700
200. Antia R, Ganusov VV, Ahmed R. The role of models in understanding CD8+ T-cell memory. *Nat Rev Immunol* (2005) **5**:101–11. doi:10.1038/nri1550
201. Thomas-Vaslin V, Six A, Bellier B, Klatzmann D. Lymphocytes dynamics repertoires, modeling. In: Dubitzky W, Wolkenhauer O, Cho K-H, Yokota H editors. *Encyclopedia of Systems Biology.* Heidelberg: Springer Verlag (2013). p. 1149–52. doi:10.1007/978-1-4419-9863-7_96
202. De Boer RJ, Homann D, Perelson AS. Different dynamics of CD4+ and CD8+ T cell responses during and after acute lymphocytic choriomeningitis virus infection. *J Immunol* (2003) **171**:3928–35.
203. Verkoczy LK, Martensson AS, Nemazee D. The scope of receptor editing and its association with autoimmunity. *Curr Opin Immunol* (2004) **16**:808–14. doi:10.1016/j.coi.2004.09.017
204. Wucherpfennig KW, Allen PM, Celada F, Cohen IR, De BR, Garcia KC, et al. Polyspecificity of T cell and B cell receptor recognition. *Semin Immunol* (2007) **19**:216–24. doi:10.1016/j.smim.2007.02.012
205. Germain RN, Meier-Schellersheim M, Nita-Lazar A, Fraser IDC. Systems biology in immunology: a computational modeling perspective. *Annu Rev Immunol* (2011) **29**:527–85. doi:10.1146/annurev-immunol-030409-101317
206. Emonet T, Altan-Bonnet G. Systems immunology: a primer for biophysicists. In: Egelman E editor. *Comprehensive Biophysics.* New York: Academic Press (2012). p. 389–413.
207. Quigley MF, Greenaway HY, Venturi V, Lindsay R, Quinn KM, Seder RA, et al. Convergent recombination shapes the clonotypic landscape of the naïve T-cell repertoire. *Proc Natl Acad Sci U S A* (2010) **107**:19414–9. doi:10.1073/pnas.1010586107
208. Martins VC, Ruggiero E, Schlenner SM, Madan V, Schmidt M, Fink PJ, et al. Thymus-autonomous T cell development in the absence of progenitor import. *J Exp Med* (2012) **209**:1409–17. doi:10.1084/jem.20120846
209. Farmer JD, Packard NH, Perelson AS. The immune system, adaptation and machine learning. *Physica D* (1986) **22**:187–204. doi:10.1016/0167-2789(86)90240-X
210. De Boer RJ, Perelson AS. Size and connectivity as emergent properties of a developing immune network. *J Theor Biol* (1991) **149**:381–424. doi:10.1016/S0022-5193(05)80313-3
211. Celada F, Seiden PE. A computer model of cellular interactions in the immune system. *Immunol Today* (1992) **13**:56–62. doi:10.1016/0167-5699(92)90135-T
212. Goldstein B, Faeder JR, Hlavacek WS. Mathematical and computational models of immune-receptor signalling. *Nat Rev Immunol* (2004) **4**:445–56. doi:10.1038/nri1374
213. Chao A, Chazdon RL, Colwell RK, Shen TJ. A new statistical approach for assessing similarity of species composition with incidence and abundance data. *Ecol Lett* (2005) **8**:148–59. doi:10.1111/j.1461-0248.2004.00707.x
214. Kosmrlj A, Jha AK, Huseby ES, Kardar M, Chakraborty AK. How the thymus designs antigen-specific and self-tolerant T cell receptor sequences. *Proc Natl Acad Sci U S A* (2008) **105**:16671–6. doi:10.1073/pnas.0808081105
215. Kosmrlj A, Chakraborty AK, Kardar M, Shakhnovich EI. Thymic selection of T-cell receptors as an extreme value problem. *Phys Rev Lett* (2009) **103**:068103. doi:10.1103/PhysRevLett.103.068103
216. Verhagen J, Genolet R, Britton GJ, Stevenson BJ, Sabatos-Peyton CA, Dyson J, et al. CTLA-4 controls the thymic development of both conventional and regulatory T cells through modulation of the TCR repertoire. *Proc Natl Acad Sci U S A* (2013) **110**:E221–30. doi:10.1073/pnas.1208573110
217. Mora T, Walczak AM, Bialek W, Callan CG. Maximum entropy models for antibody diversity. *Proc Natl Acad Sci U S A* (2010) **107**:5405–10. doi:10.1073/pnas.1001705107
218. Baum PD, Venturi V, Price DA. Wrestling with the repertoire: the promise and perils of next generation sequencing for antigen receptors. *Eur J Immunol* (2012) **42**:2834–9. doi:10.1002/eji.201242999
219. Robins H, Desmarais C, Matthis J, Livingston R, Andriesen J, Reijonen H, et al. Ultra-sensitive detection of rare T cell clones. *J Immunol Methods* (2012) **375**:14–9. doi:10.1016/j.jim.2011.09.001
220. Zipf GK. *Human Behaviour and the Principle of Least Effort: An Introduction to Human Ecology.* Cambridge, MA: Addison-Wesley (1949).
221. Sepulveda N, Paulino CD, Carneiro J. Estimation of T-cell repertoire diversity and clonal size distribution by Poisson abundance models. *J Immunol Methods* (2009) **353**:124–37. doi:10.1016/j.jim.2009.11.009
222. Rempala GA, Seweryn M, Ignatowicz L. Model for comparative analysis of antigen receptor repertoires. *J Theor Biol* (2011) **269**:1–15. doi:10.1016/j.jtbi.2010.10.001
223. Ben-Hamo R, Efroni S. The whole-organism heavy chain B cell repertoire from Zebrafish self-organizes into distinct network features. *BMC Syst Biol* (2011) **5**:27. doi:10.1186/1752-0509-5-27
224. Bleakley K, Lefranc MP, Biau G. Recovering probabilities for nucleotide trimming processes for T cell receptor TRA and TRG V-J junctions analyzed with IMGT tools. *BMC Bioinformatics* (2008) **9**:408. doi:10.1186/1471-2105-9-408
225. Kleinstein SH, Louzoun Y, Shlomchik MJ. Estimating hypermutation rates from clonal tree data. *J Immunol* (2003) **171**:4639–49.
226. Anderson SM, Khalil A, Uduman M, Hershberg U, Louzoun Y, Haberman AM, et al. Taking advantage: high-affinity B cells in the germinal center have lower death rates, but similar rates of division, compared to low-affinity cells. *J Immunol* (2009) **183**:7314–25. doi:10.4049/jimmunol.0902452
227. Uduman M, Yaari G, Hershberg U, Stern JA, Shlomchik MJ, Kleinstein SH. Detecting selection in immunoglobulin sequences. *Nucleic Acids Res* (2011) **39**:W499–504. doi:10.1093/nar/gkr413
228. Yaari G, Uduman M, Kleinstein SH. Quantifying selection in high-throughput Immunoglobulin sequencing data sets. *Nucleic Acids Res* (2012) **40**:e134. doi:10.1093/nar/gks457
229. Rock EP, Sibbald PR, Davis MM, Chien Y. CDR3 length in antigen-specific immune receptors. *J Exp Med* (1994) **179**:323–8. doi:10.1084/jem.179.1.323
230. Hyatt G, Melamed R, Park R, Seguritan R, Laplace C, Poirot L, et al. Gene expression microarrays: glimpses of the immunological genome. *Nat Immunol* (2006) **7**:686–91. doi:10.1038/ni0706-686
231. Han Q, Bagheri N, Bradshaw EM, Hafler DA, Lauffenburger DA, Love JC. Polyfunctional responses by human T cells result from sequential release of cytokines. *Proc Natl Acad Sci U S A* (2012) **109**:1607–12. doi:10.1073/pnas.1117194109
232. Bendall SC, Simonds EF, Qiu P, Amir E, Krutzik PO, Finck R, et al. Single-cell mass cytometry of differential immune and drug responses across a human hematopoietic continuum. *Science* (2011) **332**:687–96. doi:10.1126/science.1198704
233. Newell EW, Sigal N, Bendall SC, Nolan GP, Davis MM. Cytometry by time-of-flight shows combinatorial cytokine expression and virus-specific cell niches within a continuum of CD8+ T cell phenotypes. *Immunity* (2012) **36**:142–52. doi:10.1016/j.immuni.2012.01.002
234. Schepers K, Swart E, van Heijst JW, Gerlach C, Castrucci M, Sie D, et al. Dissecting T cell lineage relationships by cellular barcoding. *J Exp Med* (2008) **205**:2309–18. doi:10.1084/jem.20072462
235. Sumen C, Mempel TR, Mazo IB, von Andrian UH. Intravital microscopy: visualizing immunity in context. *Immunity* (2004) **21**:315–29. doi:10.1016/j.immuni.2004.08.006
236. Marangoni F, Murooka TT, Manzo T, Kim EY, Carrizosa E, Elpek NM, et al. The transcription factor NFAT exhibits signal memory during serial T cell interactions with antigen-presenting cells. *Immunity* (2013) **38**:237–49. doi:10.1016/j.immuni.2012.09.012

237. Flatz L, Roychoudhuri R, Honda M, Filali-Mouhim A, Goulet JP, Kettaf N, et al. Single-cell gene-expression profiling reveals qualitatively distinct CD8 T cells elicited by different gene-based vaccines. *Proc Natl Acad Sci U S A* (2011) **108**:5724–9. doi:10.1073/pnas.1013084108

238. Mehr R. Modeling and analysis of the meta-population dynamics of lymphocyte repertoires. *J Comput Appl Math* (2005) **184**:223–41. doi:10.1016/j.cam.2004.07.033

239. Ciupe SM, Devlin BH, Markert ML, Kepler TB. The dynamics of T-cell receptor repertoire diversity following thymus transplantation for DiGeorge anomaly. *PLoS Comput Biol* (2009) **5**:e1000396. doi:10.1371/journal.pcbi.1000396

240. Stirk ER, Molina-Paris C, van den Berg HA. Stochastic niche structure and diversity maintenance in the T cell repertoire. *J Theor Biol* (2008) **255**:237–49. doi:10.1016/j.jtbi.2008.07.017

241. Benoist C, Germain RN, Mathis D. A plaidoyer for 'systems immunology.' *Immunol Rev* (2006) **210**:229–34. doi:10.1111/j.0105-2896.2006.00374.x

242. Cohen IR. Autoantibody repertoires, natural biomarkers, and system controllers. *Trends Immunol* (2013). doi:10.1016/j.it.2013.05.003

243. Petrausch U, Haley D, Miller W, Floyd K, Urba WJ, Walker E. Polychromatic flow cytometry: a rapid method for the reduction and analysis of complex multiparameter data. *Cytometry* (2006) **69A**:1162–73. doi:10.1002/cyto.a.20342

244. Hofmann M, Zerwes HG. Identification of organ-specific T cell populations by analysis of multiparameter flow cytometry data using DNA-chip analysis software. *Cytometry A* (2006) **69**:533–40.

245. Lugli E, Pinti M, Troiano L, Nasi M, Patsekin V, Robinson JP, et al. Subject classification obtained by cluster analysis and principal component analysis applied to flow cytometric data. *Cytometry A* (2007) **71A**:334–44. doi:10.1002/cyto.a.20387

5

Differences in the composition of the human antibody repertoire by B cell subsets in the blood

Eva Szymanska Mroczek[1], Gregory C. Ippolito[2], Tobias Rogosch[3], Kam Hon Hoi[4,5], Tracy A. Hwangpo[6], Marsha G. Brand[6], Yingxin Zhuang[6], Cun Ren Liu[6], David A. Schneider[7], Michael Zemlin[3], Elizabeth E. Brown[8], George Georgiou[2,4,5] and Harry W. Schroeder Jr.[1,6]*

[1] *Department of Microbiology, University of Alabama at Birmingham, Birmingham, AL, USA*
[2] *Department of Molecular Biosciences, University of Texas at Austin, Austin, TX, USA*
[3] *Laboratory for Neonatology and Pediatric Immunology, Department of Pediatrics, Philipps-University, Marburg, Germany*
[4] *Department of Chemical Engineering, University of Texas at Austin, Austin, TX, USA*
[5] *Department of Biomedical Engineering, University of Texas at Austin, Austin, TX, USA*
[6] *Department of Medicine, University of Alabama at Birmingham, Birmingham, AL, USA*
[7] *Department of Biochemistry and Molecular Genetics, University of Alabama at Birmingham, Birmingham, AL, USA*
[8] *Department of Epidemiology, University of Alabama at Birmingham, Birmingham, AL, USA*

Edited by:
Ignacio Sanz, University of Rochester, USA

Reviewed by:
I-Hsin Su, Nanyang Technological University, Singapore
Masaki Hikida, Kyoto University, Japan

****Correspondence:***
Harry W. Schroeder Jr., Department of Medicine, University of Alabama at Birmingham, SHEL 176, 1530 3rd Avenue South, Birmingham, AL 35294-2182, USA
e-mail: hwsj@uab.edu

The vast initial diversity of the antibody repertoire is generated centrally by means of a complex series of V(D)J gene rearrangement events, variation in the site of gene segment joining, and TdT catalyzed N-region addition. Although the diversity is great, close inspection has revealed distinct and unique characteristics in the antibody repertoires expressed by different B cell developmental subsets. In order to illustrate our approach to repertoire analysis, we present an in-depth comparison of V(D)J gene usage, hydrophobicity, length, D_H reading frame, and amino acid usage between heavy chain repertoires expressed by immature, transitional, mature, memory IgD$^+$, memory IgD$^-$, and plasmacytes isolated from the blood of a single individual. Our results support the view that in both human and mouse, the H chain repertoires expressed by individual, developmental B cell subsets appear to differ in sequence content. Sequencing of unsorted B cells from the blood is thus likely to yield an incomplete or compressed view of what is actually happening in the immune response of the individual. Our findings support the view that studies designed to correlate repertoire expression with diseases of immune function will likely require deep sequencing of B cells sorted by subset.

Keywords: human antibody repertoire, CDR-H3, B cells subsets

INTRODUCTION

Production of a highly diverse, polyclonal immunoglobulin repertoire plays a central role in the ability of B cells to produce antibodies specific to a diverse range of foreign and self-antigens (1, 2). The antigen-binding sites of these antibodies are created by the juxtaposition of six hypervariable loops, termed complementarity determining regions (CDRs): three from the heavy (H) and three from the light (L) chain V domains. Because the third CDR of the H chain, termed CDR-H3 (2–5), is the direct product of V(D)J joining and N-region addition, it is the most variable component of the pre-immune immunoglobulin repertoire. The location of CDR-H3 at the center of the antigen-binding site allows this interval to play a key role in antigen recognition and binding (6–8).

Developing B cells pass through a series of checkpoints designed to test the functionality and antigen specificity of the immunoglobulin (9–14). In adults, this process begins in the bone marrow, and then continues in the periphery where it is heavily influenced by exposure to both self and foreign antigens. Immature B cells are released into the blood and in the periphery pass through a transitional stage prior to entering specific anatomic sites, such as the splenic marginal zone and the splenic and lymph node follicles (15, 16). Maturation is associated with the co-expression of IgM and IgD (17). Mature cells exposed to antigen can become either memory cells or plasmacytes. Both types of cells circulate through the blood on their way to their specific anatomic niches (18–21). IgM bearing memory cells can be divided into two populations, those that express IgD concurrently and those that do not (22–25). The IgM$^+$IgD$^-$ memory B cell population includes conventional, follicular B cells, whereas the IgM$^+$IgD$^+$memory B cell population includes marginal zone-like B cells that play a more immediate role in response to foreign antigens (26–28).

Recent studies in mice have shown that the composition of CDR-H3 exhibits preferred patterns in amino acid composition, length, and charge distribution that differ by developmental stage and B cell subset (29–33). These categorical constraints are initially imposed by natural selection of the germline V, D, and J gene sequence; and alteration of the sequence of these gene segments can give rise to dramatically different CDR-H3 repertoires (34–36). D gene sequence-specific changes in CDR-H3 content lead to altered patterns of B cell development, antigen-specific antibody production, and levels of protection against infectious agents (31, 37, 38), which underscores the important role played by the composition of the CDR-H3 repertoire in the regulation and function of the humoral immune response.

Given the importance of CDR-H3 to antigen recognition and antibody specificity, and the observation that CDR-H3 content can differ by peripheral developmental stage in the mouse; we sought to test whether V(D)J usage and CDR-H3 content would also differ by developmental stage in human. We used surface expression of CD19, CD27, IgD, CD24, and CD38 expression to identify and sort immature, transitional, mature, memory IgD$^+$, memory IgD$^-$ B cell subsets, and plasmacytes from the blood of a healthy female subject. We then used RT-PCR followed by Roche GS-FLX 454 deep sequencing to clone and sequence Cμ and Cγ-containing transcripts from the sorted cells. As in the mouse, we found that the distribution of V, D, and J utilization, and CDR-H3 length, amino acid usage, and average hydrophobicity differed between developmentally and functionally distinct B cell subsets. We conclude that studies of differences between healthy individuals and patients with diseases referable to the humoral immune response will likely require comparisons of the B cell repertoire by subset.

MATERIALS AND METHODS

SUBJECT DESCRIPTION AND ISOLATION OF B CELL SUBSETS

One healthy female subject, age 56, was recruited for antibody repertoire high throughput sequencing using the 454 platform. The subject is Caucasian, a lifelong native of the state of Alabama, and was without a history of illness or repeated infection that could be related to abnormal immune function. The complete blood count was well within normal limits. Serum immunoglobulin levels were IgM 382, IgG 1,680, and IgA 368 mg/dL, respectively. Venous blood (100 cm^3) was drawn by routine venipuncture and mononuclear cells were isolated using Ficoll-Paque Plus (GE Healthcare). CD19$^+$ magnetic beads (Miltenyi Biotec MACS) were used to enrich for B cells. These CD19$^+$ cells were further fractionated by CD27$^\pm$ populations using CD27 magnetic beads (Miltenyi Biotec MACS) according to the manufacturer's protocol. CD19$^+$CD27$^+$ B cells were stained with CD19 APC$_{780}$ (eBioscience), CD27 PE–Cy7 (BD Pharmingen), CD24 APC (BioLegend), and IgD FITC (Southern Biotech), and sorted into IgD$^+$ memory B cells (CD19$^+$/CD27$^+$/IgD$^+$/CD24$^+$), IgD$^-$ memory B cells (CD19$^+$/CD27$^+$/IgD$^-$/CD24$^+$), and plasmacytes (CD19$^+$/CD27$^+$/CD24$^-$) using a high speed sorting cytometer (FACSAria III; Becton Dickinson). CD19$^+$/CD27$^-$ B cells were stained with CD19 APC$_{780}$ (eBioscience), CD24 APC (BioLegend), CD38 PE (BioLegend), and IgD FITC (Southern Biotech) and sorted into mature/naïve (CD19$^+$/CD27$^-$/IgD$^+$/CD38$^+$/CD24$^+$), transitional (CD19$^+$/CD27$^-$/IgD$^+$/CD38^{+++}/CD24^{+++}), and immature (CD19$^+$/CD27$^-$/IgD$^-$) B cell subsets. Each B cell subset was then individually resuspended in 1 mL TRI reagent (Ambion) and archived at −80°C until processed for total RNA extraction. This work was performed in accordance with an Institutional Review Board approved protocol and informed consent was obtained from the subject at the University of Alabama at Birmingham, Birmingham, AL, USA.

GENERATION OF IgH LIBRARIES

For RNA extraction, 0.2 mL chloroform was added to the 1 mL sample, vortexed for 15 s, left to stand at room temperature for 5 min, then spun at 12,000 × g for 10 min at 4°C. The aqueous phase (~400 μL) was removed and to this an equal volume of 70% ethanol was added and then mixed by pipetting. This was applied immediately to an RNA-binding silica spin-column and subsequently processed according to the manufacturer's protocol (Qiagen RNeasy micro column; catalog no. 74004). Purified total RNA was eluted in 14 μL RNase-free water. Oligo-dT primer was used to generate first-strand cDNA from ~100 ng input RNA using the SuperScript RT II synthesis kit (Invitrogen; catalog no. 11904-018) per the manufacturer's protocol.

FastStart high fidelity PCR system (Roche; catalog no. 03-553-361-001) and an equimolar mix of eight optimized VH-FWD primers previously described for human IgH amplification (39, 40) coupled with a multiplex of 10-nucleotide uniquely barcoded CH-REV primers: IgM-rev, 5′-10 nt ID-GGTTGGGGCGGATGCACTCC-3′, and IgG-all-rev, 5′-10 nt ID-SGATGGGCCCTTGGTGGARGC-3′ were used to amplify V(D)JCμ and V(D)JCγ cDNAs from the cDNA template. Cycling conditions were as follows: 95°C denaturation for 3 min; 92°C for 1 min, 50°C for 1 min, 72°C for 1 min for 4 cycles; 92°C for 1 min, 55°C for 1 min, 72°C for 1 min for 4 cycles; 92°C for 1 min, 63°C for 1 min, 72°C for 1 min for 22 cycles; 72°C for 7 min. PCR amplicons were gel-purified (Zymo Research) before sequencing.

HIGH-THROUGHPUT SEQUENCING OF IgH REPERTOIRES AND BIOINFORMATIC ANALYSIS

The University of Texas Genomics Sequencing and Analysis Facility performed Roche GS-FLX 454 deep sequencing. CH-REV barcodes were examined to verify the integrity of each library after filtering raw data for read quality. Sequences were submitted to the ImMunoGeneTics (IMGT) database and IMGT/high V-QUEST web-based analysis tool (version 1.0.3) (41). The 11 CSV text files outputted by IMGT/highV-QUEST were then imported into IgAT immunoglobulin analysis tool for further deconstruction (42). Differences between populations were assessed, where appropriate, by Student's t-test, two tailed; Fisher's exact test, two tailed and d; χ^2, or Levene's test for the homogeneity of variance. Analysis was performed with PRISM version 5 (Graph Pad). The standard deviation accompanies mean. Raw 454 sequence files were deposited to the NCBI Sequence Read Archive (Accession SRP037774).

RESULTS

ISOLATION OF B LINEAGE CELLS AND 454 HIGH-THROUGHPUT SEQUENCING OF IgH TRANSCRIPTS FROM PERIPHERAL BLOOD

CD19$^+$ cells bearing the cell surface markers characteristic of immature, transitional, mature, memory IgD$^+$, memory IgD$^-$, and plasmacytes were isolated from the blood of a healthy female subject (43–47) (**Figure 1**). Following total RNA extraction, PCR was used to amplify cDNA copies of V(D)JCμ and V(D)JCγ transcripts using optimized VH-FWD primers previously described for human IgH amplification (39, 40). We obtained a total of 15,433 immature, 37,396 transitional, 47,781 mature, 43,558 memory IgD$^+$, 28,142 memory IgD$^-$, and 43,824 plasmacyte unique and in-frame IgH heavy chain reads. Of these, we obtained 1,240 immature, 1,354 transitional, 1,250 mature, 1,244 memory IgD$^+$, 833 memory IgD$^-$, and 1,714 plasmacyte reads that were of sufficient length to be identified as Igμ sequences, and 1,879

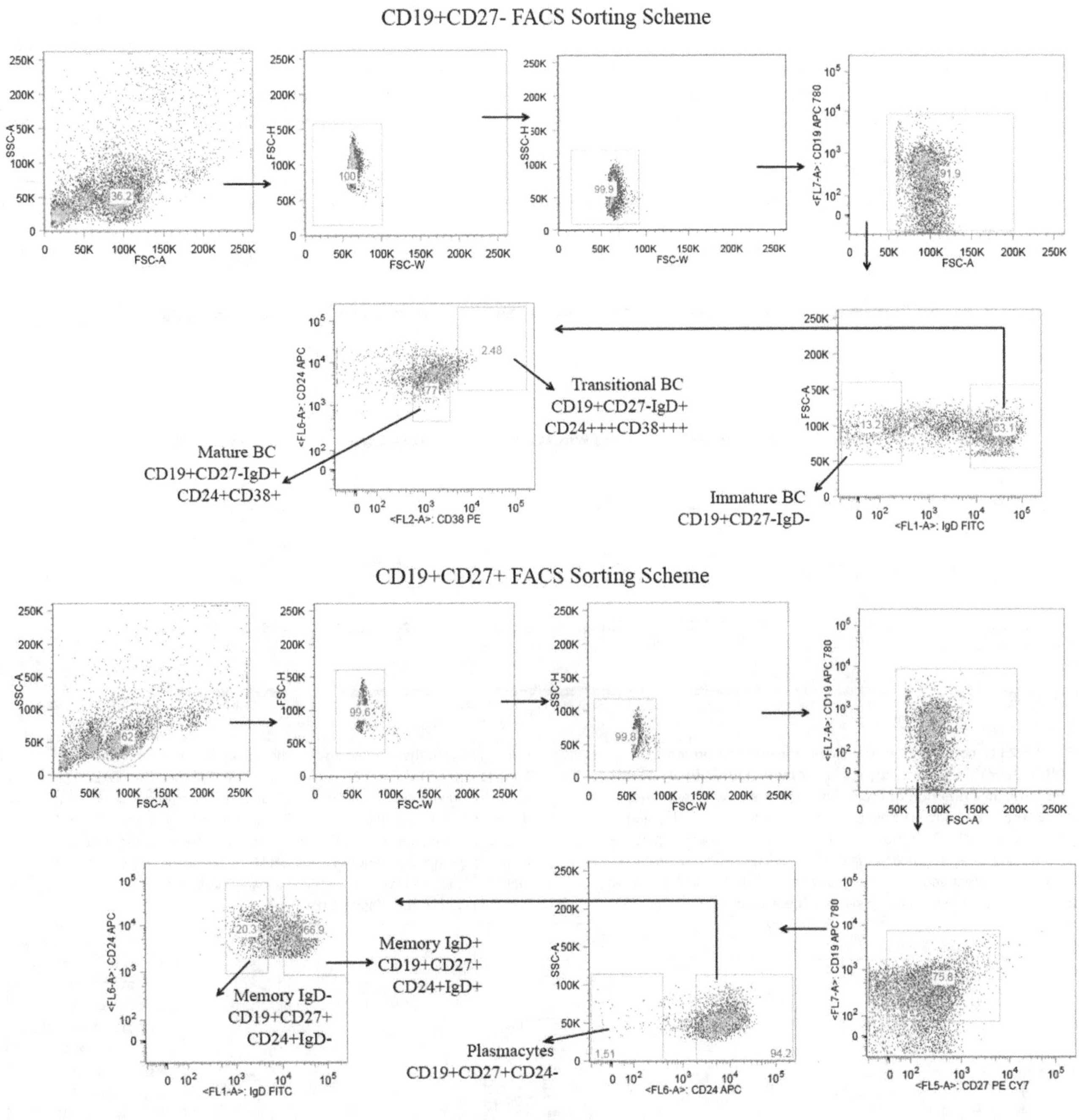

FIGURE 1 | Flow cytometric gates for the collection of six distinct B cell lineage populations from the peripheral blood of a healthy adult human subject. B cells were separated from the total lymphocytes using $CD19^+$ magnetic beads and further separated into $CD27^{\pm}$ populations using CD27 magnetic beads. The $CD19^+CD27^+$ B cells were stained with CD19 APC_{780}, CD27 PE-Cy7, CD24 APC, and IgD FITC and sorted into IgD+ memory B cells ($CD19^+/CD27^+/IgD^+/CD24^+$), IgD^- memory B cells ($CD19^+/CD27^+/IgD^-/CD24^+$), and plasmacytes ($CD19^+/CD27^+/CD24^-$) using the high speed sorting cytometer. The $CD19^+/CD27^-$ B cells were stained with CD19, APC 780, CD24 APC, CD38 PE, and IgD FITC, and sorted into mature ($CD19^+/CD27^-/IgD^+/CD38^+/CD24^+$), transitional ($CD19^+/CD27^-/IgD^+/CD38^{+++}/CD24^{+++}$), and immature ($CD19^+/CD27^-/IgD^-$) B cell subsets.

memory IgD^- and 3,347 plasmacyte reads that were of sufficient length to be identified as Igγ sequences. All of the unique Igμ and Igγ reads were deconstructed to assess the presence and extent of changes in these repertoires that had occurred as B cells progressed through the various developmental checkpoints.

THE IMMATURE B CELL RECEPTOR REPERTOIRE UTILIZES SHORTEST CONTRIBUTION OF GERMLINE GENE VJ SEGMENTS AND FAVORS V1–18, D2–15, D4–23, AND D5–12

The immature B cell subset is primarily composed of recent bone marrow emigrants. It expressed a highly diverse repertoire that differed from the subsequent transitional stage in that it contained the smallest contribution of germline V and J gene sequence to the CDR-H3 region (**Figure 2**). By family, V_H4 gene segments contributed the most, followed by V_H3, V_H1, V_H5, V_H2, and V_H6 (**Figure 3**). By individual V gene segments, V1–18, V1–69, V3–73, and V4–59 were most common. Across subsets, the immature B cell subset was enriched for V1–18, V3–30–3, and V3–74 (**Figure 4**). By D_H family, D_H3 was the most common, followed by D_H2 and D_H6 (**Figure 5**). By individual D gene segment, D2–2, D3–3, D3–22, D6–13, and D6–19 were favored. Across subsets, D1–26, D2–15, D3–10, D4–23, and D5–12 were more commonly used in the immature B cell lineage (**Figure 6**). By J_H gene segment,

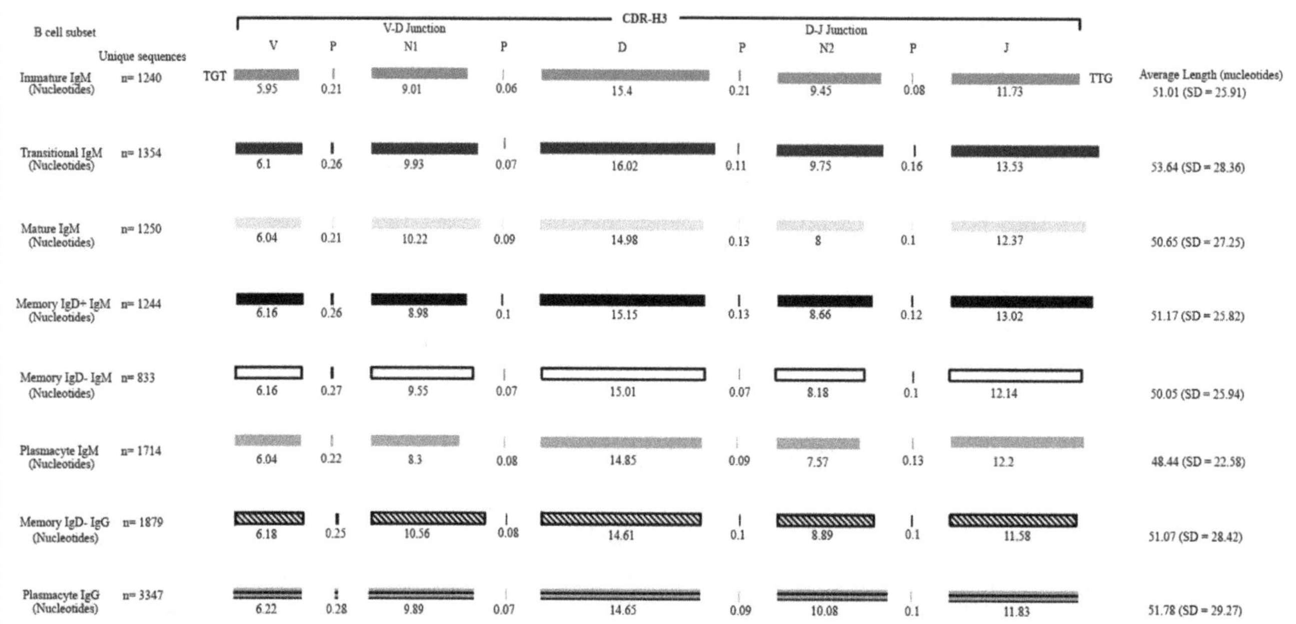

FIGURE 2 | Deconstruction of the contributing components to CDR-H3 length in Igμ and Igγ reads containing identifiable D_H gene segments as a function of B cell development in the peripheral blood. The contributions of nucleotides provided by the V_H, D_H, and J_H gene segments, by P junctions, and by the extent of N addition at the $V_H \rightarrow D_H$ and $D_H \rightarrow J_H$ junctions to the CDR-H3 length are illustrated. The IgAT (42) identified the CDR-H3 as amino acids 105–117, according to the IMGT unique numbering system. The average length was calculated with the components of the CDR-H3, namely the V length, P-nucleotides 3′ of the V, N1 nucleotides, P-nucleotides 5′ of D, D length, P-nucleotides 3′ of D, N2 nucleotides, P-nucleotides 3′ of J, and J length. The deconstructed CDR-H3 segments shown are of CDR-H3 sequences with identifiable D_H gene segments. The reported average length is the average length of all CDR-H3 sequences (with the identifiable D_H and without identifiable D_H gene segments) accompanied by the standard deviation.

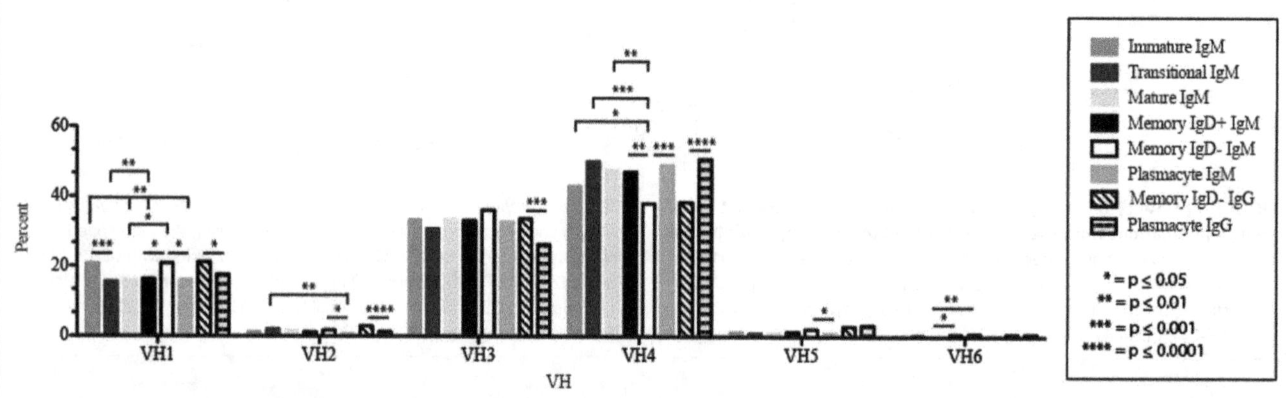

FIGURE 3 | V_H gene segment usage in Igμ and Igγ transcripts from selected B cell populations in the blood of a normal, healthy human. V_H gene segments are arranged according to their position relative to the J_H locus in the genome. Percent of unique, in-frame sequences using the V_H gene segment specified in the peripheral blood from immature, transitional, mature, memory IgD+, memory IgD− B cells, and plasmacytes are displayed. All comparisons were made using χ^2-test or Fisher's exact test as appropriate. Significant differences among each fraction in the different mice are indicated by asterisks: $*p \leq 0.05$, $**p \leq 0.01$, $***p \leq 0.001$, $****p \leq 0.0001$.

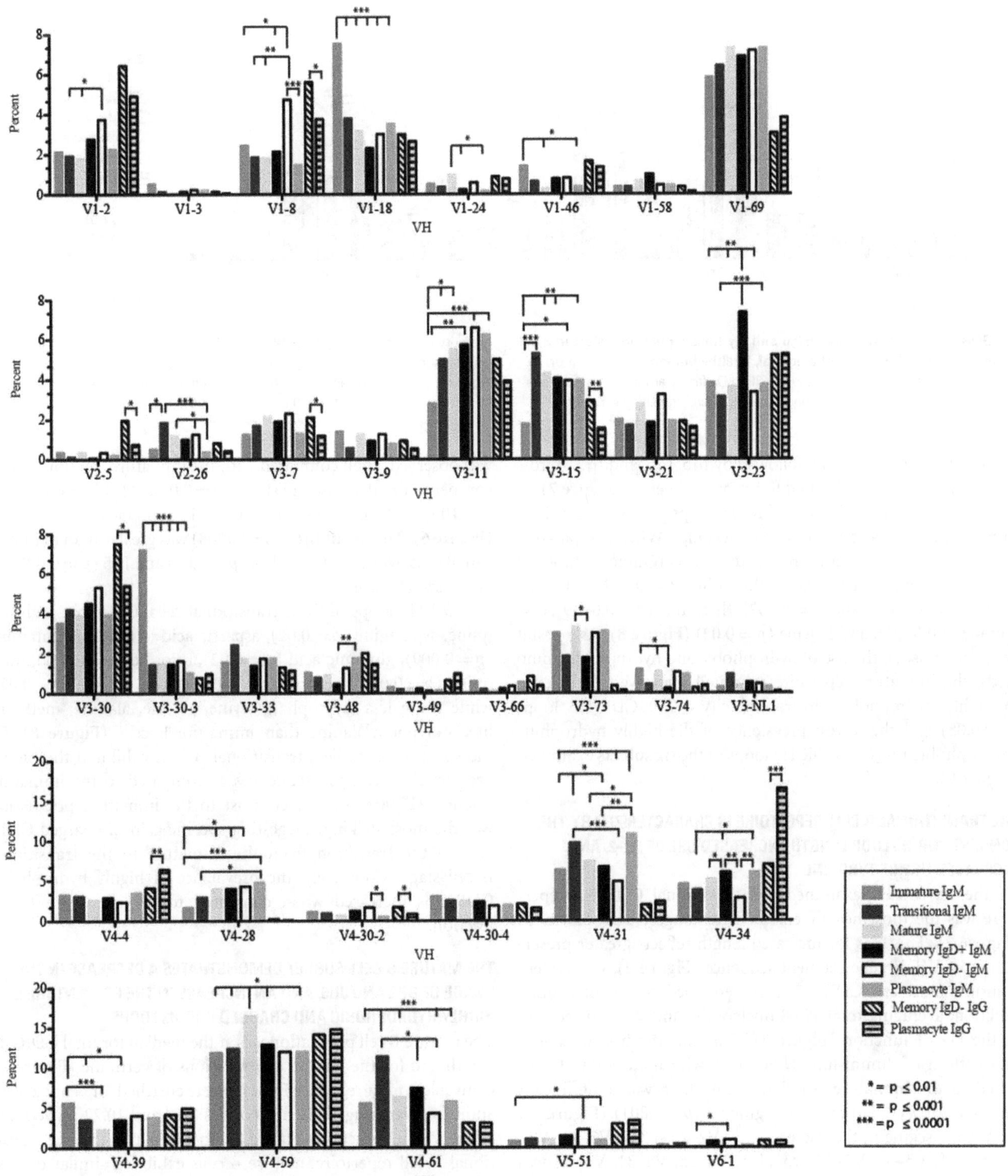

FIGURE 4 | Individual V_H gene segment usage in Igμ and Igγ transcripts from selected B cell populations in the blood of a normal, healthy human. Percent of unique, in-frame sequences using the individual V_H gene segments specified in the peripheral blood from immature, transitional, mature, memory IgD+, memory IgD− B cells, and plasmacytes are displayed. All comparisons were made using χ^2-test or Fisher's exact test as appropriate. Significant differences among each fraction in the different mice are indicated by asterisks: $*p \leq 0.01$, $**p \leq 0.001$, $***p \leq 0.0001$.

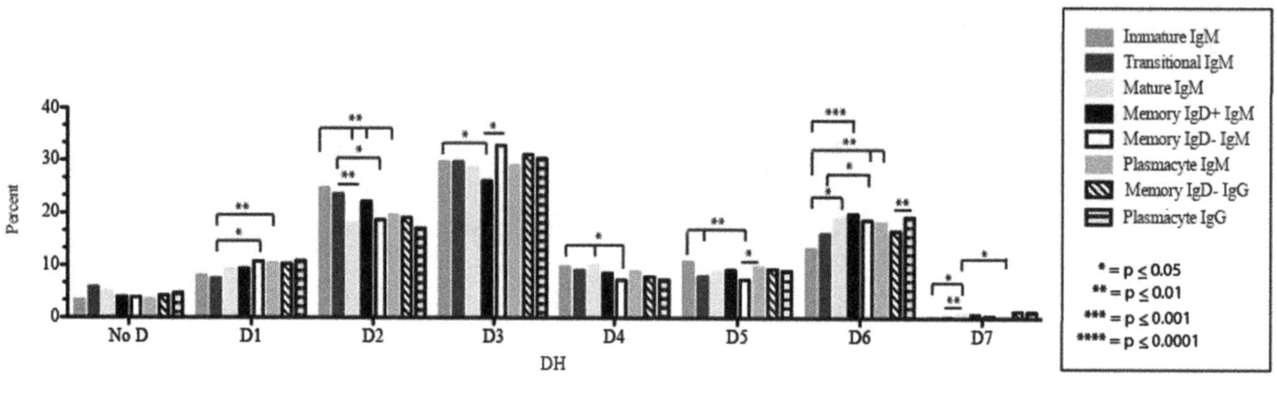

FIGURE 5 | D_H family usage in Igμ and Igγ transcripts from selected B cell populations in the blood of a normal, healthy human. The percent of sequences using members of the specified D_H family among in-frame reads obtained from the peripheral blood from immature, transitional, mature, memory IgD$^+$, memory IgD$^-$ B cells, and plasmacytes are displayed. All comparisons were made using χ^2-test or Fisher's exact test as appropriate. Significant differences among each fraction in the different mice are indicated by asterisks: *$p \leq 0.05$, **$p \leq 0.01$, ***$p \leq 0.001$, ****$p \leq 0.0001$.

J_H4 was the most common, followed by J_H6, J_H5, and J_H3. Across subsets, immature B cells used J_H5 more frequently (**Figure 7**).

Amino acid usage in the CDR-H3 loops expressed by these immature B cells varied within a narrow range. When compared to transitional cells, immature B cells used less arginine, asparagine ($p = 0.02$), aspartic acid (0.04), glutamine ($p = 0.009$), glutamic acid ($p = 0.02$), tyrosine ($p = 0.002$), threonine ($p = 0.0039$), cysteine ($p < 0.0001$), and leucine ($p = 0.02$) (**Figure 8**). As a result of the decrease in the use of hydrophobic and hydrophilic amino acids, the immature repertoire exhibited the lowest prevalence of highly hydrophobic (hydrophobicity >0.7) CDR-H3 loops ($p < 0.05$) and the lowest prevalence of the highly hydrophilic (hydrophobicity ≤0.7) CDR-H3 loops of the six subsets examined (**Figure 9**).

THE TRANSITIONAL B CELL REPERTOIRE IS CHARACTERIZED BY THE LONGEST CDR-H3 LOOP LENGTH, INCREASED USE OF D2–2, AND INCREASED USE OF TYROSINE

Of the six subsets examined, the transitional CDR-H3 repertoire was the most heavily enriched for longest CDR-H3 loops (**Figure 2**). This bias for increased length reflects greater preservation of V(D)J gene segment sequence (**Figure 2**). Conversely, transitional B cell CDR-H3s were enriched for N nucleotide addition, averaging total 19.68 nucleotides and 9.75 nucleotides at the D→J junction (**Figure 2**). This was the first in a general pattern of diminishing N addition with maturation. Compared to the immature B cell fraction, there was a significant decrease for V_H1 family gene segments ($p < 0.001$) (**Figure 3**). By V gene segment, the use of V1–69,V2–26, V3–7, V3–11, V3–15, V3–21, V3–30, V3–33, V3–NL1, V4–28, V4–31, V4–61 was greater than in immature B cells, whereas use of V1–2, V1–3, V1–8, V1–18, V1–24, V1–46, V1–58, V2–5, V3–9, V3–21, V3–23, V3–30–3, V3–48, V3–66, V3–73, V3–74, V4–34, and V4–39 was decreased (**Figure 4**). The transitional B cell CDR-H3 loop utilized higher levels of D_H6 gene segments (not significant), with lower levels of D_H5 ($p = 0.005$) than immature B cells (**Figure 5**). By D gene assignment, a significant increase in D1–1 ($p = 0.09$) and D2–2 ($p = 0.0002$) usage in transitional B cells was observed when compared with the immature fraction, with a compensatory decrease in D1–26 ($p = 0.01$), D2–15 ($p < 0.0001$), D3–10 ($p = 0.005$), D4–23 ($p = 0.0026$), and D5–12 ($p = 0.0004$) (**Figure 6**). The use of J_H6 ($p = 0.0008$) was greater than in immature B cells, while the use of J_H4 ($p = 0.01$) and J_H5 ($p = 0.09$) was decreased (**Figure 7**).

CDR-H3 loops of these transitional cells used more arginine, lysine, asparagine ($p = 0.02$), aspartic acid ($p = 0.04$), glutamine ($p = 0.009$), glutamic acid ($p = 0.02$), tyrosine ($p = 0.001$), threonine ($p = 0.003$), cysteine ($p < 0.0001$), and leucine ($p = 0.02$), while using less tryptophan, serine, glycine, alanine, methionine, and phenylalanine than immature B cells (**Figure 8**). Of the six subsets studied, transitional B cells exhibited the higher prevalence of charged sequences as compared to the immature fraction (**Figure 9**). The contrast to the immature population was the most striking, suggesting specific gain of charged CDR-H3s in the transition from the immature to the transitional B cell stage. Conversely, the prevalence of highly hydrophobic CDR-H3s increased when compared to the immature B cell fraction.

THE MATURE B CELL SUBSET DEMONSTRATES A DECREASE IN THE USAGE OF DH2 AND JH6, AND AN INCREASE IN THE PERCENTAGE OF HIGHLY HYDROPHOBIC AND CHARGED CDR-H3 LOOPS

The mature B cell population was at the median for total CDR-H3 length and for the relative contributions of germline (**Figure 2**). Conversely, mature B cell CDR-H3s were enriched for N nucleotide addition, averaging 18.22 nucleotides total and 10.22 nucleotides at the V→D junction (**Figure 2**). In comparison to the transitional B cell repertoire, mature B cells exhibited similar expression of V_H family gene usage (**Figure 3**). An increase in V4–59 ($p = 0.01$) and a decrease in the use of V4–61 ($p < 0.0001$), respectively, were observed when compared to the transitional and mature fractions (**Figure 4**). Use of the D_H2 ($p = 0.01$) family in general, and the D2–2 gene segment ($p = 0.01$) in particular, was lower than in transitional cells (**Figures 5** and **6**). There was an increase in the use of J_H1 ($p = 0.0004$) with a decrease in the use of J_H6 ($p = 0.002$) (**Figure 7**).

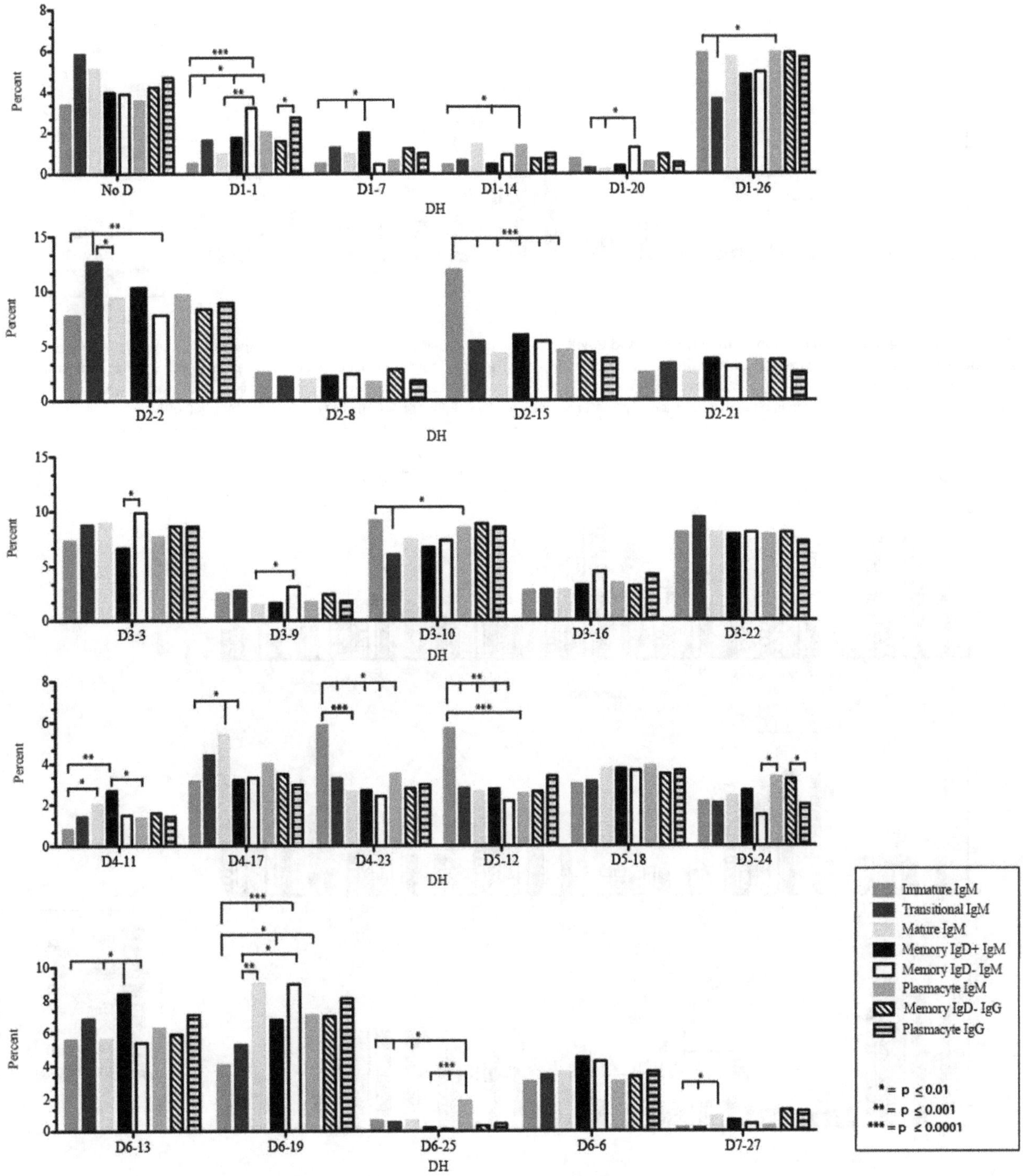

FIGURE 6 | Individual D_H gene segment usage in Igμ and Igγ transcripts from selected B cell populations in the blood of a normal, healthy human. Percent of unique, in-frame reads using the individual D_H gene segments specified in the peripheral blood from immature, transitional, mature, memory IgD^+, memory IgD^- B cells, and plasmacytes are displayed. All comparisons were made using χ^2-test or Fisher's exact test as appropriate. Significant differences among each fraction in the different mice are indicated by asterisks: $*p \leq 0.01$, $**p \leq 0.001$, $***p \leq 0.0001$.

CDR-H3 loops demonstrated an increase in the use of glutamine ($p = 0.007$), with a decrease in tyrosine ($p = < 0.0001$), cysteine ($p = 0.0001$), and valine ($p = 0.04$) (**Figure 8**). As a result, the mature B cell repertoire was enriched for the use of hydrophobic and charged CDR-H3 loops when compared with immature and transitional subsets (**Figure 9**).

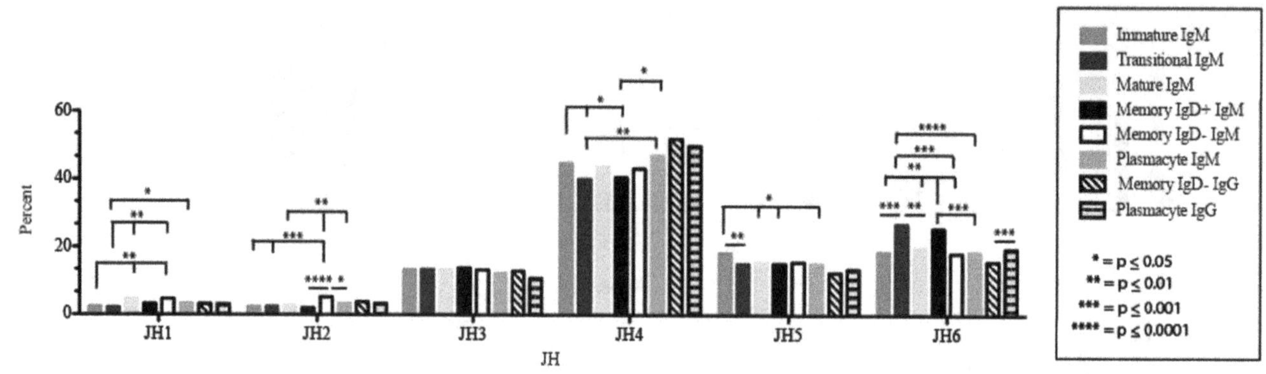

FIGURE 7 | J_H usage in Igμ and Igγ transcripts from selected B cell populations in the blood of a normal, healthy human. The percent of sequences using J_H1 through J_H6 among in-frame reads cloned from the peripheral blood from immature, transitional, mature, memory IgD+, memory IgD− B cells, and plasmacytes are displayed. All comparisons were made using χ^2-test or Fisher's exact test as appropriate. Significant differences among each fraction in the different mice are indicated by asterisks: $*p \leq 0.05$, $**p \leq 0.01$, $***p \leq 0.001$, $****p \leq 0.0001$.

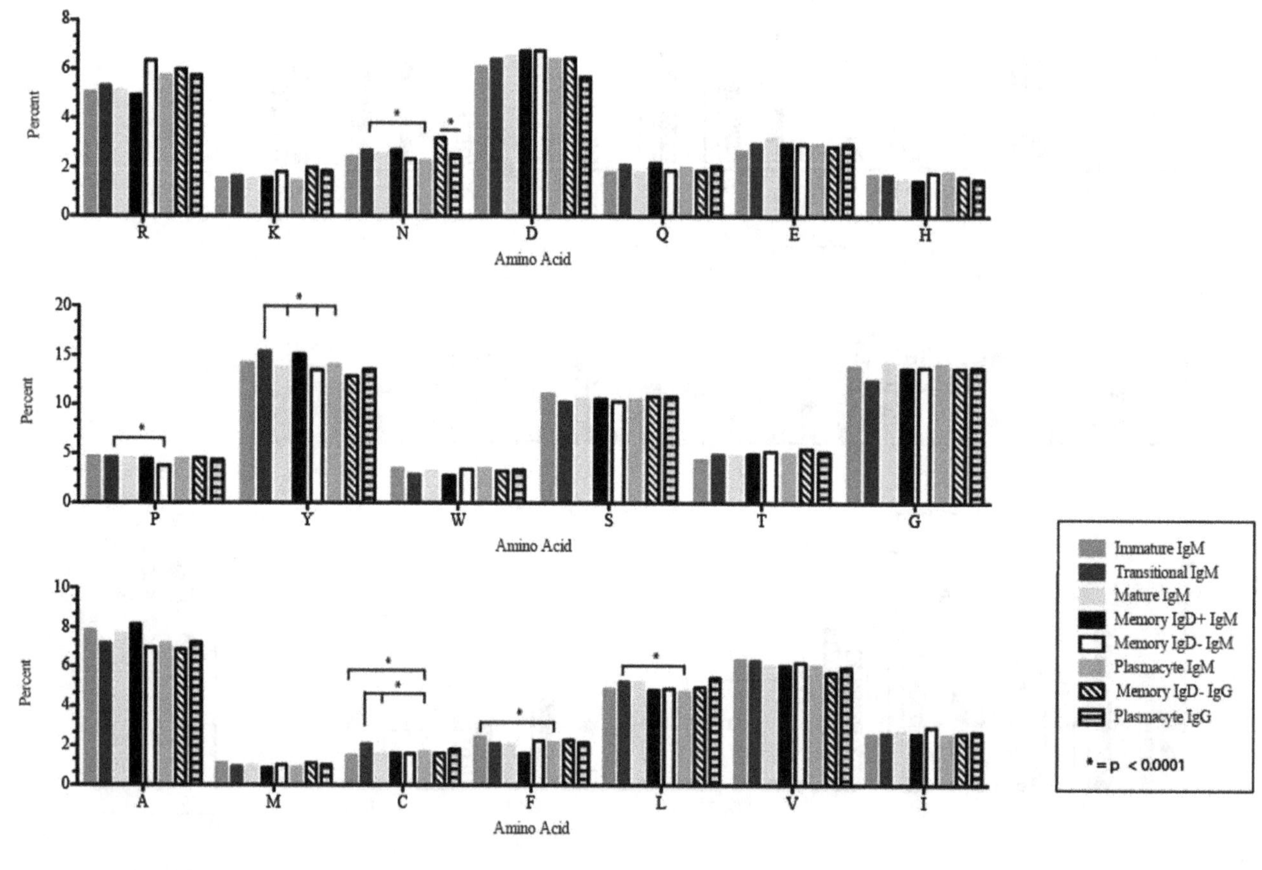

FIGURE 8 | Amino acid usage in the CDR-H3 loop of Igμ and Igγ transcripts from selected B cell populations in the blood of a normal, healthy human. The distribution of individual amino acids is displayed. All comparisons were made using χ^2-test or Fisher's exact test as appropriate. Significant differences among each fraction in the different mice are indicated by asterisk: $*p < 0.0001$.

MEMORY IgD+ AND IgD− B CELLS DISPLAY DIVERGENT Igμ REPERTOIRES

The Igμ repertoires of the memory IgD+ and memory IgD− blood B cells were distinguishable and divergent from both mature B cells and from each other. The memory IgD+B cell CDR-H3 region exhibited a greater contribution of germline D_H and J_H gene sequences than memory IgD− (**Figure 2**). Memory IgD+ B cells used V_H4 ($p = 0.008$) family gene segments more frequently than

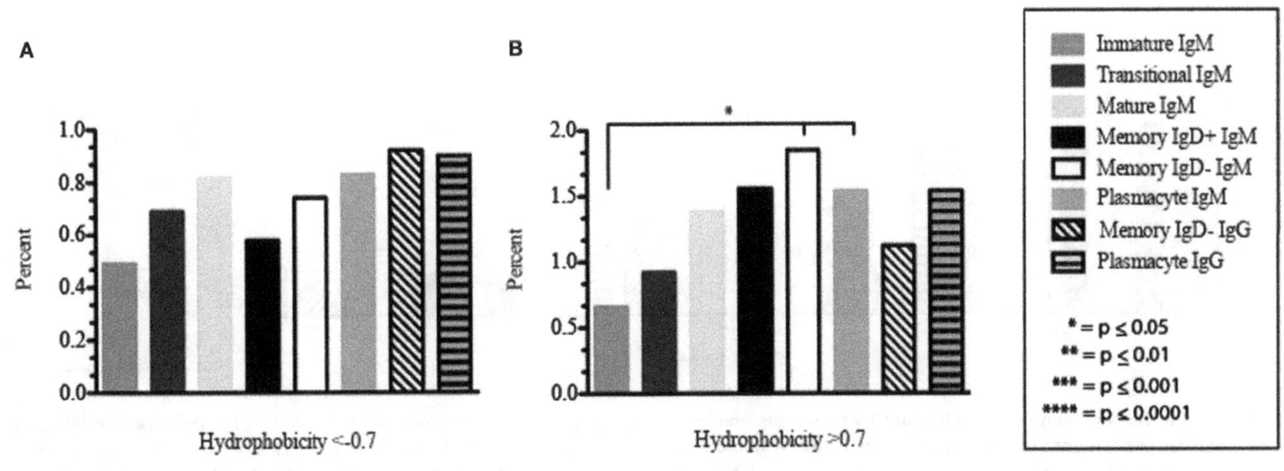

FIGURE 9 | The prevalence of highly charged and highly hydrophobic CDR-H3 loops of Igμ and Igγ transcripts from selected B cell populations in the blood of a normal, healthy human. (A) Prevalence of CDR-H3 loops with an average hydrophobicity of ≤0.7 is displayed. **(B)** Prevalence of CDR-H3 loops with an average hydrophobicity of >0.7 is displayed. The normalized Kyte–Doolittle hydrophobicity scale (48) and normalized by Eisenberg (49) has been used to calculate average hydrophobicity (23). Prevalence is reported as the percent of the sequenced population of unique, in-frame, open transcripts from each B lineage fraction. All comparisons were made using χ^2-test or Fisher's exact test as appropriate. Significant differences among each fraction in the different mice are indicated by asterisks: *$p \leq 0.05$, **$p \leq 0.01$, ***$p \leq 0.001$, ****$p \leq 0.0001$.

memory IgD$^-$ B cells, and V_H1 ($p = 0.03$) family gene segments less frequently. The memory IgD$^-$ B cells used V_H1 ($p = 0.03$) gene segments more frequently and V_H4 ($p = 0.03$) gene segments less frequently than mature B cells (**Figure 3**). By individual gene V_H gene segment, the most prominent differences between memory IgD$^+$and IgD$^-$ reflected increased use of V3–23 ($p = 0.0003$), V4–34 ($p = 0.001$), V4–61 ($p = 0.004$) in the former, and decreased use of V1–8 ($p = 0.002$) and V4–74 ($p = 0.02$) in the latter ($p < 0.0001$) (**Figure 4**), with the exception of V4–31 ($p = 0.02$, memory IgD$^-$) and V4–59 ($p = 0.02$, memory IgD$^+$ and $p = 0.01$, memory IgD$^-$), which was increased among mature B cells (**Figure 4**).

Igμ from memory IgD$^+$ B cells used D3 ($p = 0.01$) family D_H gene segments less frequently than memory IgD$^-$ cells (**Figure 5**). When compared with mature B cells, the memory IgD$^+$ Igμ repertoire also used D2 and family D_H gene segments more frequently and D3 family D_H gene segments less frequently (not significant). Finally, memory IgD$^-$ B cells appeared to use D3 family D_H gene segments more frequently than mature B cells, although this preference did not achieve statistical significance. By individual D_H gene segment, the memory IgD$^+$ Igμ repertoire displayed increased use of D6–13 ($p = 0.01$); and a decrease in use of D3–3 ($p = 0.01$) (**Figure 6**). Divergent usage of J_H2 and J_H6 was also observed (**Figure 7**). The memory IgD$^+$ Igμ repertoire used J_H6 more frequently than the memory IgD$^-$ ($p = 0.001$) or mature B cell Igμ repertoire ($p = 0.009$); and J_H2 ($p < 0.0001$) less frequently than memory IgD$^-$. J_H usage in the memory IgD$^-$ Igμ repertoire was very similar to that observed in mature B cells, with the exception of an increase in memory IgD$^-$ J_H2 usage as compared to the mature B cells ($p = 0.007$) (**Figure 7**).

The CDR-H3 loop of the memory IgD$^+$ B Igμ repertoire contained more proline ($p = 0.01$), tyrosine ($p = 0.01$), and alanine ($p = 0.005$); but less arginine ($p = 0.001$), and tryptophan ($p = 0.04$) than memory IgD$^-$ B cells (**Figure 8**). The increase in tyrosine reflected increased use of J_H6, rather than increased use of reading frame 1. Indeed, use of reading frame 1, 2, and 3 were similar between the memory fractions (**Figure 10**). When compared to mature B cells, the memory IgD$^+$ Igμ repertoire was similarly enriched for glutamine ($p = 0.02$) and tyrosine ($p = 0.03$), and depleted of phenylalanine ($p = 0.01$). The memory IgD$^-$ Igμ repertoire also contained more arginine ($p = 0.005$) and less proline ($p = 0.01$) than the mature B cell Igμ repertoire. The memory IgD$^-$ Igμ repertoire relatively contained a higher percentage of highly charged CDR-H3s (hydrophobicity >0.7) (1.85%) when compared to the Igμ repertoires of subsequent B cell fractions (**Figure 9**).

THE PLASMACYTE Igμ REPERTOIRE DIVERGED FROM BOTH THE MEMORY IgD$^+$ AND IgD$^-$ Igμ REPERTOIRE, AS WELL AS FROM THE MATURE B CELL Igμ REPERTOIRE

In comparison to the other Igμ and Igγ repertoires, the CDR-H3 component of the plasmacyte Igμ repertoire exhibited the fewest N nucleotides at both the V → D and D → J junctions, respectively. As a result, not only the Igμ repertoire relatively enriched for germline V(D)J sequence, but also exhibited the shortest average length (**Figure 2**).

By V_H family, plasmacytes exhibited higher usage of V_H4 than either memory B cell population, and lower usage of V_H2, V_H3, and V_H5 (**Figure 3**). These differences were most affected by increased use of V4–34 ($p = 0.007$, $p < 0.0001$) when compared to both the memory IgD$^-$ and IgD$^+$Igμ repertoires and decreased use of V5–51 ($p = 0.01$) when compared to the memory IgD$^-$ Igμ repertoire (**Figure 4**).

The distribution of D_H gene family usage among the plasmacyte Igμ repertoire was similar to that of the mature B cell Igμ repertoire, but differed for individual families with the two memory B cell Igμ repertoires. There were no statistically significant

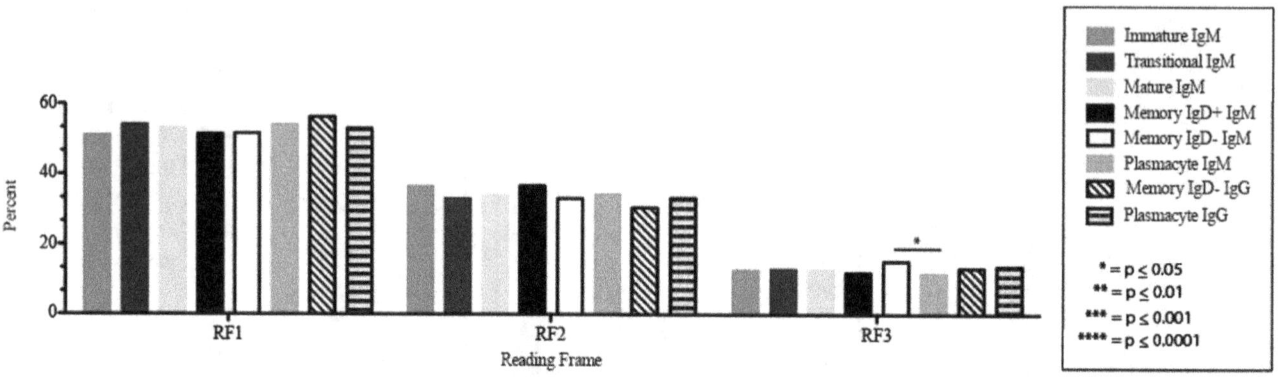

FIGURE 10 | D_H reading frame usage in Igμ and Igγ transcripts from selected B cell populations in the blood of a normal, healthy human. The percent of sequences using members of the specified D_H family members in reading frames 1, 2, or 3 among in-frame sequences cloned from the peripheral blood from immature B cells through plasmacytes are displayed. All comparisons were made using χ^2-test or Fisher's exact test as appropriate. Significant differences among each fraction in the different mice are indicated by asterisks: $*p \leq 0.05$, $**p \leq 0.01$, $***p \leq 0.001$, $****p \leq 0.0001$.

differences in the use of D_H gene segments between the memory IgD^+ and the plasmacyte Igμ repertoires. When compared to the memory IgD^- Igμ repertoire, the plasmacyte Igμ repertoire used D_H5 gene segments more frequently ($p = 0.04$) (**Figure 5**). By individual D_H gene segment, plasmacytes used D6–25 more frequently ($p = 0.006$) and D7–27 less frequently ($p = 0.03$) than mature B cells. Plasmacytes used D6–25 more frequently ($p < 0.0001$), and D4–11 ($p = 0.01$), D6–13 ($p = 0.04$), and D6–6 ($p = 0.03$) less frequently than the IgD^+ memory Igμ repertoire. Finally, plasmacytes used D5–24 ($p = 0.007$) and D6–25 ($p = 0.0001$) more frequently, and D3–9 ($p = 0.03$) less frequently than the memory IgD^- Igμ repertoire (**Figure 6**).

By J_H gene segment, the plasmacyte Igμ repertoire displayed similar levels of J gene segments when compared to the mature B cell Igμ repertoire. Plasmacytes expressed higher levels of J_H2 ($p = 0.01$), J_H4 ($p = 0.01$); and lower levels of J_H6 than memory IgD^+ B cells ($p = 0.0004$). Finally, plasmacytes expressed lower levels of J_H2 ($p = 0.04$) than memory IgD^- B cells (**Figure 7**).

When compared with the mature B cell Igμ repertoire, plasmacytes expressed lower levels of asparagine ($p = 0.02$), alanine ($p = 0.01$), and leucine ($p = 0.007$) in the CDR-H3 loop. When compared with memory IgD^+ B cells, plasmacytes expressed lower levels of asparagine ($p = 0.001$), aspartic acid ($p = 0.02$), glutamine ($p = 0.04$), tyrosine ($p = 0.001$), and alanine ($p = 0.0002$); and higher levels of tryptophan ($p = 0.02$) and phenylalanine ($p = 0.01$). When compared with the memory IgD^- Igμ repertoire, plasmacytes expressed lower levels of arginine ($p = 0.02$), lysine ($p = 0.009$), and isoleucine ($p = 0.02$) (**Figure 8**).

When comparing the relative prevalence of either highly charged or highly hydrophobic CDR-H3 loops, plasmacytes were enriched for charged CDR-H3 loops (0.84%) in comparison to the five other Igμ repertoires (**Figures 9** and **11**). The distribution of highly hydrophobic CDR-H3 loops decreased in plasmacytes (1.54%) as compared to memory IgD^- B cells (1.85%), and returned to the comparable levels of memory IgD^+ B cells (1.56%) (**Figure 9**).

THE PLASMACYTE Igγ REPERTOIRE DIVERGED FROM IgD^- IgD^+ MEMORY B CELLS

The *Igγ* repertoires expressed by memory IgD^- B cells and plasmacytes were distinguishable and uniquely different from each other. While the average length and V(D)J gene segment length was very similar between the memory IgD^- and plasmacytes, differences in the N-region additions were observed. The memory IgD^- B cell CDR-H3 region exhibited a greater number of N nucleotide addition at the V-D junction (10.56 nucleotides) as compared to the plasmacytes. Conversely, plasmacytes contained more N nucleotide addition at the D–J junction than memory IgD^- B cells (10.08 nucleotides) (**Figure 2**). Memory IgD^- B cells used V_H1 ($p = 0.03$), V_H2 ($p = 0.0001$), and V_H3 ($p = 0.0003$) family gene segments more frequently than plasmacyte; and V_H4 ($p < 0.0001$) family gene segments less frequently (**Figure 3**). This pattern is due to an increase in individual gene V_H gene segment, the most prominent differences between memory IgD^- and plasmacytes reflected increased use of V1–2 ($p = 0.03$), V1–8 ($p = 0.003$), V2–5 ($p = 0.0003$), V3–7 ($p = 0.01$), V3–15 ($p = 0.001$), V3–30 ($p = 0.005$), and V4–40–2 ($p = 0.01$), in the former, and decreased use of V4–4 ($p = 0.0007$) and V4–34 ($p < 0.0001$) in the latter (**Figure 4**).

The memory IgD^- Igγ repertoire used D6 ($p = 0.01$) family D_H gene segments less frequently than plasmacyte Igγ (**Figure 5**). By individual D_H gene segment, the memory IgD^- Igγ repertoire displayed increased use of D5–24 ($p = 0.005$) and decreased use of D2–21 ($p = 0.03$) (**Figure 6**). The memory IgD^- Igγ repertoire used J_H6 less frequently than plasmacytes ($p = 0.0006$) (**Figure 7**).

The CDR-H3 loop of the memory IgD^- Igγ repertoire contained more asparagine ($p < 0.0001$) and aspartic acid ($p = 0.01$); but less tyrosine ($p = 0.04$), cysteine ($p = 0.03$), and leucine ($p = 0.01$) than plasmacyte Igγ (**Figure 8**). The plasmacyte Igγ repertoire was relatively enriched for hydrophobic amino acids, which was reflected by a higher percentage of hydrophobic CDR-H3s (hydrophobicity > 0.7) (1.54%) when compared to the memory IgD^- (1.12%) (**Figure 9**).

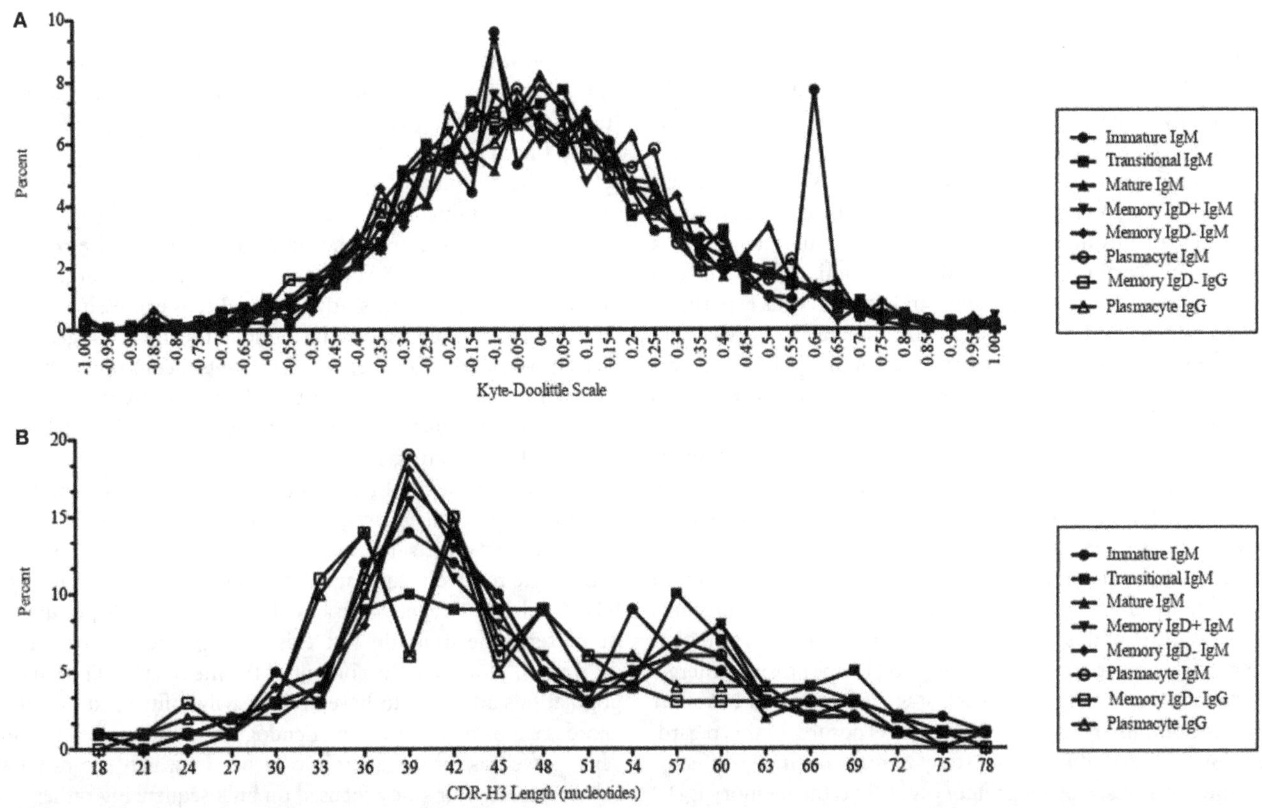

FIGURE 11 | CDR-H3 loop charge and length as a function of B cell development in the peripheral blood of this adult subject. (A) Distribution of CDR-H3 hydrophobicities in Igμ and Igγ transcripts from peripheral blood as a function of B cell development. The Kyte–Doolittle hydrophobicity scale (48) as normalized by Esienberg (49) has been used to calculate average hydrophobicity (30). Although this scale ranges from −1.3 to +1.7, only the range from −1.0 (charged) to +1.0 (hydrophobic) is shown. Prevalence is reported as the percent of the sequenced population of unique, in-frame, open transcripts from each B lineage fraction. **(B)** Distribution of CDR-H3 lengths in nucleotides of μ and γ H chain transcripts is displayed.

The Igμ and Igγ repertoires of analyzed cell types expressed similar distribution of D_H reading frames, with reading frame 1 having greatest preference, followed by reading frame 2 and reading frame 3 (**Figure 10**), while the μH chain plasmacytes used reading frame 3 less likely than memory IgD^- B cells ($p = 0.03$) (**Figure 10**).

DISCUSSION

In both mice and humans, the composition of the antibody repertoire varies by ontogeny and by developmental stage (29, 37, 50). In order to study this process in detail, we developed a series of tools to evaluate the development of the repertoire in mice. This approach enabled us to identify constraints on V(D)J gene segment preference and CDR-H3 composition that are first established in early B cell progenitors, and then focused as the B lineage cells pass through various developmental checkpoints. The constraints are a reflection of the specific sequence from the contributing gene segments that vary in usage as a function of development (29, 30, 51–55).

Differences in the individual V–D–J gene usage, length, and amino acid composition of the adult human germline repertoires from peripheral blood and specific tissues have been previously reported (37, 50, 56–62), but comparative studies of repertoire development in human blood have been sparse. The difficulty of study is compounded by the enhanced variability of the human repertoire when compared to mice, especially in CDR-H3. This reflects both a greater diversity of the germline sequence of the D_H gene segment sequences and an increase in the extent of N addition when compared to mouse. In this work, we sought to use the same tools we had developed for the study of the mouse repertoire to perform a comparative analysis of the expressed in both the Igμ and Igγ repertoires in the blood of a normal, healthy human female in order to gain insight into the forces that shape the repertoire during its passage through the different stages of B cell ontogeny.

While similarities have been reported between the frequency of naïve and memory B cell repertoire usage of the V–D–J gene segments (58, 61, 62), our analysis focuses on a more detailed examination of the repertoires. Our results of low J_H1 and J_H2 usage across B cell development is consistent with previous published reports of low J_H1 and J_H2 usage in transitional, naïve, switched, and IgM memory B cell repertoires (**Figure 7**) (61). Altered expression of individual V_H gene segments have been previously also reported in the transitional, naïve, switched, and IgM memory B cell antibody repertoires (61). As in mice, we found changes in V(D)J gene segment usage and CDR-H3 hydrophobicity in the progression from immature to transitional to mature (**Figures 3**, **5**, **7**, **9**, and **11**). These observations support the view that the B cell receptor repertoire continues to be selected throughout early and late B cell development in the peripheral blood. Unlike mice, however, the prevalence of highly charged CDR-H3 loops increased during maturation from the immature to mature cell subsets and memory IgD^- to plasmacyte subsets (**Figure 9**). Also unlike mice, the prevalence of highly hydrophobic CDR-H3 loops also increased in our human study subject. This may reflect a greater tolerance or preference for the use of amino acids encoded by hydrophobic D_H reading frame 2 in human B cells exposed to self and non-self antigens (35%) when compared to mice (10%), or a property specific to this particular individual, since patterns of regulation have been shown to differ in mouse strains (**Figure 10**) (34, 63).

We observed a decrease in the length of CDR-H3 during maturation (**Figures 2** and **11**). This appears to be part of a continuum of focusing CDR-H3 length in developing B cells in the bone marrow (50) and has been observed by others, as well (61). The use of long CDR-H3 loops has been previously associated with enhanced autoreactivity and polyreactivity (38, 64–66), which are presumably the features of this component of the antibody repertoire that somatic selection are designed to minimize by apoptosis or anergy.

Selection past the mature B cell stage is considered to reflect both endogenous and exogenous antigen exposure. In this regard, the most striking findings of our study were the distinctly different repertoires expressed by the memory $IgD^+Ig\mu$, the memory IgD^- $Ig\mu$, and $Ig\gamma$ repertoires; and the plasmacyte $Ig\mu$ and $Ig\gamma$ repertoires. We did not sort memory B cells or plasmacytes by $Ig\mu$ or $Ig\gamma$ expression, but were able to identify unique $Ig\mu$ or $Ig\gamma$ reads through the use of $Ig\mu$ and $Ig\gamma$ specific primers.

The memory IgD^+ and memory IgD^- $Ig\mu$ repertoires displayed differences in virtually all of the features of the repertoire that we evaluated, including V(D)J usage, N addition, D_H reading frame usage, CDR-H3 length, CDR-H3 loop amino acid content, and CDR-H3 hydrophobicity (**Figures 3–11**). Differences in IgD^+ and IgD^- $Ig\mu$ repertoires in V_H1 gene family usage ($p = 0.03$) (**Figure 3**) have been reported previously (61). We observed a similar decrease in usage of V_H3–23 ($p = 0.0003$) between the memory IgD^+ and memory IgD^- $Ig\mu$ repertoires (**Figure 4**) (61). Differences between these two memory $Ig\mu$ repertoires were further enhanced by altered amino acid usage, especially an increase in arginine ($p = 0.001$) and decrease of tyrosine ($p = 0.01$) in the memory IgD^- $Ig\mu$ cell subset as compared to the memory IgD^+ $Ig\mu$ cell subset (**Figure 8**) (61). The memory IgD^- $Ig\mu$ repertoire exhibited enhanced use of charged amino acids and hydrophobic amino acids (**Figure 8**). As a result, there was a higher percentage of CDR-H3s with excess charge when compared to the memory IgD^+ $Ig\mu$ repertoire (**Figure 9**). These observations are consistent with a previous report showing that IgD^+ memory cells had levels of negatively charged amino acids comparable to transitional and naïve B cells, while switched memory had more negatively charged residues (**Figures 8** and **9**) (61).

The vast majority of the IgD^+ memory B cell pool also expresses IgM, whereas the IgD^- pool expresses class-switched Ig in addition to IgM. Memory B cells expressing both IgM and IgD are considered to be the circulating equivalents of the marginal zone B cell subset in mice; whereas memory B cells restricted to IgM production are considered to represent the more conventional B cell pool, which also is the primary source for class-switched B cells. Thus, our observations regarding the differences in repertoire between the IgD^+ and IgD^- memory B cell pools fit well within the view that the IgM^+IgD^+ and IgM^+IgD^- memory subsets are the products of very different immune responses. In this regard, the marginal zone-like repertoire expressed by our female study subject diverges from the marginal zone repertoire expressed in BALB/c mice in that BALB/c appears tolerant for charged CDR-H3s (35), whereas in our study subject B cells expressing charged CDR-H3s were more likely to be found in the memory IgD^- population. Whether this difference represents a common difference between human and mouse, or reflects variation within the outbred human population is unclear and will require analysis of additional study subjects.

The plasmacyte pool represents the products of recently activated mature B cells as well as memory IgD^+ and IgD^- B cells that have been reactivated. This observation may explain why the plasmacyte repertoire appears intermediate between the memory IgD^+ and IgD^- repertoires and the mature B cell population. At present, the tools do not exist to separate plasmacytes by derivation. Moreover, the content of the memory and plasmacyte populations are likely to have been heavily influenced by several decades exposure to a variety of endogenous and exogenous antigens as well as by the anatomic niches in which the disparate subsets reside. Our study focused on bulk sequencing rather than analysis of repertoire in cells that were isolated by specific antigen reactivity, thus we cannot define the precise nature of the response to specific antigens. However, the most striking difference between the plasmacyte population and the other subsets in bulk was the decrease in the contribution of N nucleotides to the final product. Coupled with the observation that the greatest contribution of non-germline encoded nucleotides among the six subsets studied was found in the immature B cell fraction, final enrichment for germline V(D)J sequence among plasmacytes supports the view that the germline V domain repertoire has been selected by evolution for maximal advantage in responding to antigen (34–36).

As in mouse, the repertoires expressed by distinct B cell subset appear to differ in human. Sequencing of unsorted B cells from the blood is thus likely to yield an incomplete view of what is actually happening in the immune response of the individual. Our findings support the view that determination of whether diseases of immune function reflect abnormal regulation of these various B cell subsets will require considerable effort to perform deep sequencing of sorted cells from a variety of healthy individuals and patients with immune-mediated disorders (14, 38).

ACKNOWLEDGMENTS

This work was supported in part by AI090902 and AI007051.

REFERENCES

1. Hozumi N, Tonegawa S. Evidence for somatic rearrangement of immunoglobulin genes coding for variable and constant regions. *Proc Nat Acad Sci U S A* (1976) **73**:3628–32. doi:10.1073/pnas.73.10.3628
2. Tonegawa S. Somatic generation of antibody diversity. *Nature* (1983) **302**:575–81. doi:10.1038/302575a0

3. Yancopoulos GD, Desiderio SV, Paskind M, Kearney JF, Baltimore D, Alt FW. Preferential utilization of the most JH-proximal VH gene segments in pre-B cell lines. *Nature* (1984) **311**:727–33. doi:10.1038/311727a0
4. Alt FW, Baltimore D. Joining of immunoglobulin heavy chain gene segments: implications from a chromosome with evidence of three D-J heavy fusions. *Proc Natl Acad Sci U S A* (1982) **79**:4118–22. doi:10.1073/pnas.79.13.4118
5. Rajewsky K. Clonal selection and learning in the antibody system. *Nature* (1996) **381**:751–8. doi:10.1038/381751a0
6. Kabat EA, Wu TT. Identical V region amino acid sequences and segments of sequences in antibodies of different specificities: relative contributions of VH and VL genes, minigenes, and complementarity-determining regions to binding of antibody-combining sites. *J Immunol* (1991) **147**:1709–19.
7. Padlan EA. Anatomy of the antibody molecule. *Mol Immunol* (1994) **31**:169–217. doi:10.1016/0161-5890(94)90001-9
8. Xu JL, Davis MM. Diversity in the CDR3 region of V(H) is sufficient for most antibody specificities. *Immunity* (2000) **13**:37–45. doi:10.1016/S1074-7613(00)00006-6
9. Burrows PD, Stephan RP, Wang YH, Lassoued K, Zhang Z, Cooper MD. The transient expression of pre-B cell receptors governs B cell development. *Semin Immunol* (2002) **14**:343–9. doi:10.1016/S1044-5323(02)00067-2
10. Hardy RR, Hayakawa K. B cell development pathways. *Annu Rev Immunol* (2001) **19**:595–621. doi:10.1146/annurev.immunol.19.1.595
11. Keyna U, Beck-Engeser GB, Jongstra J, Applequist SE, Jack HM. Surrogate light chain-dependent selection of Ig heavy chain V regions. *J Immunol* (1995) **155**:5536–42.
12. Kline GH, Hartwell L, Beck-Engeser GB, Keyna U, Zaharevitz S, Klinman NR, et al. Pre-B cell receptor-mediated selection of pre-B cells synthesizing functional mu heavy chains. *J Immunol* (1998) **161**:1608–18.
13. Martin DA, Bradl H, Collins TJ, Roth E, Jack HM, Wu GE. Selection of Ig mu heavy chains by complementarity-determining region 3 length and amino acid composition. *J Immunol* (2003) **171**:4663–71.
14. Meffre E, Casellas R, Nussenzweig MC. Antibody regulation of B cell development. *Nat Immunol* (2000) **1**:379–85. doi:10.1038/80816
15. Kraus M, Alimzhanov MB, Rajewsky N, Rajewsky K. Survival of resting mature B lymphocytes depends on BCR signaling via the Ig α/β heterodimer. *Cell* (2004) **117**:787–800. doi:10.1016/j.cell.2004.05.014
16. Zikherman J, Parameswaran R, Weiss A. Endogenous antigen tunes the responsiveness of naive B cells but not T cells. *Nature* (2012) **489**:160–4. doi:10.1038/nature11311
17. Loder F, Mutschler B, Ray RJ, Paige CJ, Sideras P, Torres R, et al. B cell development in the spleen takes place in discrete steps and is determined by the quality of B cell receptor-derived signals. *J Exp Med* (1999) **190**:75–89. doi:10.1084/jem.190.1.75
18. Liu YJ, Zhang J, Lane PJ, Chan EY, MacLennan IC. Sites of specific B cell activation in primary and secondary responses to T cell-dependent and T cell-independent antigens. *Eur J Immunol* (1991) **21**:2951–62. doi:10.1002/eji.1830211209
19. Jacob J, Kassir R, Kelsoe G. In situ studies of the primary immune response to (4-hydroxy-3-nitrophenyl)acetyl. I. The architecture and dynamics of responding cell populations. *J Exp Med* (1991) **173**:1165–75. doi:10.1084/jem.173.5.1165
20. Garside P, Ingulli E, Merica RR, Johnson JG, Noelle RJ, Jenkins MK. Visualization of specific B and T lymphocyte interactions in the lymph node. *Science* (1998) **281**:96–9. doi:10.1126/science.281.5373.96
21. Jacob J, Kelsoe G. In situ studies of the primary immune response to (4-hydroxy-3-nitrophenyl)acetyl. II. A common clonal origin for periarteriolar lymphoid sheath-associated foci and germinal centers. *J Exp Med* (1992) **176**:679–687. doi:10.1084/jem.176.3.679
22. Klein U, Küppers R, Rajewsky K. Evidence for a large compartment of IgM-expressing memory B cells in humans. *Blood* (1997) **89**:1288–98.
23. Klein U, Rajewsky K, Küppers R. Human immunoglobulin (Ig)M+ IgD+ peripheral blood B cells expressing the CD27 cell surface antigen carry somatically mutated variable region genes: CD27 as a general marker for somatically mutated (memory) B cells. *J Exp Med* (1998) **188**:1679–89. doi:10.1084/jem.188.9.1679
24. Tangye SG, Liu YJ, Aversa G, Phillips JH, de Vries JE. Identification of functional human splenic memory B cells by expression of CD148 and CD27. *J Exp Med* (1998) **188**:1691–703. doi:10.1084/jem.188.9.1691
25. Shi Y, Agematsu K, Ochs HD, Sugane K. Functional analysis of human memory B-cell subpopulations: IgD+ CD27+ B cells are crucial in secondary immune response by producing high affinity IgM. *Clin Immunol* (2003) **108**:128–37. doi:10.1016/S1521-6616(03)00092-5
26. Paus D, Pham RG, Chan TD, Gardam S, Basten A, Brink R. Antigen recognition strength regulates the choice between extrafollicular plasma cell and germinal center B cell differentiation. *J Exp Med* (2006) **203**:1081–91. doi:10.1084/jem.20060087
27. Berek C, Berger A, Apel M. Maturation of the immune response in germinal centers. *Cell* (1991) **67**:1121–9. doi:10.1016/0092-8674(91)90289-B
28. Dal Porto JM, Haberman AM, Shlomchik MJ, Kelsoe G. Antigen drives very low affinity B cells to become plasmacytes and enter germinal centers. *J Immunol* (1998) **161**:5373–81.
29. Schroeder HW Jr, Ippolito GC, Shiokawa S. Regulation of the antibody repertoire through control of HCDR3 diversity. *Vaccine* (1998) **16**:1383–90. doi:10.1016/S0264-410X(98)00096-6
30. Ippolito GC, Schelonka RL, Zemlin M, Ivanov II, Kobayashi R, Zemlin C, et al. Forced usage of positively charged amino acids in immunoglobulin CDR-H3 impairs B cell development and antibody production. *J Exp Med* (2006) **203**:1567–78. doi:10.1084/jem.20052217
31. Ivanov II, Schelonka RL, Zhuang Y, Gartland GL, Zemlin M, Schroeder HW Jr. Development of the expressed immunoglobulin CDR-H3 repertoire is marked by focusing of constraints in length, amino acid utilization, and charge that are first established in early B cell progenitors. *J Immunol* (2005) **174**:7773–80.
32. Schelonka RL, Ivanov II, Jung DH, Ippolito GC, Nitschke K, Zhuang Y, et al. A single DH gene segment creates its own unique CDR-H3 repertoire and is sufficient for B cell development and immune function. *J Immunol* (2005) **175**(10):6624–32.
33. Schelonka RL, Zemlin M, Kobayashi R, Szalai A, Ippolito GC, Zhuang Y, et al. Preferential use of DH reading frame 2 alters B cell development and antigen-specific antibody production. *J Immunol* (2008) **181**:8409–15.
34. Khass M, Buckley K, Kapoor P, Schelonka RL, Watkins LS, Zhuang Y, et al. Recirculating bone marrow B cells in C57BL/6 mice are more tolerant of highly hydrophobic and highly charged CDR-H3s than those in BALB/c mice. *Eur J Immunol* (2013) **43**(3):629–40. doi:10.1002/eji.201242936
35. Raaphorst FM, Raman CS, Tami J, Fischbach M, Sanz I. Human Ig heavy chain CDR3 regions in adult bone marrow pre-B cells display an adult phenotype of diversity: evidence for structural selection of DH amino acid sequences. *Int Immunol* (1997) **9**:1503–15. doi:10.1093/intimm/9.10.1503
36. Schroeder HW Jr, Zemlin M, Khass M, Nguyen HH, Schelonka RL. Genetic control of DH reading frame and its effect on B-cell development and antigen-specific antibody production. *Crit Rev Immunol* (2010) **30**:327–44. doi:10.1615/CritRevImmunol.v30.i4.20
37. Ivanov II, Link JM, Ippolito GC, Schroeder HW Jr. Constraints on hydropathicity and sequence composition of HCDR3 are conserved across evolution. In: Zanetti M, Capra JD, editors. *The Antibodies*. London: Taylor and Francis Group (2002). p. 43–67.
38. Wardemann H, Yurasov S, Schaefer A, Young JW, Meffre E, Nussenzweig MC. Predominant autoantibody production by early human B cell precursors. *Science* (2003) **301**:1374–7. doi:10.1126/science.1086907
39. Lim PS, Shannon MF, Hardy K. Epigenetic control of inducible gene expression in the immune system. *Epigenomics* (2010) **2**:775–95. doi:10.2217/epi.10.55
40. Ippolito GC, Hoi KH, Reddy ST, Carroll SM, Ge X, Rogosch T, et al. Antibody repertoires in humanized NOD-SCID-IL2Rγ(null) mice and human B cells reveals human-like diversification and tolerance checkpoints in the mouse. *PLoS One* (2012) **7**:e35497. doi:10.1371/journal.pone.0035497
41. Brochet X, Lefranc MP, Giudicelli V. IMGT/V-QUEST: the highly customized and integrated system for IG and TR standardized V-J and V-D-J sequence analysis. *Nucleic Acids Res* (2008) **36**:W503–8. doi:10.1093/nar/gkn316
42. Rogosch T, Kerzel S, Hoi KH, Zhang Z, Maier RF, Ippolito GC, et al. Immunoglobulin analysis tool: a novel tool for the analysis of human and mouse heavy and light chain transcripts. *Front Immunol* (2012) **3**:1–14. doi:10.3389/fimmu.2012.00176
43. Foerster C, Voelxen N, Rakhmamov M, Keller B, Gutenberger S, Goldacker S, et al. B cell receptor mediated calcium signaling is impaired in B lymphocytes of Type Ia patients with common variable immunodeficiency. *J Immunol.* (2010) **184**:7305–13. doi:10.4049/jimmunol.1000434

44. Manjarrez-Orduno N, Quach TD, Sanz I. B cells and immunological tolerance. *J Invest Dermatol* (2009) **129**:278–88. doi:10.1038/jid.2008.240
45. Palanichamy A, Barnard J, Zheng B, Owen T, Quach T, Wei C, et al. Novel human transitional B cell populations revealed by B cell depletion therapy. *J Immunol* (2009) **182**:7982–3. doi:10.4049/jimmunol.0801859
46. Sanz I, Wei C, Lee FEH, Anolik J. Phenotypic and functional heterogeneity of human memory B cells. *Semin Immunol* (2008) **20**:67–82. doi:10.1016/j.smim.2007.12.006
47. Warnatz K, Denz A, Drager R, Braun M, Groth C, Wolff-Vorbeck G, et al. Severe deficiency of switched memory B cells (CD27+IgM-IgD-) in subgroups of patients with common variable immunodeficiency: a new approach to classify a heterogeneous disease. *Blood* (2002) **99**(5):1544–51. doi:10.1182/blood.V99.5.1544
48. Kyte J, Doolittle RF. A simple method for displaying the hydropathic character of a protein. *J Mol Biol* (1982) **157**:105–32. doi:10.1016/0022-2836(82)90515-0
49. Eisenberg D. Three-dimensional structure of membrane and surface proteins. *Annu Rev Biochem* (1984) **53**:595–623. doi:10.1146/annurev.bi.53.070184.003115
50. Schroeder HW Jr. Similarity and divergence in the development and expression of the mouse and human antibody repertoires. *Dev Comp Immunol* (2005) **30**:119–35. doi:10.1016/j.dci.2005.06.006
51. Asma GE, van den Bergh RL, Vossen JM. Characterization of early lymphoid precursor cells in the human fetus using monoclonal antibodies and anti-terminal deoxynucleotidyl transferase. *Clin Exp Immunol* (1986) **64**:356–63.
52. Logtenberg T, Schutte MEM, Ebeling SB, Gmelig-Meyling FHJ, Van Es JH. Molecular approaches to the study of human B-cell and (auto)antibody repertoire generation and selection. *Immunol Rev* (1992) **128**:23–47. doi:10.1111/j.1600-065X.1992.tb00831.x
53. Schelonka RL, Ivanov II, Jung D, Ippolito GC, Nitschke L, Zhuang Y, et al. A single DH gene segment is sufficient for B cell development and immune function. *J Immunol* (2005) **175**:6624–32.
54. Terrell TG, Holmberg CA, Osburn BI. Immunologic surface markers on nonhuman primate lymphocytes. *Am J Vet Res* (1977) **38**:503–7.
55. Zemlin M, Schelonka RL, Ippolito GC, Zemlin C, Zhuang Y, Gartland GL, et al. Regulation of repertoire development through genetic control of DH reading frame preferences. *J Immunol* (2008) **181**:8416–24.
56. Arnaout R, Lee W, Cahill P, Honan T, Sparrow T, Weiand M, et al. High-resolution description of antibody heavy chain repertoires in humans. *PLoS One* (2011) **6**:e22365. doi:10.1371/journal.pone.0022365
57. Boyd SD, Gaeta BA, Jackson KJ, Fire AZ, Marshall EL, Merker JD, et al. Individual variation in the germline Ig gene repertoire inferred from variable region gene rearrangements. *J Immunol* (2010) **184**:6986–92. doi:10.4049/jimmunol.1000445
58. Briney BS, Willis JR, McKinney BA, Crowe JE Jr. High-throughput antibody sequencing reveals genetic evidence of global regulation of the naïve and memory repertoires that extends across individuals. *Genes Immun* (2012) **13**:469–73. doi:10.1038/gene.2012.20
59. Kraj P, Friedman DF, Stevenson F, Silberstein LE. Evidence for the overexpression of the VH4-34 (VH4.21) Ig gene segment in the normal adult human peripheral blood B cell repertoire. *J Immunol* (1995) **154**:6406–20.
60. Stewart AK, Huang C, Stollar BD, Schwartz RS. High-frequency representation of a single VH gene in the expressed human B cell repertoire. *J Exp Med* (1993) **177**:409–18. doi:10.1084/jem.177.2.409
61. Wu YC, Kipling D, Leong HS, Martin V, Ademokun AA, Dunn-Walters DK. High-throughput immunoglobulin repertoire analysis distinguishes between human IgM memory and switched memory B cell populations. *Blood* (2010) **116**:1070–8. doi:10.1182/blood-2010-03-275859
62. Larimore K, McCormick MW, Robins HS, Greenberg PD. Shaping of human germline IgH repertoires revealed by deep sequencing. *J Immunol* (2012) **189**:3221–30. doi:10.4049/jimmunol.1201303
63. Zemlin M, Ippolito GC, Zemlin C, Link J, Monestier M, Schroeder HW Jr. Adult lupus-prone MRL/MpJ2+ mice express a primary antibody repertoire that differs in CDR-H3 length distribution and hydrophobicity from that expressed in the C3H parental strain. *Mol Immunol* (2005) **42**(7):789–98. doi:10.1016/j.molimm.2004.07.049
64. Aguilera I, Melero J, Nunez-Roldan A, Sanchez B. Molecular structure of eight human autoreactive monoclonal antibodies. *Immunology* (2001) **102**:273–80. doi:10.1046/j.1365-2567.2001.01159.x
65. Ichiyoshi Y, Casali P. Analysis of the structural correlates for antibody polyreactivity by multiple reassortments of chimeric human immunoglobulin heavy and light chain V segments. *J Exp Med* (1994) **180**:885–95. doi:10.1084/jem.180.3.885
66. Klonowki KD, Primiano LL, Monestier M. Atypical VH-D-JH rearrangements in newborn autoimmune MRL mice. *J Immunol* (1999) **162**:1566–72.

6

How do CD4+ T cells detect and eliminate tumor cells that either lack or express MHC class II molecules?

Ole Audun Werner Haabeth[1†], Anders Aune Tveita[1†], Marte Fauskanger[1], Fredrik Schjesvold[1], Kristina Berg Lorvik[1], Peter O. Hofgaard[2], Hilde Omholt[1], Ludvig A. Munthe[1], Zlatko Dembic[3], Alexandre Corthay[1,4,5] and Bjarne Bogen[1,2]*

Department of Immunology, Centre for Immune Regulation, Oslo University Hospital, University of Oslo, Oslo, Norway
KG Jebsen Centre for Research on Influenza Vaccines, Institute of Immunology, Oslo University Hospital, University of Oslo, Oslo, Norway
[3] Faculty of Dentistry, Molecular Genetics Laboratory, Department of Oral Biology, University of Oslo, Oslo, Norway
[4] Department of Biosciences, University of Oslo, Oslo, Norway
[5] Tumor Immunology Group, Department of Pathology, Oslo University Hospital, University of Oslo, Oslo, Norway

Edited by:
Fang-Ping Huang, Imperial College London, UK

Reviewed by:
Luca Gattinoni, National Cancer Institute, USA
Junko Matsuzaki, Roswell Park Cancer Institute, USA
William J. Magner, Roswell Park Cancer Institute, USA

***Correspondence:**
Bjarne Bogen, Institute of Immunology, University of Oslo, OUS Rikshospitalet HF, A2/A3, Sognsvannsveien 20, Oslo N-0027, Norway
e-mail: bjarne.bogen@medisin.uio.no

† Ole Audun Werner Haabeth and Anders Aune Tveita have contributed equally to this work.

CD4+ T cells contribute to tumor eradication, even in the absence of CD8+ T cells. Cytotoxic CD4+ T cells can directly kill MHC class II positive tumor cells. More surprisingly, CD4+ T cells can indirectly eliminate tumor cells that lack MHC class II expression. Here, we review the mechanisms of direct and indirect CD4+ T cell-mediated elimination of tumor cells. An emphasis is put on T cell receptor (TCR) transgenic models, where anti-tumor responses of naïve CD4+ T cells of defined specificity can be tracked. Some generalizations can tentatively be made. For both MHCII^{POS} and MHCII^{NEG} tumors, presentation of tumor-specific antigen by host antigen-presenting cells (APCs) appears to be required for CD4+ T cell priming. This has been extensively studied in a myeloma model (MOPC315), where host APCs in tumor-draining lymph nodes are primed with secreted tumor antigen. Upon antigen recognition, naïve CD4+ T cells differentiate into Th1 cells and migrate to the tumor. At the tumor site, the mechanisms for elimination of MHCII^{POS} and MHCII^{NEG} tumor cells differ. In a TCR-transgenic B16 melanoma model, MHCII^{POS} melanoma cells are directly killed by cytotoxic CD4+ T cells in a perforin/granzyme B-dependent manner. By contrast, MHCII^{NEG} myeloma cells are killed by IFN-γ stimulated M1-like macrophages. In summary, while the priming phase of CD4+ T cells appears similar for MHCII^{POS} and MHCII^{NEG} tumors, the killing mechanisms are different. Unresolved issues and directions for future research are addressed.

Keywords: tumor immunology, CD4+ T cells, MHC class II, T cell receptor transgenic, transgenic mouse models, tumor antigen, T helper 1, multiple myeloma

RECENT ADVANCES IN TUMOR IMMUNOLOGY

The field of tumor immunology has come a long way since the formulation of the tumor immunosurveillance hypothesis by Thomas and Burnet (1–4). Although still debated, increasing evidence suggests that the immune system can detect and reject incipient tumors, and that CD4+ and CD8+ T cells play an important role as mediators of immunosurveillance (5). Furthermore, there is accumulating evidence that the immune system is not completely tolerant even to established tumors, based on the observation that tumor-infiltrating T cells, when expanded *in vitro* and injected back to lymphopenic patients, have a clinical effect in some patients (6). Further supporting the notion of ongoing immune responses to tumors, antibodies that block inhibitory molecules on T cells induce long-term remission in a subset of cancer patients (7). Finally, parameters that indicate immune activation in tumors are associated with improved prognosis (8).

Abbreviations: APC, antigen-presenting cell; CIITA, class II trans-activator; FasL, Fas ligand; HA, hemagglutinin; Id, idiotype; IFN-γ, interferon gamma; Ig, immunoglobulin; MHC, major histocompatibility complex; MM, multiple myeloma; MOPC, mineral oil-induced plasmacytoma; OVA, ovalbumin; s.c., subcutaneous; TCR-Tg, T cell receptor transgenic; TIL, tumor-infiltrating lymphocyte; Trp1, tyrosinase-related protein 1; SCID, severe combined immunodeficiency.

CD4+ VERSUS CD8+ T CELLS IN TUMOR IMMUNOLOGY

Traditionally, CD8+ T cells have been thought to be the major mediators of effective anti-tumor T cell responses. Such a view is supported by the pronounced cytotoxic activity of CD8+ T cells *in vitro*, and the observation that tumors that escape CD8+ T cells onslaught may have altered or downregulated MHC class I antigen expression (9–11). Moreover, studies done in an MHC class I-restricted T cell receptor (TCR) transgenic mouse showed that CD8+ T cells, in the absence of CD4+ T cells, maintained their anti-tumor effect (12). Despite these observations, several studies indicate limited anti-tumor effects of CD8+ T cells alone (13–16).

The helper function of tumor-reactive CD4+ T cells improves the efficacy of tumor-reactive CD8+ T cells (17–20). Similarly, treatment of a patient with metastatic melanoma with autologous CD4+ T cells specific for the tumor-associated antigen NY-ESO-1 resulted in sustained clinical remissions with evidence of endogenous immune responses against other tumor-derived antigens (21). In support of these findings, transfection of tumor cells with MHC class II genes resulted in increased protective immune responses against tumors (22, 23). Collectively, these results indicate an augmenting effect of $CD4^+$ T cells on $CD8^+$ T cell responses against tumors.

On the other hand, $CD4^+$ T cells alone, in the absence of $CD8^+$ T cells, have also been demonstrated to eliminate tumor cells. Thus, adoptive transfer experiments using primed $CD4^+$ T cells generated by immunization with tumor cells conferred protection against a subsequent tumor challenge (24, 25). Moreover, naïve $CD4^+$ T cells in TCR-transgenic mice conferred protection against tumor development upon subcutaneous (s.c.) injection of tumor cells (26, 27). Finally, using MHC class I-molecule and MHC class II-molecule restricted TCR-transgenic mice specific for the Dby H–Y antigen, $CD4^+$ T cells were found to be more efficient at eradicating cancer cells than $CD8^+$ T cells in a side-by-side comparison (28). Here, we will focus on the anti-tumor properties of $CD4^+$ T cells in the absence of $CD8^+$ T cells.

PIONEERING EXPERIMENTS ON THE ROLE OF CD4+ T CELLS IN ERADICATION OF TUMORS

The role of $CD4^+$ T cells was initially investigated in experiments where tumor-bearing mice were treated by adoptive transfer of T cells obtained from syngeneic mice immunized with irradiated tumor cells (25, 29), or with living tumor cells followed by surgical resection (24). It was shown that when T cells from tumor-immunized donors were purified prior to adoptive transfer, $Lyt1^+ 2^-$ ($CD4^+$) T cells had a superior ability to cure FBL-3 erythroleukemic tumors compared to $Lyt1^- 2^+$ ($CD8^+$) T cells (29). Treatment with cyclophosphamide was required for the curative effect of $CD4^+$ T cells to be observed. However, in the first reported experiments (29), a role of endogenous $CD8^+$ T cells in the tumor-bearing host was not ruled out. In follow-up experiments, this possibility was formally excluded by the use of T cell deficient tumor-bearing recipients (25). Similar results were obtained using the X5563 plasmacytoma model (24), where transfer of purified $Lyt1^+ 2^-$ ($CD4^+$) T cells had superior therapeutic potential. In the following decades, experimental evidence supporting the anti-tumor properties of tumor-specific $CD4^+$ T cells alone has accumulated (27, 28, 30–39).

TCR-TRANSGENIC MODELS FOR CD4+ T CELL-MEDIATED REJECTION OF TUMORS

The experiments referred to in the preceding section had features that prohibited detailed studies of the mechanisms of $CD4^+$ T cell-mediated tumor protection. First, the $CD4^+$ T cells were polyclonal. Second, $CD4^+$ T cells were pre-primed cells obtained after immunization, making it impossible to study naïve $CD4^+$ T cells in primary anti-tumor responses. Third, the relevant tumor-specific antigens were often not known.

The generation of TCR-transgenic mice that recognize tumor antigens presented on MHC class II molecules (**Table 1**) offered a novel approach to bypass these difficulties. In two models, these antigens are *bona fide* cancer antigens; the tumor-specific myeloma protein V region idiotype (Id) (26, 27) and the melanoma-associated tyrosinase-related protein 1 (Trp1) (35). In other TCR-transgenic models, the antigens are either minor histocompatibility antigen Dby (H-Y) (28), viral antigens such as the hemagglutinin (HA) (40–42), or xenogeneic proteins such as ovalbumin (OVA) (17, 43, 44). While the transgenic TCR specific for the mutated myeloma antigen was obtained after immunization of mice syngeneic to the tumor (45, 46), the transgenic TCR specific for the non-mutated antigen was obtained after immunization of Trp1-deficient mice. Thus, in the latter model, Trp1 represents a foreign antigen to which high-affinity TCRs are induced (due to a lack of T cell tolerance) (35).

Table 1 | TCR-transgenic models employed in studies of anti-tumor $CD4^+$ T cell responses.

TCR-Tg model	Antigen	Classification of antigen	Antigen location	MHC II restriction	Peptide	Reference
4B2A1 ($\lambda 2^{315}$)	Light chain idiotype (Id) of mouse M315 myeloma protein	Mutated tumor-specific antigen	Secreted, plasma membrane (52, 53)	$I\text{–}E^d$	aa91–101	(46)
7A6 (Trp1)	Mouse tyrosinase-related protein 1	Melanocyte-specific differentiation antigen	Secreted, melanosome membrane (54)	$I\text{–}A^b$	aa113–125	(35)
Marilyn (H–Y)	Minor histocompatibility antigen (Dby)	Tissue antigen	Secreted, cell membrane (55, 56)	$I\text{–}A^b$	aa608–622	(47)
T2.5-5 (HA)	Influenza PR8 hemagglutinin	Viral antigen	Varying (construct dependent)[1]	$I\text{–}A^d$	aa126–138	(48)
14.3.d (HA)	Influenza PR8 hemagglutinin	Viral antigen	Varying (construct dependent)[1]	$I\text{–}E^d$	aa110–120	(49)
DO11.10 (OVA)	Chicken ovalbumin	Xenogeneic model antigen	Varying (construct dependent)[2]	$I\text{–}A^d$	aa323–339	(50)
OT-II (OVA)	Chicken ovalbumin	Xenogeneic model antigen	Varying (construct dependent)[2]	$I\text{–}A^b$	aa323–339	(51)

[1]*Varyingly expressed by fusion to other proteins, which control cellular distribution. The viral protein, as such, localizes to the cell surface (57).*

[2]*Varyingly expressed as full-length cDNA [containing signal sequence for secretion (58)] or fused to other proteins, which control cellular distribution.*

MHC CLASS II STATUS OF TUMOR CELLS USED IN TUMOR IMMUNOLOGY STUDIES FOCUSED ON THE ROLE OF CD4+ T CELLS

$CD4^+$ T cells recognize peptides (about 13–17aa long) bound to the groove of MHC class II molecules (59) on professional antigen-presenting cells (APCs) (B cells, dendritic cells, macrophages, in addition to thymic epithelial cells) (60–62). However, in certain cells, MHC class II molecules may be induced by interferon gamma (IFN-γ) stimulation (63, 64). Thus, in $CD4^+$ T cell immune responses to tumors, the MHC class II status of the tumor cells is of importance. The MHC II expression status of tumor cells used in studies with $CD4^+$ TCR-transgenic mice is summarized in **Table 2.**

DIRECT AND INDIRECT KILLING OF TUMOR CELLS BY CD4+ T CELLS

The antigen-specific interaction between $CD4^+$ T cells and MHC II^{POS} tumor cells is conceptually easy to grasp. On the other hand, the basis for antigen presentation and anti-tumor effector mechanisms are less obvious in the context of MHC II^{NEG} tumors (25, 26, 31, 70) – simply because such cancer cells cannot directly stimulate MHC class II-restricted $CD4^+$ T cells (**Figure 1**). In the following sections, we discuss mechanism of $CD4^+$ T cell-mediated direct killing of MHC II^{POS} tumor cells and indirect killing of MHC II^{NEG} tumor cells. Emphasis is put on observations from TCR-transgenic models, where the T cell specificity is known and both naïve and primed $CD4^+$ T cells are readily available.

Table 2 | Use of TCR-Tg models for studies of anti-tumor CD4+ T cell immune responses.

TCR-Tg model (antigen)	Tumor cell line	Ectopic antigen expr.[a]	MHC II expr.	Antigen secreted?	T cell source	Reference
4B2A1 ($\lambda2^{315}$)	MOPC315 (plasmacytoma)	No	–	Yes	Naïve (endogenous)[b]	(26, 27, 34, 65)
	MOPC315.37[c]	No	–	No	Naive (endogenous)	(36)
	A20 (B lymphoma)	Yes	+	Yes	Naive (endogenous) Adoptive transfer, naive	(26, 33, 66)
	A20 (B lymphoma)[d]	Yes	+	No	Naive (endogenous)	(26)
7A6 (Trp1)	B16/CIITA (melanoma)	No	+[e]	N/D	Naive (endogenous) Adoptive transfer, activated	(35)
	B16 (melanoma)	No	+[f]	N/D	Adoptive transfer, naïve Adoptive transfer, activated	(37, 38)
Marilyn (H–Y)	MB49 (bladder)	No	+[f]	N/D	Adoptive transfer, naive Adoptive transfer, activated	(28)
	TRAMP-C2 (prostate)	No	–	N/D		
	βTC-TET	No	–	N/D		
	WR21 (salivary gland)	No	–	N/D		
T2.5-5 (HA)	AB1 (mesothelioma)	Yes	–	N/D[g]	Naive (endogenous) Adoptive transfer, naive	(40)
14.3d (HA)	CT26 (colon)	Yes	N/D[h]	N/D[i]	Naive (endogenous) Adoptive transfer, naive	(41, 42)
DO11.10 (OVA)	A20 (B lymphoma)	Yes	+	N/D[j]	Adoptive transfer, activated	(17)
	A20 (B lymphoma)	Yes	+	No[k]	Naive (endogenous) Adoptive transfer, activated	(44)
OT-II (OVA)	EG-7 (thymoma)	Yes	–	Yes[l]	Adoptive transfer, activated	(43)

N/D, not determined.

[a] Ectopic antigen expression signifies that the tumor cell line was transfected for expression of the relevant antigen.

[b] The designation naive (endogenous) is used to describe tumor challenge experiments in TCR-Tg mice in which no prior priming of antigen-specific T cells was performed.

[c] MOPC315.37 contains a Gly15→ Arg15 mutation within the λ2 gene that causes intracellular retention (67).

[d] Cells were transfected with a mutated $\lambda2^{315}$ variant that causes retention within the endoplasmic reticulum, precluding secretion (67).

[e] Cells were transfected to overexpress MHC class II trans-activator (CIITA) to ensure high levels of expression of MHC II (35).

[f] Inducible expression by interferon gamma stimulation.

[g] Only cell surface expression was tested (40).

[h] A previous publication reports constitutive MHC II expression in vitro (68).

[i] Cells were transfected with HA fused to EGFP. Only surface expression was tested (41).

[j] Secretion expected; cells were transduced with constructs containing the full-length OVA cDNA sequence, which contains signal element for secretion (58).

[k] Cells were transfected with OVA fused to the trans-membrane domain of transferrin receptor, causing membrane expression (44).

[l] Earlier report demonstrates secretion from the same cell line (69).

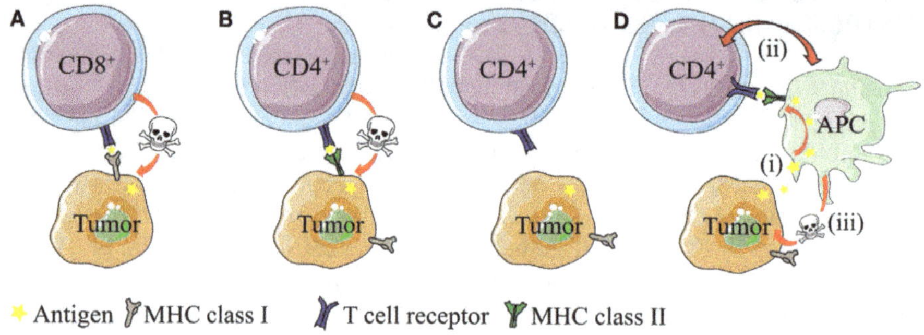

FIGURE 1 | Direct and indirect killing of tumor cells by CD4+ T cells. **(A)** CD8+ T cells can directly kill tumor cells that express MHC class I molecules, whereas **(B)** cytotoxic CD4+ T cells can kill tumor cells that express MHC class II molecules. **(C)** While most tumor types express MHC class I molecules, they often lack expression of MHC class II. How do CD4+ T cells recognize and eliminate MHCII^{NEG} tumor cells? **(D)** CD4+ T cells may kill MHC class II negative (MHC II^{NEG}) tumors by a mechanism where (i) tumor antigen secreted by tumor cells is processed and presented by MHCII^{POS} macrophages to CD4+ T cells. (ii) Bi-directional interaction/activation of macrophages and CD4+ T cells (iii) activates tumoricidal macrophages that in turn kill the tumor cells (In addition, activated CD4+ T cells themselves could possibly directly kill tumor cell in a TCR/MHC II-independent manner.).

DIRECT KILLING OF MHC CLASS II^{POS} TUMOR CELLS

The existence of CD4$^+$ T cells with cytotoxic properties has been increasingly recognized throughout the last three decades. Such cells are thought to function in a fashion analogous to cytotoxic CD8$^+$ T cells, with antigen recognition triggering the release of cytotoxic mediators. CD4$^+$ T cells displaying direct cytotoxicity *in vitro* toward MHC II^{POS} targets, including tumor cells, have been described by several authors (37, 45, 70, 71). Correspondingly, efficient elimination of MHC II^{POS} tumors by T cells with such properties is also observed *in vivo* (26, 28, 33, 35, 37, 38, 72).

Several effector mechanisms have been implicated for tumor-specific cytotoxic CD4$^+$ T cells. In a model of Id-specific CD4$^+$ T cell responses against an MHC II^{POS} B lymphoma, *in vitro* cytotoxicity was shown to be dependent on signaling mediated by binding of Fas ligand (FasL) on CD4$^+$ T cells to the death receptor Fas on tumor cells (66). Naïve T cells showed little killing activity, whereas Th1 differentiation greatly enhanced cytotoxicity. However, *in vivo* elimination of tumor cells was not affected in FasL-deficient ($gld^{-/-}$) Id-specific TCR-Tg mice, suggesting that signaling through the Fas pathway is dispensable for tumor killing and that additional mechanisms are operational *in vivo* (66). Indeed, if the tumor antigen is secreted as is the case in the studies of Lundin et al. (33, 66), the indirect mechanism via Th1/M1 macrophages described below could also be active, and might play a prominent role in tumor rejection. In the Trp1-specific TCR-transgenic model, it was demonstrated that the rejection of B16 melanoma cells was abrogated in mice deficient for either granzyme B or perforin, indicating that these molecules are important for CD4$^+$ T cell-mediated killing of MHC II^{POS} tumor cells (37). In summary, different MHC II^{POS} tumors may vary in susceptibility to various effector mechanisms of CD4$^+$ T cells, as indicated by the observations addressed above.

INDIRECT KILLING OF MHC CLASS II^{NEG} TUMOR CELLS

In general, antibody-secreting plasma cells are MHC class II negative due to silencing of the MHC Class II trans-activator (CIITA) occurring during plasma cell differentiation (73, 74). Multiple myeloma (MM) is the malignant counterpart of plasma cells and usually express little if any MHC class II molecules. MHC class II negativity due to loss of CIITA expression appears to be a stable phenotype, although some studies have reported MHC II upregulation in MM cells exposed to retinoic acid (75) or IFN-γ (76, 77).

The work of our research group is based on experiments using the mineral oil-induced BALB/c plasmacytoma (MOPC)315 (52, 70). MOPC315 cells secrete a highly mutated and unique monoclonal IgA (myeloma protein). The λ2 light chain of the myeloma protein contains somatic mutations in positions 38, 50, 94, 95, and 96 that are unique to MOPC315 (78). Thus, the myeloma protein light chain is referred to as $\lambda 2^{315}$ (**Figure 2A**).

By immunization of BALB/c mice with free $\lambda 2^{315}$ L chain, known from previous studies to stimulate T cells (81), I-E^d-restricted, Id-specific CD4$^+$ T cell clones were generated (**Figure 2A**) (45). These clones recognize a unique Id-epitope, which depends on the somatic mutations in codons 94, 95, and 96 within the CDR3 loop of the $\lambda 2^{315}$ light chain (79). As would be expected, MOPC315 derived $\lambda 2^{315}$-immunoglobulin has to be endocytosed and processed by APCs prior to MHC class II presentation of the Id-peptide (80).

MOPC315 is found to be MHC class II negative by a number of criteria: (i) Negative staining with anti-MHC class II antibodies both *in vitro*, *ex vivo* (70), and *in vivo* (65). Lack of expression of MHC II molecules on MOPC315 was independently reported by others (82). (ii) Exposure to high amounts (500 ng/ml) of IFN-γ IL-4, or supernatant from activated Th1 cells, all failed to induce any detectable expression of MHC class II *in vitro* (70). (iii) Both *in vitro*-cultured (70) and *ex vivo* (65) MOPC315 cells failed to stimulate Id-specific MHC class II-restricted T cells in proliferation and cytokine secretion assays.

IDIOTYPE-SPECIFIC CD4$^+$ T CELL CLONES INDUCE KILLING OF MHC CLASS II NEGATIVE MYELOMA CELLS *IN VITRO* – BUT ONLY IN THE PRESENCE OF MHC-COMPATIBLE APCs

A weak cytotoxicity that was greatly augmented by addition of high amounts of myeloma protein was observed when Id-specific CD4$^+$

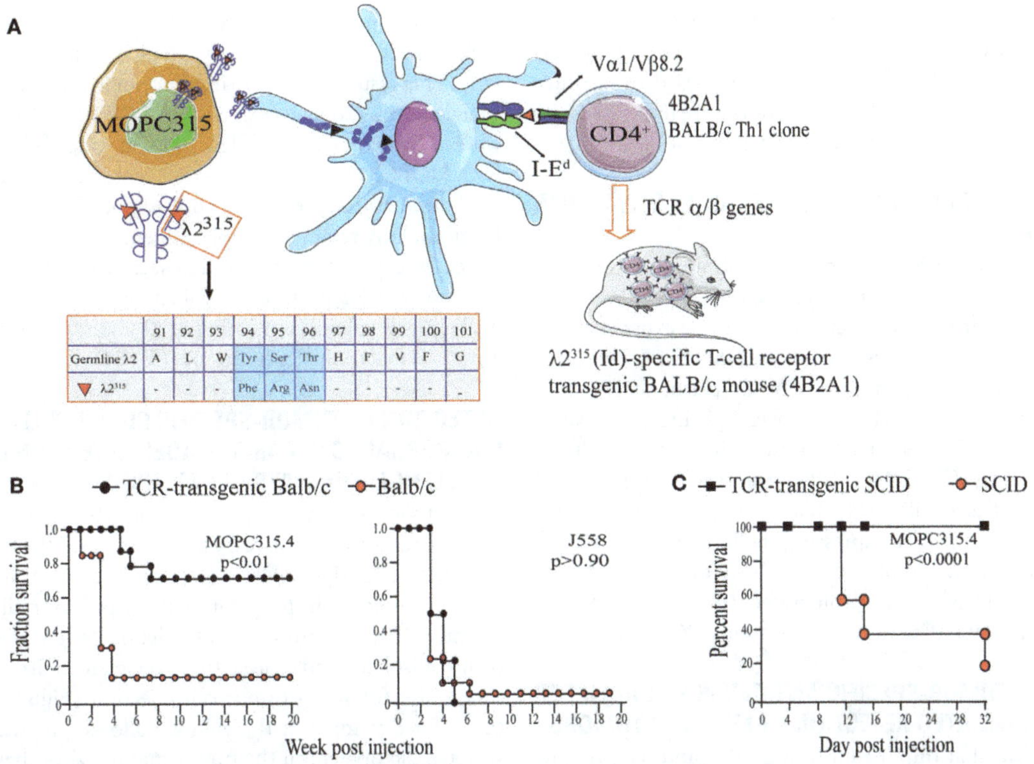

FIGURE 2 | The MOPC315 myeloma model. Naïve tumor-specific CD4+ T cells protect against MHC II^{NEG} tumor challenge in the absence of other T cells and B cells. **(A)** MOPC315 myeloma cells of BALB/c origin secrete an IgA M315 myeloma protein with a mutated λ2 light chain referred to as λ2^{315}. M315 is endocytosed and processed by BALB/c APCs, and a CDR3 sequence that includes residues 91–101 of λ2^{315} is presented on the MHC class II molecule I-E^d to Id-specific CD4+ T cells. The peptide that is recognized by Id-specific CD4+ T cells contains somatic mutations in positions 94, 95, and 96 (45, 79, 80). Based on the αβ TCR of the Id-recognizing 4B2A1 clone, a TCR-transgenic mouse was generated (46). Most CD4+ T cells in this mouse express a transgenic TCR that can be tracked by a clonotype-specific mAb [Nomenclature: antigenic determinants in immunoglobulin variable (V) regions are called idiotopes (Id). The 91–101 peptide is thus an Id-peptide, and the CD4+ T cells that recognize this Id-peptide presented by I-E^d are called Id-specific]. **(B)** Id-specific TCR-transgenic mice on an immunosufficient background (BALB/c) are resistant to a challenge with Id^{POS} MOPC315 cells but succumb to Id^{NEG} J558 myeloma cells [reproduced with permission from Proc Natl Acad Sci (26), U.S.A.]. **(C)**. Id-specific TCR-transgenic mice on an immunodeficient background (SCID), lacking other T and B cells than Id-specific CD4+ T cells, are also resistant to MOPC315 tumor development [reproduced with permission from Immunity (34)]. Tumor resistance could be transferred with purified Id-specific CD4+ T cells to SCID mice (27).

T cells were co-cultured with MHC-compatible spleen cells from BALB/c (H-2^d) MHC II^{NEG} MOPC315. Importantly, MHC II incompatible spleen cells from C57BL/6 failed to support cytotoxicity (70). Moreover, the cytotoxic effect could not be transferred by supernatants of activated T cells. It was suggested that some of the spleen cells, e.g., macrophages (Mϕ) stimulated by activated T cells, were important as cytotoxic effector cells in the *in vitro* cultures (70).

NAÏVE Id-SPECIFIC CD4$^+$ T CELLS IN T CELL RECEPTOR TRANSGENIC MICE PROTECT AGAINST Id$^+$ MYELOMA CELLS IN THE ABSENCE OF CD8$^+$ T CELLS AND B CELLS

To facilitate studies of the role of Id-specific CD4$^+$ T cells in tumor protection against MHC II negative MOPC315, an Id-specific TCR-transgenic mouse on syngeneic BALB/c background was established (46).

In initial experiments, naïve Id-specific T cells from TCR-transgenic mice did not respond to MOPC315 *in vitro*. Despite this, Id-specific TCR-transgenic mice were specifically protected against s.c. challenge with MOPC315 cells (26) (**Figure 2B**). Eradication of MOPC315 cells resulted in a change of T cell phenotype, since T cells of surviving TCR-transgenic mice had increased cytotoxicity against Id$^+$ MHC II^{POS} B lymphomas, and since they upon stimulation produced much IFNγ and some IL-4.

By breeding the TCR-Tg mice onto a SCID background, it was demonstrated that rejection of MOPC315 was independent of CD8$^+$ T cells and B cells/antibodies (27, 34) (**Figure 2C**). Additionally, tumor protection could be transferred to SCID mice with adoptive transfer of purified Id-specific CD4$^+$ T cells (27).

Id-PRIMED APC CAN BE DETECTED IN TUMOR TISSUE OF LARGE ESTABLISHED MYELOMAS

The finding that naïve CD4$^+$ T cells could initiate rejection of a MHC II negative tumor indicated that host cells expressing MHC class II molecules were responsible for the presentation of Id to CD4$^+$ T cells. In a subsequent study, it was demonstrated that s.c.

MOPC315 tumors contained APCs that were able to stimulate Id-specific CD4$^+$ T cells *in vitro* in an MHC-restricted manner (65). The great majority of MHC II^{POS} tumor-infiltrating APCs were CD11b$^+$CD11c^{LOW}CD80$^+$CD86$^+$. These studies demonstrated that MHC class II negative MOPC315 tumors were infiltrated with Id-primed APCs with macrophage-like characteristics.

Id-SPECIFIC CD4$^+$ T CELLS ARE PRESENT AND ACTIVATED IN TUMOR TISSUE

Given that Id-primed APC could be demonstrated in MOPC315 tumors, it was investigated if Id-specific CD4$^+$ T cells were also present, and whether they were activated. In these experiments, a high amount of MOPC315 cells were injected in order to overcome the resistance of TCR-transgenic mice. A number of observations indicated that Id-specific CD4$^+$ T cells were specifically activated in small s.c. MOPC315 tumors established in Id-specific TCR-transgenic mice: (i) The CD4$^+$/CD8$^+$ ratio was skewed toward CD4$^+$ in tumor tissue. (ii) CD4$^+$ blasts within the tumor were selectively enriched for cells expressing the Id-specific TCR. (iii) Id-specific CD4$^+$ tumor-infiltrating lymphocytes (TIL) were activated (CD69$^+$ CD25$^+$), and proliferated (BrdU$^+$) in clusters associated with MHC II^{POS} tumor-infiltrating APC (65).

SECRETION OF TUMOR-SPECIFIC ANTIGEN IS REQUIRED FOR CD4$^+$ T CELL-MEDIATED REJECTION OF MHC II^{NEG} TUMORS

While it was clear that tumor-infiltrating APCs and lymph node cells take up the $\lambda2^{315}$ antigen and display the Id-peptide on MHC class II molecules (34, 65), the precise source of the priming Id antigen was not established. To address this question, we used two secretory variants of MOPC315: one that secretes the complete M315 myeloma protein composed of α H chain and $\lambda2^{315}$ L chain (MOPC315), and another that only secrets the free $\lambda2^{315}$ L chain (MOPC315.26). In addition, we used two non-secretory variants: one where the free $\lambda2^{315}$ L chain is retained intracellularly due to a point mutation (MOPC315.37) and another where no Ig is produced (MOPC315.36) (67, 83).

When Id-specific TCR-transgenic SCID mice were challenged with the four variants, protection was observed for the $\lambda2^{315}$-secreting variants MOPC315 and MOPC315.26, while there was no protection against the antigen-negative MOPC315.36. Tumor take was significantly delayed, but still complete, in mice challenged with the MOPC315.37, which retains $\lambda2^{315}$ intracellularly. This result was surprising since in MOPC315.37-containing Matrigels, macrophages were MHC II^{HI}, and Id-specific T cells were activated (CD69$^+$). The only striking deficiency observed with MOPC315.37 *in vivo* was deficient T cell activation in draining lymph nodes, presumably due to poor local availability of the intracellularly retained tumor antigen. These results indicate that the extracellular concentration of secreted tumor-specific antigen is important for protection against an MHC II^{NEG} tumor, most likely due to enhanced priming of APCs in draining lymph nodes as well as macrophages in tumors (36, 84).

DETECTION OF TUMOR-SPECIFIC CD4$^+$ T CELLS AND MACROPHAGES IN EARLY STAGES AFTER TUMOR CELL CHALLENGE: THE MATRIGEL METHOD

To study local events at the injection site at the early stages of the anti-tumor immune response, we injected the tumor cells suspended in a Matrigel solution (**Figures 3** and **4**). Matrigel is a liquid basement membrane preparation that jellifies rapidly at body temperature. Thus, a tumor bed of a defined size was generated that could be isolated and assayed to characterize infiltrating cells at any time point following tumor cell injection (**Figure 3**). Moreover, the defined volume of the gel plug allows quantitative assays of secreted factors within the tumor microenvironment (39). Initial experiments demonstrated that tumor cells embedded in Matrigel were rejected by TCR-transgenic SCID mice, although less efficiently than in the absence of Matrigel (34). Thus, events in the tumor cell-containing Matrigel most likely reflected those taking place during successful immunosurveillance of MHC II negative tumor cells by CD4$^+$ T cells.

Using this system, a longitudinal characterization of the immune response within the tumor microenvironment and draining lymph nodes was undertaken (34, 36, 39, 85). The findings are summarized in **Figure 4**. Briefly, secreted myeloma protein is presented by APC in tumor-draining lymph nodes to Id-specific CD4$^+$ T cells. Upon recognition, T cells are activated, polarize into Th1 cells, and migrate to the Matrigel/tumor. In

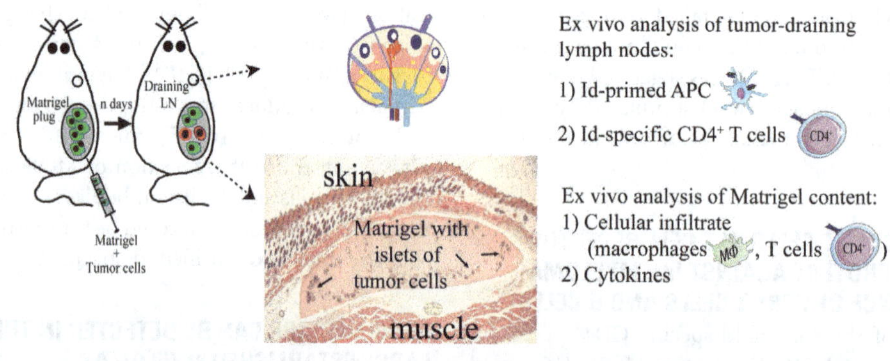

FIGURE 3 | The Matrigel assay. A novel approach to unravel the dynamics of CD4$^+$ T cell-mediated primary anti-tumor immune responses. At day 0, subcutaneous injections with MOPC315 tumor cells suspended in liquid Matrigel. When the Matrigel solution reaches body temperature, it jellifies and forms a plug containing the tumor cells. At various time points after injection (*n* days), the Matrigel plug and tumor-draining lymph nodes are dissected out and analyzed *ex vivo* for cellular content, function of cells, and cytokines (34, 36, 39, 85).

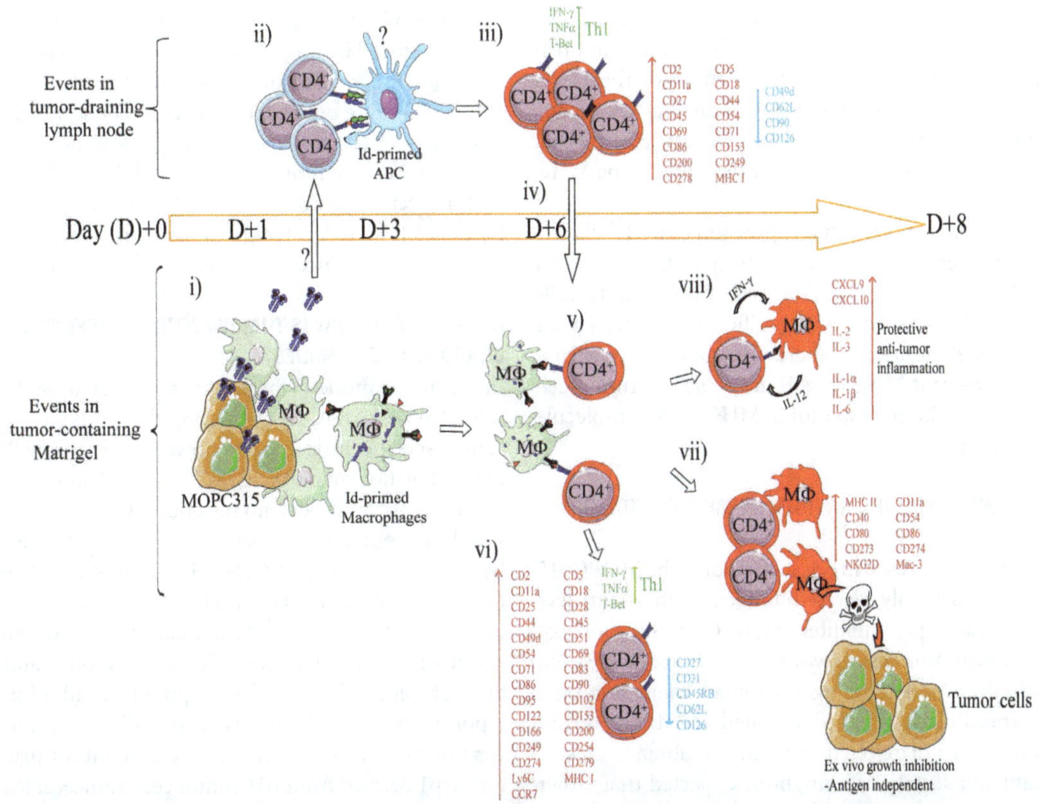

FIGURE 4 | Mechanism of rejection of MHCII^NEG myeloma cells by Id-specific CD4⁺ T cells. The following events are based on experiments where Id-secreting MOPC315 suspended in liquid Matrigel was injected subcutaneously in TCR-transgenic mice. (i–viii). (i) At the incipient tumor site, macrophages [CD11b⁺, CD11c⁻, CD80/CD86⁺ MHC II^LO, F4/80⁺] start to infiltrate the tumor/Matrigel from day +1. Tumor-infiltrating macrophages become Id-primed by extracellular myeloma protein by the conventional MHC II presentation pathway (65). (ii) Extracellular Id+ myeloma protein (or possibly Id-primed tumor APCs) drain to lymph nodes where Id-primed APCs stimulate Id-specific CD4⁺ T cells. Uncertainties as to the mechanism of Id+ Ag draining and the identity of Id-primed APCs are indicated by a question mark (?). (iii) Id-specific CD4⁺ T cells become activated by day +3, are substantially expanded by day +6 (34), and polarize into Th1 cells by day +8 (39, 85). Upon activation in the tumor-draining lymph node, a number of molecules are significantly upregulated on the surface of the Id-specific CD4⁺ T cells, while some are consistently downregulated (85). (iv) Activated CD4⁺ T cells (CD62L^LOW) leave the lymph node and accumulate at the tumor site from day +6 (34, 86). (v) At the incipient tumor site, infiltrating Id-specific CD4⁺ T cells are re-activated by Id-primed macrophages (34). (vi) Moreover, in addition to a sustained Th1 phenotype, the tumor-infiltrating CD4⁺ T cells dramatically change expression of a number of surface molecules (85). Several molecules are upregulated on both activated CD4⁺ T cells in the tumor-draining lymph node, and on tumor-infiltrating CD4⁺ T cells, although at higher levels in the latter population. (vii) IFN-γ produced by tumor-infiltrating Th1 cells activates macrophages that up-regulate MHC class II on the cell surface and show increased expression of M1-associated surface molecules (34, 39). IFN-γ-activated macrophages acquire a tumoricidal phenotype with the upregulation of cytotoxicity-associated markers including granzyme A/B, and NKG2D (39). In addition, purified activated macrophages can directly inhibit myeloma growth *in vitro* (34, 36, 39). The mechanisms underlying M1 macrophage-mediated growth inhibition is unknown, but once the macrophages are activated the growth inhibition is antigen independent (36). (viii) Analysis by gene expression profiling and Luminex multiplex cytokine analyses has revealed that the Id-specific CD4⁺ Th1-mediated anti-tumor immune response has a striking resemblance to the characteristics of acute inflammatory responses (39). Thus, we propose that Th1-mediated inflammatory responses may protect against cancer (87).

the Matrigel/tumor, Th1 cells become re-activated by tumor-infiltrating macrophages that has endocytosed and processed myeloma protein. Th1 derived IFN-γ activates macrophages into tumoricidal M1 macrophages (34, 36, 39, 65).

UNRESOLVED ISSUES AND DIRECTIONS FOR FUTURE RESEARCH

USE OF MHC CLASS II NEGATIVE TUMOR CELL LINES IN TUMOR IMMUNOLOGY

While MHC class II positivity in tumor cells is generally to be trusted, MHC class II negativity should, for obvious reasons, be viewed with a healthy skepticism. In the case of MOPC315, many attempts by others and us have consistently failed to detect expression of MHC class II molecules *in vitro* as well as *in vivo*, even when MOPC315 cells were exposed to IFN-γ (34, 70, 82, 88). In several other models, such as the use of the erythroleukemia cell line FBL-3 (25), the UV-induced fibrosarcoma 6132A-PRO (31), and the methylcholanthrene-induced Mc51.9 (32); no MHC class II was detected on tumor cells even after IFN-γ exposure, similar to MOPC315. In the B16 melanoma model, Quezada et al. showed that the cell line used in their experiments expressed MHC class II, but only when the tumor-bearing hosts were subjected to a combination of irradiation and adoptive transfer of Trp1-specific $CD4^+$ T cells together with anti-CTLA mAb (37). Xie et al. also reported that B16 cells express MHC class II by immunofluorescence staining of tumor biopsies, but the identity of the MHC class II^{POS} cells within the sections was not further characterized, complicating interpretation (38). In contrast, Hung et al. reports the use of B16 tumor cells that were described to be MHC II^{NEG} (30).

Peres-Diez et al. (28) reported that expression of MHC class II molecules on tumor cells was not required for rejection mediated by $CD4^+$ cells. In note, they found that: H-2^k H-Y^+ tumor cells were rejected by I–A^b-restricted, H–Y-specific $CD4^+$ T cells in an immunodeficient H-2^b mouse. An alternative approach to ensure the absence of the relevant MHC class II molecule in a tumor cell line would be to delete the corresponding MHC class II molecule genes from the tumor cells.

IS SECRETION OF TUMOR-SPECIFIC ANTIGEN BY MHC II^{NEG} TUMORS REQUIRED?

The tumor-specific antigen used in our own studies, the MOPC315 myeloma protein, is a highly secreted antigen, with serum levels reaching milligrams per milliliter levels. Concentrations of myeloma protein in tumor tissues would be expected to be even higher. Surprisingly, a non-secreting myeloma variant that only expresses an intracellularly retained mutated Id^+ L chain, but in high amounts, was not rejected (36). In the absence of sufficient tumor antigen secretion, it might be expected that either spontaneous necrosis or apoptosis of tumor cells containing such high amounts of intracellular tumor antigen could prime tumor-infiltrating APC with tumor-specific antigen. This is apparently not the case for the non-secreting variant of MOPC315. It remains to be seen whether cytotoxic drug treatment of mice with tumors caused by this particular MOPC315 variant could enhance Id priming of APCs via uptake of necrotic or apoptotic cells.

In other MHC II^{NEG} models where tumor cells is reported to be rejected by $CD4^+$ T cells (28, 31, 32), there is scarce information as to whether tumor-specific antigen is secreted or not (**Table 2**). In the case of H-Y antigen, which clearly must be transferred from the tumor cells to host APC for MHC II presentation (28), there is little information about the extent of secretion of the antigen. In yet other cases, the tumor-specific antigen is simply not known (25), precluding any analysis of secretion status. It should further be noted that in some experiments [e.g., Ref. (24, 25, 37)] it has not been rigorously excluded that non-malignant normal cells could also produce the "tumor-specific" antigen. This possibility is virtually excluded in the MOPC315 model since $CD4^+$ T cells recognize a somatically mutated tumor-specific antigen unique to MOPC315 myeloma cells. By and large, it appears that secretion of tumor-specific antigen facilitates priming of host APC and stimulation of $CD4^+$ T cells. However, it is possible that the requirement of secretion could vary for distinct tumors and tumor-specific antigens, perhaps related to differences in susceptibility for cross-presentation of antigen associated with either necrotic or apoptotic tumor cells, or secreted vesicles such as exosomes.

What about MHC II^{POS} tumors – do they also require secretion of tumor-specific antigen? For MHC II^{POS} B lymphoma, a transfectant that secretes $\lambda 2^{315}$ was rejected, while another transfectant expressing a mutated intracellularly retained $\lambda 2^{315}$ was not (26). Similarly, A20 cells expressing HA, which apparently was negligibly secreted since HA was not found in serum, was not rejected (89). The Dby minor histocompatibility antigen (H–Y) (28) and Trp1 (35, 37, 38) have both been reported to be secreted by tumor cells. A strategy to test the hypothesis that secretion of tumor-specific antigen is required for rejection of MHC II^{POS} tumors would be to transfect MOPC315.37 with CIITA so that the tumor cells become MHC II^{POS}. If this transfectant is rejected in Id-specific TCR-transgenic mice, this would weaken the hypothesis.

BY WHICH PATHWAY IS TUMOR ANTIGEN PRESENTED BY APC IN DRAINING LYMPH NODES?

In the tumor models where it has been tested, be they MHC II^{NEG} (28, 34, 65) or MHC II^{POS} (37, 38), there was an apparent need for tumor-specific antigen to be presented by host APC to stimulate naïve (but not memory) $CD4^+$ T cells. Thus, in the case of the B16 MHC II^{POS} model, no rejection by naïve Trp1-specific $CD4^+$ T cells was obtained in hosts that lacked MHC class II molecules. By contrast, transfer of $CD4^+$ T cells that first had been primed *in vitro* could readily reject B16 tumors (37, 38). These findings indicate that MHC II^{POS} tumor cells themselves are incapable of stimulating naïve Trp1-specific $CD4^+$ T cells, and that priming by professional host APC is required. In addition, experiments reported by Xie et al. (38) using Trp1-deficient mice indicate that Trp1 derived from host tissue is redundant for priming APC and that Trp1 derived from B16 tumor cells suffice, at least for stimulation of memory $CD4^+$ T cells. It is still, however, unclear how the Trp1 antigen is transferred from tumors to host APC, and in which anatomical compartment priming of $CD4^+$ T cells take place.

The conclusions of the above experiments are supported by previous observations in the MOPC315 model, which directly demonstrate activation of Id-specific $CD4^+$ T cells in draining lymph nodes (34, 36, 85). Moreover, treatment with the sphingosine phosphate receptor modulator fingolimod that abrogates egress of T cells from lymph nodes led to a decreased number of Id-specific $CD4^+$ T cells within the tumor, resulting in failure of tumor rejection (86). Consistent with these findings, the non-secreting MOPC315.37 variant caused little activation of $CD4^+$ T cells in draining lymph nodes, and tumor rejection did not occur.

Idiotype-primed APCs are readily found in lymph nodes that drain MOPC315 tumors (Dembic and Bogen, unpublished experiments). It should therefore be possible by cell purifications and characterizations to reveal the identity of these Id-primed APCs in lymph nodes. Information from such experiments could help to define the mechanisms by which APC get primed by secreted tumor antigen. For example, if the predominant features of Id-primed APCs are that of a residential dendritic cell, this may signify priming by soluble antigen arriving to the lymph node via afferent lymphatic vessels.

ELIMINATION OF MHC II^{NEG} TUMOR CELLS

It is well documented that Th1/IFN-γ-activated M1 macrophages isolated from tumors under conditions of tumor rejection can directly inhibit the growth of MHC II^{NEG} myeloma cells *in vitro* (34, 36, 39). However, the molecular mechanisms mediating the inhibition of tumor cell growth remain to be established. Possibly, reactive oxygen species could be of importance, since resistance against B16 cells [although in later work reported to be MHC class II^{POS} under conditions of rejection (37)] was reduced in $iNOS^{-/-}$ and $NOX2^{-/-}$ mice (30). Results of Perez-Diez et al. indicate that under some circumstances, NK cells activated by $CD4^{+}$ T cells are important, but the effector mechanisms employed by such NK cells have not been addressed (28).

It is also possible that $CD4^{+}$ T cells could themselves directly kill tumor cells, e.g., through FasL/Fas interactions, similar to what has been described for killing of MHC II^{POS} B lymphoma cells (33), or a perforin/granzyme B-dependent mechanism as described for killing of the MHC II^{POS} B16 cells (37). The efficacy of killing mechanisms of $CD4^{+}$ T cells could also differ for different tumors. Thus, even though Th1 cells efficiently killed transfected A20 cells *in vitro* by a FasL-dependent mechanism, the same cells could not kill MOPC315 (26, 66). Finally, it has been reported that IFN-γ produced by tumor-specific Th1 cells mediate tumor rejection by means of angiostatic effects, thus causing starvation of the tumor (32).

DO CD4+ T CELL-MEDIATED IMMUNE RESPONSES AGAINST MHC II^{NEG} TUMOR CELLS CONVEY BYSTANDER KILLING OF TUMOR CELLS THAT HAVE LOST EXPRESSION OF ANTIGEN?

In theory, macrophage-mediated killing of MHC II^{NEG} tumors could be expected to indiscriminately kill surrounding cells, including tumor cells that have lost expression of antigen ("bystander killing"). If true, this would be a clinically important asset of Th1/M1 macrophage-mediated killing of tumor cells (34, 36, 39). The previously described angiostatic properties of Th1 derived IFNγ (32) would also be expected to cause bystander killing. On the other hand, direct killing of MHC II^{POS} tumor cells by cytotoxic $CD4^{+}$ T cells was demonstrated not to induce bystander killing (37).

WHAT CD4+ T CELL PHENOTYPES SUPPORT ANTI-TUMOR IMMUNITY?

Naïve $CD4^{+}$ T cells in Id-specific TCR-transgenic mice, which eradicate injected MHC II^{NEG} tumor cells, develop into IFNγ-secreting Th1 TILs that induce macrophage polarization into tumoricidal M1 macrophages (33, 34, 39). Transfer of naïve Id-specific $CD4^{+}$ T cells could cure established MHC II^{POS} tumors (33). In the Trp1-specific TCR-transgenic model, naïve (37, 38), Th1 (35), and Th17 (35) cells have been demonstrated to eradicate MHC II^{POS} tumors. Collectively, these results indicate that the primary anti-tumor response of naïve $CD4^{+}$ T cells is followed by T cell differentiation into Th1 (or possibly Th17) cells that confer anti-tumor immunity irrespective of MHC class II expression on tumor cells. While Th1 cells are clearly associated with anti-tumor immunity, variable effects have been observed with other $CD4^{+}$ T cell subsets, reviewed in Ref. (90). Moreover, recent studies suggest that effector $CD4^{+}$ T cells retain some degree of functional plasticity (91, 92). The plasticity of effector Th populations may explain the differential effects of the various Th cell populations in tumor immunity. In addition, exploiting the plasticity of Th cell subsets may be utilized in immune therapy.

TOLERANCE INDUCTION OF TUMOR-SPECIFIC CD4+ T CELLS

Use of TCR-transgenic mice offers the possibility of studying tolerance development by following the fate and function of tumor-reactive $CD4^{+}$ T cells. When Id-specific TCR-transgenic mice failed to reject high amounts of injected MHC II^{NEG} MOPC315 cells, $CD4^{+}$ T cells in peripheral lymphoid organs and in the tumor became deleted (93). The extent of deletion became more profound as tumor size increased. The deletion of peripheral tumor-specific $CD4^{+}$ T cells seen in this model for a highly secreted tumor antigen resembles that of exhaustion observed in chronic viral diseases. In addition to peripheral deletion of Id-specific $CD4^{+}$ T cells, progressive MOPC315 tumors also caused thymocyte deletion. It was demonstrated that circulatory myeloma protein gained access to the thymus and was presented in an MHC class II context by thymic APCs, thus causing negative selection of thymocytes (94).

In a recent paper, T cell characteristics in Trp1-specific TCR-transgenic mice developing B16 tumor recurrence following adoptive therapy were studied. Recurrence was associated with increased $FoxP3^{+}$ T_{reg} cell numbers, and increased expression of inhibitory ligands, including PD-1 and CTLA-4 inhibitory receptors on both T_{reg} and effector $CD4^{+}$ cells (95). Tumor recurrence could be prevented by concomitant depletion of T_{regs} and administration of checkpoint blockade antibodies. Collectively, these results indicate that $CD4^{+}$ T cells must eliminate tumor antigen-secreting tumor cells efficiently within a short timeframe. If the elimination is incomplete, T cell tolerance is induced by multiple mechanisms.

It has been shown that MHC II^{POS} A20 cells, are not rejected after i.v. injection in HA-specific TCR-transgenic mice, but induce anergy in $CD4^{+}$ T cells via priming of bone marrow derived APCs (89, 96). Interestingly, when presentation by bone marrow derived APCs was prevented by the use of bone marrow chimeras, anergy did not occur, and tumor cells were rejected (72). Thus, it might seem that tumor cells that poorly secrete tumor antigen could favor anergy development by induction tolerogenic APCs. The above results are consistent with previous observations that A20 cells expressing a non-secreted $\lambda 2^{315}$ were not rejected in Id-specific TCR-transgenic mice (26) (although it was not tested if anergy was induced). These results, obtained with non-secreting MHC II^{POS} A20 transfectants in two different TCR-transgenic models, are in support of the notion that tumor-specific antigen, perhaps via presentation of apoptotic or necrotic tumor cells by a special type of APC, favor induction of T cell anergy. In contrast, secretion of tumor-specific antigen and presentation (perhaps by another type of host APCs) in lymph nodes, may favor induction of potent primary anti-tumor $CD4^{+}$ T cell responses.

DICHOTOMOUS ROLE OF Th CELLS IN B CELL CANCERS

This review paper has focused on $CD4^{+}$ T cell-mediated eradication of tumor cells. However, $CD4^{+}$ T cells may also induce tumors. This dichotomy may especially apply to B cell tumors since B cells are known to proliferate in response to help from $CD4^{+}$ T cells. Extensive and prolonged B cell proliferation could indeed predispose to genetic instability and malignant transformation. In fact, B lymphoma development has been associated with continuous antigenic exposure in chronic infectious diseases caused by *Helicobacter pylori*, EBV, and hepatitis C. Moreover, chronic immune responses to self antigens in autoimmune diseases such as systemic lupus erythematosus, Sjögren's syndrome and rheumatoid arthritis have also been linked to development of B cell lymphomas, reviewed in Ref. (97, 98). Further supporting a role for chronic antigen stimulation, diffuse large B cell lymphomas (98, 99) and follicular B cell lymphomas (98, 100, 101) are frequently infiltrated with T cells. In Ig- and TCR-transgenic mice, chronic stimulation of Id^+ B cells by Id-specific $CD4^+$ Th2 cells results in the induction of Id^+ B lymphomas (102). Moreover, two separate studies have shown that proliferation of B lymphomas (103) and MM (104) was augmented by the presence of $CD4^+$ T cells.

The MOPC315 model, reviewed herein, was used in the experiments were Id^+ lymphomas were induced. Interestingly, when such induced lymphoma cells were injected s.c into naïve Id-specific TCR-transgenic mice, the lymphoma cells were promptly rejected (102). Thus, Id^+ B lymphoma cells were eliminated by mice having naïve $CD4^+$ T cells with an identical Id-specific TCR to that of the B lymphoma-inducing Th2 cells. If naïve T cells in the protected mice differentiated into tumor-eliminating Th1 cells was not investigated. However, analogous experiments indicate that Th1 is the primary response to subcutaneously inoculated B lymphomas (34, 39). These results suggest that B lymphoma cells induced by Th2 cells are rejected by Th1 cells expressing an identical TCR. The finding has obvious implications for T cell therapy: if a B cell tumor is initiated by Th2 cells, it may be treated by Th1 cells of the same specificity (and possibly *vice versa*). The same may apply to other combinations of Th cells such as Th17/Th1 etc. Thus, re-education of T cell phenotype may become part of the tumor immunotherapy armamentarium. Given the plasticity of $CD4^+$ subsets (91, 92), such re-education may become a real possibility.

CONCLUDING REMARKS

HOW DISPARATE ARE THE MECHANISMS FOR REJECTION OF MHC II^{POS} AND MHC II^{NEG} TUMORS?

The data reviewed herein suggest that the difference between direct and indirect killing of tumors relates predominantly to the effector stage of tumor cell killing. Thus, $CD4^+$ T cells can kill MHC II^{POS} cells directly, while killing of MHC II^{NEG} occurs indirectly via macrophages or possibly NK cells, angiostatic effects, or all of these. In contrast, the primary activation of naïve tumor-specific $CD4^+$ T cells appears to be similar for the direct and indirect mechanisms, in that presentation of tumor-specific antigen by host APC seems to be required. However, the evidence for this in the context of MHC II^{POS} tumors is largely circumstantial. In an MHC II^{NEG} myeloma model, secretion of tumor-specific myeloma protein clearly facilitates priming of APC in lymph nodes and stimulation of naive $CD4^+$ T cells that subsequently infiltrate the tumor site. Thus, the nature of the antigen, by virtue of its cellular localization and accessibility to APCs, might determine the ability of the antigen to serve as an efficient tumor-specific antigen in $CD4^+$ T cell responses. A more in-depth analysis of such factors might be of value in reconciling observations made in the various TCR-transgenic models.

ACKNOWLEDGMENTS

The authors would like to thank everyone in Bogen lab who, over the years, have contributed to the work described in this review. The work has been generously supported by the Norwegian Cancer Society, The Multiple Myeloma Research Foundation, The Research Council of Norway, The South-Eastern Norway Regional Health Authority, and numerous funds and legacies mentioned in the original research reports. The authors apologize for any omissions of publications that could not be included due to space constraints.

REFERENCES

1. Burnet M. Cancer; a biological approach. I. The processes of control. *Br Med J* (1957) **1**:779–86. doi:10.1136/bmj.1.5022.779
2. Thomas L. *Discussion in Cellular and Humoral Aspects of the Hypersensitive State*. New York: Hoebner-Harper (1959). p. 529–32.
3. Burnet FM. The evolution of bodily defence. *Med J Aust* (1963) **2**:817–21.
4. Burnet FM. The concept of immunological surveillance. *Prog Exp Tumor Res* (1970) **13**:1–27.
5. Koebel CM, Vermi W, Swann JB, Zerafa N, Rodig SJ, Old LJ, et al. Adaptive immunity maintains occult cancer in an equilibrium state. *Nature* (2007) **450**:903–7. doi:10.1038/nature06309
6. Dudley ME, Wunderlich JR, Robbins PF, Yang JC, Hwu P, Schwartzentruber DJ, et al. Cancer regression and autoimmunity in patients after clonal repopulation with antitumor lymphocytes. *Science* (2002) **298**:850–4. doi:10.1126/science.1076514
7. Page DB, Postow MA, Callahan MK, Allison JP, Wolchok JD. Immune modulation in cancer with antibodies. *Annu Rev Med* (2013). doi:10.1146/annurev-med-092012-112807
8. Galon J, Angell HK, Bedognetti D, Marincola FM. The continuum of cancer immunosurveillance: prognostic, predictive, and mechanistic signatures. *Immunity* (2013) **39**:11–26. doi:10.1016/j.immuni.2013.07.008
9. Khong HT, Restifo NP. Natural selection of tumor variants in the generation of "tumor escape" phenotypes. *Nat Immunol* (2002) **3**:999–1005. doi:10.1038/ni1102-999
10. Garrido F, Cabrera T, Aptsiauri N. "Hard" and "soft" lesions underlying the HLA class I alterations in cancer cells: implications for immunotherapy. *Int J Cancer* (2010) **127**:249–56. doi:10.1002/ijc.25270
11. Matsushita H, Vesely MD, Koboldt DC, Rickert CG, Uppaluri R, Magrini VJ, et al. Cancer exome analysis reveals a T-cell-dependent mechanism of cancer immunoediting. *Nature* (2012) **482**:400–4. doi:10.1038/nature10755
12. Hanson HL, Donermeyer DL, Ikeda H, White JM, Shankaran V, Old LJ, et al. Eradication of established tumors by CD8+ T cell adoptive immunotherapy. *Immunity* (2000) **13**:265–76. doi:10.1016/S1074-7613(00)00026-1
13. Lee KH, Wang E, Nielsen MB, Wunderlich J, Migueles S, Connors M, et al. Increased vaccine-specific T cell frequency after peptide-based vaccination correlates with increased susceptibility to in vitro stimulation but does not lead to tumor regression. *J Immunol* (1999) **163**:6292–300.
14. Dudley ME, Wunderlich JR, Yang JC, Hwu P, Schwartzentruber DJ, Topalian SL, et al. A phase I study of nonmyeloablative chemotherapy and adoptive transfer of autologous tumor antigen-specific T lymphocytes in patients with metastatic melanoma. *J Immunother* (2002) **25**:243–51. doi:10.1097/00002371-200205000-00007
15. Peterson AC, Harlin H, Gajewski TF. Immunization with melan-A peptide-pulsed peripheral blood mononuclear cells plus recombinant human interleukin-12 induces clinical activity and T-cell responses in advanced melanoma. *J Clin Oncol* (2003) **21**:2342–8. doi:10.1200/JCO.2003.12.144
16. Boon T, Coulie PG, Van Den Eynde BJ, Van Der Bruggen P. Human T cell responses against melanoma. *Annu Rev Immunol* (2006) **24**:175–208. doi:10.1146/annurev.immunol.24.021605.090733
17. Nishimura T, Iwakabe K, Sekimoto M, Ohmi Y, Yahata T, Nakui M, et al. Distinct role of antigen-specific T helper type 1 (Th1) and Th2 cells in tumor eradication in vivo. *J Exp Med* (1999) **190**:617–27. doi:10.1084/jem.190.5.617
18. Gao FG, Khammanivong V, Liu WJ, Leggatt GR, Frazer IH, Fernando GJ. Antigen-specific CD4+ T-cell help is required to activate a memory CD8+ T cell to a fully functional tumor killer cell. *Cancer Res* (2002) **62**:6438–41.
19. Janssen EM, Lemmens EE, Wolfe T, Christen U, Von Herrath MG, Schoenberger SP. CD4+ T cells are required for secondary expansion and memory in CD8+ T lymphocytes. *Nature* (2003) **421**:852–6. doi:10.1038/nature01441

20. Antony PA, Piccirillo CA, Akpinarli A, Finkelstein SE, Speiss PJ, Surman DR, et al. CD8+ T cell immunity against a tumor/self-antigen is augmented by CD4+ T helper cells and hindered by naturally occurring T regulatory cells. *J Immunol* (2005) **174**:2591–601.
21. Hunder NN, Wallen H, Cao J, Hendricks DW, Reilly JZ, Rodmyre R, et al. Treatment of metastatic melanoma with autologous CD4+ T cells against NY-ESO-1. *N Engl J Med* (2008) **358**:2698–703. doi:10.1056/NEJMoa0800251
22. Ostrand-Rosenberg S, Thakur A, Clements V. Rejection of mouse sarcoma cells after transfection of MHC class II genes. *J Immunol* (1990) **144**: 4068–71.
23. Ostrand-Rosenberg S, Roby CA, Clements VK. Abrogation of tumorigenicity by MHC class II antigen expression requires the cytoplasmic domain of the class II molecule. *J Immunol* (1991) **147**:2419–22.
24. Fujiwara H, Fukuzawa M, Yoshioka T, Nakajima H, Hamaoka T. The role of tumor-specific Lyt-1+2– T cells in eradicating tumor cells in vivo. I. Lyt-1+2– T cells do not necessarily require recruitment of host's cytotoxic T cell precursors for implementation of in vivo immunity. *J Immunol* (1984) **133**: 1671–6.
25. Greenberg PD, Kern DE, Cheever MA. Therapy of disseminated murine leukemia with cyclophosphamide and immune Lyt-1+,2– T cells. Tumor eradication does not require participation of cytotoxic T cells. *J Exp Med* (1985) **161**:1122–34. doi:10.1084/jem.161.5.1122
26. Lauritzsen GF, Weiss S, Dembic Z, Bogen B. Naive idiotype-specific CD4+ T cells and immunosurveillance of B-cell tumors. *Proc Natl Acad Sci U S A* (1994) **91**:5700–4. doi:10.1073/pnas.91.12.5700
27. Bogen B, Munthe L, Sollien A, Hofgaard P, Omholt H, Dagnaes F, et al. Naive CD4+ T cells confer idiotype-specific tumor resistance in the absence of antibodies. *Eur J Immunol* (1995) **25**:3079–86. doi:10.1002/eji.1830251114
28. Perez-Diez A, Joncker NT, Choi K, Chan WFN, Anderson CC, Lantz O, et al. CD4 cells can be more efficient at tumor rejection than CD8 cells. *Blood* (2007) **109**:5346–54. doi:10.1182/blood-2006-10-051318
29. Greenberg PD, Cheever MA, Fefer A. Eradication of disseminated murine leukemia by chemoimmunotherapy with cyclophosphamide and adoptively transferred immune syngeneic Lyt-1+2– lymphocytes. *J Exp Med* (1981) **154**:952–63. doi:10.1084/jem.154.3.952
30. Hung K, Hayashi R, Lafond-Walker A, Lowenstein C, Pardoll D, Levitsky H. The central role of CD4(+) T cells in the antitumor immune response. *J Exp Med* (1998) **188**:2357–68. doi:10.1084/jem.188.12.2357
31. Mumberg D, Monach PA, Wanderling S, Philip M, Toledano AY, Schreiber RD, et al. CD4(+) T cells eliminate MHC class II-negative cancer cells in vivo by indirect effects of IFN-gamma. *Proc Natl Acad Sci U S A* (1999) **96**:8633–8. doi:10.1073/pnas.96.15.8633
32. Qin Z, Blankenstein T. CD4+ T cell – mediated tumor rejection involves inhibition of angiogenesis that is dependent on IFN gamma receptor expression by nonhematopoietic cells. *Immunity* (2000) **12**:677–86. doi:10.1016/S1074-7613(00)80218-6
33. Lundin KU, Hofgaard PO, Omholt H, Munthe LA, Corthay A, Bogen B. Therapeutic effect of idiotype-specific CD4+ T cells against B-cell lymphoma in the absence of anti-idiotypic antibodies. *Blood* (2003) **102**:605. doi:10.1182/blood-2002-11-3381
34. Corthay A, Skovseth DK, Lundin KU, Rosjo E, Omholt H, Hofgaard PO, et al. Primary antitumor immune response mediated by CD4+ T cells. *Immunity* (2005) **22**:371–83. doi:10.1016/j.immuni.2005.02.003
35. Muranski P, Boni A, Antony PA, Cassard L, Irvine KR, Kaiser A, et al. Tumor-specific Th17-polarized cells eradicate large established melanoma. *Blood* (2008) **112**:362–73. doi:10.1182/blood-2007-11-120998
36. Corthay A, Lundin KU, Lorvik KB, Hofgaard PO, Bogen B. Secretion of tumor-specific antigen by myeloma cells is required for cancer immunosurveillance by CD4+ T cells. *Cancer Res* (2009) **69**:5901–7. doi:10.1158/0008-5472.CAN-08-4816
37. Quezada SA, Simpson TR, Peggs KS, Merghoub T, Vider J, Fan X, et al. Tumor-reactive CD4(+) T cells develop cytotoxic activity and eradicate large established melanoma after transfer into lymphopenic hosts. *J Exp Med* (2010) **207**:637–50. doi:10.1084/jem.20091918
38. Xie Y, Akpinarli A, Maris C, Hipkiss EL, Lane M, Kwon EKM, et al. Naive tumor-specific CD4+ T cells differentiated in vivo eradicate established melanoma. (2010) **207**:651–67. doi:10.1084/jem.20091921
39. Haabeth OA, Lorvik KB, Hammarstrom C, Donaldson IM, Haraldsen G, Bogen B, et al. Inflammation driven by tumour-specific Th1 cells protects against B-cell cancer. *Nat Commun* (2011) **2**:240. doi:10.1038/ncomms1239
40. Marzo AL, Lake RA, Robinson BW, Scott B. T-cell receptor transgenic analysis of tumor-specific CD8 and CD4 responses in the eradication of solid tumors. *Cancer Res* (1999) **59**:1071–9.
41. Klein L, Trautman L, Psarras S, Schnell S, Siermann A, Liblau R, et al. Visualizing the course of antigen-specific CD8 and CD4 T cell responses to a growing tumor. *Eur J Immunol* (2003) **33**:806–14. doi:10.1002/eji.200323800
42. Zhou G, Drake CG, Levitsky HI. Amplification of tumor-specific regulatory T cells following therapeutic cancer vaccines. *Blood* (2006) **107**:628–36. doi:10.1182/blood-2005-07-2737
43. Chamoto K, Wakita D, Narita Y, Zhang Y, Noguchi D, Ohnishi H, et al. An essential role of antigen-presenting cell/T-helper type 1 cell-cell interactions in draining lymph node during complete eradication of class II-negative tumor tissue by T-helper type 1 cell therapy. *Cancer Res* (2006) **66**:1809–17. doi:10.1158/0008-5472.CAN-05-2246
44. Marabelle A, Kohrt H, Sagiv-Barfi I, Ajami B, Axtell RC, Zhou G, et al. Depleting tumor-specific Tregs at a single site eradicates disseminated tumors. *J Clin Invest* (2013) **123**:2447–63. doi:10.1172/JCI64859
45. Bogen B, Malissen B, Haas W. Idiotope-specific T cell clones that recognize syngeneic immunoglobulin fragments in the context of class II molecules. *Eur J Immunol* (1986) **16**:1373–8. doi:10.1002/eji.1830161110
46. Bogen B, Gleditsch L, Weiss S, Dembic Z. Weak positive selection of transgenic T cell receptor-bearing thymocytes: importance of major histocompatibility complex class II, T cell receptor and CD4 surface molecule densities. *Eur J Immunol* (1992) **22**:703–9. doi:10.1002/eji.1830220313
47. Lantz O, Grandjean I, Matzinger P, Di Santo JP. Gamma chain required for naive CD4+ T cell survival but not for antigen proliferation. *Nat Immunol* (2000) **1**(1):54–8. doi:10.1038/76917
48. Scott B, Liblau R, Degermann S, Marconi LA, Ogata L, Caton AJ, et al. A role for non-MHC genetic polymorphism in susceptibility to spontaneous autoimmunity. *Immunity* (1994) **1**(1):73–83. doi:10.1016/1074-7613(94)90011-6
49. Kirberg J, Baron A, Jakob S, Rolink A, Karjalainen K, von Boehmer H. Thymic selection of CD8+ single positive cells with a class II major histocompatibility complex-restricted receptor. *J Exp Med* (1994) **180**(1):25–34. doi:10.1084/jem.180.1.25
50. Murphy KM, Heimberger AB, Loh DY. Induction by antigen of intrathymic apoptosis of CD4+CD8+TCRlo thymocytes in vivo. *Science* (1990) **250**(4988):1720–23.
51. Barnden MJ, Allison J, Heath WR, Carbone FR. Defective TCR expression in transgenic mice constructed using cDNA-based alpha- and beta-chain genes under the control of heterologous regulatory elements. *Immunol Cell Biol* (1998) **76**(1):34–40. doi:10.1046/j.1440-1711.1998.00709.x
52. Eisen HN, Simms ES, Potter M. Mouse myeloma proteins with antihapten antibody activity. The protein produced by plasma cell tumor MOPC-315. *Biochemistry* (1968) **7**:4126–34. doi:10.1021/bi00851a048
53. Hannestad K, Kao MS, Eisen HN. Cell-bound myeloma proteins on the surface of myeloma cells: potential targets for the immune system. *Proc Natl Acad Sci U S A* (1972) **69**(8):2295–9.
54. Xu Y, Setaluri V, Takechi Y, Houghton AN. Sorting and secretion of a melanosome membrane protein, gp75/TRP1. *J Invest Dermatol* (1997) **109**(6):788–95. doi:10.1111/1523-1747.ep12340971
55. Zenzes MT, Müller U, Aschmoneit I, Wolf U. Studies on H-Y antigen in different cell fractions of the testis during pubescence: immature germ cells are H-Y antigen negative. *Hum Genet* (1978) **45**(3):297–303. doi:10.1007/BF00278727
56. Müller U. H-Y antigens. *Hum Genet* (1996) **97**(6):701–4. doi:10.1007/BF02346175
57. Copeland CS, Doms RW, Bolzau EM, Webster RG, Helenius A. Assembly of influenza hemagglutinin trimers and its role in intracellular transport. *J Cell Biol* (1986) **103**(4):1179–91. doi:10.1083/jcb.103.4.1179
58. Meek RL, Walsh KA, Palmiter RD. The signal sequence of ovalbumin is located near the NH2 terminus. *J Biol Chem* (1982) **257**(20):12245–51.
59. Rudensky A, Preston-Hurlburt P, Hong SC, Barlow A, Janeway CA Jr. Sequence analysis of peptides bound to MHC class II molecules. *Nature* (1991) **353**:622–7. doi:10.1038/353622a0

60. Benoist C, Mathis D. Regulation of major histocompatibility complex class-II genes: X, Y and other letters of the alphabet. *Annu Rev Immunol* (1990) **8**:681–715. doi:10.1146/annurev.immunol.8.1.681
61. Glimcher LH, Kara CJ. Sequences and factors: a guide to MHC class-II transcription. *Annu Rev Immunol* (1992) **10**:13–49. doi:10.1146/annurev.iy.10.040192.000305
62. Ting JP, Baldwin AS. Regulation of MHC gene expression. *Curr Opin Immunol* (1993) **5**:8–16. doi:10.1016/0952-7915(93)90074-3
63. Steimle V, Siegrist CA, Mottet A, Lisowska-Grospierre B, Mach B. Regulation of MHC class II expression by interferon-gamma mediated by the transactivator gene CIITA. *Science* (1994) **265**:106–9. doi:10.1126/science.8016643
64. Mach B, Steimle V, Martinez-Soria E, Reith W. Regulation of MHC class II genes: lessons from a disease. *Annu Rev Immunol* (1996) **14**:301–31. doi:10.1146/annurev.immunol.14.1.301
65. Dembic Z, Schenck K, Bogen B. Dendritic cells purified from myeloma are primed with tumor-specific antigen (idiotype) and activate CD4+ T cells. *Proc Natl Acad Sci U S A* (2000) **97**:2697–702. doi:10.1073/pnas.050579897
66. Lundin KU, Screpanti V, Omholt H, Hofgaard PO, Yagita H, Grandien A, et al. CD4+ T cells kill Id+ B-lymphoma cells: FasLigand-Fas interaction is dominant in vitro but is redundant in vivo. *Cancer Immunol Immunother* (2004) **53**:1135–45. doi:10.1007/s00262-004-0538-4
67. Wu GE, Hozumi N, Murialdo H. Secretion of a lambda 2 immunoglobulin chain is prevented by a single amino acid substitution in its variable region. *Cell* (1983) **33**:77–83. doi:10.1016/0092-8674(83)90336-7
68. Esumi N, Hunt B, Itaya T, Frost P. Reduced tumorigenicity of murine tumor cells secreting gamma-interferon is due to nonspecific host responses and is unrelated to class I major histocompatibility complex expression. *Cancer Res* (1991) **51**(4):1185–9.
69. Moore MW, Carbone FR, Bevan MJ. Introduction of soluble protein into the class I pathway of antigen processing and presentation. *Cell* (1988) **54**(6):777–85.
70. Lauritzsen GF, Bogen B. The role of idiotype-specific, CD4+ T cells in tumor resistance against major histocompatibility complex class II molecule negative plasmacytoma cells. *Cell Immunol* (1993) **148**:177–88. doi:10.1006/cimm.1993.1100
71. Tite JP, Janeway CA Jr. Cloned helper T cells can kill B lymphoma cells in the presence of specific antigen: Ia restriction and cognate vs. noncognate interactions in cytolysis. *Eur J Immunol* (1984) **14**:878–86. doi:10.1002/eji.1830141004
72. Horna P, Cuenca A, Cheng F, Brayer J, Wang HW, Borrello I, et al. In vivo disruption of tolerogenic cross-presentation mechanisms uncovers an effective T-cell activation by B-cell lymphomas leading to antitumor immunity. *Blood* (2006) **107**:2871–8. doi:10.1182/blood-2005-07-3014
73. Silacci P, Mottet A, Steimle V, Reith W, Mach B. Developmental extinction of major histocompatibility complex class II gene expression in plasmocytes is mediated by silencing of the transactivator gene CIITA. *J Exp Med* (1994) **180**:1329–36. doi:10.1084/jem.180.4.1329
74. Reith W, Mach B. The bare lymphocyte syndrome and the regulation of MHC expression. *Annu Rev Immunol* (2001) **19**:331–73. doi:10.1146/annurev.immunol.19.1.331
75. Sanda T, Iida S, Kayukawa S, Ueda R. Induction of class II major histocompatibility complex expression in human multiple myeloma cells by retinoid. *Haematologica* (2007) **92**:115–20. doi:10.3324/haematol.10300
76. Yi Q, Dabadghao S, Osterborg A, Bergenbrant S, Holm G. Myeloma bone marrow plasma cells: evidence for their capacity as antigen-presenting cells. *Blood* (1997) **90**:1960–7.
77. Zhao M, Flynt FL, Hong M, Chen H, Gilbert CA, Briley NT, et al. MHC class II transactivator (CIITA) expression is upregulated in multiple myeloma cells by IFN-gamma. *Mol Immunol* (2007) **44**:2923–32. doi:10.1016/j.molimm.2007.01.009
78. Bothwell AL, Paskind M, Reth M, Imanishi-Kari T, Rajewsky K, Baltimore D. Somatic variants of murine immunoglobulin lambda light chains. *Nature* (1982) **298**:380–2. doi:10.1038/298380a0
79. Bogen B, Lambris JD. Minimum length of an idiotypic peptide and a model for its binding to a major histocompatibility complex class II molecule. *EMBO J* (1989) **8**:1947–52.
80. Weiss S, Bogen B. B-lymphoma cells process and present their endogenous immunoglobulin to major histocompatibility complex-restricted T cells. *Proc Natl Acad Sci U S A* (1989) **86**:282–6. doi:10.1073/pnas.86.1.282
81. Jorgensen T, Hannestad K. Helper T cell recognition of the variable domains of a mouse myeloma protein (315). Effect of the major histocompatibility complex and domain conformation. *J Exp Med* (1982) **155**:1587–96. doi:10.1084/jem.155.6.1587
82. Foy TM, Lynch RG, Waldschmidt TJ. Ontogeny and distribution of the murine B cell Fc gamma RII. *J Immunol* (1992) **149**:1516–23.
83. Winberry L, Marks A, Baumal R. Immunoglobulin production and secretion by variant clones of the MOPC 315 mouse myeloma cell line. *J Immunol* (1980) **124**:1174–82.
84. Corthay A, Lorvik KB, Bogen B. Is secretion of tumour-specific antigen important for cancer eradication by CD4(+) T cells? – Implications for cancer immunotherapy by adoptive T cell transfer. *Scand J Immunol* (2011) **73**:527–30. doi:10.1111/j.1365-3083.2011.02558.x
85. Lorvik KB, Haabeth OA, Clancy T, Bogen B, Corthay A. Molecular profiling of tumor-specific T1 cells activated in vivo. *Oncoimmunology* (2013) **2**:e24383. doi:10.4161/onci.24383
86. Lorvik KB, Bogen B, Corthay A. Fingolimod blocks immunosurveillance of myeloma and B-cell lymphoma resulting in cancer development in mice. *Blood* (2012) **119**:2176–7. doi:10.1182/blood-2011-10-388892
87. Haabeth OA, Bogen B, Corthay A. A model for cancer-suppressive inflammation. *Oncoimmunology* (2012) **1**:1146–55. doi:10.4161/onci.21542
88. Bogen B, Schenck K, Munthe LA, Dembic Z. Deletion of idiotype (Id)-specific T cells in multiple myeloma. *Acta Oncol* (2000) **39**:783–8. doi:10.1080/028418600750063505
89. Staveley-O'Carroll K, Sotomayor E, Montgomery J, Borrello I, Hwang L, Fein S, et al. Induction of antigen-specific T cell anergy: an early event in the course of tumor progression. *Proc Natl Acad Sci U S A* (1998) **95**:1178–83. doi:10.1073/pnas.95.3.1178
90. Fridman WH, Pages F, Sautes-Fridman C, Galon J. The immune contexture in human tumours: impact on clinical outcome. *Nat Rev Cancer* (2012) **12**:298–306. doi:10.1038/nrc3245
91. Murphy KM, Stockinger B. Effector T cell plasticity: flexibility in the face of changing circumstances. *Nat Immunol* (2010) **11**:674–80. doi:10.1038/ni.1899
92. O'Shea JJ, Paul WE. Mechanisms underlying lineage commitment and plasticity of helper CD4+ T cells. *Science* (2010) **327**:1098–102. doi:10.1126/science.1178334
93. Bogen B. Peripheral T cell tolerance as a tumor escape mechanism: deletion of CD4+ T cells specific for a monoclonal immunoglobulin idiotype secreted by a plasmacytoma. *Eur J Immunol* (1996) **26**:2671–9. doi:10.1002/eji.1830261119
94. Lauritzsen GF, Hofgaard PO, Schenck K, Bogen B. Clonal deletion of thymocytes as a tumor escape mechanism. *Int J Cancer* (1998) **78**:216–22. doi:10.1002/(SICI)1097-0215(19981005)78:2<216::AID-IJC16>3.0.
95. Goding SR, Wilson KA, Xie Y, Harris KM, Baxi A, Akpinarli A, et al. Restoring immune function of tumor-specific CD4+ T cells during recurrence of melanoma. *J Immunol* (2013) **190**:4899–909. doi:10.4049/jimmunol.1300271
96. Sotomayor EM, Borrello I, Rattis FM, Cuenca AG, Abrams J, Staveley-O'carroll K, et al. Cross-presentation of tumor antigens by bone marrow-derived antigen-presenting cells is the dominant mechanism in the induction of T-cell tolerance during B-cell lymphoma progression. *Blood* (2001) **98**:1070–7. doi:10.1182/blood.V98.4.1070
97. Morse HC III, Kearney JF, Isaacson PG, Carroll M, Fredrickson TN, Jaffe ES. Cells of the marginal zone – origins, function and neoplasia. *Leuk Res* (2001) **25**:169–78. doi:10.1016/S0145-2126(00)00107-7
98. Kuppers R. Mechanisms of B-cell lymphoma pathogenesis. *Nat Rev Cancer* (2005) **5**:251–62. doi:10.1038/nrc1589
99. Monti S, Savage KJ, Kutok JL, Feuerhake F, Kurtin P, Mihm M, et al. Molecular profiling of diffuse large B-cell lymphoma identifies robust subtypes including one characterized by host inflammatory response. *Blood* (2005) **105**:1851–61. doi:10.1182/blood-2004-07-2947
100. Ansell SM, Stenson M, Habermann TM, Jelinek DF, Witzig TE. CD4+ T-cell immune response to large B-cell non-Hodgkin's lymphoma predicts patient outcome. *J Clin Oncol* (2001) **19**:720–6.
101. Dave SS, Wright G, Tan B, Rosenwald A, Gascoyne RD, Chan WC, et al. Prediction of survival in follicular lymphoma based on molecular features of tumor-infiltrating immune cells. *N Engl J Med* (2004) **351**:2159–69. doi:10.1056/NEJMoa041869

102. Zangani MM, Froyland M, Qiu GY, Meza-Zepeda LA, Kutok JL, Thompson KM, et al. Lymphomas can develop from B cells chronically helped by idiotype-specific T cells. *J Exp Med* (2007) **204**:1181–91. doi:10.1084/jem.20061220
103. Os A, Burgler S, Ribes AP, Funderud A, Wang D, Thompson KM, et al. Chronic lymphocytic leukemia cells are activated and proliferate in response to specific T helper cells. *Cell Rep* (2013) **4**:566–77. doi:10.1016/j.celrep.2013.07.011
104. Ostad M, Andersson M, Gruber A, Sundblad A. Expansion of immunoglobulin autoreactive T-helper cells in multiple myeloma. *Blood* (2008) **111**:2725–32. doi:10.1182/blood-2006-11-056242

7

Harnessing the heterogeneity of T cell differentiation fate to fine-tune generation of effector and memory T cells

Chang Gong[1], **Jennifer J. Linderman**[2] **and Denise Kirschner**[3]*

[1] *Department of Computational Medicine and Bioinformatics, University of Michigan, Ann Arbor, MI, USA*
[2] *Department of Chemical Engineering, University of Michigan, Ann Arbor, MI, USA*
[3] *Department of Microbiology and Immunology, University of Michigan Medical School, Ann Arbor, MI, USA*

Edited by:
Veronika Zarnitsyna, Emory University, USA

Reviewed by:
Rustom Antia, Emory University, USA
Thomas Höfer, German Cancer Research Center, Germany

****Correspondence:***
Denise Kirschner, 6730 Medical Science Building II, Ann Arbor, MI, USA
e-mail: kirschne@umich.edu

Recent studies show that naïve T cells bearing identical T cell receptors experience heterogeneous differentiation and clonal expansion processes. The factors controlling this outcome are not well characterized, and their contributions to immune cell dynamics are similarly poorly understood. In this study, we develop a computational model to elaborate mechanisms occurring within and between two important physiological compartments, lymph nodes and blood, to determine how immune cell dynamics are controlled. Our multi-organ (multi-compartment) model integrates cellular and tissue level events and allows us to examine the heterogeneous differentiation of individual precursor cognate naïve T cells to generate both effector and memory T lymphocytes. Using this model, we simulate a hypothetical immune response and reproduce both primary and recall responses to infection. Increased numbers of antigen-bearing dendritic cells (DCs) are predicted to raise production of both effector and memory T cells, and distinct "sweet spots" of peptide-MHC levels on those DCs exist that favor CD4+ or CD8+ T cell differentiation toward either effector or memory cell phenotypes. This has important implications for vaccine development and immunotherapy.

Keywords: two-compartment model, lymph nodes, blood, agent-based, circulation, systems biology, dendritic cells, cognate

INTRODUCTION

Antigen-presenting cells (APCs), especially dendritic cells (DCs), process antigens and carry information from sites of infection to secondary lymphoid organs, such as lymph nodes (LNs) (1). T cells are produced in the thymus and are deployed into blood circulation to recognize millions of different epitopes from pathogenic organisms; each T cell is hardwired to have one type of T cell receptor (TCR) that recognizes a single pattern (i.e., "cognate" with respect to a specific antigen) (2). The frequency of particular cognate T cells is as low as 10^{-5}–10^{-6} (3, 4). Through high endothelial venules (HEVs), T cells are recruited to LNs, where they are exposed to antigenic peptides presented by MHC molecules expressed on DCs – this initiates the adaptive immune response (5–9). LNs are organized such that when T cells travel through they can be efficiently scanned by DCs to identify that rare cognate encounter (10–12). Such encounters result in binding of cognate T cells to DCs and subsequent activation and proliferation of the T cells. The expanded T cell population differentiates into two classes: effector cells, which perform immediate killing and cytokine secretion functions, and memory cells, which are reserved for long-term protection (13, 14). These cells move out of LNs via efferent lymphatics (ELs) into blood circulation (15). Through the blood, effector T cells reach sites of infection while memory T cells continue to recirculate and await a potential secondary infection for which they will wage a faster and stronger recall response (16, 17). A snapshot of the trafficking of these cells is shown in **Figure 1**. The immune system responds differently to different antigenic materials; however, the same set of machinery is engaged to face each challenge. Thus, there should be a general program adaptively guiding the behavior of this system. In this study, we focus on cellular-mediated events shared among immune responses during the initiation of adaptive immunity and generation of immune memory.

Differentiation of T cells during generation of adaptive and memory responses is highly heterogeneous, and this heterogeneity is may be dependent on the environmental context that each cell experiences (18, 19). However, the cause of such heterogeneity is poorly understood. If mechanisms other than mere stochasticity contribute to heterogeneity, it could be possible to more precisely direct the differentiation to favor the production of the desired output from an immune response (e.g., effectors in an immune therapy or memory cells in vaccination) by manipulating the mechanisms involved. We are interested in which mechanisms could provide handles for such manipulation. Since T cell priming occurs in LNs, and blood circulation conveys effector and memory T cells to locations where they perform their specific functions, mechanisms in these two organs could be responsible for the heterogeneous differentiation. The dynamics of T cells in these compartments will also reflect progression of infection or effectiveness of vaccinations. Thus, understanding how different LN and blood mechanisms affect the dynamics of infection and treatment could help guide immunotherapy and vaccine design.

Computational and mathematical models are widely used in biological systems to assess hypotheses and generate predictions

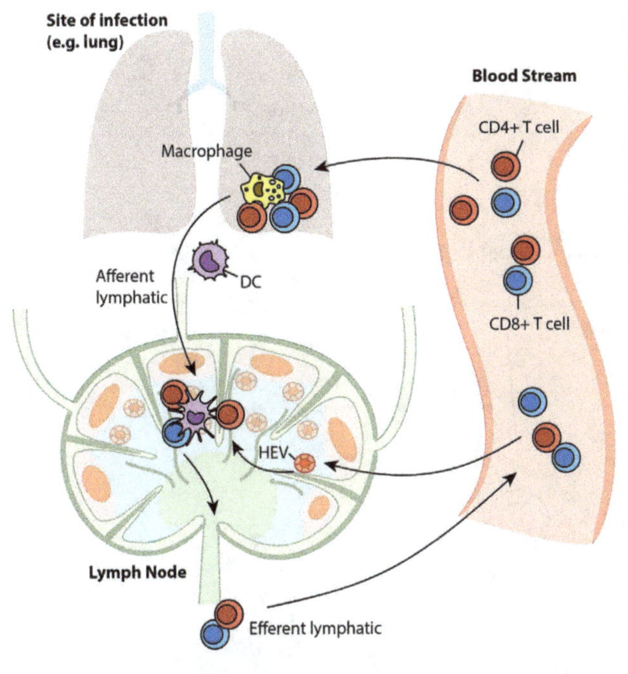

FIGURE 1 | T cell trafficking between compartments. Naïve T cells circulate between LNs and blood. Upon infection, APCs present antigen to cognate T cells in LNs to initiate their proliferation and differentiation to generate effector and memory cells. After entering the blood, effector cells are recruited to sites to fight ongoing infection, while memory cells recirculate, awaiting secondary infections.

for experimental validation. Deterministic equation-based models have been developed to understand the dynamics of T cells responding to immunogenic antigens, and these models helped with estimating parameters, determining alternative hypothesis, and predicting the outcomes of immune responses (20, 21). Agent-based models (ABMs) have proven convenient in assessing roles of cellular and molecular level interactions during infection (22–27). However, because of the extremely low cognate frequency that exists in primates, these models usually require large numbers of cells to be simulated and thus are very computationally intensive. In order to capture both heterogeneous stimuli-sensitive short-term activation events as well as average long-term dynamics, a model needs to be capable of adapting itself to both situations.

In this study, we present a hybrid computational model that uses an agent-based modeling to capture events occurring in a LN and a non-linear ordinary differential equation (ODE) model to capture events occurring in the well-mixed compartment of blood. This model allows us to track a highly stochastic immune response operating during the first few weeks of an immune response (with time resolution around seconds), as well as long-term dynamics afterward (at a time scale of months to years). Using this model, we assess which mechanisms in both LN and blood compartments control the differentiation and clonal expansion processes of T cells and also direct the immune response toward potent effector T cell output and/or robust memory generation. These findings could bring insights to vaccine design strategies.

MATERIALS AND METHODS

LN ABM MODEL

Agent-based models are computational models in which individual agents are represented on an explicitly formulated grid and they interact with each other according to a defined set of rules implemented in discrete time steps. As these types of models can account for spatial-sensitive interactions between DC and cognate T cells, they are ideal for studying heterogeneous priming and differentiation of T cells in LNs (23–25, 28, 29).

We previously developed *LymphSim*, a three-dimensional (3D) LN computational model capturing dynamics of CD4+ T cells, CD8+ T cells, and DCs during both steady state and infection (30). Briefly, cells move on a 3D grid that is shaped like a truncated cone and represents ~1/200 of a primate LN. T cells enter the LN via HEVs, search for DCs, activate and proliferate to generate effector cells that exit via ELs. In *LymphSim*, cell motility and steady state values in a LN are calibrated to experimental data with model antigens such as OVA (31), and the dynamics during an immune response are not quantitatively fit to any specific infection. For simplicity, we only include one type of cognate T cell each for CD4+ and CD8+ T cells in current model, and DCs present the corresponding antigens on pMHC (peptide-MHC)-II and pMHC-I for both primary and secondary infections. The model can be adapted to account for multiple sub-antigens. For the work herein, this single antigen study is sufficient to address the key questions under study. A complete list of rules can be found at: http://malthus.micro.med.umich.edu/lab/movies/3dLN/.

EFFECTOR AND MEMORY T CELL DIFFERENTIATION RULES

In the present study, we modified *LymphSim* to include two additional T cell differentiation states: central memory (CM) and effector memory (EM), for both CD4+ and CD8+ T cells. We also added rules that govern generation of these memory cells, and their interaction with other cells (**Figure 2**).

We based the cell differentiation process on a version of a "signal-strength model," in which the overall strength of signal received by a naïve T cell during DC contact will determine the fate of cell differentiation (**Figure 3**) (32–35). A definitive differentiation scheme after T cell priming occurs has not been determined by experimentation. Previous modeling studies based on experimental data reject memory to effector differentiation in favor of effector to memory differentiation (20); however, more recent work showed that differentiation has as its backbone differentiation from naïve to CM precursor to EM precursor to effector (18). The scheme we use in this study considers effector to EM differentiation, but is still topologically similar to the scheme from (18), with precursors of both EM and effectors differentiating into these two subtypes (**Figure 3**). The difference between the two schemes is that "effectors" in our model are cells that have differentiated toward effector phenotype sufficiently so as not to enter into the CM population, nor have they entered into the EM pool. They are allowed to exit the LN due to the loss of early activation markers (CD69), even though these cells do not perform effector functions until they would reach sites of infection, which is not studied in this current work.

In our model, a series of probabilistic checkpoints are established to determine to which state a cell will proceed (36–39).

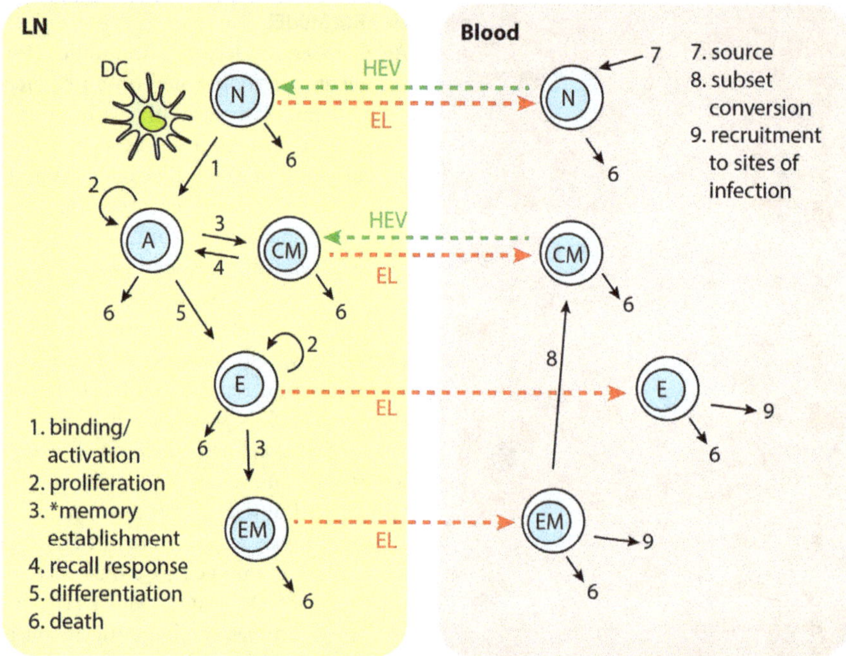

FIGURE 2 | T cell subsets in two-compartments of LNs and blood: N, naïve; A, activated; CM, central memory; E, effector; EM, effector memory. Each number indicates a collection of processes occurring in that step and in different cell types. Naïve T cells are recruited to LN from blood. In the LN, cognate T cells bind with Ag-DCs and get activated. Activated T cells proliferate and differentiate into central memory (CM) and effector cells. CM in the LN can bind to DC and be activated again. Effector T cells can further differentiate to effector memory (EM) cells. Naïve, effector, CM, and EM exit LN from EL. Naïve and CM cells recirculate between LN and blood. Effector and EM are recruited to sites of infection. EM can covert to CMs. *Memory establishment for CD8+ T cells requires LDCs.

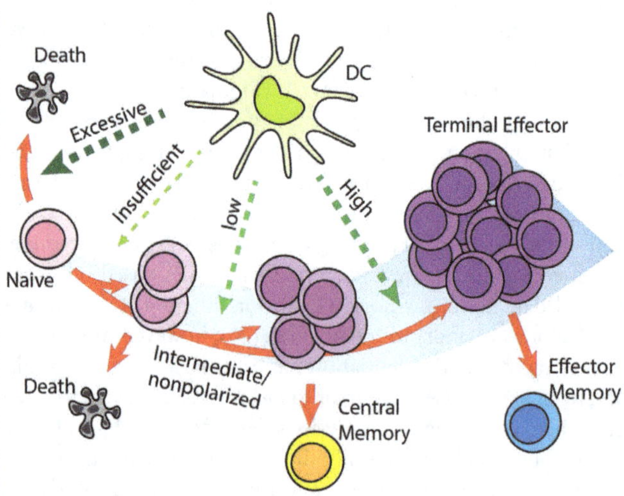

FIGURE 3 | "Signal-strength model" of T cell differentiation. T cells receive antigenic, co-stimulatory, and inflammatory signals from DC during priming. In concert, these of stimulations determine the fate of T cell clonal expansion and differentiation. Greater proliferation correlates with stronger signal. However, insufficient stimulation results in death by neglect, while excessive stimulation causes activation induced cell death. Stronger stimulation also drives T cells toward terminal differentiation and reduces their memory-forming potential. Please see Section "Effector and Memory T Cell Differentiation Rules" for a description of differentiation models and how this was selected.

When a cognate T cell finds an Ag-bearing DC (Ag-DC) or licensed DC (LDC) in its binding area, the corresponding pMHC value of the DC is checked to see if a successful binding can be established. If bound, a T cell continuously accumulates signals from the DC (40), represented by pMHC levels at each time point. Here, pMHC level is used as a proxy for the strength of antigenic stimulation from the DC or LDC. When a T cell unbinds from a DC or LDC, the accumulated signal value is used to determine whether a T cell proceeds to an activated state, or returns to a resting state (naïve). Activated cells go through a set number of rounds of divisions, after which the accumulated signal level is checked again to decide if the cell can further differentiate into an effector state. Effector cells will divide a few more rounds. With given probabilities, the cells with intermediate differentiation status do not proceed to effector status, but become CM cells, while those effector cells with sufficient signals will become EM cells (41–43). The probability of effector cell converting to EM is estimated between 0.1 and 0.4. CM T cells can be recruited to LNs from HEVs. These cells act similarly to cognate naïve T cells. When they detect Ag-DCs or LDCs, CMs will bind to DC and accumulate signal more efficiently in comparison with naïve cells (44, 45). The rules above apply to both CD4+ and CD8+ T cells. Because we developed some of these rules based on LCMV studies, one difference we captured between these two cell types is that CD8+ T cells can bind only to LDCs to generate functional memory cells in the primary response, whereas CD4+ T cells do not have this restriction and can generate memory cells after binding to both Ag-DCs and LDCs (46).

Other models of T cell differentiation exist, and some of these models are not mutually exclusive. We also integrated features from these models into our rule set, and excluded those that are inconsistent with current findings or are not applicable to our model at this stage. A single naïve T cell can produce both effector and memory progenies (19, 47), so we excluded the possibility that effector and memory arise from separate precursors. In the decreasing-potential model (13), the stimulation that T cells receive during infection drives greater clonal expansion but reduces their potential to differentiate into memory cells. Some studies show T cells are committed to massive proliferation after initial encounters with APCs, and can differentiate into both memory and effector subsets even if adoptively transferred into hosts absent of antigen (48). Thus, we limited the signal accumulation stage to the period of time when a T cell is bound to a DC before its first division, similar to findings made in B cell expansion (49). In the asymmetric cell fate model (50), heterogeneity arises from the unequal distribution of differentiation factors into daughter cells during division. We will further study this hypothesis as we incorporate dynamics at molecular level, but currently account for these asymmetries using phenomenological probabilities.

BLOOD COMPARTMENT SUB-MODEL: ODE AND PARAMETER ESTIMATION

We developed a blood compartment model by assuming the blood is a well-mixed, homogenous compartment. We use a system of non-linear ODEs to capture the dynamics of T cells therein. Equations for CD4+ T cells are:

$$\frac{dN_4}{dt} = S_{N4}(t) - \delta_{N4}N_4 + e_{N4}^{\mathrm{LN}} \tag{1}$$

$$\frac{dE_4}{dt} = -\delta_{E4}E_4 - \xi_{E4}E_4 + e_{E4}^{\mathrm{LN}} \tag{2}$$

$$\frac{d\mathrm{CM}_4}{dt} = -\delta_{\mathrm{CM4}}\mathrm{CM}_4 + \alpha_{\mathrm{EM4}}\mathrm{EM}_4 + e_{\mathrm{EM4}}^{\mathrm{LN}} \tag{3}$$

$$\frac{d\mathrm{EM}_4}{dt} = -\delta_{\mathrm{EM4}}\mathrm{EM}_4 - \xi_{\mathrm{EM4}}\mathrm{EM}_4 - \alpha_{\mathrm{EM4}}\mathrm{EM}_4 + e_{\mathrm{EM4}}^{\mathrm{LN}} \tag{4}$$

N_4, E_4, CM_4, and EM_4 represent the blood concentrations of naïve, effector, CM, and EM CD4+ T cells, respectively. $S_{N4}(t)$ is the time-dependent thymus output of naïve CD4+ T cells (51). The initial output is estimated from healthy 30-year-old individuals, and declines by 5% per year (52). δ_{N4} is the overall death rate constant for naïve cells, including homeostatic proliferation and death. We estimated this parameter by assuming a quasi-equilibrium between thymus output and peripheral loss. δ_{E4}, δ_{CM4}, and δ_{EM4} are the death rate constants for effector, CM, and EM CD4+ T cells, respectively. δ_{E4} and δ_{EM4} account for the death of circulating effector and EM cells, excluding those recruited to sites of infection (53). δ_{CM4} reflects the overall loss of CM cells, including self-renewal and death (53). ξ_{E4} and ξ_{EM4} are the rate constants for recruitment of CD4+ effectors and EM cells from blood to sites of infection. As the dynamics at a site of infection are not considered in this study, these recruitment terms serve as a sink for the corresponding cell species in the blood compartment. α_{EM4} is the rate constant for EM cell differentiation into CM cells (54). The terms e_{N4}^{LN}, e_{E4}^{LN}, $e_{\mathrm{CM4}}^{\mathrm{LN}}$, and $e_{\mathrm{EM4}}^{\mathrm{LN}}$ represent rates of LN net output of corresponding cells. These terms are converted to the changes in concentration in the blood per time step. For naïve and CM cells, this is calculated as the difference between the number of exited and recruited cells. For effector and EM cells, this is calculated as the number of exited cells. These four terms are not solved directly in the ODE system but rather are added as an initial condition before each blood time step is processed in the computational model. We show them in the equations for completeness. Similar equations and parameter estimates are written for CD8+ T cells (see Supplementary Material). Because the CM CD8+ T cells population is maintained for life, we assume a very small value for the loss rate constant δ_{CM8}, corresponding to half-life of 20 years (53). See Table S3 in Supplementary Material for a complete list of parameters, definitions, values, units, and source references.

TWO-COMPARTMENT HYBRID MODEL

Our goal is to develop a two-compartment computational model that combines *LymphSim* and the blood ODE model described above. Recently, we published other models linking ODEs and ABMs (55–57). For this study, we use the implementation method we employed successfully to link a LN compartment with a lung (56). The LN and blood compartment models are processed sequentially during each time step of simulation (**Figure 4**). During the T cell recruitment subroutine of the LN ABM model, the probability of recruiting T cells of each type/state is calculated based on their blood concentration levels. At the end of LN compartment simulation time step, the LN net output is calculated as the difference between exited and recruited number of each cell type and is multiplied by a factor that accounts for physiological compartment-size scaling from 0.5% back to the entire paracortex and unit conversion from cell number to blood concentration. This net output is then added to the corresponding variables in blood compartment ODEs. We have made a few assumptions regarding how we capture the LN to blood dynamics. First, we are only modeling dynamics of T cells and DCs within a single LN. There are ~700 LNs in the human body and they are connected via an intricate lymphoreticular network. T cells travel between multiple LNs via these lymphatics and eventually enter the blood via the superior vena cava. We assume that cells exit the LN and enter the blood compartment immediately, coarse-graining the time spent in the lymphatic system. However, our cells travel through the LN and blood in time frames consistent with experimental data [<24 h; Ref. (58)], accounting for the delay.

For computational efficiency, we use a method we term *tunable resolution* (TR) (manuscript submitted). One of the goals of TR is to develop multi-scale models with sub-models of different resolutions, so that models can be run with coarse- or fine-grained alternative versions of sub-models during simulation to save resources without sacrificing accuracy. Here, for each physiological compartment (blood or LN), there is a computational switch that allows the model in an automated fashion to bypass simulation of a given compartment. In this two-compartment model, we do not have an alternate version of each compartment *per se*; instead, each compartment can be suspended when specific criteria are met. For example, during the pre-simulation,

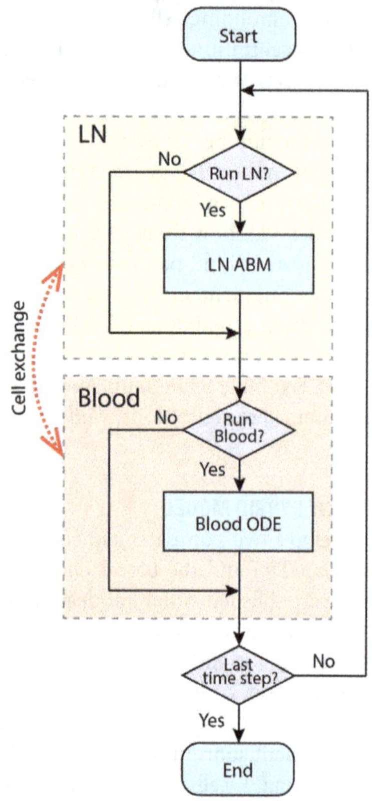

FIGURE 4 | Simulation procedure using tunable resolution. LN and blood compartment are processed sequentially in each time step. LNs recruit cells from blood and put exiting cells into it. The recruitment probabilities are modified by blood concentration of corresponding cell types. Each compartment has a switch to determine whether this compartment is processed in current time step, or will it be bypassed.

the blood compartment is turned off, and the LN is simulated until a baseline steady state is reached. When an immune response is occurring, LN and blood compartments are both running to simulate the immune response in fine-grained, spatially explicit detail for a time scale of a few weeks. When an active immune response finishes and there are no Ag-DCs, LDCs, bound, active, effector, or EM cells in the LN compartment, the LN compartment is suspended to allow rapid simulation of the blood compartment at longer time scales (months to years). When a secondary infection begins, the LN compartment is switched on again (**Figure 4**).

MODEL CALIBRATION

The hybrid model contains 103 parameters that govern mechanisms occurring in both physiological compartments and the interactions between them (see Table S3 in Supplementary Material for a complete list of the parameters). For the LN compartment model, parameters governing T cell motility and trafficking are calibrated to data as described previously (30). Parameter estimates for the ODE model in the blood compartment are discussed in Section "Blood Compartment Sub-Model: ODE and Parameter Estimation" and Supplementary Material.

To use our model for memory T cell differentiation dynamics, we estimated parameters in our model using the limited data available in the literature for memory cell generation in LNs. We estimated parameters governing total production of expanded cognate CD8+ cells generated in the LN model (Table S3 in Supplementary Material, parameters marked with ‡) to data from T cell clonal expansion studies in mice using OVA as a stimulating antigen (59). In that study, DCs are ablated at different time points to show that the duration of antigen presentation correlates with magnitude of T cell expansion, but a short exposure is sufficient to program CD8+ T cells to differentiate into both effector and memory subsets (59). We adapted our model to reflect experimental methods used in these studies. DCs are removed from the LN grid at indicated time points after the recruitment during primary challenge (**Figure 5A**), as was done experimentally by injecting diptheria toxin (DT) (59). Unlike rules for LCMV as previously discussed, CD8+ naïve T cells are allowed to bind both Ag-DC and LDC to be primed and the enter memory state. This is because in these experiments, DCs are activated from LPS pulsing or *Listeria monocytogenes*-OVA. From our *in silico* experiments terminating antigen presentation from DCs at various time points after Ag-DC recruitment, we predict that the magnitude of the primary response is dependent of the duration of DC presence (**Figure 5B**). However, a very short period of stimulation is capable of generating memory cells, as we see a potent production of antigen-specific CD8+ T cells after a secondary challenge (**Figure 5C**). Moreover, it takes only 3 days for the recall response to exceed the magnitude of primary response on day 5, indicating a faster reaction to previously experienced antigens, as observed *in vivo*. Our simulation results are comparable to data from the Prlic study (59). The parameter set we obtained is used as our baseline for simulating infection scenarios (see below and Table S3 in Supplementary Material).

SIMULATED INFECTION AND MODEL VALIDATION

We next validated our model with data sets from experimental studies using LCMV or OVA as stimulating antigens. For each simulated infection, a 3-day pre-simulation of the ABM LN sub-model precedes the actual experiment to allow cells to reach a steady state in terms of quantity and spatial distribution. During this period, the blood sub-model is suspended, with the naïve CD4+ and CD8+ T cells concentrations fixed at 450 and 320/mm^3, respectively (51, 60). Then Ag-DCs are introduced to stimulate the T cell response. We represent this by introducing antigen-bearing DCs in such a way as to mimic an acute infection (23, 25, 30). Ag-DCs carry and present a unique antigen and are recruited to the LN compartment for 2 days. These DCs will prime cognate T cells (cognate frequency is set to 10^{-4}) for about 5 days before they die, mimicking a hypothetical acute infection. To mimic a hypothetical secondary infection, Ag-DCs are recruited to the LN again from day 600 to 602. Each experiment is simulated five times to reduce aleatory uncertainty.

To confirm that our model produces reasonable dynamics in the blood compartment, we qualitatively compare the time course of blood antigen-specific cells to data sets from LCMV studies, where the measurements are performed in spleen (61–63).

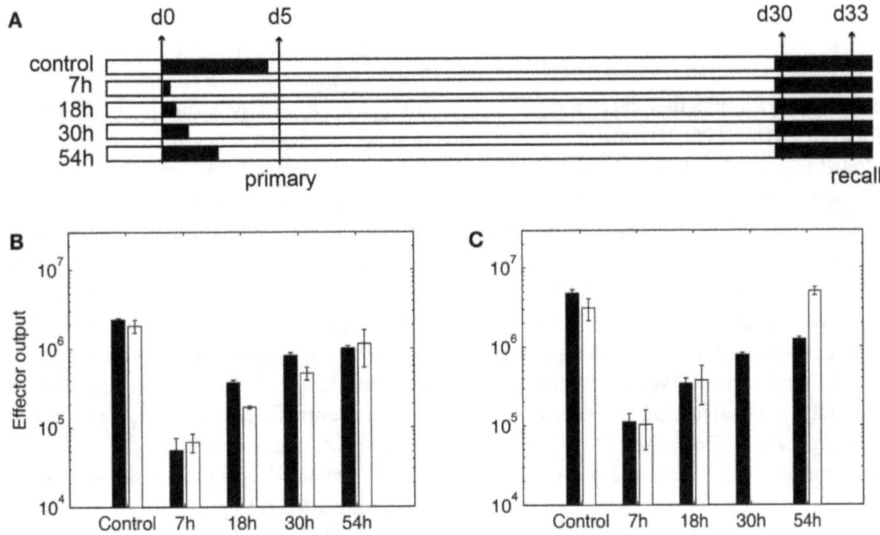

FIGURE 5 | Expansion of CD8+ T cells in simulation. **(A)** *In silico* experimental schemes. Black bars show the duration of Ag-DC presence. In primary challenge, DC antigen presentation is terminated at time points indicated on the left. "Control" indicates no termination and DC are allowed to live their natural lifespan. Recall challenge is given from day 30. Measurements are taken on day 5 for primary response and day 33 for recall response, respectively. **(B,C)** CD8+ T cell population in simulated responses (black bars) and experimental data (white bars) (59). **(B)** Size of expanded CD8+ T cell population in primary response. Values are measured from day 5 after Ag-DC are recruited to the LN. **(C)** Size of expanded CD8+ T cell population during recall response on day 33. *X*-axis value indicates antigen presentation times in the primary challenge.

For lineage tracing simulations (see Cognate Naïve Cells Undergo Heterogeneous Expansion), every cognate naïve T cell recruited to the LN is assigned a unique serial number. This number is passed to the daughter cells when these labeled T cells proliferate and differentiate, so T cells sharing the same serial number belong to the same single-cell derived progeny. When each differentiated cell exits the LN, its serial number is recorded. For each individual cognate precursor, the number of descendant cells and their differentiation states are calculated. Cell progenies are ranked by the abundance of their progenies, from largest to smallest. Five replications are performed for this simulation.

We calculate the Index of disparity D between the expanded populations of different single-cell derived progenies (19), which is the inverse Simpson diversity index mapped to a 0–1 interval:

$$D = \frac{N - \frac{1}{\sum_{i=1}^{N} f_i^2}}{N - 1}, \qquad (5)$$

where N is the number of progenies and f is the frequency of each single-cell derived progeny in the total population.

UNCERTAINTY AND SENSITIVITY ANALYSIS

In this study, our goal is to reproduce patterns of generalized immune responses. In addition to using parameters estimated from previous work (see above and Table S3 in Supplementary Material) and experimental data, we use global uncertainty and sensitivity analysis (U/SA) to study how particular biological mechanisms affect simulation outputs (64).

For each set of sensitivity analysis, a list of parameters is chosen, and for each parameter of interest, a range is specified. Latin hypercube sampling (LHS) is applied to generate the matrix of parameter values, where each experiment represents one combination of sampled parameter values. LHS is a stratified sampling method that requires fewer samples compared with random sampling method but achieves the same accuracy (65). This technique is particularly helpful for our ABM model where parameter values need to be estimated from a high-dimensional space (64). The parameter space is sampled completely and accurately, with a large sampling size. Each experiment is replicated five times to reduce aleatory uncertainty from inherent stochastic variations (64). After the simulation, model readouts are chosen and partial rank correlation coefficients (PRCCs) are calculated between each readout-parameter pair to assess global sensitivity and detect monotonic relationship between mechanisms and output of interests.

To study how various mechanisms affect the generation of memory from within each compartment (blood and LN) as well as how they influence the other compartment (LN and blood, respectively), we performed intra- and inter-compartment sensitivity analysis (64). We choose two sets of parameters governing mechanisms in each sub-model and estimated a range for each parameter (see Table S3 in Supplementary Material). We use LHS to sample the parameter space and generate 100 or 408 experiments for blood and LN experiments, respectively. Here we performed 2540 simulations, which provides ample coverage of the space. Sensitivities of outputs to mechanisms are assessed with PRCCs.

COMPUTATIONAL SIMULATIONS AND IMPLEMENTATION

Our hybrid model is implemented in C++ and runs on Linux/Mac OS/windows. Documentation and pseudo code are available in the online Supplement. A Forward Euler method is used to solve the ODEs. Each time step of the ABM simulation is further divided into 100 pieces (step size of 0.25 s) to reduce error. Each simulation of 350 days (LN sub-model is active for ~40 days) takes 30–40 h to run.

RESULTS

HEALTHY UNINFECTED BASELINE DYNAMICS OF T CELLS ARE REACHED WITHOUT SIMULATED ANTIGEN PRESENTATION

Without Ag-DC introduced to the LN, all T cells remain naïve. The cell dynamics in LN in the absence of any infection present show that over a short time scale (days to weeks), cells remain at the steady state of ~170,000, or 4.0×10^6 cells/mm^3. There is an equal input/output flow of ~1000 cells per million cells per minute, and an average transit time of 16 h, which is consistent with previous data (30). The population of both CD4+ and CD8+ T cells in the blood declines long-term (20 years). By the end of year 20, the blood concentration of naïve CD4+ T cells drops to 210 mm^{-3}, and that of naïve CD8+ T cell drops to 170 mm^{-3}. Such long-term decline of naïve T cell number is comparable to clinical observations (66, 67).

EFFECTOR AND MEMORY T CELL POPULATIONS ARE GENERATED IN A SIMULATED ACUTE INFECTION

We simulated immune responses to a hypothetical acute infection by introducing Ag-DCs into the LN compartment to activate cognate T cells as shown in **Figure 6A**. The cognate frequency is set to 10^{-4}. **Figures 6B–E** show simulated immune cell dynamics in the LN and blood compartments.

In the LN compartment, the Ag-DC population increases first. These DCs scan surrounding CD4+ and CD8+ T cells and bind to their cognate matches. After this binding event, CD4+ and CD8+ T cells begin to proliferate and differentiate into active and effector T cells. After day 2, the influx of Ag-DCs to LN stops, and the number of Ag-DCs begins to decline (**Figure 6A**). At the same time, differentiated effector CD4+ T cells license Ag-DCs, further increasing their surface pMHC levels and stimulation strength, enabling them to allow CD8+ T cell memory potential. Because we assume that CD8+ T cell memory establishment requires LDCs, the appearance of CM and EM CD8+ T cells is delayed as compared with corresponding CD4+ T cells. After differentiation from the active state, effector, CM, and EM cells can exit the LN from ELs, resulting in the decline of these populations within the LN. The system eventually returns to baseline, but CMs can still recirculate through LN (**Figures 6B,C**).

In the blood compartment, the concentrations of effector, CM, and EM cell populations increase as they exit the LN (**Figures 6D,E**). The total concentration of both CD4+ and CD8+ Ag-specific T cell (effector, EM, and CM) peaks at about day 6 and 8, respectively (0.91 mm^{-3} for CD4+ T cells and 2.49 mm^{-3} for CD8+ T cells). The lifespans of effector cells are relatively short. These cells either die, or are recruited to sites of infection, bringing about a contraction phase characterized by a decline of total blood Ag-specific T cells. However, about 5% of the peak level is maintained in the memory cell class, especially CM cells in the

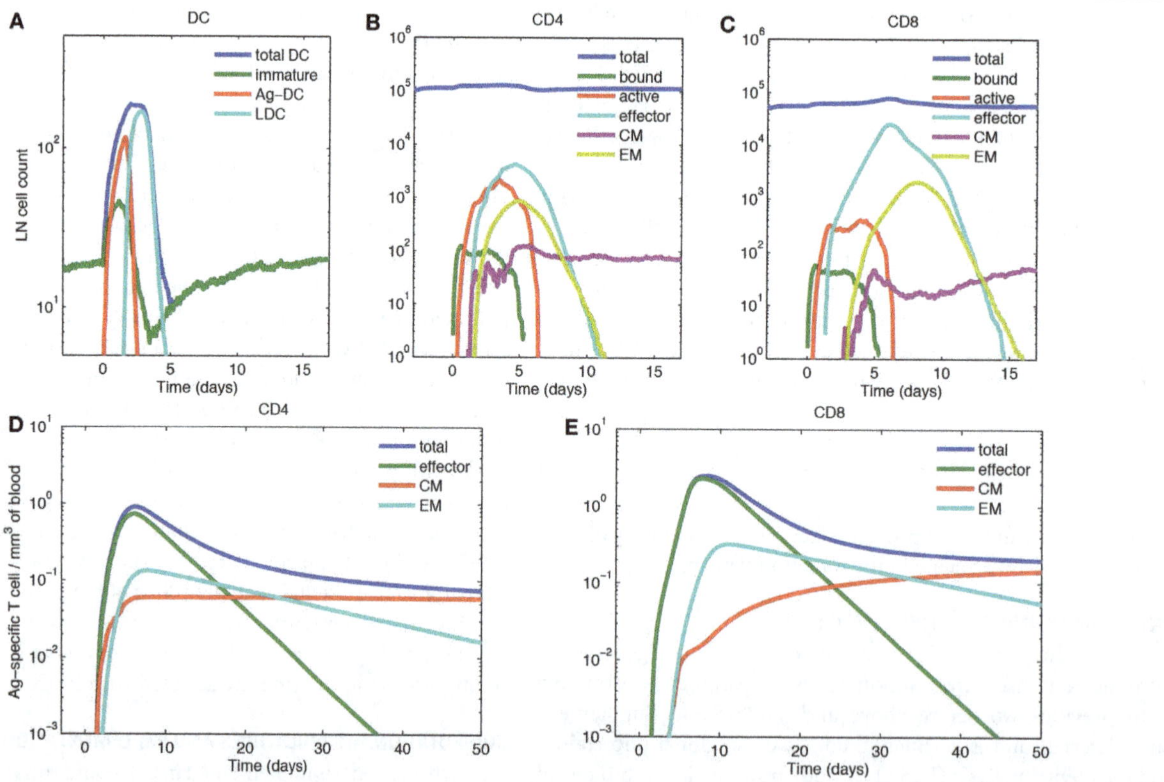

FIGURE 6 | Primary response dynamics of immune cells in LN and blood during a hypothetical acute infection (log scale). (A–C) Number of dendritic cells, CD4+ and CD8+ T cells of different subsets in the LN compartment. **(D,E)** Concentration of CD4+ and CD8+ T cells of different subsets in the blood compartment. **(A)** Model input of DCs representing a hypothetical acute infection, such as LCMV and **(B–E)** output.

long-term as their lifespan is longer than EM cells. In the blood, some of the EM cells convert to CM cells, while others are recruited away to sites of infection (**Figures 6D,E**). While there are no data from primates on these dynamics, our results are qualitatively in accordance with experimental data from mouse LCMV studies (61–63).

IMMUNE CELLS REACH HIGHER LEVELS DURING A RECALL RESPONSE AS COMPARED TO A PRIMARY RESPONSE

To understand the dynamics of a recall response, we simulated a scenario where Ag-DCs are introduced from day 0 to 2 in an initial round of infection (the same as that of Section "Effector and Memory T Cell Populations are Generated in a Simulated Acute Infection"). Once that infection dampens and immune cells return to a resting state, we introduce a second round of challenge by recruiting Ag-DCs from day 600 to 602. We challenge with the same antigen and use the same cognate frequency for naïve cells, but CM populations are maintained in the blood after the primary response. The resulting dynamics of Ag-specific T cells occurring in blood are shown in **Figure 6**.

As above, the primary response is initiated after the first round of Ag-DC input. Blood Ag-specific T cell numbers rise as the response continues and peak at day 6 and 8. After the peak, effector and EM T cells decline while the CM cell population is maintained. On day 600, the blood concentration of CM CD4+ T cells has dropped from 0.059 to 0.023 mm^{-3}, while the CM CD8+ T cell population remains at 0.16 mm^{-3}. The stable maintenance of CD8+ memory and decline of CD4+ memory is in agreement with mouse LCMV infection data (53). During the recall response, because of a memory cell population generated during the primary response that can faster and more strongly respond to the same antigen, both CD4+ and CD8+ T cells in the blood exceed peak levels of their primary response, peaking at 1.07 mm^{-3} for CD4+ and 6.05 mm^{-3} for CD8+ T cells. The recall response is more than twice as large as primary response for CD8+ T cells, but only marginally increased (18%) for CD4+ T cells. Such differences in CD4+ and CD8+ recall responses have been observed in LCMV experiments as well (68). After the recall response, higher levels of CM cells are maintained as compared to following the primary response (**Figure 7**). After the recall response ceases, the

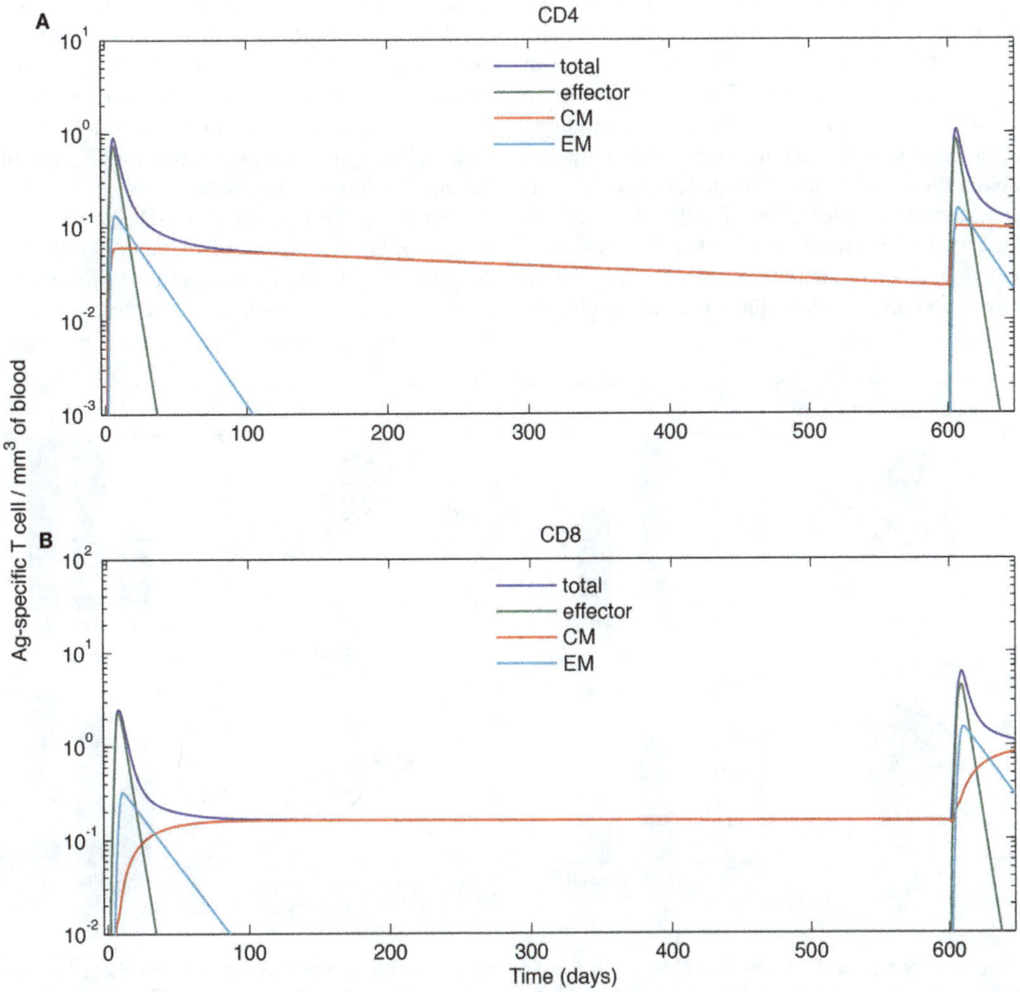

FIGURE 7 | Simulated cell dynamics in the blood compartment during a primary and recall response to a hypothetical acute infection (log scale). (A) Concentration of CD4+T cells of different subsets in the blood. **(B)** Concentration of CD8+T cells of different subsets in the blood. The left parts of the graphs are identical to those of **Figure 6**.

blood concentrations of CM cells are 0.094 and 0.84 mm^{-3} for CD4+ and CD8+ T cells, respectively. These results indicate that the antigen-specific immune memory is reinforced after the second round of challenge, as the central memory population formed in the primary challenge gets further expanded during the second round of challenge.

COGNATE NAÏVE CELLS UNDERGO HETEROGENEOUS EXPANSION

Recent lineage tracing studies showed that CD8+ T cells have a heterogeneous differentiation pattern (18, 19). Because the LN compartment of our model is agent-based, it is possible to track the fate of each individual cell during a simulated infection. We take advantage of this feature to validate our model using data from these recent studies.

Figure 8 shows our lineage tracing analysis for the primary response. The fraction of each single-cell derived progeny in the total population is shown in **Figure 8A** for CD8+ and **Figure 8E** for CD4+ T cells. For both CD4+ and CD8+ T cells, a small number of progenies have a large expanded population. The average size of the largest population is ~2000 for CD4+ T cells and ~8000 for CD8+ T cells. However, the majority of derived progenies have intermediate to small population sizes, with about 50 for CD4+ T cells and 200 for CD8+ T cells. The maximum population size of CD8+ T cell is 50-fold larger than the median. The index of disparity in our simulations is 0.81 for CD8+ T cells, close to the range of 0.85–0.95 shown in Ref. (19). These results indicate our model matches well with the heterogeneous differentiation experimental observations. While the corresponding experimental studies were performed only for CD8+ T cells, we are able to use our model to simulate the dynamics of CD4+ T cells as well. Our model predicts less heterogeneity for CD4+ T cells, with an index of disparity of 0.82 and a 50-fold difference between largest and median progenies (**Figure 8F**).

We also assessed the composition of these sub-populations. In **Figures 8C,G**, the proportion of CM cells of each single-cell derived progeny is plotted against the population size. These results suggest that progenies with a higher proportion of CM cells tend to have a smaller expanded population during the primary response. We calculated the Spearman correlation coefficients between each subtype and the total number of expanded cells (**Figures 8D,H**). The correlations are strong between effectors and overall total population size, but weak between CM and the overall population size. This is comparable to the results from Ref. (18). Thus, in addition to our other findings, these results confirm those previously identified (18, 19) that the magnitude of the primary response for single-cell derived progenies might not be the sole predictor of immune memory. We next study, which mechanisms influence the heterogeneous differentiation and clonal expansion processes of T cells.

ANTIGEN PRESENTATION BY DCs INFLUENCES OUTCOME OF AN IMMUNE RESPONSE

It is no surprise that antigen stimulation plays a crucial role in T cell activation and differentiation (35, 69). However, it is difficult to conduct experiments that quantitatively determine the mechanism of dependency. Here we varied the number of Ag-DCs recruited to LN in a range of 50–300 and the levels of pMHC molecules on the surface Ag-DCs from 100 to 300, and analyzed how they influence production of effector and CM cells. Model pMHC levels are used as a proxy for DC stimulation strength. Results are shown in **Figure 9**.

Increasing the number of Ag-DC recruitment promotes the output of both effector and memory T cells from the LN. The number of Ag-DC has a larger impact when the pMHC molecule levels are low. This result indicates that more Ag-DCs are beneficial for the production of higher levels of effector and memory

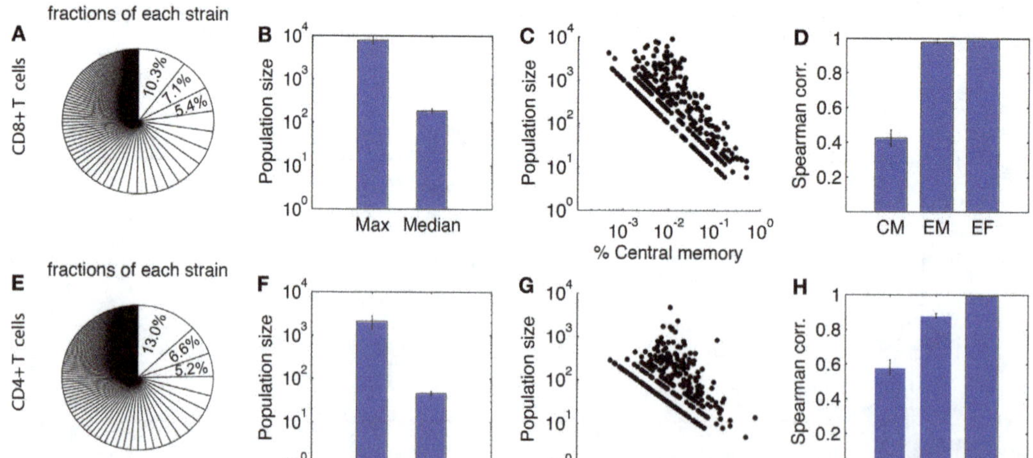

FIGURE 8 | Heterogeneity of expanded T cell families. Upper panel: CD8+ T cells. **(A)** Sizes of expanded CD4+ T cell population from each single-cell derived progeny (strain), represented as fraction of total expanded population as done in Buchholz et al. (18) and Gerlach et al. (19). **(B)** Maximum and median size of CD4+ T cell progenies. **(C)** Correlation between population size and the percentage of central memory cells. Each dot represents progeny of a single-cell derived progeny. **(D)** Spearman correlation of CM, EM, and effector CD4+ T cell number versus total expanded population. **(E–H)** Prediction of CD4+ T cell heterogeneity in clonal expansion. The four panels correspond to the same readouts as for panels **A–D**.

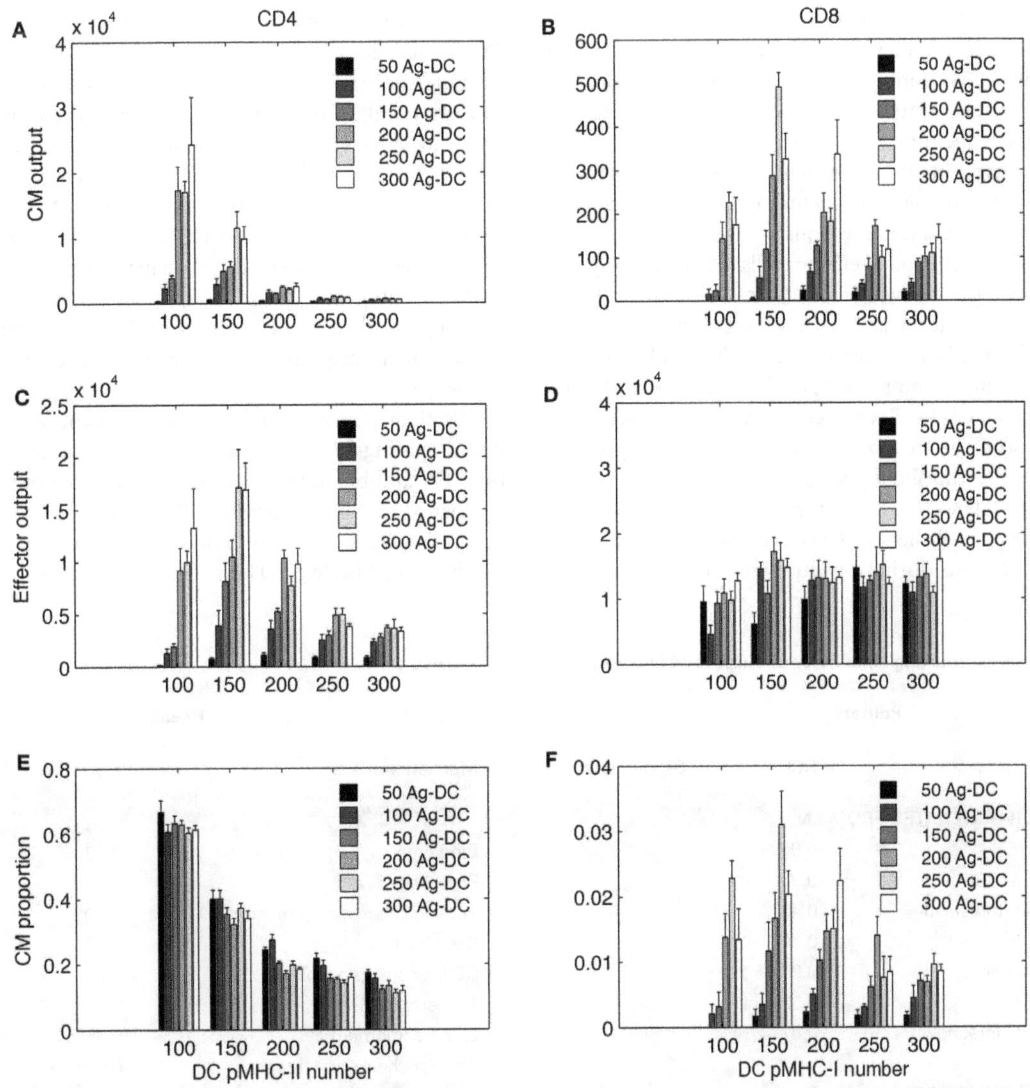

FIGURE 9 | Simulated T cell differentiation is influenced by number of DCs and number of pMHC molecules displayed. *X*-axis: number of pMHC molecules on an Ag-DC. Bar color: number of Ag-DCs recruited to the grid. **(A,B)** Number of central memory (CM) cells produced. **(C,D)** Number of effector cells produced. **(E,F)** Fraction of CM cells in the expanded population.

cells, but this benefit is diminished when pMHC molecule levels are high.

Interestingly, for each subset of cells, the effects of increased pMHC molecule levels on the surface of DCs are different. pMHC levels are always negatively correlated with CM output of CD4+ T cells (**Figure 9A**). However, the highest numbers of effector CD4+ T cell output are reached at intermediate levels of pMHC (**Figure 9C**). CD8+ T cells are affected in a different pattern. Intermediate levels of pMHC are required for higher CM production (**Figure 9B**). Our explanation for this difference is that we defined our rules based on LCMV experiments and other studies suggesting that CD8+ T cell memory establishment is dependent on DC licensing by effector CD4+ T cells, and intermediate levels of pMHC are required so that LDC numbers will not be the bottleneck for memory CD8+ T cell production. Also different than CD4+ T cells, effector CD8+ T cell output first increases with pMHC levels on DCs and then remains relatively stable (**Figure 9D**). The fraction of CM among total expanded population is shown in **Figures 9E,F**.

In general, our simulations suggest that in order to obtain high CD4+ T CM cell production, DCs with lower pMHC levels should be provided. However, DCs with high pMHC levels maximize CD8+ effector output. CD4+ effectors and CD8+ CM T cells require intermediate pMHC levels. Increased recruitment of Ag-DC boosts all four subsets to different extents.

SENSITIVITY ANALYSIS DETECTS MECHANISMS CORRELATED WITH STRENGTH OF RECALL RESPONSES

We also studied how other mechanisms, such as thresholds of different checkpoints in the LN, conversion rates of EM to CM, and recruitment rate to sites of infection from the blood, shape model outputs (see Table S3 in Supplementary Material for parameters varied. The mechanisms they control are explained in the column "description"). We performed intra- and inter-compartment sensitivity analysis (see Materials and Methods), and PRCCs were calculated to assess the monotonic correlation between values of the parameters governing these mechanisms, and outputs including: LN production and blood concentration of effector and CM cells in both primary and recall responses (**Tables 1–3**).

We found that production of effector cells in primary responses is most sensitive to the following mechanisms: binding time (negatively correlated, **Tables 1** and **2**), the probability of effectors differentiating into EM (negatively correlated, **Tables 1** and **2**), and extra recruitment in inflammation (positively correlated, **Tables 1** and **2**). In addition, CD4+ T cell effector output negatively correlates with the stimulation threshold for priming but positively correlates with the threshold for differentiation into effectors (**Tables 1** and **2**); CD8+ T cell effector cell output negatively correlates with extra recruitment of CD4+ T cells (**Tables 1** and **2**). Generation of CM cells during a primary response is sensitive to a similar set of mechanisms, along with some additional ones: CD4+ T cell CM output is negatively affected by the efficiency of CM cells to accumulate stimulation signal; CD8+ T cell CM output is positively correlated with threshold to become effectors (**Tables 1** and **2**). Interestingly, in the recall response, the mechanisms to which effector cell production are sensitive are consistent with that of those affecting effector cells and CM cells during primary responses. For instance, the LN output of effectors in the recall response has a more significant negative correlation with EM differentiation probability than in the primary response, blood CM concentration. This is in accordance with the intuition that a strong recall response requires both memory generation during a primary response and priming efficiency during secondary challenge.

We then perform an inter-compartment sensitivity analysis by comparing how the readouts for the same cell types from both LN and blood are affected by corresponding LN and blood mechanisms. LN mechanisms affect both LN and blood outputs in similar ways, but only blood outputs are sensitive to blood mechanisms (**Table 3**). The recruitment rates of effector cells to

Table 1 | PRCC results: tracking sensitivity of outputs of LN cells to LN mechanisms.

Primary			Recall		
Mechanism	**PRCC**	**Significance**	**Mechanism**	**PRCC**	**Significance**
CD4+ EFFECTOR GENERATED FROM LN					
Bind time	−0.90	−−−	Bind time	−0.82	−−−
Probability EM	−0.73	−−−	Probability EM	−0.64	−−−
Priming checkpoint threshold	−0.42	−−−	Priming checkpoint threshold	−0.40	−−−
CM bind time	−0.29	−−	CM bind time	−0.37	−−−
DC licensing probability	−0.26	−−	DC licensing probability	−0.29	−−
Extra recruitment	0.38	+++	Efficiency CM	−0.27	−−
Effector checkpoint threshold	0.67	+++	Extra recruitment	0.35	+++
			Effector checkpoint threshold	0.61	+++
CD4+ CM GENERATED FROM LN					
Bind time	−0.88	−−−	Bind time	−0.62	−−−
Priming checkpoint threshold	−0.70	−−−	Priming checkpoint threshold	−0.48	−−−
Efficiency CM	−0.29	−−	CM bind time	−0.44	−−−
CM bind time	−0.26	−−	Efficiency CM	−0.33	−−−
Extra recruitment	0.33	+++	Extra recruitment	0.26	++
Effector checkpoint threshold	0.81	+++	Effector checkpoint threshold	0.61	+++
CD8+ EFFECTOR GENERATED FROM LN					
Extra recruitment (CD4)	−0.56	−−−	Probability EM	−0.74	−−−
Bind time	−0.41	−−−	Extra recruitment (CD4)	−0.56	−−−
DC licensing prob.	−0.25	−−	Bind time (CD8)	−0.37	−−−
Probability EM	−0.25	−−	DC licensing probability	−0.21	−−
CD8+ CM GENERATED FROM LN					
Bind time	−0.71	−−−	Efficiency CM	−0.42	−−−
Priming checkpoint threshold	−0.71	−−−	CM bind time	−0.35	−−−
CM bind time	−0.19	−	Priming checkpoint threshold	−0.22	−
Extra recruitment	0.30	++	Bind time	−0.18	−
Effector checkpoint threshold	0.77	+++	Prob. EM	0.33	+++
			Effector checkpoint threshold	0.35	+++

−/+, $p < 0.001$, with negative or positive correlation; −−/++, $p < 10^{-6}$, with negative or positive correlation; −−−/+++, $p < 10^{-9}$, with negative or positive correlation.

Table 2 | PRCC results: tracking sensitivity of concentrations of cells in Blood to LN mechanisms.

Primary			Recall		
Mechanism	**PRCC**	**Significance**	**Mechanism**	**PRCC**	**Significance**
CD4+ EFFECTOR CONCENTRATION					
Bind time	−0.83	−−−	Bind time	−0.71	−−−
Probability EM	−0.74	−−−	Probability EM	−0.67	−−−
Priming checkpoint threshold	−0.42	−−−	DC licensing probability	−0.39	−−−
DC licensing probability	−0.41	−−−	CM bind time	−0.38	−−−
CM bind time	−0.29	−−	Priming checkpoint threshold	−0.35	−−−
Extra recruitment	0.32	+++	Efficiency CM	−0.25	−−
Effector checkpoint threshold	0.64	+++	Extra recruitment	0.27	++
			Effector checkpoint threshold	0.53	+++
CD4+ CM CONCENTRATION					
Bind time	−0.89	−−−	Bind time	−0.70	−−−
Priming checkpoint threshold	−0.71	−−−	Priming checkpoint threshold	−0.53	−−−
Efficiency CM	−0.30	−−	CM bind time	−0.43	−−−
CM bind time	−0.26	−−	Efficiency CM	−0.33	−−−
Extra recruitment	0.33	+++	Extra recruitment	0.26	++
Effector checkpoint threshold	0.81	+++	Effector checkpoint threshold	0.66	+++
CD8+ EFFECTOR CONCENTRATION					
Extra recruitment (CD4+)	−0.57	−−−	Probability EM	−0.72	−−−
Bind time	−0.31	−−−	Extra recruitment (CD4+)	−0.55	−−−
DC licensing probability	−0.28	−−	Bind time (CD8+)	−0.28	−−
Probability EM	−0.27	−−	DC licensing probability	−0.23	−
			Bind time (CD4+)	0.18	+
CD8+ CM CONCENTRATION					
Probability EM	−0.78	−−−	Probability EM	−0.82	−−−
Bind time	−0.53	−−−	Extra recruitment (CD4+)	−0.42	−−−
Priming checkpoint threshold	−0.39	−−−	Bind time	−0.38	−−−
Extra recruitment (CD4+)	−0.37	−−−	Efficiency CM	−0.30	−−
Effector checkpoint threshold	0.52	+++	CM bind time	−0.27	−−
			Priming checkpoint threshold	−0.25	−−
			Effector checkpoint threshold	0.39	+++

−/+, $p < 0.001$, with negative or positive correlation; −−/++, $p < 10^{-6}$, with negative or positive correlation; −−−/+++, $p < 10^{-9}$, with negative or positive correlation.

Table 3 | PRCC results: tracking sensitivity of concentrations of cells in blood to blood mechanisms.

Primary			Recall		
Mechanism	**PRCC**	**Significance**	**Mechanism**	**PRCC**	**Significance**
CD4+ EFFECTOR CONCENTRATION					
Recruit to site of infection (ξ_{E4})	−0.79	−−−	Recruit to site of infection (ξ_{E4})	−0.54	−−
CD4+ CM					
Recruit to site of infection (ξ_{EM4})	−0.39	−	Probability EM	0.44	+
Probability EM	−0.80	+++			
CD8+ EFFECTOR CONCENTRATION					
Recruit to site of infection (ξ_{E8})	−0.39	−	Recruit to site of infection (ξ_{E8})	−0.43	−
			Recruit to site of infection (ξ_{EM8})	−0.36	−
			Probability EM	0.72	+++
CD8+ CM CONCENTRATION					
Recruit to site of infection (ξ_{EM8})	−0.41	−	Recruit to site of infection (ξ_{EM8})	−0.45	−
Probability EM	0.93	+++	Probability EM	0.83	+++

−/+, $p < 0.001$, with negative or positive correlation; −−/++, $p < 10^{-6}$, with negative or positive correlation; −−−/+++, $p < 10^{-9}$, with negative or positive correlation.

sites of infection reduce blood effector levels. Conversion rates from EM to CM induce both blood CD4+ and CD8+ T cell CM levels. Also, our predictions suggest that dynamics occurring in blood do not significantly affect dynamics occurring in LNs during both primary or recall responses, as no significant correlation is detected.

DISCUSSION

Single cognate naïve T cells have been known to be able to generate both memory and effector progenies. Moreover, recent studies further demonstrated that the fate of identical naïve cells is heterogeneous. By understanding which mechanisms contribute to this heterogeneity and in which way they are contributing, it is possible to manipulate the priming environment so that differentiation of activated precursor cells can be routed to favor generation of a desired population toward specific needs. For example, in the context of vaccination, establishing a significant antigen-specific CM population has a high priority. On the other hand, massive production of effector cells could be the key issue considered when using immunotherapies against active diseases. Our new findings suggest that pMHC number on the surface of APCs provides such a handle; and using our model we can enhance the production of specific T cell types (CD4+/CD8+, effector/memory) in different ideal ranges. By fitting our model to data collected from experiments designed for a specific antigen, we will be capable of making quantitative predictions of DC stimulation levels that maximize the generation of particular subsets of T cells, which are most relevant to the circumstances.

In order to study how mechanisms in LN and blood influence the generation of effector and memory T cells, we developed a hybrid model with both LN and blood compartments to simulate immune responses in both primary and recall challenges. Using this model, we generated T cell dynamics in blood and LN during infections that are similar to murine models (61–63) and also can capture heterogeneous differentiation observations of individual cognate naïve T cells (18, 19). Furthermore, our model predicts that the outputs of different subsets of T cells that arise during immune responses, including effector and memory, CD4+, and CD8+ T cells, respond differently to the amount of stimulation they receive from antigen-bearing DCs during priming. Simulations showed that CD4+ CM T cell generation is maximized at low pMHC-II levels, and intermediate pMHC-II levels result in the highest number of effector CD4+ T cell generation. However, further increases in pMHC-II levels reduce generation of both effector and CM CD4+ T cells. On the other hand, intermediate pMHC-I level is required to generate the highest levels of CD8+ CM cells, and high pMHC-I level favors CD8+ T effector cell generation.

Results from our previous study using a 2D model showed pMHC levels always compensate for DC numbers to induce effector T cell production (25) in a trade-off fashion. We find a similar trend herein for CD8+ T cells, and for CD4+ T cells, when DC numbers are small. But when DC numbers are large, high pMHC levels are playing an opposite (for CD4+ T cell) or insignificant (for CD8+ T cell) role. This can be explained by the findings from our 3D LN model (30), that DC searching time for T cells is far more efficient in a 3D model environment than 2D. Thus, even for high total DC numbers in the 2D study, there are likely insufficient DCs, suggesting what we observed in the 2D model represents only the case with relatively low DC numbers in 3D.

While our model is able to make some important predictions, further development to include more detail regarding events during antigen presentation is called for. First, DCs are known to be a heterogeneous population, with subsets of cells diversified in origin and function. Different DC subsets are differentially involved in T cell priming. For example, lymphoid organ-resident DCs are specialized for cross-presentation, while inflammatory DCs stimulate T_H17 polarization (70, 71). Furthermore, the stimulation that T cells receive from DCs are also combinations of multiple signals, including TCR avidity, co-stimulation regulation, and environmental, such as inflammatory cytokine profiles. Reducing these signals to a general stimulation signal package represented with pMHC levels as done here helps conceptualize the question and generate theoretical insights; nonetheless, adding these details will confer power for predicting more precise manipulations of the immune response. Harnessing the power of both mathematical and computational modeling and wet-lab investigation, our systems biology approach can eventually provide guidance for clinical practices in an era of personalized medicine.

ACKNOWLEDGMENTS

This research used resources of the National Energy Research Scientific Computing Center, which is supported by the Office of Science of the US Department of Energy under Contract No. DE-AC02-05CH11231. This research was supported by the following grants: NIH R01 HL106804 (awarded to Denise Kirschner), R01 EB012579 (awarded to Denise Kirschner and Jennifer J. Linderman), and R01 HL 110811 (awarded to Denise Kirschner and Jennifer J. Linderman) and by a University of Michigan Rackham International Student Fellowship awarded to Chang Gong.

REFERENCES

1. Randolph GJ, Angeli V, Swartz MA. Dendritic-cell trafficking to lymph nodes through lymphatic vessels. *Nat Rev Immunol* (2005) **5**:617–28. doi:10.1038/nri1670
2. Arstila TP, Casrouge A, Baron V, Even J, Kanellopoulos J, Kourilsky P. A direct estimate of the human alphabeta T cell receptor diversity. *Science* (1999) **286**:958–61. doi:10.1126/science.286.5441.958
3. Casrouge A, Beaudoing E, Dalle S, Pannetier C, Kanellopoulos J, Kourilsky P. Size estimate of the αβ TCR repertoire of naive mouse splenocytes. *J Immunol* (2000) **164**:5782–7.
4. Blattman JN, Antia R, Sourdive DJ, Wang X, Kaech SM, Murali-Krishna K, et al. Estimating the precursor frequency of naive antigen-specific CD8 T cells. *J Exp Med* (2002) **195**:657–64. doi:10.1084/jem.20001021
5. Chicz RM, Urban RG, Lane WS, Gorga JC, Stern LJ, Vignali DA, et al. Predominant naturally processed peptides bound to HLA-DR1 are derived from MHC-related molecules and are heterogeneous in size. *Nature* (1992) **358**:764–8. doi:10.1038/358764a0

6. Butcher EC, Picker LJ. Lymphocyte homing and homeostasis. *Science* (1996) **272**:60–6. doi:10.1126/science.272.5258.60
7. Banchereau J, Steinman RM. Dendritic cells and the control of immunity. *Nature* (1998) **392**:245–52. doi:10.1038/32588
8. Girard JP, Moussion C, Forster R. HEVs, lymphatics and homeostatic immune cell trafficking in lymph nodes. *Nat Rev Immunol* (2012) **12**:762–73. doi:10.1038/nri3298
9. Masopust D, Schenkel JM. The integration of T cell migration, differentiation and function. *Nat Rev Immunol* (2013) **13**:309–20. doi:10.1038/nri3442
10. Bajenoff M, Granjeaud S, Guerder S. The strategy of T cell antigen-presenting cell encounter in antigen-draining lymph nodes revealed by imaging of initial T cell activation. *J Exp Med* (2003) **198**:715–24. doi:10.1084/jem.20030167
11. Mempel TR, Henrickson SE, Von Andrian UH. T-cell priming by dendritic cells in lymph nodes occurs in three distinct phases. *Nature* (2004) **427**:154–9. doi:10.1038/nature02238
12. Grigorova IL, Panteleev M, Cyster JG. Lymph node cortical sinus organization and relationship to lymphocyte egress dynamics and antigen exposure. *Proc Natl Acad Sci U S A* (2010) **107**:20447–52. doi:10.1073/pnas.1009968107
13. Ahmed R, Gray D. Immunological memory and protective immunity: understanding their relation. *Science* (1996) **272**:54–60. doi:10.1126/science.272.5258.54
14. Sallusto F, Lenig D, Forster R, Lipp M, Lanzavecchia A. Two subsets of memory T lymphocytes with distinct homing potentials and effector functions. *Nature* (1999) **401**:708–12. doi:10.1038/44385
15. Cyster JG. Chemokines, sphingosine-1-phosphate, and cell migration in secondary lymphoid organs. *Annu Rev Immunol* (2005) **23**:127–59. doi:10.1146/annurev.immunol.23.021704.115628
16. Mackay CR. Homing of naive, memory and effector lymphocytes. *Curr Opin Immunol* (1993) **5**:423–7. doi:10.1016/0952-7915(93)90063-X
17. Dutton RW, Bradley LM, Swain SL. T cell memory. *Annu Rev Immunol* (1998) **16**:201–23. doi:10.1146/annurev.immunol.16.1.201
18. Buchholz VR, Flossdorf M, Hensel I, Kretschmer L, Weissbrich B, Graf P, et al. Disparate individual fates compose robust CD8+ T cell immunity. *Science* (2013) **340**:630–5. doi:10.1126/science.1235454
19. Gerlach C, Rohr JC, Perie L, Van Rooij N, Van Heijst JW, Velds A, et al. Heterogeneous differentiation patterns of individual CD8+ T cells. *Science* (2013) **340**:635–9. doi:10.1126/science.1235487
20. Antia R, Ganusov VV, Ahmed R. The role of models in understanding CD8+ T-cell memory. *Nat Rev Immunol* (2005) **5**:101–11. doi:10.1038/nri1550
21. De Boer RJ, Perelson AS. Quantifying T lymphocyte turnover. *J Theor Biol* (2013) **327**:45–87. doi:10.1016/j.jtbi.2012.12.025
22. Beltman JB, Maree AF, De Boer RJ. Spatial modelling of brief and long interactions between T cells and dendritic cells. *Immunol Cell Biol* (2007) **85**:306–14. doi:10.1038/sj.icb.7100054
23. Riggs T, Walts A, Perry N, Bickle L, Lynch JN, Myers A, et al. A comparison of random vs. chemotaxis-driven contacts of T cells with dendritic cells during repertoire scanning. *J Theor Biol* (2008) **250**:732–51. doi:10.1016/j.jtbi.2007.10.015
24. Bogle G, Dunbar PR. T cell responses in lymph nodes. *Wiley Interdiscip Rev Syst Biol Med* (2010) **2**:107–16. doi:10.1002/wsbm.47
25. Linderman JJ, Riggs T, Pande M, Miller M, Marino S, Kirschner DE. Characterizing the dynamics of CD4+ T cell priming within a lymph node. *J Immunol* (2010) **184**:2873–85. doi:10.4049/jimmunol.0903117
26. Bogle G, Dunbar PR. On-lattice simulation of T cell motility, chemotaxis, and trafficking in the lymph node paracortex. *PLoS One* (2012) **7**:e45258. doi:10.1371/journal.pone.0045258
27. Vroomans RM, Maree AF, De Boer RJ, Beltman JB. Chemotactic migration of T cells towards dendritic cells promotes the detection of rare antigens. *PLoS Comput Biol* (2012) **8**:e1002763. doi:10.1371/journal.pcbi.1002763
28. Kirschner DE, Linderman JJ. Mathematical and computational approaches can complement experimental studies of host-pathogen interactions. *Cell Microbiol* (2009) **11**:531–9. doi:10.1111/j.1462-5822.2008.01281.x
29. Mirsky HP, Miller MJ, Linderman JJ, Kirschner DE. Systems biology approaches for understanding cellular mechanisms of immunity in lymph nodes during infection. *J Theor Biol* (2011) **287**:160–70. doi:10.1016/j.jtbi.2011.06.037
30. Gong C, Mattila JT, Miller M, Flynn JL, Linderman JJ, Kirschner D. Predicting lymph node output efficiency through systems biology. *J Theor Biol* (2013) **335**:169–84. doi:10.1016/j.jtbi.2013.06.016
31. Miller MJ, Wei SH, Parker I, Cahalan MD. Two-photon imaging of lymphocyte motility and antigen response in intact lymph node. *Science* (2002) **296**:1869–73. doi:10.1126/science.1070051
32. Constant S, Pfeiffer C, Woodard A, Pasqualini T, Bottomly K. Extent of T cell receptor ligation can determine the functional differentiation of naive CD4+ T cells. *J Exp Med* (1995) **182**:1591–6. doi:10.1084/jem.182.5.1591
33. Lanzavecchia A, Sallusto F. Dynamics of T lymphocyte responses: intermediates, effectors, and memory cells. *Science* (2000) **290**:92–7. doi:10.1126/science.290.5489.92
34. Gett AV, Sallusto F, Lanzavecchia A, Geginat J. T cell fitness determined by signal strength. *Nat Immunol* (2003) **4**:355–60. doi:10.1038/ni908
35. Kaech SM, Cui W. Transcriptional control of effector and memory CD8+ T cell differentiation. *Nat Rev Immunol* (2012) **12**:749–61. doi:10.1038/nri3307
36. Viola A, Lanzavecchia A. T cell activation determined by T cell receptor number and tunable thresholds. *Science* (1996) **273**:104–6. doi:10.1126/science.273.5271.104
37. Itoh Y, Germain RN. Single cell analysis reveals regulated hierarchical T cell antigen receptor signaling thresholds and intraclonal heterogeneity for individual cytokine responses of CD4+ T cells. *J Exp Med* (1997) **186**:757–66. doi:10.1084/jem.186.5.757
38. Iezzi G, Karjalainen K, Lanzavecchia A. The duration of antigenic stimulation determines the fate of naive and effector T cells. *Immunity* (1998) **8**:89–95. doi:10.1016/S1074-7613(00)80461-6
39. Lanzavecchia A, Sallusto F. Progressive differentiation and selection of the fittest in the immune response. *Nat Rev Immunol* (2002) **2**:982–7. doi:10.1038/nri959
40. Gett AV, Hodgkin PD. A cellular calculus for signal integration by T cells. *Nat Immunol* (2000) **1**:239–44. doi:10.1038/79782
41. Jacob J, Baltimore D. Modelling T-cell memory by genetic marking of memory T cells in vivo. *Nature* (1999) **399**:593–7. doi:10.1038/21208
42. Opferman JT, Ober BT, Ashton-Rickardt PG. Linear differentiation of cytotoxic effectors into memory T lymphocytes. *Science* (1999) **283**:1745–8. doi:10.1126/science.283.5408.1745
43. Pepper M, Jenkins MK. Origins of CD4(+) effector and central memory T cells. *Nat Immunol* (2011) **12**:467–71. doi:10.1038/ni.2038
44. Byrne JA, Butler JL, Cooper MD. Differential activation requirements for virgin and memory T cells. *J Immunol* (1988) **141**:3249–57.
45. Bachmann MF, Gallimore A, Linkert S, Cerundolo V, Lanzavecchia A, Kopf M, et al. Developmental regulation of Lck targeting to the CD8 coreceptor controls signaling in naive and memory T cells. *J Exp Med* (1999) **189**:1521–30. doi:10.1084/jem.189.10.1521
46. Wiesel M, Oxenius A. From crucial to negligible: functional CD8(+) T-cell responses and their dependence on CD4(+) T-cell help. *Eur J Immunol* (2012) **42**:1080–8. doi:10.1002/eji.201142205
47. Stemberger C, Huster KM, Koffler M, Anderl F, Schiemann M, Wagner H, et al. A single naive CD8+ T cell precursor can develop into diverse effector and memory subsets. *Immunity* (2007) **27**:985–97. doi:10.1016/j.immuni.2007.10.012
48. Kaech SM, Ahmed R. Memory CD8+ T cell differentiation: initial antigen encounter triggers a developmental program in naïve cells. *Nat Immunol* (2001) **2**:415–22. doi:10.1038/87720
49. Hawkins ED, Markham JF, McGuinness LP, Hodgkin PD. A single-cell pedigree analysis of alternative stochastic lymphocyte fates. *Proc Natl Acad Sci U S A* (2009) **106**:13457–62. doi:10.1073/pnas.0905629106
50. Chang JT, Palanivel VR, Kinjyo I, Schambach F, Intlekofer AM, Banerjee A, et al. Asymmetric T lymphocyte division in the initiation of adaptive immune responses. *Science* (2007) **315**:1687–91. doi:10.1126/science.1139393
51. Bajaria SH, Webb G, Cloyd M, Kirschner D. Dynamics of naive and memory CD4+ T lymphocytes in HIV-1 disease progression. *J Acquir Immune Defic Syndr* (2002) **30**:41–58. doi:10.1097/00126334-200205010-00006
52. Steinmann GG, Klaus B, Muller-Hermelink HK. The involution of the ageing human thymic epithelium is independent of puberty. A morphometric study. *Scand J Immunol* (1985) **22**:563–75. doi:10.1111/j.1365-3083.1985.tb01916.x
53. Homann D, Teyton L, Oldstone MB. Differential regulation of antiviral T-cell immunity results in stable CD8+ but declining CD4+ T-cell memory. *Nat Med* (2001) **7**:913–9. doi:10.1038/90950
54. Wherry EJ, Teichgraber V, Becker TC, Masopust D, Kaech SM, Antia R, et al. Lineage relationship and protective immunity of memory CD8 T cell subsets. *Nat Immunol* (2003) **4**:225–34. doi:10.1038/ni889
55. Fallahi-Sichani M, El-Kebir M, Marino S, Kirschner DE, Linderman JJ. Multiscale computational modeling reveals a critical role for TNF-alpha receptor 1

dynamics in tuberculosis granuloma formation. *J Immunol* (2011) **186**:3472–83. doi:10.4049/jimmunol.1003299
56. Marino S, El-Kebir M, Kirschner D. A hybrid multi-compartment model of granuloma formation and T cell priming in Tuberculosis. *J Theor Biol* (2011) **280**:50–62. doi:10.1016/j.jtbi.2011.03.022
57. Fallahi-Sichani M, Kirschner DE, Linderman JJ. NF-kappaB signaling dynamics play a key role in infection control in tuberculosis. *Front Physiol* (2012) **3**:170. doi:10.3389/fphys.2012.00170
58. Sprent J, Tough DF. T cell death and memory. *Science* (2001) **293**:245–8. doi:10.1126/science.1062416
59. Prlic M, Hernandez-Hoyos G, Bevan MJ. Duration of the initial TCR stimulus controls the magnitude but not functionality of the CD8+ T cell response. *J Exp Med* (2006) **203**:2135–43. doi:10.1084/jem.20060928
60. Roederer M, Dubs JG, Anderson MT, Raju PA, Herzenberg LA. CD8 naive T cell counts decrease progressively in HIV-infected adults. *J Clin Invest* (1995) **95**:2061–6. doi:10.1172/JCI117892
61. De Boer RJ, Oprea M, Antia R, Murali-Krishna K, Ahmed R, Perelson AS. Recruitment times, proliferation, and apoptosis rates during the CD8(+) T-cell response to lymphocytic choriomeningitis virus. *J Virol* (2001) **75**:10663–9. doi:10.1128/JVI.75.22.10663-10669.2001
62. Antia R, Bergstrom CT, Pilyugin SS, Kaech SM, Ahmed R. Models of CD8+ responses: 1. What is the antigen-independent proliferation program. *J Theor Biol* (2003) **221**:585–98. doi:10.1006/jtbi.2003.3208
63. De Boer RJ, Homann D, Perelson AS. Different dynamics of CD4+ and CD8+ T cell responses during and after acute lymphocytic choriomeningitis virus infection. *J Immunol* (2003) **171**:3928–35.
64. Marino S, Hogue IB, Ray CJ, Kirschner DE. A methodology for performing global uncertainty and sensitivity analysis in systems biology. *J Theor Biol* (2008) **254**:178–96. doi:10.1016/j.jtbi.2008.04.011
65. McKay MD, Beckman RJ, Conover WJ. Comparison of 3 methods for selecting values of input variables in the analysis of output from a computer code. *Technometrics* (1979) **21**:239–45. doi:10.2307/1268522
66. Erkeller-Yuksel FM, Deneys V, Yuksel B, Hannet I, Hulstaert F, Hamilton C, et al. Age-related changes in human blood lymphocyte subpopulations. *J Pediatr* (1992) **120**:216–22. doi:10.1016/S0022-3476(05)80430-5
67. Douek DC, McFarland RD, Keiser PH, Gage EA, Massey JM, Haynes BF, et al. Changes in thymic function with age and during the treatment of HIV infection. *Nature* (1998) **396**:690–5. doi:10.1038/25374
68. Ravkov EV, Williams MA. The magnitude of CD4+ T cell recall responses is controlled by the duration of the secondary stimulus. *J Immunol* (2009) **183**:2382–9. doi:10.4049/jimmunol.0900319
69. Zehn D, King C, Bevan MJ, Palmer E. TCR signaling requirements for activating T cells and for generating memory. *Cell Mol Life Sci* (2012) **69**:1565–75. doi:10.1007/s00018-012-0965-x
70. Segura E, Durand M, Amigorena S. Similar antigen cross-presentation capacity and phagocytic functions in all freshly isolated human lymphoid organ-resident dendritic cells. *J Exp Med* (2013) **210**:1035–47. doi:10.1084/jem.20121103
71. Segura E, Touzot M, Bohineust A, Cappuccio A, Chiocchia G, Hosmalin A, et al. Human inflammatory dendritic cells induce Th17 cell differentiation. *Immunity* (2013) **38**:336–48. doi:10.1016/j.immuni.2012.10.018

8

Human plasmacytoid dendritic cells: from molecules to intercellular communication network

Till S. M. Mathan, Carl G. Figdor and Sonja I. Buschow*

Department of Tumor Immunology, Nijmegen Centre for Molecular Life Sciences, Radboud University Nijmegen Medical Centre, Nijmegen, Netherlands

Edited by:
Lisa Helene Butterfield, University of Pittsburgh, USA

Reviewed by:
Cheol-Heui Yun, Seoul National University, South Korea
Daniel Benitez-Ribas, CIBERehd, Spain
Marc Gregoire, Institut national de la santé et de la recherche médicale, France

****Correspondence:***
Sonja I. Buschow, Department of Tumor Immunology, Nijmegen Centre for Molecular Life Sciences, Radboud University Nijmegen Medical Centre, Route 278, P.O. Box 9101, 6500 HB, Nijmegen, Netherlands
e-mail: s.buschow@ncmls.ru.nl

Plasmacytoid dendritic cells (pDCs) are a specific subset of naturally occurring dendritic cells, that secrete large amounts of Type I interferon and play an important role in the immune response against viral infection. Several studies have highlighted that they are also effective antigen presenting cells, making them an interesting target for immunotherapy against cancer. However, the modes of action of pDCs are not restricted to antigen presentation and IFN secretion alone. In this review we will highlight a selection of cell surface proteins expressed by human pDCs that may facilitate communication with other immune cells, and we will discuss the implications of these molecules for pDC-driven immune responses.

Keywords: cross talk, surface markers, T lymphocytes, viral infection, pDC migration

INTRODUCTION

Within the heterogeneous dendritic cell (DC) family, two main subsets of naturally occurring blood DCs can be discriminated based on their phenotype and functional characteristics: myeloid DCs (mDCs) and plasmacytoid dendritic cells (pDCs). The mDC subset can be further divided in $CD1c^+$ and $CD141^+$, which show a high level of similarity in protein expression yet have also specific functions in the initiation of adaptive immune responses. $CD1c^+$ mDCs have been shown to readily stimulate naïve $CD4^+$ T cells and to secrete high amounts of IL-12 in response to toll-like receptor (TLR) ligation, whereas $CD141^+$ DCs do not secrete much IL-12 but are well equipped to take up dead and necrotic cells for subsequent cross presentation of derived antigens to $CD8^+$ T cells (1–4). In contrast to mDCs, pDCs have a very different protein expression profile reflecting their important and unique function in the secretion of IFN-α and anti-viral immune response (1, 2, 5). We and others have however recently demonstrated that like mDCs, pDCs are also very well capable of presenting both soluble and particulate exogenous antigens on both major histocompatibility complex (MHC) class I and II (6). In recent years, numerous studies have been performed to characterize the expression of pathogen recognition receptors (PRRs), TLRs, Fc receptors, C-type lectin (CTL) receptors, and other surface receptors on these cells (7–13). Furthermore, these studies have emphasized both similarities and differences between DC subtypes in their cytokine release profiles, and their ability to acquire, process, and present antigens (5, 14–17). These characteristics of the different DC subtypes have recently been reviewed extensively elsewhere (2, 4, 6, 18). Here, we will focus our attention specifically on pDCs, their role in immunity and, more specifically, their (potential) direct interactions with cells of the innate and adaptive immune system via cell surface molecules. Before going into detail about these cell surface receptors and how they mediate intercellular communication, we will first give a brief summary on general pDC function and localization to provide a context in which these intercellular communications take place. Although studies on murine pDCs are numerous, and commonalities between human and murine pDCs certainly exist, major differences between pDC of both species have also been reported. Therefore, in order to prevent confusion we limited ourselves to human pDCs unless explicit stated otherwise.

pDC FUNCTION

A perturbation of the homeostatic condition that sets off the immune system can trigger either an immunogenic (immunostimulatory) or a tolerogenic (immunosuppressive) response, depending on the local circumstances and type of disease. By default, immature pDCs are tolerogenic, whereas activated (mature) pDCs can have both immunogenic and tolerogenic capacities depending on the local environment in which they are activated (19–21). pDCs are characterized as Lin^- MHC-II^+ CD123 $(IL3R)^+$ $CD4^+$ CD303$(BDCA\text{-}2)^+$ CD304(BDCA4; Neuropilin-1$)^+$ and are mostly known for their ability to quickly produce large amounts of the Type I interferons (IFNs), IFN-α, and IFN-β, following viral infection, implicating pDCs as an important contributor during the early phase of anti-viral response (2, 22, 23).

The most important documented enveloped viruses known to stimulate Type I IFN release by pDCs are human immunodeficiency virus type 1 (HIV-1), herpes simplex virus (HSV), and influenza virus (24–27). Furthermore, parasites and bacteria containing DNA with unmethylated CpG sequences can trigger pDC activation (28–31). In addition to the anti-viral capacity,

Type I IFN release by pDCs has also been reported to be important for pDC survival, (m)DC-mediated CD4$^+$ and CD8$^+$ T cell responses, mDC differentiation, cross presentation, upregulation of co-stimulatory MHC molecules and activation of natural killer (NK), and B cells (32–34).

Because of their expression of the endosomal TLRs TLR7 and 9, pDCs, in contrast to other (immune) cells, do not need to become infected to respond to viruses or intracellular bacteria (35, 36). TLR7 recognizes guanosine or uridine-rich, single-stranded RNA from viruses or synthetic products like guanosine analogs such as R848. TLR9 senses single stranded DNA containing unmethylated CpG motifs, which are usually found in bacterial and viral genomes, and additionally senses for synthetic oligonucleotides, such as CpG-ODN (37, 38). pDCs show differential responses based on the type of virus/bacteria that is recognized, which has been suggested to be attributed to a different site of TLR activation within the endosomal system (39). For example, depending on the subtype of CpG recognized (CpG-A, CpG-B, CpG-C) the outcome of the response can be different. While CpG-A, that triggers TLR9 in early endosomes, induces IFN-α release, CpG-B, signaling from late endosomes, leads to tumor necrosis factor α (TNF-α) and IL-6 production by pDCs (40). In addition, the interplay of the various PRRs tailors the pDC response to a specific pathogenic threat. In addition to TLRs, pDCs express several CLRs, including BDCA-2, DEC-205, dectin-1 and DCIR, and Fc receptor CD32, but they lack for instance DC-SIGN (22, 41–45). Although the full repertoire of receptors is still under investigation, most of these receptors drive antigen uptake, and in concert with TLR7 and 9, coordinate pDC-mediated immune responses.

pDC LOCALIZATION

Immature pDCs circulate in the blood but have been equipped with migratory capacities as they are found within lymph nodes (LNs), tumors, and near sites of viral/bacterial infection (46, 47). At all these sites pDCs are able to promote inflammatory responses by attracting other immune cells through chemokine release, and the subsequent modulation of these cells via cytokines or direct cell–cell interactions (48–51). However, in contrast to human myeloid mDCs or murine pDCs studies, reports addressing which inflammatory chemokines and adhesion receptors specifically drive migration of human pDCs are scarce (52). Human pDCs express chemotactic receptors C-C chemokine receptor type 7 (CCR7), chemokine (C-X-C motif) receptor 3 (CXCR3), CXCR4, and ChemR23 (CMKLR1) that likely mediate migration of pDCs into lymphoid organs and/or into inflamed tissue (48, 52–55). However, due to conflicting reports the role of classical lymphoid tissue CCR7$^-$ Chemokine (C-C motif) ligand 21 (CCL21)/CCL19 pathways in resting human pDCs, is not conclusive yet (53, 56). Several studies show a high expression of CCR7 on "resting" blood DCs while others have reported a very low or a lack of expression on resting pDCs (53, 57–60). Similar to mDCs and murine pDCs, human pDCs upregulate expression of CCR7 upon TLR stimulation and migrate toward CCL21 molecules, suggesting an important role of CCR7 at least for the migration of mature pDCs to the LN (55). Furthermore IL-3 produced by T cells in the LN or by activated endothelial cells can lead to the upregulation of chemokine receptor 6 (CCR6) and CCR10 that may drive migration of activated IFN producing pDCs to inflamed skin or mucosa (61).

In contrast to mDCs, which migrate from peripheral tissue to secondary lymphoid organs via afferent lymphatic vessels, pDCs have been described to migrate to the LN mostly directly from the blood via high endothelial venules (HEVs) (62, 63). Since pDCs first need to engage and traverse the endothelial cells lining of the blood vessels, endothelial cells likely represent the first cellular contact pDCs will engage in after leaving the blood stream. pDC would require a similar migration capacity to enter into inflamed or tumor tissue, which also requires interaction with endothelial cells and extravasation. Next, within the LN, or at the site of infectious or cancerous lesions, pDCs may encounter various immune cells. In the LN, pDC have been found in close contact with T lymphocytes, Invariant Natural Killer T (iNKT) cells, B lymphocytes, and NK cells (21, 24, 42, 64–66). At sites of infection pDCs might activate or get activated by mDCs and NK cells, whereas within the tumor microenvironment pDCs are known to interact predominantly with tumor cells and regulatory T (Treg) cells (67, 68). Below we have summarized the evidence reported thus far for each of these (potential) interactions, and the circumstances under which they occur (**Figure 1**).

ENDOTHELIAL CELLS

Depending on their location (peripheral tissue or LN) and activation state, endothelial cells have been shown to express distinct cell surface molecules and to secrete a variety of chemokines and cytokines that may aid leukocyte transmigration and regulate the activation state of the migrating cells (69). Endothelial cells thus not only facilitate pDC transmigration into the site of infection, the tumor lesion, or the LN but may also have the potency to influence pDCs mediated immune responses trough pro- or anti-inflammatory cytokines as well as growth factors (69). Indeed, endothelial cells also produce IL-3 and VEGF that bind and trigger pDC marker proteins CD123 and BDCA4 respectively, and likely will promote pDC survival and migration after crossing the endothelial barrier. Documentation however of the crosstalk between human pDCs and endothelia is scarce and limited to a few recent studies that we will discuss. Intriguingly, and in contrast to murine pDCs, both resting and matured human pDCs (stimulated by influenza virus) uniquely express the receptor for chemerin, ChemR23 (48). Chemerin is present on the surface of endothelial cells in the lumen of HEVs as well as in blood vessels of inflamed tissue. The interaction between endothelial cell-bound chemerin and pDC ChemR23 seems to play a crucial role in the migration of pDC from the blood both into LNs and into inflamed tissue (**Figure 2**) (48, 70, 71). Like pDCs, T cells also migrate from the blood to the LN via HEVs and thus pDCs may exploit a similar set of molecules as used by T cells. Indeed, pDCs express adhesion molecules CD31, CD43, CD44, CD47, CD62L, CD99, and CD162 (SELPLG, CLA) that may play an important role in the tethering and rolling of pDCs on endothelial cells, but for most of these molecules, functional data for a role on human pDCs is lacking (54, 72, 73). The Lymphocyte function-associated antigen 1 (LFA-1) and very late antigen 1 (VLA-1) (CD49a/CD29) molecules might play an important role in subsequent firm adhesion and transmigration of pDCs (72). Although the expression of all these molecules was

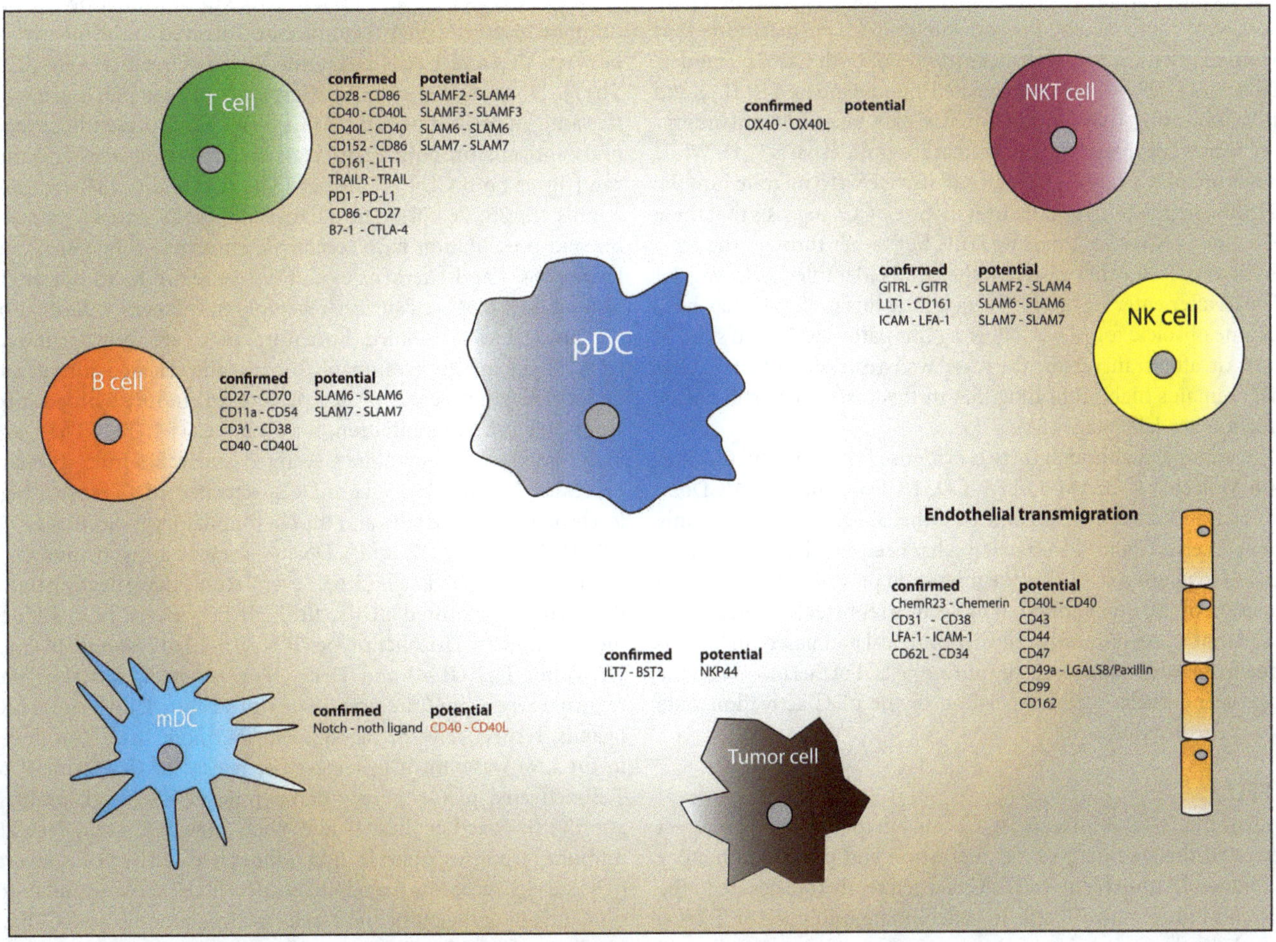

FIGURE 1 | Plasmacytoid dendritic cell have the capacity to interact with various immune cells through an array of surface molecules. The expressed surface molecules of each cell type are divided into confirmed and potential interactions. The "confirmed" molecules have been reported to have a functional effect. Molecules listed in the "potential" column are molecules that have been found on human pDC but without functional data reported in literature. Molecules playing a potential role in humans, but already confirmed with functional studies in mouse are depicted in red.

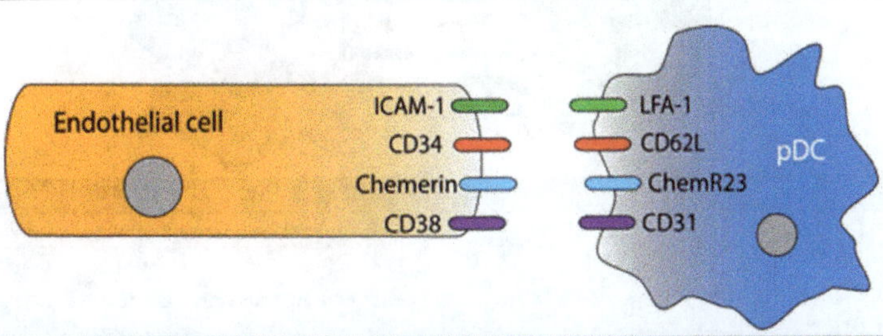

Ligand/receptor	pDC activation state	effect upon the interaction
ICAM-1 - LFA-1	resting, IL-3, HSV	Transmigration of the pDC
CD34 - CD62L	resting, downregulation upon IL-3 and HSV	Transmigration of the pDC
Chemerin - ChemR23	resting, IL-3, HSV	Transmigration of the pDC
CD38 - CD31	resting, IL-3 and HSV	Transmigration of the pDC

FIGURE 2 | Ligand/receptor paring of a pDC with an endothelial cell and the maturation state/activation stimuli associated with ligand or receptor expression on the pDC surface.

initially only detected by microarray, with the exception of CD44, most were confirmed by flow cytometry (74). Furthermore, flow cytometry demonstrated that expression of both CD62L (moderately) and CD99 was downregulated upon exposure to IL-3 and HSV, indicating that activated pDCs may take different migratory routes compared to their immature counterparts (74). While immature pDCs express CD62L and use HEVs to migrate into the LN, downregulation of CD62L on mature pDCs suggests that these cells enter LN without passing HEV, but rather through the lymphatic vessels. Furthermore, another study identified a cleavage of CD62L after entering the HEV suggesting this molecule may have become obsolete for pDCs following this pathway (75). In skin, in contrast, after transversing the vessel wall expression of CD62L on pDC remains high, indicating that in this case it may still have a function at a later stage (54).

In summary, although there is evidence for Intercellular Adhesion Molecule 1 (ICAM-1)/LFA, CD31/CD38, and CD34/CD62L interaction between pDCs and endothelial cells, until now, only the chemerin/ChemR23 interaction has been conclusively demonstrated to play a role during the migration process. The migratory function of the other adhesion molecules reportedly expressed by human pDC are currently only hypothetical and based on knowledge from other leukocytes or murine cells. Furthermore also the role of endothelia in the regulation of the pDC activation state awaits further study.

T CELLS

During infection, immature DCs located in the inflamed tissue get activated through pathogenic interaction and pro-inflammatory cytokines. Mature (activated) DCs subsequently translocate to the LN and induce naïve T cells to differentiate into effector T cells. Based on the repertoire of danger signals, effector T cells will have different characteristics and will evoke a different immune response. pDCs have an important role in coordinating such an immune response, since the molecules involved in the interaction between DCs and T cells determine T cell polarization (Th1, Th2, Th17). Numerous studies have established that pDCs are *bona fide* antigen presenting cells (APCs), capable of presenting exogenous antigens on both MHC class I and II molecules and thus can trigger both $CD4^+$ T helper (Th) cells and $CD8^+$ cytotoxic T cells (5, 26, 76–78). The nuances of pDCs antigen processing and presentation have recently been reviewed by Guery and Hugues (42) and Nierkens et al. (79). Here, we focus our attention on how pDC cell surface receptors may skew T cell function (**Figure 3**). Freshly isolated (immature) pDCs are known to induce $CD4^+$ T cell anergy presumably because they lack co-stimulatory molecules; conversely, activated pDC clearly induce a broad spectrum of T cell differentiation, for example, Th1, Th2, Th17, and Treg, based on the cytokines secreted and cell surface proteins expressed (21, 80–84). Like mDCs, activated pDC express high levels of MHC molecules and the co-stimulatory molecules CD80 (B7-1), CD86 (B7-2), and CD83 to present antigens and fully license and activate T cells (5, 6). Several studies have demonstrated that (virally) matured pDCs, through the release of cytokines, mostly induce a Th1 phenotype (IFN-γ/Il-12 in response to CpG, virus) but Th2 (IL-4) and Th17 (IL-17) skewing has also been reported when pDC are activated with IL-3 or CD40 and TLR7 ligands, respectively (82, 85–87). Furthermore IL-21 (produced in the LN) was shown to trigger the release of Granzyme B by TLR-activated pDCs thereby dampening $CD4^+$ T cell proliferation (88). Together these studies show how pDCs may regulate immune responses. Apart from cytokines released by pDCs, several pDC surface receptors may directly affect T cell skewing and function, including the inducible T-cell co-stimulator ligand (ICOSL). pDCs express ICOSLG when activated by CpG-(A, B, and C) IL-3/CD40L or virus (Flu/HSV) (83). ICOSLG is the ligand for the

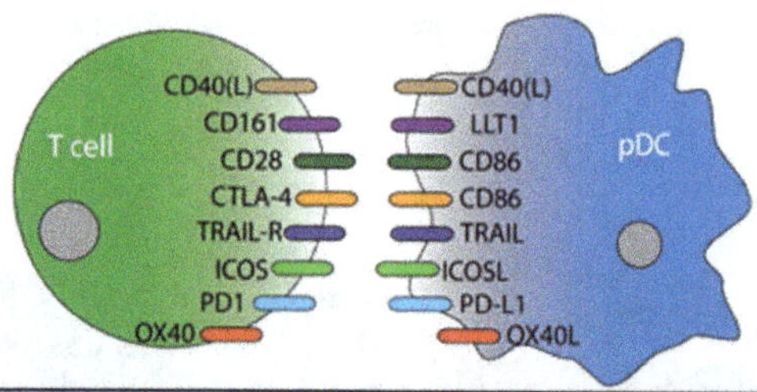

Ligand/receptor	pDC activation state	effect upon the interaction
TRAIL-R - TRAIL	HIV, influenza virus, HSVuv	TRAIL-dependent pDC-mediated killing
CD40L - CD40 (pDC)	Virus	B cell differentiation (indirect)
CD40 - CD40L (pDC)	IL-3	T cells: anti-inflammatory Th2 cytokines IL-4, IL-5, IL-10 and IL-13 pDC: no IFN-α
CD28 - CD86	CpG	T cell activation
CTLA-4 (CD152) - CD86	CpG	Th17 cell inhibition
ICOS - ICOSL	CpG-B, CpG-A HSV	IL-10 release by naive CD4+ T cells
CD161 (NKR-P1A) - LLT1	TLR activated	IFN-γ release by T cells (in combination with TCR signaling)
PD1 - PD-L1	TLR activated	IFN-γ and IL10 release by T cells
OX40 - OX40L	CpG activated, IL-3	priming of Th2 cells

FIGURE 3 | Ligand/receptor paring of a pDC with a T cell and the maturation state/activation stimuli associated with ligand or receptor expression on the pDC surface.

T-cell-specific cell surface receptor inducible costimulator (ICOS) and has been shown to trigger naive $CD4^+$ T cells to produce IL-10 during both pDC Th1 or Th2 skewing in response to CpG/virally or IL-3/CD40L-matured pDCs, respectively (83, 84). It has been suggested that ICOSL-activated pDCs generate IL-10 producing Tregs to dampen immune responses, preventing excessive inflammation (83). Furthermore TLR activated, but not resting pDCs and mDCs, express programed death receptor-ligand 1 (PD-L1), which may induce T cells anergy/suppresses T cell activation by binding to its receptor, program death ligand 1 (PD1), which is expressed by T cells (89, 90). The immunosuppressive effect of PD-L1 has been confirmed by using blocking antibodies on DCs, and additionally in follow-up studies where blocking the PD-L1/PD1 interaction lead to "enhanced tumor-specific T cell expansion and activation" (6, 91, 92). The surface receptor OX40, which is expressed on IL-3 activated pDCs, can induce a Th2 T cell response resulting in IL-4, IL-5, and IL-13 release by $CD4^+$ T cells (93, 94).

Furthermore, after stimulation either with synthetic TLR7 and 9 agonists or with the natural TLR7 agonists, like influenza virus or UV-inactivated HSV type 1(HSV_{UV}) pDCs can induce programed cell death/apoptosis, by expressing tumor necrosis factor-related apoptosis-inducing ligand (TRAIL) (74, 95, 96). TRAIL expression on pDCs uniquely correlates with viral load, and the capacity to kill HIV-infected $CD4^+$ T cells by binding to the TRAIL receptor, a process described as "TRAIL-dependent pDC-mediated killing" (97). However, given the very limited cell numbers, it remains to be seen how important $TRAIL^+$ pDCs are in clearing a viral infection via the direct killing of infected cells (97, 98).

Another surface molecule expressed on TLR-activated pDCs that may affect T cell function is the lectin-like transcript 1 (LLT1), which in addition to activated pDCs, is expressed by most activated lymphocytes (including B cells, T cells, and NK cells) and mature monocyte-derived DCs (99). LLT1 is a ligand of CD161 (NKR-P1A), which is expressed by subsets of T cells (e.g., Th1, Th17, and a subpopulation of $CD8^+$ T cells) and NK cells. When ligated LLT1 triggers T cell proliferation and IFN-γ secretion as well as inhibition of NK cell cytotoxicity (99–102). Thus, LLT1 on pDCs may serve as a co-stimulatory molecule, and after binding to CD161 expressing T cells, could drive proliferation and IFN-γ secretion (51).

So far, we discussed how pDC receptors may affect T cell function but of course, conversely, T cells may also influence pDC function. In a multicellular immune cell signaling cascade the presentation of viral antigens by pDCs brings about IL-2 release by T cells as well as CD40L expression. T cell CD40L upon binding to CD40 on pDCs, triggers IL-6 release by pDC, which in turn enables B cell plasma blasts to become antibody-secreting plasma cells (**Figure 8**) (21, 64).

In summary, while immature pDCs predominantly induce T cell anergy, their activated counterparts may have either inhibitory or activating effects on T cells. Which of the latter in the case depends on stimuli that trigger pDC maturation and which cytokines and surface molecules are expressed as a result. Thus pDCs play pivotal role in T cell activation and fine tuning of the adaptive immune response.

iNKT CELLS

Natural Killer T (NKT) cells form a specialized T cell subset expressing a semi-invariant T cell receptor (TCR-αβ) and surface antigens traditionally associated with NK cells. The unique TCR on their cell surface enables NKT cells to recognize glycolipid antigens rather than peptides, presented in the context of the MHC class I-like molecule, CD1d (103). The most well characterized subset of NKT cells are called iNKT cells, since they express an invariant TCR-α chain, and are reactive to the potent NKT cell agonists α-galactosylceramide (α-GalCer) (103).

Studies have shown that pDCs interact with iNKT cells directly, both via cell–cell interactions and by cytokine release (104). In contrast to the mDCs, pDCs lack the expression of CD1d, which is an important molecule for crosstalk with iNKT cells (105). Nonetheless, over the past few years the ability of iNKT cell to "sense" subtle changes within their microenvironment in a CD1d-independent mechanism, uncovered that cytokines released by pDCs are essential (106, 107). Indeed, CpG activated pDCs upregulate activation markers on iNKT cells via TNF-α and IFN-α release, and selectively enhance double-negative iNKT cell survival but not that of other NKT cell populations (104). However, the interplay of iNKT cells with pDCs alone is not sufficient for iNKT expansion and does not lead to a cytokine release by iNKT cells. Rather, the CpG activated pDCs enables the iNKT cells to productively interact with CD1d expressing mDCs, thus initiating an immune response (61). Both iNKT cells and mDCs lack expression of TLR9 and are therefore unresponsive to CpG; hence, cytokines released upon ligation of TLR9 on pDCs modulate the tissue microenvironment. Not only cytokines, but also a direct interaction between pDCs and iNKT cells may be of importance; CpG-stimulated pDCs express the ligand CD252 (OX40L), which binds CD134 (OX40) present on the surface of iNKT cells, and augments IFN-γ release by iNKT cells in response to lipid antigen presentation by mDCs (**Figure 4**) (66). Further support for such a direct interaction between pDCs and iNKT cells via OX40L/OX40 comes from murine studies (108–110).

In summary, the interaction between iNKT cells and pDCs can be both via cytokines and via direct cell interaction. The role so far seems to facilitate the activation of iNKT by CD1d expressing mDCs. This may become important particularly in situation when TLR9 ligands are available. So far, only OX40L/OX40 are known to play a role in the direct pDC/iNKT cell cross talk.

B CELLS

B cells are the only cells that produce antibodies, and therefore, have a critical role in the humoral immune response. Release of Type I IFNs by pDCs leads to an increase of TLR7 and several activation markers on B cells (111, 112). Moreover, as outlined above, pDCs, in concert with T cells, control B cell differentiation into plasma cells via the secretion of IFN-α and IL-6 (64). In addition, pDCs can affect B cells via direct cell–cell contact. Several studies have shown the importance of CD40-CD40L interactions between B cells and pDCs (**Figure 5**) (24, 64, 65). In addition, upon activation with CpG, pDCs were demonstrated to interact with B cells via CD70/CD27 molecules. This interaction results in B cell growth, differentiation, and immunoglobulin secretion (113).

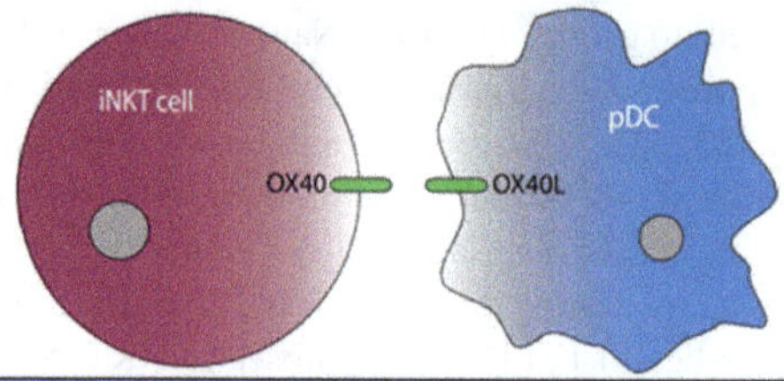

Ligand/receptor	pDC activation state	effect upon the interaction
OX40 - OX40L	CpG activated, IL-3	augment IFN-γ release by iNKT cells upon additional mDC binding

FIGURE 4 | Ligand/receptor paring of a pDC with an iNKT cell and the maturation state/activation stimuli associated with ligand or receptor expression on the pDC surface.

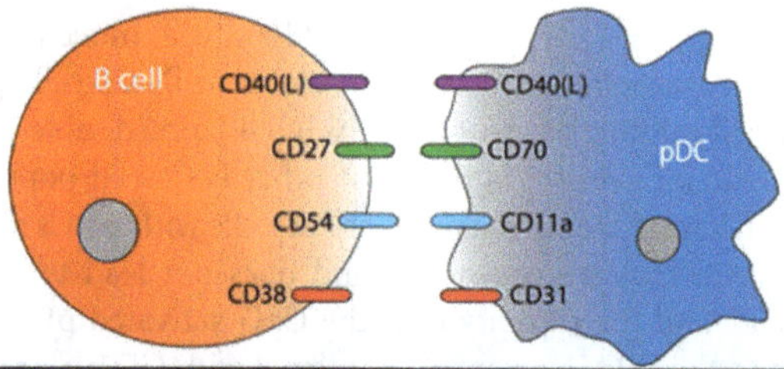

Ligand/receptor	pDC activation state	effect upon the interaction
CD40L - CD40	HIV-1 infection	inhibition of IFN-α production
CD40 - CD40L	HIV-1 infection	inhibition of IFN-α production
CD27 - CD70	CpG	B cell growth, differentiation and immunoglobin secretion
CD38 - CD31	resting, RNA-containing IC-stimulation	IFN-α production by pDCs
CD54 - CD11a	resting, IL-3 and HSV	IFN-α production by pDCs

FIGURE 5 | Ligand/receptor paring of a pDC with a B cell and the maturation state/activation stimuli associated with ligand or receptor expression on the pDC surface.

Furthermore, recent *in vitro* studies have shown that activated B cells are able to stimulate matured pDC to produce IFN-α by direct cell–cell contact (114). Blocking the surface molecules OX40L, CD27, CD40, or CD40L with monoclonal antibodies did not influence the effect of B cells on pDC-derived IFN-α production. However, the IFN-α production by pDCs was significantly reduced when blocking LFA-1 or PECAM-1 (CD31) by 50% and 80%, respectively, indicating that these molecules are at least partially responsible for B cell mediated pDCs activation (114).

Taken together, pDCs and B cells are able to induce reciprocal cytokine release and activation by both soluble mediators and direct cell–cell interaction, and so far have been found to be predominantly stimulatory in nature (64, 113, 114).

mDCs

Synergism of mDCs and pDCs are not restricted to the activation of NKT cells. pDCs and mDCs have been demonstrated to be in close contact *in vivo* at steady state as well as under inflammatory conditions, and it has been suggested that they act synergistically to induce more potent immune responses (115–117). Upon stimulation both mDCs and pDCs function as APCs and follow a similar maturation program, and express the co-stimulatory markers CD40, CD80, CD83, and CD86 to interact with T cells (17, 118). However, there are complementary differences especially in the expression of PRRs (e.g., TLRs, CLRs) and thus in their response to pathogenic triggers. Whereas mDC subtypes express TLR1, 2, 3, 4, 5, 6, 8, and 10, but no TLR7 and 9, the expression of these TLRs on pDCs is the exactly opposite except from TLR2 and 10, which are shared (7, 8, 35, 119–122). pDCs respond to TLR7 and 9 ligands with large amounts of IFN-α and TNF-α (123). In contrast, mDCs release very different cytokines, primarily IL-1β, IL-8, IL-6, IL-10, IL-12p70, TNF-α to variable extents, upon triggering of their TLRs (7, 118, 122). Upon viral infection pDCs are known to respond quicker and with larger amounts of cytokines than mDCs (124). Thus pDCs and mDCs have non-overlapping sensitivities to invading pathogens, and accumulating reports suggest that pDC and CD1c-mDC may cross-activate each other for a more effective immune response. Crosstalk may occur in a paracrine fashion through cytokines like Type I IFNs and TNF-α but also via direct cell contact (118, 125). In a paracrine fashion TNF-α expressed by pDC can cross-activate co-cultured CD1c-mDCs (126). However, there is clear evidence to suggest that CD1c-mDCs and pDCs in other cases require close contact for some parts of this crosstalk, until now it is unclear what molecules are involved (118).

Recent studies by Piccioli et al. implies that several members of the TNF family, CD40L/CD40, OX40L, HEVML, RANKL, CD27, CD30L, glucocorticoid-induced tumor necrosis factor receptor-ligand (GITRL), and 4-1BB are redundant in the CD1c-mDC/pDC cross talk (9). Experimental evidence for the absence of a role for any of these interactions however was so far not reported but only came from unpublished blocking experiments mentioned in these studies, making it extremely hard to deduce whether these interactions can and should be excluded completely (9, 118). Interestingly, murine models do suggest that the TNF member CD40/CD40L may have a crucial role in the CD1c-mDC/pDC cross talk, yet this result needs to be recapitulated in human CD1c-mDC/pDC assays (9).

So far only for the NOTCH receptor-ligand interaction evidence is provided for a role in the communication between pDCs and CD1c-mDCs but again experimental evidence is scant (**Figure 6**) (117). With co-culture experiments they demonstrated that LPS-activated CD1c-mDCs caused an upregulation of maturation marker (CD25, CD86) on the pDC surface and increased IL-6 and CCL19 release in the supernatant. To confirm the involvement of NOTCH pathway, experiments with γ-secretase/NOTCH inhibitor DAPT and soluble NOTCH ligands were preformed and showed a reduced effect on Notch target genes. Activation of the NOTCH pathway upon CD1c-mDC/pDC interaction suggests that this intercellular contact promotes an immune stimulatory response, however, further experiments are needed to unravel the exact mechanism and other molecules potentially involved in this CD1c-mDC/pDC cross talk (117).

Another possible candidate for the interaction between pDC and CD1c-mDC is ICAM-1, expressed on both, pDCs and mDCs, and known as an widespread adhesion molecule with co-stimulatory activity on other immune cells (127). ICAM-1 was found to be strongly upregulated on pDC upon stimulation with TLR9 ligand CpG, while its matching receptor LFA-1 (CD11a/CD18) is constitutively expressed on CD1c-mDCs (9).

Taken together, there is clear evidence that direct cellular interactions are indeed important for CD1c-mDC/pDC cross talk in humans, similar to what was observed in murine studies. However, besides NOTCH receptor-ligand interactions, any experimental evidence that argues in favor of or against the involvement of other specific receptor-ligand interactions is so far lacking (9, 118).

NK CELLS

Natural killer cells belong to the innate immune system and are able to respond rapidly to virally infected cells and to tumor formation. This is due to their unique ability to recognize stressed cells or the absence of MHC on the surface of infected or malignantly transformed cells, and their subsequent ability to lyse these cells. The bi-directional pDC-NK cell interaction is known to play an important role in host defense, and again is mediated both by cytokines and via direct cell contact (128, 129). Type I IFNs secreted by pDCs have long been known to enhance the cytolytic potential of NK cells, and NK cells co-cultured with pDCs are more activated, and have increased cytolytic activity (49, 50, 130–133). pDCs and NK cells have been found in close proximity in the T cells areas of human tonsils (50). In addition, during infection or in case of a malignancy, pDCs and NK cells may migrate simultaneously to the site of the lesion, for example during Herpes simplex infection (25). These reports demonstrate the ample opportunities for these cells to engage in direct interactions, which is further supported by the findings that, when co-cultured, pDCs and NKs cells readily interact (134). Upon stimulation by a virus or CpG, pDCs express GITRL that can bind GITR expressed by NK cells (**Figure 7**). Via the (GITRL)-GITR interaction mature pDCs enhance NK cell mediated killing as well as IFN-γ production. To affect NK cells, however, pDCs expressing GITRL do require the simultaneous presence of IFN-α (50). Furthermore, while the upregulation of CD69 on the surface of NK cells depends on the release of IFN-α and TNF-α by mature pDCs, upregulation of HLA-DR on the surface of a subpopulation of NK cells depends on direct pDC-NK cells contact (49). HLA-DR expressed on NK cells is thought to play an important role in handling bacterial infections such as *Mycobacterium bovis* (BCG) (135). Although the interaction responsible for HLA-DR upregulation remains to be elucidated, it is known that the maturation state of the pDC is not important for the induction of HLA-DR expression on NK cells, indicating the HLA-DR inducing factor is not affected by pDC maturation (49, 130, 132, 136).

The bi-directional crosstalk between pDCs and NK cells also affects pDC function; IL-2, immune complex or IL-12/IL18-stimulated NK cells induce pDCs to release IFN-α which was shown to depend largely on LFA-1-mediated interactions between NK cells and pDCs, and to a lesser extent on NK cell secreted

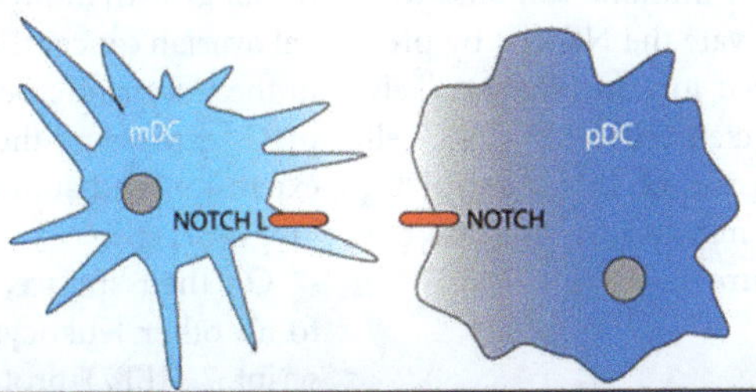

Ligand/receptor	pDC activation state	effect upon the interaction
NOTCH ligand - NOTCH	IL-3	possible T cell recruitment and activation

FIGURE 6 | Ligand/receptor paring of a pDC with a mDC and the maturation state/activation stimuli associated with ligand or receptor expression on the pDC surface.

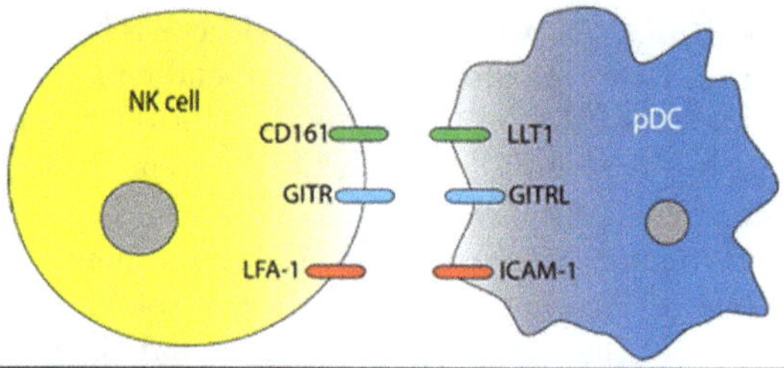

Ligand/receptor	pDC activation state	effect upon the interaction
CD161 (NKR-P1A) - LLT1	TLR activated	LLT1 on target cells inhibits NK cell cytotoxity
GITR - GITRL	CpG	NK cell mediated killing and IFN-γ release
LFA-1 - ICAM-1	RNA contain. imm. complexes	IFN-α production by pDCs

FIGURE 7 | Ligand/receptor paring of a pDC with an NK cell and the maturation state/activation stimuli associated with ligand or receptor expression on the pDC surface.

MIP1α (132, 134). LFA-1 and FcγRIIIA on the pDC also increase cytokine release by NK cells (137). Furthermore, IL-2 stimulated NK cells induced pDCs to express the maturation marker CD83, but not CD80 and CD86, in a contact dependent manner, which also indicates the existence of different stimulatory pathways that can induce expression of different maturation markers on pDCs (132).

Contact with NK cells potentially puts pDCs in danger of becoming lysed. However, immature pDCs are protected from NK cell mediated lysis, and this is at least partly due to the high expression of HLA class I, and the absence of Nectin-2, the ligand for NK cell activating receptors DNAM-1 (132, 138). Culture of pDCs with IL-3 however causes the upregulation of Nectin-2 on pDCs, and makes them more susceptible to DNAM-1 and NKp30-mediated killing (138). Activation of pDCs by TLR7 and 9 may help to prevent NK cells lysis as they express the LLT1 (LLT1 or CLEC2D; above), which is a ligand of NK cell surface protein P1A (NKR-P1A; CD161). P1A is expressed by both NK and NKT cells and when ligated inhibits NK cell cytolytic function and IFN-γ release (51, 99, 101, 139). Taken together, pDCs in various modes of action, seem to be differentially susceptible to NK cell-mediated lysis through the absence of activating NK cell receptor-ligands, as well as the regulated expression of ligands for NK cell inhibitory receptors. Also, high MHC I expression is protective.

In summary, non-lethal pDC/NK cell interactions seem to play an important role in enhancing the early immune response to a viral or bacterial infection as pDCs activate the NK cell by producing IFN-α and via GITRL. This feed-forward system likely promotes NK cells to rapidly lyse infected cells (132). NK cell activity in turn induces a further increase of IFN-α by pDCs and promotes their maturation, which may in turn increase the recruitment and survival of mDCs (**Figure 8**).

TUMOR CELLS

Several early studies have reported decreased numbers of pDCs and mDCs in the blood of patients suffering from various types of cancers (140–143). However, a recent study with melanoma patients detected no significant difference between the levels of immature pDCs in healthy donors and patients (144). Compared to healthy volunteers, pDCs derived from melanoma patients did, however, show a higher expression of CCR6, and increased ability to migrate toward Chemokine (C-C motif) ligand 20 (CCL20), a ligand for CCR6 (144). CCL20 is expressed by keratinocytes in the skin and by melanoma cells, suggesting that the CCL20/CCR6 interaction is involved in the pDC migration process from the blood to the tumor (145–147). Indeed, high pDC infiltration have been observed in many types of cancer including melanoma, head and neck cancer, ovarian and prostate cancer, and these infiltrates mostly negatively correlate with patient survival. On the other hand, an increase of pDCs in tumor-draining LN may be beneficial [reviewed in (143, 148)]. pDCs infiltrated in tumor microenvironment are mainly immature, and therefore seem to be predominantly immunosuppressive/tolerogenic (148). In recent years, evidence has accumulated that tumors may block anti-tumor response by maintaining pDCs in an inactive/tolerogenic state. Mechanisms responsible for keeping the pDC in this state include the secretion of prostaglandin 2 (PGE_2) and TGF-β, which, in a synergistic manner inhibit pDC-derived IFN-α and TNF-α production in response to TLR7 and 9 ligands, as well as inhibiting CCR7 expression, thereby impairing the migration of pDCs to the tumor-draining LN to prime T cells with tumor antigens (148–150). In addition, there is evidence that PGE_2-stimulated pDCs indirectly support tumor cell proliferation, migration, and invasion, as well as tumor angiogenesis, via the release of IL-6 and IL-8 (151–158). Furthermore, tumor-resident pDCs may also influence tumor growth indirectly through the induction of Tregs. In epithelial ovarian cancer the majority of $Foxp3^+$ Treg cells accumulating in the tumor microenvironment expressed the ICOS, and tumor pDCs expressing the ICOSL were shown to be essential for the expansion and suppressive function of these regulatory $Foxp3^+$ Tregs (67, 68).

On their surface, unstimulated pDCs (uniquely with respect to all other leukocytes) express the immunoglobulin-like transcript 7 (ILT7) protein, which is activated by binding to bone marrow stromal cell antigen 2 (BST2, CD317; reviewed in (159)). BST2 is expressed on human cancer cells, monocytes, and vascular endothelium in response to IFN-α (**Figure 9**) (160–162). Similar to BDCA-2, ILT7 forms a complex with FcεRIγ, which, when ligated activates an immunoreceptor tyrosine-based activation motif (ITAM)-mediated signaling pathway that dampens

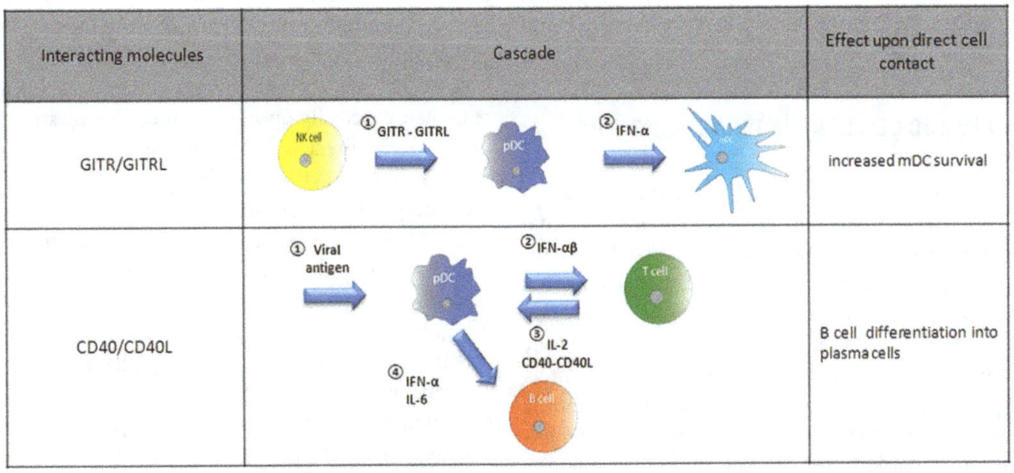

FIGURE 8 | Direct cell interaction dependent on GITR/GITRL or CD40/CD40L binding and their effect on a certain cell type.

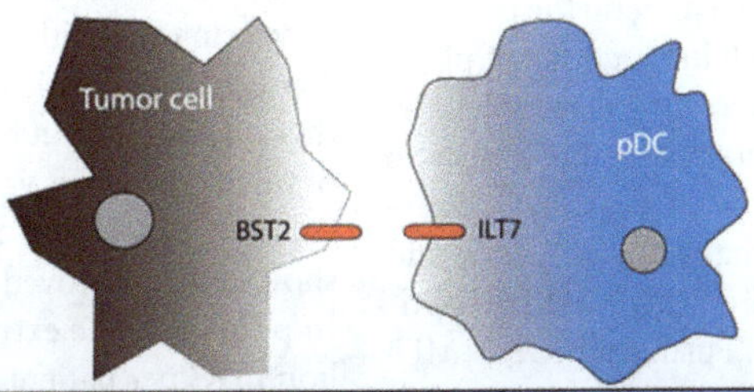

Ligand/receptor	pDC activation state	effect upon the interaction
BST2 - ILT7	resting downregulation upon IL-3, HSV and CpG	immune tolerance

FIGURE 9 | Ligand/receptor paring of a pDC with a tumor cell and the maturation state/activation stimuli associated with ligand or receptor expression on the pDC surface.

TLR-7 and 9-induced IFN-α and TNF-α production (163, 164). ILT7 is downregulated upon stimulation of the pDCs by CpG, HSV, or IL-3, suggesting that pDC maturation prior to entering the tumor site may partly protect it from this suppressive mechanism (159, 164, 165). In addition to ILT7, immature pDCs also express the ITIM motif containing receptors ILT2 and ILT3 that bind to MHC class I molecules, and an unknown ligand, respectively. Both receptors are associated with immune tolerance, probably through the suppression of T cell responses, and in agreement with this notion, these receptors are downregulated upon pDC activation (166–168). Whether these molecules may also have an active role in the pDC-tumor cell interaction, or rather regulate pDC-T cell activation, remains to be investigated. Likewise, there may be a yet unappreciated role for pDC expression of NKp44, which has been demonstrated to down modulate pDC IFN-α responses upon ligation, and may be utilized by the tumor to dampen pDC-mediated immune responses (169). Indeed, an inhibitory NKp44 ligand complex containing HLA I and PCNA was recently reported to be expressed by several tumor cells (159, 165, 170).

So far, most studies point out an immune suppressive role for pDCs favoring tumor progression, however several other studies demonstrate that the situation may be very different if pDCs are properly activated. In this case pDCs may trigger anti-tumor T cell-mediated immune responses (above) or even actively kill tumor cells (171, 172). As previously discussed, in relation to the T cell/pDC interaction, activated pDCs express TRAIL, which induces an apoptotic process by binding to the TRAIL receptors. Tumor cells are known to be sensitive to TRAIL, and via this interaction could directly induce tumor cell apoptosis (171). Avoiding this apoptotic pathway by downregulation of TRAIL has been reported for several cancers by numerous studies (173).

Taken together, the suppressive tumor microenvironment decreases the immune stimulatory functions of pDCs resulting in tumor progression. Preventing these processes, while at the same time activating pDCs, forms a promising target for anti-tumor therapies. Moreover, in a recent clinical feasibility study in our department, we demonstrated that the administration of autologous *ex vivo*-matured tumor antigen loaded pDCs proved to be successful and induced objective clinical responses in several patients (60).

LESS EXPLORED IN pDC CELLULAR INTERACTIONS: THE SLAM FAMILY

Above we have provided an overview of the interactions pDCs likely engage in during their lifecycle, as based on experimental evidence and *in vivo* proximity. In addition we discussed the molecules likely to participate in these interactions. There is, however, a poorly understood family of proteins which are highly expressed pDCs, and which deserve more attention. This is the SLAM family of receptors, for which a role in a diverse range of cellular interactions is highly suspected, yet currently unexplored. Five family members are expressed on the pDC surface (largely) independent of its activation state: SLAMF2 (CD48; BLAST1), SLAMF5 (CD84), SLAMF3 (CD229; Ly9), SLAM7 (CD319, CRACC), and NTBA (CD352) (74, 102). Except for SLAMF2 (below), these proteins have in common that they engage mostly in homotypic interactions; such interactions may occur between homotypic cells, but also between different cell types, opening up the possibility that these molecules mediated direct cell interactions of pDCs with each other, or with others cells also expressing these receptors (174). Homotypic SLAM family interactions have the ability to regulate cell activation and proliferation as well as cytolytic activity (174). SLAMF5 is highly expressed by many immune cells, and has been shown to play a role in T cell-B cell adhesion, and for optimal germinal center formation (175, 176). Furthermore SLAMF5 was detected on leukemic pDCs, and can work as an inhibitor for FcεRI-mediated signaling in mast cells (177, 178). SLAMF3 is also expressed on T cells. Here it reduces IFN-γ production and ERK activation upon stimulation, and thus via this molecule pDCs might trigger a similar response (175, 179). SLAM7, in contrast, is widely expressed on activated B lymphocytes, NK cells, and $CD8^+$ T lymphocytes (74, 180–182) and has been shown to promote B cell proliferation, activate NK cell cytotoxicity (but not NK cell proliferation) (180, 182, 183). Finally, NTBA in addition to pDCs, is present on NK, T, and B cells where it may affect cytotoxicity as well as the IFN-γ and TNF-α release (174, 184, 185). Interactions between NTBA on pDCs and NK cells may therefore have the potential to positively regulate both NK cells and pDCs.

In contrast to the other family members, SLAMF2 which is also present on the surface of pDCs, engages in a heterotypic interaction with family member 2B4 (CD244), and could thus play a role in the interaction of pDCs with 2B4-expressing NK or T cells (74, 175, 186). SLAMF2 via 2B4 can activate NK cells (186).

Overall, although experiments are largely lacking, the presence of such a high number of SLAM family members on pDCs, their homotypic interactions, as well as the known effects of their triggering on other immune cells makes us speculate that pDCs may very well exploit these receptors to communicate with other immune cells.

CONCLUSION AND OUTLOOK

In this review we summarized the existing data which supports the idea that during their life cycle, human pDCs interact with numerous immune cells. Additionally, we have attempted to provide a contemporary overview of the molecules that drive these interactions, and the consequences of their expression on pDCs. It is clear that pDCs play a pivotal role in ensuring a rapid immune response, especially upon viral infection, by strong IFN-α release, but also via direct cell–cell interaction. Depending on the pDC activation state, cytokines released by pDCs and direct pDCs surface receptors may inhibit or activate other immune cells. This large influential capacity of pDCs suggest that they are master regulators of both innate and adaptive immune responses. Besides secretion of the highly potent yet broadly acting IFN-α, pDCs have a highly versatile repertoire of cell surface molecules to further fine tune immune responses. These characteristics make them an interesting and potential highly valuable therapeutic target to be exploited or targeted in cancer therapy, infectious or autoimmune disease. Importantly, controlling cytokine secretion and the surface expression of specific receptors is essential to steer the immune response into the desired direction. In cancer therapy, lifting the suppressive actions of tumor-resident pDCs may greatly enhance existing/endogenous anti-tumor immune response (187). In addition, anti-cancer immune responses may be initiated or boosted by vaccination with autologous tumor antigen loaded pDCs (60). A preliminary clinical trial using pDCs in melanoma vaccination therapy, carried out by our department, has demonstrated the use of thick born virus vaccine (FSME)-matured pDCS in cancer vaccination is safe and feasible, and despite low patients numbers, showed an improved survival of pDCs vaccinated patients (60). In particular, the extremely low doses ranging from 0.5 to 3 million pDC per patient demonstrate the potency of these cells. The exact reason for the success of pDCs however is not yet completely understood, but in addition to IFN-α production and the induction of tumor-specific T cells, we envision there may also be a significant role for the effective combination of surface receptors expressed by the pDCs and their resulting interaction with other immune cells.

In conclusion, research over the past few years has greatly increased our knowledge of the repertoire of pDC-expressed surface receptors and cellular interaction partners, and has emphasized that there is more to the pDCs than IFN-α alone. Importantly, however, further studies are required to identify the role of these molecules and interactions in pDC function and immune responses in general.

ACKNOWLEDGMENTS

The authors would like to thank Dr. Jurjen Tel (Radboud University Nijmegen), Dr. John-Paul Jukes (University of Oxford), Rosanna McEwen-Smith (University of Oxford), and Sandhya Ramalingam Venkateswari Subbammal (London School of Economics, London) for the critical reading of our manuscript. This work was supported by a RUNMC-NCMLS JO grant and grant KUN2009-4402 from the Dutch Cancer Society. Carl G. Figdor was awarded with an NWO Spinoza prize and an ERC Advanced grant (ERC-2010-AdG-269019-PATHFINDER).

REFERENCES

1. Robbins SH, Walzer T, Dembele D, Thibault C, Defays A, Bessou G, et al. Novel insights into the relationships between dendritic cell subsets in human and

mouse revealed by genome-wide expression profiling. *Genome Biol* (2008) **9**(1):R17. doi:10.1186/gb-2008-9-1-r17

2. Merad M, Sathe P, Helft J, Miller J, Mortha A. The dendritic cell lineage: ontogeny and function of dendritic cells and their subsets in the steady state and the inflamed setting. *Annu Rev Immunol* (2013) **31**:563–604. doi:10.1146/annurev-immunol-020711-074950
3. Crozat K, Guiton R, Guilliams M, Henri S, Baranek T, Schwartz-Cornil I, et al. Comparative genomics as a tool to reveal functional equivalences between human and mouse dendritic cell subsets. *Immunol Rev* (2010) **234**(1):177–98. doi:10.1111/j.0105-2896.2009.00868.x
4. Collin M, McGovern N, Haniffa M. Human dendritic cell subsets. *Immunology* (2013) **140**(1):22–30. doi:10.1111/imm.12117
5. Tel J, Schreibelt G, Sittig SP, Mathan TS, Buschow SI, Cruz LJ, et al. Human plasmacytoid dendritic cells efficiently cross-present exogenous Ags to CD8+ T cells despite lower Ag uptake than myeloid dendritic cell subsets. *Blood* (2013) **121**(3):459–67. doi:10.1182/blood-2012-06-435644
6. Tel J, Hato SV, Torensma R, Buschow SI, Figdor CG, Lesterhuis WJ, et al. The chemotherapeutic drug oxaliplatin differentially affects blood DC function dependent on environmental cues. *Cancer Immunol Immunother* (2012) **61**(7):1101–11. doi:10.1007/s00262-011-1189-x
7. Schreibelt G, Tel J, Sliepen KH, Benitez-Ribas D, Figdor CG, Adema GJ, et al. Toll-like receptor expression and function in human dendritic cell subsets: implications for dendritic cell-based anti-cancer immunotherapy. *Cancer Immunol Immunother* (2010) **59**(10):1573–82. doi:10.1007/s00262-010-0833-1
8. Kadowaki N, Ho S, Antonenko S, Malefyt RW, Kastelein RA, Bazan F, et al. Subsets of human dendritic cell precursors express different toll-like receptors and respond to different microbial antigens. *J Exp Med* (2001) **194**(6):863–9. doi:10.1084/jem.194.6.863
9. Cantisani R, Sammicheli C, Tavarini S, D'Oro U, Wack A, Piccioli D. Surface molecules on stimulated plasmacytoid dendritic cells are sufficient to cross-activate resting myeloid dendritic cells. *Hum Immunol* (2011) **72**(11):1018–21. doi:10.1016/j.humimm.2011.08.008
10. McGreal EP, Miller JL, Gordon S. Ligand recognition by antigen-presenting cell C-type lectin receptors. *Curr Opin Immunol* (2005) **17**(1):18–24. doi:10.1016/j.coi.2004.12.001
11. Blomberg S, Eloranta ML, Magnusson M, Alm GV, Ronnblom L. Expression of the markers BDCA-2 and BDCA-4 and production of interferon-alpha by plasmacytoid dendritic cells in systemic lupus erythematosus. *Arthritis Rheum* (2003) **48**(9):2524–32. doi:10.1002/art.11225
12. Schreibelt G, Klinkenberg LJ, Cruz LJ, Tacken PJ, Tel J, Kreutz M, et al. The C-type lectin receptor CLEC9A mediates antigen uptake and (cross-)presentation by human blood BDCA3+ myeloid dendritic cells. *Blood* (2012) **119**(10):2284–92. doi:10.1182/blood-2011-08-373944
13. Geijtenbeek TB, van Vliet SJ, Engering A, t Hart BA, van Kooyk Y. Self- and nonself-recognition by C-type lectins on dendritic cells. *Annu Rev Immunol* (2004) **22**:33–54. doi:10.1146/annurev.immunol.22.012703.104558
14. Colonna M, Trinchieri G, Liu YJ. Plasmacytoid dendritic cells in immunity. *Nat Immunol* (2004) **5**(12):1219–26. doi:10.1038/ni1141
15. Liu YJ. IPC: professional type 1 interferon-producing cells and plasmacytoid dendritic cell precursors. *Annu Rev Immunol* (2005) **23**:275–306. doi:10.1146/annurev.immunol.23.021704.115633
16. Gilliet M, Cao W, Liu YJ. Plasmacytoid dendritic cells: sensing nucleic acids in viral infection and autoimmune diseases. *Nat Rev Immunol* (2008) **8**(8):594–606. doi:10.1038/nri2358
17. Manh TP, Alexandre Y, Baranek T, Crozat K, Dalod M. Plasmacytoid, conventional, and monocyte-derived dendritic cells undergo a profound and convergent genetic reprogramming during their maturation. *Eur J Immunol* (2013) **43**(7):1706–15. doi:10.1002/eji.201243106
18. Pulendran B. Variegation of the immune response with dendritic cells and pathogen recognition receptors. *J Immunol* (2005) **174**(5):2457–65.
19. Martin-Gayo E, Sierra-Filardi E, Corbi AL, Toribio ML. Plasmacytoid dendritic cells resident in human thymus drive natural Treg cell development. *Blood* (2010) **115**(26):5366–75. doi:10.1182/blood-2009-10-248260
20. Hanabuchi S, Ito T, Park WR, Watanabe N, Shaw JL, Roman E, et al. Thymic stromal lymphopoietin-activated plasmacytoid dendritic cells induce the generation of FOXP3+ regulatory T cells in human thymus. *J Immunol* (2010) **184**(6):2999–3007. doi:10.4049/jimmunol.0804106
21. Fonteneau JF, Gilliet M, Larsson M, Dasilva I, Munz C, Liu YJ, et al. Activation of influenza virus-specific CD4+ and CD8+ T cells: a new role for plasmacytoid dendritic cells in adaptive immunity. *Blood* (2003) **101**(9):3520–6. doi:10.1182/blood-2002-10-3063
22. Reizis B, Bunin A, Ghosh HS, Lewis KL, Sisirak V. Plasmacytoid dendritic cells: recent progress and open questions. *Annu Rev Immunol* (2011) **29**:163–83. doi:10.1146/annurev-immunol-031210-101345
23. Swiecki M, Gilfillan S, Vermi W, Wang Y, Colonna M. Plasmacytoid dendritic cell ablation impacts early interferon responses and antiviral NK and CD8(+) T cell accrual. *Immunity* (2010) **33**(6):955–66. doi:10.1016/j.immuni.2010.11.020
24. Donhauser N, Pritschet K, Helm M, Harrer T, Schuster P, Ries M, et al. Chronic immune activation in HIV-1 infection contributes to reduced interferon alpha production via enhanced CD40:CD40 ligand interaction. *PLoS One* (2012) **7**(3):e33925. doi:10.1371/journal.pone.0033925
25. Donaghy H, Bosnjak L, Harman AN, Marsden V, Tyring SK, Meng TC, et al. Role for plasmacytoid dendritic cells in the immune control of recurrent human herpes simplex virus infection. *J Virol* (2009) **83**(4):1952–61. doi:10.1128/JVI.01578-08
26. Lui G, Manches O, Angel J, Molens JP, Chaperot L, Plumas J. Plasmacytoid dendritic cells capture and cross-present viral antigens from influenza-virus exposed cells. *PLoS One* (2009) **4**(9):e7111. doi:10.1371/journal.pone.0007111
27. Tel J, Torensma R, Figdor CG, de Vries IJ. IL-4 and IL-13 alter plasmacytoid dendritic cell responsiveness to CpG DNA and herpes simplex virus-1. *J Invest Dermatol* (2011) **131**(4):900–6. doi:10.1038/jid.2010.410
28. Pichyangkul S, Endy TP, Kalayanarooj S, Nisalak A, Yongvanitchit K, Green S, et al. A blunted blood plasmacytoid dendritic cell response to an acute systemic viral infection is associated with increased disease severity. *J Immunol* (2003) **171**(10):5571–8.
29. Svensson H, Cederblad B, Lindahl M, Alm G. Stimulation of natural interferon-alpha/beta-producing cells by *Staphylococcus aureus*. *J Interferon Cytokine Res* (1996) **16**(1):7–16.
30. Bauer M, Redecke V, Ellwart JW, Scherer B, Kremer JP, Wagner H, et al. Bacterial CpG-DNA triggers activation and maturation of human CD11c-, CD123+ dendritic cells. *J Immunol* (2001) **166**(8):5000–7.
31. Moseman EA, Liang X, Dawson AJ, Panoskaltsis-Mortari A, Krieg AM, Liu YJ, et al. Human plasmacytoid dendritic cells activated by CpG oligodeoxynucleotides induce the generation of CD4+CD25+ regulatory T cells. *J Immunol* (2004) **173**(7):4433–42.
32. Montoya M, Schiavoni G, Mattei F, Gresser I, Belardelli F, Borrow P, et al. Type I interferons produced by dendritic cells promote their phenotypic and functional activation. *Blood* (2002) **99**(9):3263–71. doi:10.1182/blood.V99.9.3263
33. Le Bon A, Etchart N, Rossmann C, Ashton M, Hou S, Gewert D, et al. Cross-priming of CD8+ T cells stimulated by virus-induced type I interferon. *Nat Immunol* (2003) **4**(10):1009–15. doi:10.1038/ni978
34. Le Bon A, Schiavoni G, D'Agostino G, Gresser I, Belardelli F, Tough DF. Type i interferons potently enhance humoral immunity and can promote isotype switching by stimulating dendritic cells in vivo. *Immunity* (2001) **14**(4):461–70. doi:10.1016/S1074-7613(01)00126-1
35. Krug A, Towarowski A, Britsch S, Rothenfusser S, Hornung V, Bals R, et al. Toll-like receptor expression reveals CpG DNA as a unique microbial stimulus for plasmacytoid dendritic cells which synergizes with CD40 ligand to induce high amounts of IL-12. *Eur J Immunol* (2001) **31**(10):3026–37. doi:10.1002/1521-4141(2001010)31:10<3026::AID-IMMU3026>3.0.CO;2-H
36. Hemmi H, Kaisho T, Takeuchi O, Sato S, Sanjo H, Hoshino K, et al. Small anti-viral compounds activate immune cells via the TLR7 MyD88-dependent signaling pathway. *Nat Immunol* (2002) **3**(2):196–200. doi:10.1038/ni758
37. Lund JM, Alexopoulou L, Sato A, Karow M, Adams NC, Gale NW, et al. Recognition of single-stranded RNA viruses by toll-like receptor 7. *Proc Natl Acad Sci U S A* (2004) **101**(15):5598–603. doi:10.1073/pnas.0400937101
38. Bauer S, Kirschning CJ, Hacker H, Redecke V, Hausmann S, Akira S, et al. Human TLR9 confers responsiveness to bacterial DNA via species-specific CpG motif recognition. *Proc Natl Acad Sci U S A* (2001) **98**(16):9237–42. doi:10.1073/pnas.161293498
39. Kerkmann M, Rothenfusser S, Hornung V, Towarowski A, Wagner M, Sarris A, et al. Activation with CpG-A and CpG-B oligonucleotides reveals two distinct regulatory pathways of type I IFN synthesis in human plasmacytoid dendritic cells. *J Immunol* (2003) **170**(9):4465–74.

40. Kerkmann M, Costa LT, Richter C, Rothenfusser S, Battiany J, Hornung V, et al. Spontaneous formation of nucleic acid-based nanoparticles is responsible for high interferon-alpha induction by CpG-A in plasmacytoid dendritic cells. *J Biol Chem* (2005) **280**(9):8086–93. doi:10.1074/jbc.M410868200
41. Tel J, Benitez-Ribas D, Hoosemans S, Cambi A, Adema GJ, Figdor CG, et al. DEC-205 mediates antigen uptake and presentation by both resting and activated human plasmacytoid dendritic cells. *Eur J Immunol* (2011) **41**(4):1014–23. doi:10.1002/eji.201040790
42. Guery L, Hugues S. Tolerogenic and activatory plasmacytoid dendritic cells in autoimmunity. *Front Immunol* (2013) **4**:59. doi:10.3389/fimmu.2013.00059
43. Meyer-Wentrup F, Benitez-Ribas D, Tacken PJ, Punt CJ, Figdor CG, de Vries IJ, et al. Targeting DCIR on human plasmacytoid dendritic cells results in antigen presentation and inhibits IFN-alpha production. *Blood* (2008) **111**(8):4245–53. doi:10.1182/blood-2007-03-081398
44. Tel J, Beenhakker N, Koopman G, Hart B, Mudde GC, de Vries IJ. Targeted delivery of CpG ODN to CD32 on human and monkey plasmacytoid dendritic cells augments IFNalpha secretion. *Immunobiology* (2012) **217**(10):1017–24. doi:10.1016/j.imbio.2012.01.016
45. Benitez-Ribas D, Adema GJ, Winkels G, Klasen IS, Punt CJ, Figdor CG, et al. Plasmacytoid dendritic cells of melanoma patients present exogenous proteins to CD4+ T cells after Fc gamma RII-mediated uptake. *J Exp Med* (2006) **203**(7):1629–35. doi:10.1084/jem.20052364
46. Conrad C, Meller S, Gilliet M. Plasmacytoid dendritic cells in the skin: to sense or not to sense nucleic acids. *Semin Immunol* (2009) **21**(3):101–9. doi:10.1016/j.smim.2009.01.004
47. Sozzani S, Vermi W, Del Prete A, Facchetti F. Trafficking properties of plasmacytoid dendritic cells in health and disease. *Trends Immunol* (2010) **31**(7):270–7. doi:10.1016/j.it.2010.05.004
48. Vermi W, Riboldi E, Wittamer V, Gentili F, Luini W, Marrelli S, et al. Role of ChemR23 in directing the migration of myeloid and plasmacytoid dendritic cells to lymphoid organs and inflamed skin. *J Exp Med* (2005) **201**(4):509–15. doi:10.1084/jem.20041310
49. Benlahrech A, Donaghy H, Rozis G, Goodier M, Klavinskis L, Gotch F, et al. Human NK cell up-regulation of CD69, HLA-DR, interferon gamma secretion and cytotoxic activity by plasmacytoid dendritic cells is regulated through overlapping but different pathways. *Sensors* (2009) **9**(1):386–403. doi:10.3390/s90100386
50. Hanabuchi S, Watanabe N, Wang YH, Wang YH, Ito T, Shaw J, et al. Human plasmacytoid predendritic cells activate NK cells through glucocorticoid-induced tumor necrosis factor receptor-ligand (GITRL). *Blood* (2006) **107**(9):3617–23. doi:10.1182/blood-2005-08-3419
51. Rosen DB, Cao W, Avery DT, Tangye SG, Liu YJ, Houchins JP, et al. Functional consequences of interactions between human NKR-P1A and its ligand LLT1 expressed on activated dendritic cells and B cells. *J Immunol* (2008) **180**(10):6508–17.
52. Banchereau J, Pascual V, Palucka AK. Autoimmunity through cytokine-induced dendritic cell activation. *Immunity* (2004) **20**(5):539–50. doi:10.1016/S1074-7613(04)00108-6
53. Kohrgruber N, Groger M, Meraner P, Kriehuber E, Petzelbauer P, Brandt S, et al. Plasmacytoid dendritic cell recruitment by immobilized CXCR3 ligands. *J Immunol* (2004) **173**(11):6592–602.
54. Bangert C, Friedl J, Stary G, Stingl G, Kopp T. Immunopathologic features of allergic contact dermatitis in humans: participation of plasmacytoid dendritic cells in the pathogenesis of the disease? *J Invest Dermatol* (2003) **121**(6):1409–18. doi:10.1111/j.1523-1747.2003.12623.x
55. Penna G, Sozzani S, Adorini L. Cutting edge: selective usage of chemokine receptors by plasmacytoid dendritic cells. *J Immunol* (2001) **167**(4):1862–6.
56. Seth S, Oberdorfer L, Hyde R, Hoff K, Thies V, Worbs T, et al. CCR7 essentially contributes to the homing of plasmacytoid dendritic cells to lymph nodes under steady-state as well as inflammatory conditions. *J Immunol* (2011) **186**(6):3364–72. doi:10.4049/jimmunol.1002598
57. de la Rosa G, Longo N, Rodriguez-Fernandez JL, Puig-Kroger A, Pineda A, Corbi AL, et al. Migration of human blood dendritic cells across endothelial cell monolayers: adhesion molecules and chemokines involved in subset-specific transmigration. *J Leukoc Biol* (2003) **73**(5):639–49. doi:10.1189/jlb.1002516
58. Krug A, Uppaluri R, Facchetti F, Dorner BG, Sheehan KC, Schreiber RD, et al. IFN-producing cells respond to CXCR3 ligands in the presence of CXCL12 and secrete inflammatory chemokines upon activation. *J Immunol* (2002) **169**(11):6079–83.
59. Vanbervliet B, Bendriss-Vermare N, Massacrier C, Homey B, de Bouteiller O, Briere F, et al. The inducible CXCR3 ligands control plasmacytoid dendritic cell responsiveness to the constitutive chemokine stromal cell-derived factor 1 (SDF-1)/CXCL12. *J Exp Med* (2003) **198**(5):823–30. doi:10.1084/jem.20020437
60. Tel J, Aarntzen EH, Baba T, Schreibelt G, Schulte BM, Benitez-Ribas D, et al. Natural human plasmacytoid dendritic cells induce antigen-specific T-cell responses in melanoma patients. *Cancer Res* (2013) **73**(3):1063–75. doi:10.1158/0008-5472.CAN-12-2583
61. Sisirak V, Vey N, Vanbervliet B, Duhen T, Puisieux I, Homey B, et al. CCR6/CCR10-mediated plasmacytoid dendritic cell recruitment to inflamed epithelia after instruction in lymphoid tissues. *Blood* (2011) **118**(19):5130–40. doi:10.1182/blood-2010-07-295626
62. Banchereau J, Pulendran B, Steinman R, Palucka K. Will the making of plasmacytoid dendritic cells in vitro help unravel their mysteries? *J Exp Med* (2000) **192**(12):F39–44. doi:10.1084/jem.192.12.F39
63. Facchetti F, Vermi W, Mason D, Colonna M. The plasmacytoid monocyte/interferon producing cells. *Virchows Arch* (2003) **443**(6):703–17. doi:10.1007/s00428-003-0918-8
64. Jego G, Palucka AK, Blanck JP, Chalouni C, Pascual V, Banchereau J. Plasmacytoid dendritic cells induce plasma cell differentiation through type I interferon and interleukin 6. *Immunity* (2003) **19**(2):225–34. doi:10.1016/S1074-7613(03)00208-5
65. Garcia-Marquez M, Shimabukuro-Vornhagen A, von Bergwelt-Baildon M. Complex interactions between B cells and dendritic cells. *Blood* (2013) **121**(12):2367–8. doi:10.1182/blood-2012-12-468017
66. Marschner A, Rothenfusser S, Hornung V, Prell D, Krug A, Kerkmann M, et al. CpG ODN enhance antigen-specific NKT cell activation via plasmacytoid dendritic cells. *Eur J Immunol* (2005) **35**(8):2347–57. doi:10.1002/eji.200425721
67. Conrad C, Gregorio J, Wang YH, Ito T, Meller S, Hanabuchi S, et al. Plasmacytoid dendritic cells promote immunosuppression in ovarian cancer via ICOS costimulation of Foxp3(+) T-regulatory cells. *Cancer Res* (2012) **72**(20):5240–9. doi:10.1158/0008-5472.CAN-12-2271
68. Faget J, Bendriss-Vermare N, Gobert M, Durand I, Olive D, Biota C, et al. ICOS-ligand expression on plasmacytoid dendritic cells supports breast cancer progression by promoting the accumulation of immunosuppressive CD4+ T cells. *Cancer Res* (2012) **72**(23):6130–41. doi:10.1158/0008-5472.CAN-12-2409
69. Mai J, Virtue A, Shen J, Wang H, Yang XF. An evolving new paradigm: endothelial cells – conditional innate immune cells. *J Hematol Oncol* (2013) **6**:61. doi:10.1186/1756-8722-6-61
70. Zabel BA, Silverio AM, Butcher EC. Chemokine-like receptor 1 expression and chemerin-directed chemotaxis distinguish plasmacytoid from myeloid dendritic cells in human blood. *J Immunol* (2005) **174**(1):244–51.
71. Albanesi C, Scarponi C, Pallotta S, Daniele R, Bosisio D, Madonna S, et al. Chemerin expression marks early psoriatic skin lesions and correlates with plasmacytoid dendritic cell recruitment. *J Exp Med* (2009) **206**(1):249–58. doi:10.1084/jem.20080129
72. Schuster P, Boscheinen JB, Tennert K, Schmidt B. The role of plasmacytoid dendritic cells in innate and adaptive immune responses against alpha herpes virus infections. *Adv Virol* (2011) **2011**:679271. doi:10.1155/2011/679271
73. Fuhlbrigge RC, King SL, Sackstein R, Kupper TS. CD43 is a ligand for E-selectin on CLA+ human T cells. *Blood* (2006) **107**(4):1421–6. doi:10.1182/blood-2005-05-2112
74. Schuster P, Donhauser N, Pritschet K, Ries M, Haupt S, Kittan NA, et al. Co-ordinated regulation of plasmacytoid dendritic cell surface receptors upon stimulation with herpes simplex virus type 1. *Immunology* (2010) **129**(2):234–47. doi:10.1111/j.1365-2567.2009.03176.x
75. Cella M, Jarrossay D, Facchetti F, Alebardi O, Nakajima H, Lanzavecchia A, et al. Plasmacytoid monocytes migrate to inflamed lymph nodes and produce large amounts of type I interferon. *Nat Med* (1999) **5**(8):919–23. doi:10.1038/11360
76. Guillerme JB, Boisgerault N, Roulois D, Menager J, Combredet C, Tangy F, et al. Measles virus vaccine-infected tumor cells induce tumor antigen cross-presentation by human plasmacytoid dendritic cells. *Clin Cancer Res* (2013) **19**(5):1147–58. doi:10.1158/1078-0432.CCR-12-2733

77. Tel J, Lambeck AJ, Cruz LJ, Tacken PJ, de Vries IJ, Figdor CG. Human plasmacytoid dendritic cells phagocytose, process, and present exogenous particulate antigen. *J Immunol* (2010) **184**(8):4276–83. doi:10.4049/jimmunol.0903286
78. Di Pucchio T, Chatterjee B, Smed-Sorensen A, Clayton S, Palazzo A, Montes M, et al. Direct proteasome-independent cross-presentation of viral antigen by plasmacytoid dendritic cells on major histocompatibility complex class I. *Nat Immunol* (2008) **9**(5):551–7. doi:10.1038/ni.1602
79. Nierkens S, Tel J, Janssen E, Adema GJ. Antigen cross-presentation by dendritic cell subsets: one general or all sergeants? *Trends Immunol* (2013) **34**(8):361–70. doi:10.1016/j.it.2013.02.007
80. Kuwana M, Kaburaki J, Wright TM, Kawakami Y, Ikeda Y. Induction of antigen-specific human CD4(+) T cell anergy by peripheral blood DC2 precursors. *Eur J Immunol* (2001) **31**(9):2547–57. doi:10.1002/1521-4141(200109)31:9<2547::AID-IMMU2547>3.0.CO;2-J
81. Grouard G, Rissoan MC, Filgueira L, Durand I, Banchereau J, Liu YJ. The enigmatic plasmacytoid T cells develop into dendritic cells with interleukin (IL)-3 and CD40-ligand. *J Exp Med* (1997) **185**(6):1101–11. doi:10.1084/jem.185.6.1101
82. Kadowaki N, Antonenko S, Lau JY, Liu YJ. Natural interferon alpha/beta-producing cells link innate and adaptive immunity. *J Exp Med* (2000) **192**(2):219–26. doi:10.1084/jem.192.2.219
83. Ito T, Yang M, Wang YH, Lande R, Gregorio J, Perng OA, et al. Plasmacytoid dendritic cells prime IL-10-producing T regulatory cells by inducible costimulator ligand. *J Exp Med* (2007) **204**(1):105–15. doi:10.1084/jem.20061660
84. Ogata M, Ito T, Shimamoto K, Nakanishi T, Satsutani N, Miyamoto R, et al. Plasmacytoid dendritic cells have a cytokine-producing capacity to enhance ICOS ligand-mediated IL-10 production during T-cell priming. *Int Immunol* (2013) **25**(3):171–82. doi:10.1093/intimm/dxs103
85. Ito T, Amakawa R, Inaba M, Ikehara S, Inaba K, Fukuhara S. Differential regulation of human blood dendritic cell subsets by IFNs. *J Immunol* (2001) **166**(5):2961–9.
86. Rissoan MC, Soumelis V, Kadowaki N, Grouard G, Briere F, de Waal Malefyt R, et al. Reciprocal control of T helper cell and dendritic cell differentiation. *Science* (1999) **283**(5405):1183–6. doi:10.1126/science.283.5405.1183
87. Cella M, Facchetti F, Lanzavecchia A, Colonna M. Plasmacytoid dendritic cells activated by influenza virus and CD40L drive a potent TH1 polarization. *Nat Immunol* (2000) **1**(4):305–10. doi:10.1038/79747
88. Karrich JJ, Jachimowski LC, Nagasawa M, Kamp A, Balzarolo M, Wolkers MC, et al. IL-21-stimulated human plasmacytoid dendritic cells secrete granzyme B, which impairs their capacity to induce T-cell proliferation. *Blood* (2013) **121**(16):3103–11. doi:10.1182/blood-2012-08-452995
89. Flies DB, Chen L. The new B7s: playing a pivotal role in tumor immunity. *J Immunother* (2007) **30**(3):251–60. doi:10.1097/CJI.0b013e31802e085a
90. Keir ME, Butte MJ, Freeman GJ, Sharpe AH. PD-1 and its ligands in tolerance and immunity. *Annu Rev Immunol* (2008) **26**:677–704. doi:10.1146/annurev.immunol.26.021607.090331
91. Iwai Y, Ishida M, Tanaka Y, Okazaki T, Honjo T, Minato N. Involvement of PD-L1 on tumor cells in the escape from host immune system and tumor immunotherapy by PD-L1 blockade. *Proc Natl Acad Sci U S A* (2002) **99**(19):12293–7. doi:10.1073/pnas.192461099
92. Hirano F, Kaneko K, Tamura H, Dong H, Wang S, Ichikawa M, et al. Blockade of B7-H1 and PD-1 by monoclonal antibodies potentiates cancer therapeutic immunity. *Cancer Res* (2005) **65**(3):1089–96.
93. Ito T, Amakawa R, Inaba M, Hori T, Ota M, Nakamura K, et al. Plasmacytoid dendritic cells regulate Th cell responses through OX40 ligand and type I IFNs. *J Immunol* (2004) **172**(7):4253–9.
94. Delespesse G, Ohshima Y, Yang LP, Demeure C, Sarfati M. OX40-Mediated cosignal enhances the maturation of naive human CD4+ T cells into high IL-4-producing effectors. *Int Arch Allergy Immunol* (1999) **118**(2–4):384–6. doi:10.1159/000024143
95. Beignon AS, McKenna K, Skoberne M, Manches O, DaSilva I, Kavanagh DG, et al. Endocytosis of HIV-1 activates plasmacytoid dendritic cells via toll-like receptor-viral RNA interactions. *J Clin Invest* (2005) **115**(11):3265–75. doi:10.1172/JCI26032
96. Chaperot L, Blum A, Manches O, Lui G, Angel J, Molens JP, et al. Virus or TLR agonists induce TRAIL-mediated cytotoxic activity of plasmacytoid dendritic cells. *J Immunol* (2006) **176**(1):248–55.
97. Stary G, Klein I, Kohlhofer S, Koszik F, Scherzer T, Mullauer L, et al. Plasmacytoid dendritic cells express TRAIL and induce CD4+ T-cell apoptosis in HIV-1 viremic patients. *Blood* (2009) **114**(18):3854–63. doi:10.1182/blood-2009-04-217927
98. Dillon SM, Robertson KB, Pan SC, Mawhinney S, Meditz AL, Folkvord JM, et al. Plasmacytoid and myeloid dendritic cells with a partial activation phenotype accumulate in lymphoid tissue during asymptomatic chronic HIV-1 infection. *J Acquir Immune Defic Syndr* (2008) **48**(1):1–12. doi:10.1097/QAI.0b013e3181664b60
99. Germain C, Meier A, Jensen T, Knapnougel P, Poupon G, Lazzari A, et al. Induction of lectin-like transcript 1 (LLT1) protein cell surface expression by pathogens and interferon-gamma contributes to modulate immune responses. *J Biol Chem* (2011) **286**(44):37964–75. doi:10.1074/jbc.M111.285312
100. Montaldo E, Vitale C, Cottalasso F, Conte R, Glatzer T, Ambrosini P, et al. Human NK cells at early stages of differentiation produce CXCL8 and express CD161 molecule that functions as an activating receptor. *Blood* (2012) **119**(17):3987–96. doi:10.1182/blood-2011-09-379693
101. Rosen DB, Bettadapura J, Alsharifi M, Mathew PA, Warren HS, Lanier LL. Cutting edge: lectin-like transcript-1 is a ligand for the inhibitory human NKR-P1A receptor. *J Immunol* (2005) **175**(12):7796–9.
102. Bossard C, Malard F, Arbez J, Chevallier P, Guillaume T, Delaunay J, et al. Plasmacytoid dendritic cells and Th17 immune response contribution in gastrointestinal acute graft-versus-host disease. *Leukemia* (2012) **26**(7):1471–4. doi:10.1038/leu.2012.41
103. Godfrey DI, MacDonald HR, Kronenberg M, Smyth MJ, Van Kaer L. NKT cells: what's in a name? *Nat Rev Immunol* (2004) **4**(3):231–7. doi:10.1038/nri1309
104. Montoya CJ, Jie HB, Al-Harthi L, Mulder C, Patino PJ, Rugeles MT, et al. Activation of plasmacytoid dendritic cells with TLR9 agonists initiates invariant NKT cell-mediated cross-talk with myeloid dendritic cells. *J Immunol* (2006) **177**(2):1028–39.
105. Kadowaki N, Antonenko S, Ho S, Rissoan MC, Soumelis V, Porcelli SA, et al. Distinct cytokine profiles of neonatal natural killer T cells after expansion with subsets of dendritic cells. *J Exp Med* (2001) **193**(10):1221–6. doi:10.1084/jem.193.10.1221
106. Jukes JP, Wood KJ, Jones ND. Bystander activation of iNKT cells occurs during conventional T-cell alloresponses. *Am J Transplant* (2012) **12**(3):590–9. doi:10.1111/j.1600-6143.2011.03847.x
107. Brigl M, Tatituri RV, Watts GF, Bhowruth V, Leadbetter EA, Barton N, et al. Innate and cytokine-driven signals, rather than microbial antigens, dominate in natural killer T cell activation during microbial infection. *J Exp Med* (2011) **208**(6):1163–77. doi:10.1084/jem.20102555
108. Diana J, Griseri T, Lagaye S, Beaudoin L, Autrusseau E, Gautron AS, et al. NKT cell-plasmacytoid dendritic cell cooperation via OX40 controls viral infection in a tissue-specific manner. *Immunity* (2009) **30**(2):289–99. doi:10.1016/j.immuni.2008.12.017
109. Zaini J, Andarini S, Tahara M, Saijo Y, Ishii N, Kawakami K, et al. OX40 ligand expressed by DCs costimulates NKT and CD4+ Th cell antitumor immunity in mice. *J Clin Invest* (2007) **117**(11):3330–8. doi:10.1172/JCI32693
110. Shimizu K, Asakura M, Shinga J, Sato Y, Kitahara S, Hoshino K, et al. Invariant NKT cells induce plasmacytoid dendritic cell (DC) cross-talk with conventional DCs for efficient memory CD8+ T cell induction. *J Immunol* (2013) **190**(11):5609–19. doi:10.4049/jimmunol.1300033
111. Bekeredjian-Ding IB, Wagner M, Hornung V, Giese T, Schnurr M, Endres S, et al. Plasmacytoid dendritic cells control TLR7 sensitivity of naive B cells via type I IFN. *J Immunol* (2005) **174**(7):4043–50.
112. Braun D, Caramalho I, Demengeot J. IFN-alpha/beta enhances BCR-dependent B cell responses. *Int Immunol* (2002) **14**(4):411–9. doi:10.1093/intimm/14.4.411
113. Shaw J, Wang YH, Ito T, Arima K, Liu YJ. Plasmacytoid dendritic cells regulate B-cell growth and differentiation via CD70. *Blood* (2010) **115**(15):3051–7. doi:10.1182/blood-2009-08-239145
114. Berggren O, Hagberg N, Weber G, Alm GV, Ronnblom L, Eloranta ML. B lymphocytes enhance interferon-alpha production by plasmacytoid dendritic cells. *Arthritis Rheum* (2012) **64**(10):3409–19. doi:10.1002/art.34599
115. Vermi W, Lonardi S, Morassi M, Rossini C, Tardanico R, Venturini M, et al. Cutaneous distribution of plasmacytoid dendritic cells in lupus erythematosus. Selective tropism at the site of epithelial apoptotic damage. *Immunobiology* (2009) **214**(9–10):877–86. doi:10.1016/j.imbio.2009.06.013

116. Nascimbeni M, Perie L, Chorro L, Diocou S, Kreitmann L, Louis S, et al. Plasmacytoid dendritic cells accumulate in spleens from chronically HIV-infected patients but barely participate in interferon-alpha expression. *Blood* (2009) **113**(24):6112–9. doi:10.1182/blood-2008-07-170803
117. Perez-Cabezas B, Naranjo-Gomez M, Ruiz-Riol M, Bastos-Amador P, Fernandez MA, Carmona F, et al. TLR-activated conventional DCs promote gamma-secretase-mediated conditioning of plasmacytoid DCs. *J Leukoc Biol* (2012) **92**(1):133–43. doi:10.1189/jlb.0911452
118. Piccioli D, Sammicheli C, Tavarini S, Nuti S, Frigimelica E, Manetti AG, et al. Human plasmacytoid dendritic cells are unresponsive to bacterial stimulation and require a novel type of cooperation with myeloid dendritic cells for maturation. *Blood* (2009) **113**(18):4232–9. doi:10.1182/blood-2008-10-186890
119. Flacher V, Bouschbacher M, Verronese E, Massacrier C, Sisirak V, Berthier-Vergnes O, et al. Human Langerhans cells express a specific TLR profile and differentially respond to viruses and Gram-positive bacteria. *J Immunol* (2006) **177**(11):7959–67.
120. Means TK, Hayashi F, Smith KD, Aderem A, Luster AD. The toll-like receptor 5 stimulus bacterial flagellin induces maturation and chemokine production in human dendritic cells. *J Immunol* (2003) **170**(10):5165–75.
121. Jarrossay D, Napolitani G, Colonna M, Sallusto F, Lanzavecchia A. Specialization and complementarity in microbial molecule recognition by human myeloid and plasmacytoid dendritic cells. *Eur J Immunol* (2001) **31**(11):3388–93. doi:10.1002/1521-4141(200111)31:11<3388::AID-IMMU3388>3.0.CO;2-Q
122. Ito T, Amakawa R, Kaisho T, Hemmi H, Tajima K, Uehira K, et al. Interferon-alpha and interleukin-12 are induced differentially by toll-like receptor 7 ligands in human blood dendritic cell subsets. *J Exp Med* (2002) **195**(11):1507–12. doi:10.1084/jem.20020207
123. Ito T, Wang YH, Liu YJ. Plasmacytoid dendritic cell precursors/type I interferon-producing cells sense viral infection by toll-like receptor (TLR) 7 and TLR9. *Springer Semin Immunopathol* (2005) **26**(3):221–9. doi:10.1007/s00281-004-0180-4
124. Barchet W, Cella M, Colonna M. Plasmacytoid dendritic cells – virus experts of innate immunity. *Semin Immunol* (2005) **17**(4):253–61. doi:10.1016/j.smim.2005.05.008
125. Bond E, Liang F, Sandgren KJ, Smed-Sorensen A, Bergman P, Brighenti S, et al. Plasmacytoid dendritic cells infiltrate the skin in positive tuberculin skin test indurations. *J Invest Dermatol* (2012) **132**(1):114–23. doi:10.1038/jid.2011.246
126. Fonteneau JF, Larsson M, Beignon AS, McKenna K, Dasilva I, Amara A, et al. Human immunodeficiency virus type 1 activates plasmacytoid dendritic cells and concomitantly induces the bystander maturation of myeloid dendritic cells. *J Virol* (2004) **78**(10):5223–32. doi:10.1128/JVI.78.10.5223-5232.2004
127. Lebedeva T, Dustin ML, Sykulev Y. ICAM-1 co-stimulates target cells to facilitate antigen presentation. *Curr Opin Immunol* (2005) **17**(3):251–8. doi:10.1016/j.coi.2005.04.008
128. Mocikat R, Braumuller H, Gumy A, Egeter O, Ziegler H, Reusch U, et al. Natural killer cells activated by MHC class I(low) targets prime dendritic cells to induce protective CD8 T cell responses. *Immunity* (2003) **19**(4):561–9. doi:10.1016/S1074-7613(03)00264-4
129. Mailliard RB, Son YI, Redlinger R, Coates PT, Giermasz A, Morel PA, et al. Dendritic cells mediate NK cell help for Th1 and CTL responses: two-signal requirement for the induction of NK cell helper function. *J Immunol* (2003) **171**(5):2366–73.
130. Romagnani C, Della Chiesa M, Kohler S, Moewes B, Radbruch A, Moretta L, et al. Activation of human NK cells by plasmacytoid dendritic cells and its modulation by CD4+ T helper cells and CD4+ CD25hi T regulatory cells. *Eur J Immunol* (2005) **35**(8):2452–8. doi:10.1002/eji.200526069
131. Wehner R, Dietze K, Bachmann M, Schmitz M. The bidirectional crosstalk between human dendritic cells and natural killer cells. *J Innate Immun* (2011) **3**(3):258–63. doi:10.1159/000323923
132. Gerosa F, Gobbi A, Zorzi P, Burg S, Briere F, Carra G, et al. The reciprocal interaction of NK cells with plasmacytoid or myeloid dendritic cells profoundly affects innate resistance functions. *J Immunol* (2005) **174**(2):727–34.
133. Trinchieri G, Santoli D, Koprowski H. Spontaneous cell-mediated cytotoxicity in humans: role of interferon and immunoglobulins. *J Immunol* (1978) **120**(6):1849–55.
134. Hagberg N, Berggren O, Leonard D, Weber G, Bryceson YT, Alm GV, et al. IFN-alpha production by plasmacytoid dendritic cells stimulated with RNA-containing immune complexes is promoted by NK cells via MIP-1beta and LFA-1. *J Immunol* (2011) **186**(9):5085–94. doi:10.4049/jimmunol.1003349
135. Evans JH, Horowitz A, Mehrabi M, Wise EL, Pease JE, Riley EM, et al. A distinct subset of human NK cells expressing HLA-DR expand in response to IL-2 and can aid immune responses to BCG. *Eur J Immunol* (2011) **41**(7):1924–33. doi:10.1002/eji.201041180
136. Marshall JD, Heeke DS, Abbate C, Yee P, Van Nest G. Induction of interferon-gamma from natural killer cells by immunostimulatory CpG DNA is mediated through plasmacytoid-dendritic-cell-produced interferon-alpha and tumour necrosis factor-alpha. *Immunology* (2006) **117**(1):38–46. doi:10.1111/j.1365-2567.2005.02261.x
137. Fauriat C, Long EO, Ljunggren HG, Bryceson YT. Regulation of human NK-cell cytokine and chemokine production by target cell recognition. *Blood* (2010) **115**(11):2167–76. doi:10.1182/blood-2009-08-238469
138. Della Chiesa M, Romagnani C, Thiel A, Moretta L, Moretta A. Multidirectional interactions are bridging human NK cells with plasmacytoid and monocyte-derived dendritic cells during innate immune responses. *Blood* (2006) **108**(12):3851–8. doi:10.1182/blood-2006-02-004028
139. Aldemir H, Prod'homme V, Dumaurier MJ, Retiere C, Poupon G, Cazareth J, et al. Cutting edge: lectin-like transcript 1 is a ligand for the CD161 receptor. *J Immunol* (2005) **175**(12):7791–5.
140. Beckebaum S, Zhang X, Chen X, Yu Z, Frilling A, Dworacki G, et al. Increased levels of interleukin-10 in serum from patients with hepatocellular carcinoma correlate with profound numerical deficiencies and immature phenotype of circulating dendritic cell subsets. *Clin Cancer Res* (2004) **10**(21):7260–9. doi:10.1158/1078-0432.CCR-04-0872
141. Pinzon-Charry A, Ho CS, Maxwell T, McGuckin MA, Schmidt C, Furnival C, et al. Numerical and functional defects of blood dendritic cells in early- and late-stage breast cancer. *Br J Cancer* (2007) **97**(9):1251–9. doi:10.1038/sj.bjc.6604018
142. van Cruijsen H, Hoekman K, Stam AG, van den Eertwegh AJ, Kuenen BC, Scheper RJ, et al. Defective differentiation of myeloid and plasmacytoid dendritic cells in advanced cancer patients is not normalized by tyrosine kinase inhibition of the vascular endothelial growth factor receptor. *Clin Dev Immunol* (2007) **2007**:17315. doi:10.1155/2007/17315
143. Karthaus N, Torensma R, Tel J. Deciphering the message broadcast by tumor-infiltrating dendritic cells. *Am J Pathol* (2012) **181**(3):733–42. doi:10.1016/j.ajpath.2012.05.012
144. Charles J, Di Domizio J, Salameire D, Bendriss-Vermare N, Aspord C, Muhammad R, et al. Characterization of circulating dendritic cells in melanoma: role of CCR6 in plasmacytoid dendritic cell recruitment to the tumor. *J Invest Dermatol* (2010) **130**(6):1646–56. doi:10.1038/jid.2010.24
145. Hasan L, Mazzucchelli L, Liebi M, Lis M, Hunger RE, Tester A, et al. Function of liver activation-regulated chemokine/CC chemokine ligand 20 is differently affected by cathepsin B and cathepsin D processing. *J Immunol* (2006) **176**(11):6512–22.
146. Movassagh M, Spatz A, Davoust J, Lebecque S, Romero P, Pittet M, et al. Selective accumulation of mature DC-Lamp+ dendritic cells in tumor sites is associated with efficient T-cell-mediated antitumor response and control of metastatic dissemination in melanoma. *Cancer Res* (2004) **64**(6):2192–8. doi:10.1158/0008-5472.CAN-03-2969
147. Lee JR, Dalton RR, Messina JL, Sharma MD, Smith DM, Burgess RE, et al. Pattern of recruitment of immunoregulatory antigen-presenting cells in malignant melanoma. *Lab Invest* (2003) **83**(10):1457–66. doi:10.1097/01.LAB.0000090158.68852.D1
148. Demoulin S, Herfs M, Delvenne P, Hubert P. Tumor microenvironment converts plasmacytoid dendritic cells into immunosuppressive/tolerogenic cells: insight into the molecular mechanisms. *J Leukoc Biol* (2013) **93**(3):343–52. doi:10.1189/jlb.0812397
149. Bekeredjian-Ding I, Schafer M, Hartmann E, Pries R, Parcina M, Schneider P, et al. Tumour-derived prostaglandin E and transforming growth factor-beta synergize to inhibit plasmacytoid dendritic cell-derived interferon-alpha. *Immunology* (2009) **128**(3):439–50. doi:10.1111/j.1365-2567.2009.03134.x
150. Thiel A, Pries R, Jeske S, Trenkle T, Wollenberg B. Effect of head and neck cancer supernatant and CpG-oligonucleotides on migration and IFN-alpha production of plasmacytoid dendritic cells. *Anticancer Res* (2009) **29**(8):3019–25.

151. Ara T, Song L, Shimada H, Keshelava N, Russell HV, Metelitsa LS, et al. Interleukin-6 in the bone marrow microenvironment promotes the growth and survival of neuroblastoma cells. *Cancer Res* (2009) **69**(1):329–37. doi:10.1158/0008-5472.CAN-08-0613

152. Kamohara H, Takahashi M, Ishiko T, Ogawa M, Baba H. Induction of interleukin-8 (CXCL-8) by tumor necrosis factor-alpha and leukemia inhibitory factor in pancreatic carcinoma cells: impact of CXCL-8 as an autocrine growth factor. *Int J Oncol* (2007) **31**(3):627–32.

153. Brew R, Erikson JS, West DC, Kinsella AR, Slavin J, Christmas SE. Interleukin-8 as an autocrine growth factor for human colon carcinoma cells in vitro. *Cytokine* (2000) **12**(1):78–85. doi:10.1006/cyto.1999.0518

154. Araki S, Omori Y, Lyn D, Singh RK, Meinbach DM, Sandman Y, et al. Interleukin-8 is a molecular determinant of androgen independence and progression in prostate cancer. *Cancer Res* (2007) **67**(14):6854–62. doi:10.1158/0008-5472.CAN-07-1162

155. Yao C, Lin Y, Chua MS, Ye CS, Bi J, Li W, et al. Interleukin-8 modulates growth and invasiveness of estrogen receptor-negative breast cancer cells. *Int J Cancer* (2007) **121**(9):1949–57. doi:10.1002/ijc.22930

156. Fan Y, Ye J, Shen F, Zhu Y, Yeghiazarians Y, Zhu W, et al. Interleukin-6 stimulates circulating blood-derived endothelial progenitor cell angiogenesis in vitro. *J Cereb Blood Flow Metab* (2008) **28**(1):90–8. doi:10.1038/sj.jcbfm.9600509

157. Li A, Dubey S, Varney ML, Dave BJ, Singh RK. IL-8 directly enhanced endothelial cell survival, proliferation, and matrix metalloproteinases production and regulated angiogenesis. *J Immunol* (2003) **170**(6):3369–76.

158. Brat DJ, Bellail AC, Van Meir EG. The role of interleukin-8 and its receptors in gliomagenesis and tumoral angiogenesis. *Neuro Oncol* (2005) **7**(2):122–33. doi:10.1215/S1152851704001061

159. Cao W, Bover L. Signaling and ligand interaction of ILT7: receptor-mediated regulatory mechanisms for plasmacytoid dendritic cells. *Immunol Rev* (2010) **234**(1):163–76. doi:10.1111/j.0105-2896.2009.00867.x

160. Walter-Yohrling J, Cao X, Callahan M, Weber W, Morgenbesser S, Madden SL, et al. Identification of genes expressed in malignant cells that promote invasion. *Cancer Res* (2003) **63**(24):8939–47.

161. Ohtomo T, Sugamata Y, Ozaki Y, Ono K, Yoshimura Y, Kawai S, et al. Molecular cloning and characterization of a surface antigen preferentially overexpressed on multiple myeloma cells. *Biochem Biophys Res Commun* (1999) **258**(3):583–91. doi:10.1006/bbrc.1999.0683

162. Erikson E, Adam T, Schmidt S, Lehmann-Koch J, Over B, Goffinet C, et al. In vivo expression profile of the antiviral restriction factor and tumor-targeting antigen CD317/BST-2/HM1.24/tetherin in humans. *Proc Natl Acad Sci U S A* (2011) **108**(33):13688–93. doi:10.1073/pnas.1101684108

163. Cao W. Molecular characterization of human plasmacytoid dendritic cells. *J Clin Immunol* (2009) **29**(3):257–64. doi:10.1007/s10875-009-9284-x

164. Cao W, Rosen DB, Ito T, Bover L, Bao M, Watanabe G, et al. Plasmacytoid dendritic cell-specific receptor ILT7-Fc epsilonRI gamma inhibits toll-like receptor-induced interferon production. *J Exp Med* (2006) **203**(6):1399–405. doi:10.1084/jem.20052454

165. Cho M, Ishida K, Chen J, Ohkawa J, Chen W, Namiki S, et al. SAGE library screening reveals ILT7 as a specific plasmacytoid dendritic cell marker that regulates type I IFN production. *Int Immunol* (2008) **20**(1):155–64. doi:10.1093/intimm/dxm127

166. Ju XS, Hacker C, Scherer B, Redecke V, Berger T, Schuler G, et al. Immunoglobulin-like transcripts ILT2, ILT3 and ILT7 are expressed by human dendritic cells and down-regulated following activation. *Gene* (2004) **331**:159–64. doi:10.1016/j.gene.2004.02.018

167. Chang CC, Ciubotariu R, Manavalan JS, Yuan J, Colovai AI, Piazza F, et al. Tolerization of dendritic cells by T(S) cells: the crucial role of inhibitory receptors ILT3 and ILT4. *Nat Immunol* (2002) **3**(3):237–43. doi:10.1038/ni760

168. Shiroishi M, Tsumoto K, Amano K, Shirakihara Y, Colonna M, Braud VM, et al. Human inhibitory receptors Ig-like transcript 2 (ILT2) and ILT4 compete with CD8 for MHC class I binding and bind preferentially to HLA-G. *Proc Natl Acad Sci U S A* (2003) **100**(15):8856–61. doi:10.1073/pnas.1431057100

169. Fuchs A, Cella M, Kondo T, Colonna M. Paradoxic inhibition of human natural interferon-producing cells by the activating receptor NKp44. *Blood* (2005) **106**(6):2076–82. doi:10.1182/blood-2004-12-4802

170. Horton NC, Mathew SO, Mathew PA. Novel interaction between proliferating cell nuclear antigen and HLA I on the surface of tumor cells inhibits NK cell function through NKp44. *PLoS One* (2013) **8**(3):e59552. doi:10.1371/journal.pone.0059552

171. Kalb ML, Glaser A, Stary G, Koszik F, Stingl G. TRAIL(+) human plasmacytoid dendritic cells kill tumor cells in vitro: mechanisms of imiquimod- and IFN-alpha-mediated antitumor reactivity. *J Immunol* (2012) **188**(4):1583–91. doi:10.4049/jimmunol.1102437

172. Tel J, Smits EL, Anguille S, Joshi RN, Figdor CG, de Vries IJ. Human plasmacytoid dendritic cells are equipped with antigen-presenting and tumoricidal capacities. *Blood* (2012) **120**(19):3936–44. doi:10.1182/blood-2012-06-435941

173. Vigneswaran N, Baucum DC, Wu J, Lou Y, Bouquot J, Muller S, et al. Repression of tumor necrosis factor-related apoptosis-inducing ligand (TRAIL) but not its receptors during oral cancer progression. *BMC Cancer* (2007) **7** doi:10.1186/1471-2407-7-108

174. Calpe S, Wang N, Romero X, Berger SB, Lanyi A, Engel P, et al. The SLAM and SAP gene families control innate and adaptive immune responses. *Immunol* (2008) **97**:177–250. doi:10.1016/S0065-2776(08)00004-7

175. Cabezon R, Sintes J, Llinas L, Benitez-Ribas D. Analysis of HLDA9 mAbs on plasmacytoid dendritic cells. *Immunol Lett* (2011) **134**(2):167–73. doi:10.1016/j.imlet.2010.09.020

176. Cannons JL, Qi H, Lu KT, Dutta M, Gomez-Rodriguez J, Cheng J, et al. Optimal germinal center responses require a multistage T cell:B cell adhesion process involving integrins, SLAM-associated protein, and CD84. *Immunity* (2010) **32**(2):253–65. doi:10.1016/j.immuni.2010.01.010

177. Gopcsa L, Banyai A, Jakab K, Kormos L, Tamaska J, Matolcsy A, et al. Extensive flow cytometric characterization of plasmacytoid dendritic cell leukemia cells. *Eur J Haematol* (2005) **75**(4):346–51. doi:10.1111/j.1600-0609.2005.00513.x

178. Oliver-Vila I, Saborit-Villarroya I, Engel P, Martin M. The leukocyte receptor CD84 inhibits Fc epsilon RI-mediated signaling through homophilic interaction in transfected RBL-2H3 cells. *Mol Immunol* (2008) **45**(8):2138–49. doi:10.1016/j.molimm.2007.12.006

179. Romero X, Zapater N, Calvo M, Kalko SG, de la Fuente MA, Tovar V, et al. CD229 (Ly9) lymphocyte cell surface receptor interacts homophilically through its N-terminal domain and relocalizes to the immunological synapse. *J Immunol* (2005) **174**(11):7033–42.

180. Bouchon A, Cella M, Grierson HL, Cohen JI, Colonna M. Activation of NK cell-mediated cytotoxicity by a SAP-independent receptor of the CD2 family. *Immunol* (2001) **167**(10):5517–21.

181. Boles KS, Mathew PA. Molecular cloning of CS1, a novel human natural killer cell receptor belonging to the CD2 subset of the immunoglobulin superfamily. *Immunogenetics* (2001) **52**(3–4):302–7. doi:10.1007/s002510000274

182. Lee JK, Mathew SO, Vaidya SV, Kumaresan PR, Mathew PA. CS1 (CRACC, CD319) induces proliferation and autocrine cytokine expression on human B lymphocytes. *J Immunol* (2007) **179**(7):4672–8.

183. Stark S, Watzl C. 2B4 (CD244), NTB-A and CRACC (CS1) stimulate cytotoxicity but no proliferation in human NK cells. *Int Immunol* (2006) **18**(2):241–7. doi:10.1093/intimm/dxh358

184. Falco M, Marcenaro E, Romeo E, Bellora F, Marras D, Vely F, et al. Homophilic interaction of NTBA, a member of the CD2 molecular family: induction of cytotoxicity and cytokine release in human NK cells. *Eur J Immunol* (2004) **34**(6):1663–72. doi:10.1002/eji.200424886

185. Flaig RM, Stark S, Watzl C. Cutting edge: NTB-A activates NK cells via homophilic interaction. *J Immunol* (2004) **172**(11):6524–7.

186. Messmer B, Eissmann P, Stark S, Watzl C. CD48 stimulation by 2B4 (CD244)-expressing targets activates human NK cells. *J Immunol* (2006) **176**(8):4646–50.

187. Tel J, van der Leun AM, Figdor CG, Torensma R, de Vries IJ. Harnessing human plasmacytoid dendritic cells as professional APCs. *Cancer Immunol Immunother* (2012) **61**(8):1279–88. doi:10.1007/s00262-012-1210-z

Does the immune system naturally protect against cancer?

Alexandre Corthay[1,2,3] *

[1] Tumor Immunology Group, Department of Pathology, Oslo University Hospital Rikshospitalet, Oslo, Norway
[2] Department of Biosciences, University of Oslo, Oslo, Norway
[3] Centre for Immune Regulation, University of Oslo, Oslo, Norway

Edited by:
Fang-Ping Huang, Imperial College London, UK

Reviewed by:
Stephan Gasser, National University of Singapore, Singapore
Susanna Mandruzzato, Università degli Studi di Padova, Italy

***Correspondence:**
Alexandre Corthay, Tumor Immunology Group, Department of Pathology, Oslo University Hospital Rikshospitalet, PO Box 4950, Nydalen, Oslo NO-0424, Norway
e-mail: alexandre.corthay@ibv.uio.no

The importance of the immune system in conferring protection against pathogens like viruses, bacteria, and parasitic worms is well established. In contrast, there is a long-lasting debate on whether cancer prevention is a primary function of the immune system. The concept of immunological surveillance of cancer was developed by Lewis Thomas and Frank Macfarlane Burnet more than 50 years ago. We are still lacking convincing data illustrating immunological eradication of precancerous lesions *in vivo*. Here, I present eight types of evidence in support of the cancer immunosurveillance hypothesis. First, primary immunodeficiency in mice and humans is associated with increased cancer risk. Second, organ transplant recipients, who are treated with immunosuppressive drugs, are more prone to cancer development. Third, acquired immunodeficiency due to infection by human immunodeficiency virus (HIV-1) leads to elevated risk of cancer. Fourth, the quantity and quality of the immune cell infiltrate found in human primary tumors represent an independent prognostic factor for patient survival. Fifth, cancer cells harbor mutations in protein-coding genes that are specifically recognized by the adaptive immune system. Sixth, cancer cells selectively accumulate mutations to evade immune destruction ("immunoediting"). Seventh, lymphocytes bearing the NKG2D receptor are able to recognize and eliminate stressed premalignant cells. Eighth, a promising strategy to treat cancer consists in potentiating the naturally occurring immune response of the patient, through blockade of the immune checkpoint molecules CTLA-4, PD-1, or PD-L1. Thus, there are compelling pieces of evidence that a primary function of the immune system is to confer protection against cancer.

Keywords: cancer immunosurveillance, primary immunodeficiency, cancer risk, organ transplantation, immunosuppressive drugs, HIV, NKG2D, checkpoint blockade

INTRODUCTION

Lewis Thomas and Frank Macfarlane Burnet proposed the concept of immunological surveillance of cancer more than five decades ago (1–4). It was defined by Burnet as follows: "In large long-lived animals, like most of the warm-blooded vertebrates, inheritable genetic changes must be common in somatic cells and a proportion of these changes will represent a step toward malignancy. It is an evolutionary necessity that there should be some mechanism for eliminating or inactivating such potentially dangerous mutant cells and it is postulated that this mechanism is of immunological character" (1). More than 50 years after Burnet proposed his theory, the immunological scientific community remains largely divided with both proponents [e.g., Ref. (5, 6)] and opponents [e.g., Ref. (7, 8)] of the cancer immunosurveillance hypothesis. In fact, an opposite and very influential concept was proposed in 2001 by Frances Balkwill and Alberto Mantovani, who suggested that inflammatory immune cells and cytokines found in tumors may promote rather than suppress tumor growth (9, 10). Although, we are currently lacking convincing data illustrating immunological eradication of precancerous lesions *in vivo*, there are strong indications that a primary function of the immune system is indeed to prevent cancer. Here, I present eight types of evidence in support of the cancer immunosurveillance hypothesis.

PRIMARY IMMUNODEFICIENCY IN HUMANS AND MICE IS ASSOCIATED WITH INCREASED CANCER RISK

As Burnet himself pointed out, an implication of the cancer immunosurveillance hypothesis is that immunodeficiency should be associated with increased likelihood of neoplasia (1). Immunodeficiencies can be divided in two main types: primary (inborn) immunodeficiencies, which are caused by genetic defects and whose incidence is approximately 1:10,000 births; and secondary immunodeficiencies, which are induced by immunosuppressive medication or viral infection and which are much more common. In accordance with Burnet's prediction, severe primary immunodeficiencies have been reported to be associated with increased risk of malignancy (11–14). For instance, patients with defective humoral immunity due to common variable immunodeficiency (CVID) had increased incidence of lymphoma and epithelial tumors of the stomach, breast, bladder, and cervix (12, 15). Selective immunoglobulin A (IgA) deficiency was associated with a high incidence of gastric carcinomas (15). Moreover, patients with X-linked immunodeficiency with hyper-IgM, caused by mutations in the CD40 ligand molecule, had a high incidence of tumors of the pancreas and liver (16). However, it remains unclear to what extent primary immunodeficiency in humans leads to increased cancer development, due to the relatively low number of patients investigated.

Gene-targeted mice, which selectively lack key components of the immune system have been extensively used to experimentally test the effect of well-defined primary immunodeficiencies on cancer development [reviewed in Ref. (17)]. Mice which lacked both T and B cells, due to a deficiency in the recombination-activating gene 2 (RAG2), were more susceptible to spontaneous and carcinogen-induced carcinomas (18). Mice lacking γδ T cells were highly susceptible to multiple regimens of cutaneous carcinogenesis (19). The cytokines interferon-α/β (IFN-α/β) and IFN-γ were shown to protect mice against spontaneous and carcinogen-induced malignancy (18, 20–22). Moreover, the molecule perforin, which is used by cytotoxic lymphocytes to kill target cells, was reported to be important for surveillance of spontaneous lymphoma (23). Collectively, the human and mouse data reveal a consistent association between primary immunodeficiency and increased incidence of various types of cancer.

ORGAN TRANSPLANT RECIPIENTS ARE MORE PRONE TO CANCER DEVELOPMENT

A breakthrough in organ transplantation was the discovery of immunosuppressive drugs such as cyclosporine A, which prevent organ rejection by the adaptive immune system (24). Immunosuppressive medication is now standard treatment after organ transplantation. Life-long treatment of thousands of transplanted patients with immunosuppressive drugs was defined by Thomas as a "human experiment" to test the cancer immunosurveillance hypothesis (4). Already in 1973, an international registry-based study of renal-transplant recipients from 30 countries revealed that transplantation was associated with increased risk of developing cancer, in particular lymphoma (25). A large cohort investigation of cancer risk after organ transplantation was performed in the Nordic countries, in homogeneous populations with well-documented cancer incidence, on nearly 6000 kidney recipients (26). A two to fivefold excess risk was reported for cancers of the colon, larynx, lung, bladder, prostate, and testis. Strikingly high risks, 10-fold to 30-fold above normally expected levels, were observed for cancers of the lip, skin (non-melanoma), kidney, endocrine glands, cervix, and for non-Hodgkin's lymphoma (26). Another large study of kidney transplantation in 200,000 patients from 42 countries reported that the risk of developing lymphoma was 12-fold higher for transplant recipients than that in a matched non-transplanted population (27). Notably, the majority of posttransplant lymphomas were associated with infection with Epstein–Barr virus (EBV), which primarily infects B cells and is known to cause B cell transformation (28). Thus, most lymphomas arising in transplant patients were likely to be a secondary event resulting from reduced antiviral immunity, rather than a direct effect of reduced antitumor immunity. However, lymphomas not associated with EBV infection have also been reported after transplantation (29). An investigation of 175,000 solid organ transplants in the USA revealed that increased cancer risk occurred not only after kidney transplantation but also after liver, heart, and lung transplantation (30). Risk was increased for 32 different malignancies, some related to known infections (e.g., anal cancer and Kaposi sarcoma) and others unrelated to infections (e.g., lung cancer and melanoma). The most common malignancies with elevated risk were non-Hodgkin lymphoma and cancers of the lungs (30).

Very high rates of non-melanoma skin cancers have been reported for Swedish (20–40%) and Australian (70%) populations 20 years after transplantation (31–33). Cutaneous types of human papillomaviruses have been suggested to be the cause of non-melanoma skin cancers such as squamous cell carcinoma in immunosuppressed patients, but the epidemiological pieces of evidence remain inconsistent (34). Strikingly, non-melanoma skin tumors in the renal-transplant population of Queensland, Australia, were reported to arise predominantly on chronically sun-exposed skin (head, neck, and distal limbs), strongly suggesting a causative role of ultraviolet (UV) light rather than oncogenic viruses (33). Thus, life-long treatment of organ transplant recipients with immunosuppressive drugs leads to increased risk of developing many different types of cancer, some related to known infections and others unrelated.

IMMUNOSUPPRESSION INDUCED BY INFECTION BY HUMAN IMMUNODEFICIENCY VIRUS TYPE 1 LEADS TO ELEVATED RISK FOR CANCER

The HIV-1 virus causes acquired immunodeficiency by selectively infecting and killing $CD4^+$ T cells. Accordingly, HIV-infected patients, receiving or not antiviral treatments, possess reduced levels of $CD4^+$ T cells compared to non-infected individuals. HIV-infected individuals have elevated risk for cancer linked to oncogenic viruses such as Kaposi sarcoma (caused by human herpes virus 8), Hodgkin's and non-Hodgkin's lymphoma (EBV), anal and cervical cancer (human papilloma virus), and liver cancer (hepatitis B and C viruses). Kaposi sarcoma, non-Hodgkin's lymphoma and cervical cancer are particularly frequent and are considered as acquired immunodeficiency syndrome (AIDS)-defining cancers (35). However, several cancers that are not linked to oncogenic viruses, like lung cancer and multiple myeloma, are also more frequent in patients with HIV (35, 36). Lung cancer is the most common non-AIDS-defining cancer and a leading cause of mortality among HIV-infected individuals (37). For the majority of patients with lung cancer, malignant transformation is known to be caused by carcinogens present in cigarette smoke. Higher smoking rates have been reported for HIV-infected populations. After controlling for potential confounders including smoking, a large cohort study of veterans (with 37,000 HIV-infected patients and 75,000 healthy controls) concluded that HIV was an independent risk factor for incident lung cancer (37). Importantly, cancer incidence in HIV-infected individuals was found to be inversely related to $CD4^+$ T cell counts in blood, which supports the association between immunosuppression and increased cancer risk (38). For instance, the risk of lung cancer was doubled by $CD4^+$ T counts in the range of 350–499 cells per microliter blood compared to normal counts $\geq$500, and continued to increase as the $CD4^+$ T cell count fell (38). Thus, acquired immunodeficiency by HIV infection, which selectively depletes $CD4^+$ T cells, leads to increased risk of developing many different types of cancer, some related to known infections, and others unrelated.

QUANTITY AND QUALITY OF THE IMMUNE CELL INFILTRATE IN HUMAN PRIMARY TUMORS REPRESENT AN INDEPENDENT PROGNOSTIC FACTOR FOR PATIENT SURVIVAL

All solid tumors are infiltrated by a variety of immune cells. For many types of human cancers, an association has been reported between the type, density, and location of immune cells within the primary tumor and the clinical outcome [reviewed in Ref. (39)]. The number of intratumoral $CD3^+$ T cells was shown to positively correlate with longer survival of patients with epithelial ovarian and colorectal cancers (40, 41). A high number of stromal $CD4^+$ T cells were found to represent an independent positive prognostic factor in non-small cell lung cancer (42). Tumor-infiltrating $CD8^+$ cytotoxic T cells were shown to predict clinical outcome in colon, lung, and breast cancers (42–45). Concurrent infiltration by both $CD4^+$ and $CD8^+$ T cells was reported to represent a favorable prognostic factor in esophageal squamous cell carcinoma and non-small cell lung cancer, suggesting that both cell types cooperate to fight cancer (46, 47). Among all $CD4^+$ T cell subsets, Th1 cells seem to be particularly advantageous, as reported for colorectal, liver, and breast cancers (39, 40, 48, 49). In patients with gastrointestinal stromal tumors (GIST), the intratumoral density of $CD3^+$ T cells and $NKp46^+$ natural killer (NK) cells were found to represent two independent prognostic factors for progression-free survival (50). Notably, NK and T cells were detected in distinct areas of tumor sections, suggesting that both cell types contributed independently to GIST immunosurveillance (50). Furthermore, a high tumor infiltration by $CD68^+$ macrophages was associated with prolonged survival in prostate, lung, and colon cancers (43, 51–54). Thus, for various types of human cancers, the quantity and the quality of the immune response within the primary tumor appear to represent an independent predictor for patient survival. This correlation between immunological data and clinical outcome strongly suggests that the immune system of the patient had naturally mounted an antitumor immune response before any treatment had started. The efficiency of this response presumably varies from patient to patient, thereby critically influencing survival.

CANCER CELLS HARBOR MUTATIONS IN PROTEIN-CODING GENES THAT ARE SPECIFICALLY RECOGNIZED BY THE ADAPTIVE IMMUNE SYSTEM

Cancer cells originate from normal cells that have accumulated "driver" mutations, which either activate oncogenes by dominant gain of function or inactivate tumor suppressor genes by recessive loss of function. A typical tumor contains two to eight of these driver mutations (55). Cancer cells also accumulate "passenger" mutations, which do not contribute to tumorigenesis. Genome-wide sequencing studies have provided detailed information about somatic mutations in various types of cancers. For common solid tumors such as breast, colon, brain, and pancreas cancers, an average of 30–60 non-synonymous mutations in protein-coding genes was observed (56–59). Most of these mutations (95%) were single-nucleotide substitutions, whereas the remainder was deletions or insertions (55). Metastatic melanoma and non-small cell lung carcinoma, which represent two types of cancers caused by potent mutagens (UV light and cigarette smoke, respectively), had a higher mutation rate with ~150 mutations per tumor (60, 61). Pediatric tumors and leukemias had the fewest mutations with ~10 mutations per tumor on average (55). Thus, it is now established that tumor cells in most cancer types harbor numerous non-synonymous mutations in protein-coding genes.

Driver and passenger mutations, which alter the normal amino acid sequence of proteins, may potentially be recognized by the adaptive immune system. A number of studies have revealed that tumor-specific antigens created by mutations can be recognized either by the T cells or the B cells of the patient. For instance in melanoma, $CD4^+$ T cells were found that recognized a tumor-specific antigen generated by a non-synonymous point mutation in the gene coding for triosephosphate isomerase (62). Another antigen recognized by $CD4^+$ T cells in melanoma had been generated by a chromosomal rearrangement resulting in a fusion of a low density lipid receptor gene with a fucosyltransferase gene (63). In colorectal cancer with microsatellite instability phenotype, $CD4^+$ T cells were identified that recognized a frameshift mutation in the transforming growth factor β receptor II (TGFβRII) (64). In a melanoma patient, the tumor suppressor $p16^{INK4a}$ with a point mutation was specifically recognized by cytotoxic $CD8^+$ T cells (65). In non-small cell lung cancer, several $CD8^+$ T cell epitopes created by point mutations have been reported (66–68). Moreover, in chronic myeloid leukemia, cytotoxic $CD8^+$ T cells specific for a BCR-ABL fusion protein (resulting from the fusion of BCR and ABL genes) were found (69). Tumor-specific IgG antibodies are common in the serum of cancer patients, as revealed by serological identification of antigens by recombinant expression cloning (SEREX) technology (70). This powerful method has allowed the identification of over 2000 tumor antigens recognized by autologous IgG, including the p53 tumor suppressor modified by a point mutation (71). Collectively, these studies demonstrate that the adaptive immune system is able to detect cancer by specifically recognizing the mutated proteins of the malignant cells.

CANCER CELLS SELECTIVELY ACCUMULATE MUTATIONS TO EVADE IMMUNE DESTRUCTION

Recognition of cancer cells by tumor-specific $CD8^+$ T cells is achieved by the presentation of antigenic peptides from mutated proteins on major histocompatibility complex (MHC) class I molecules on the surface of cancer cells. In order to avoid recognition and the resulting elimination by $CD8^+$ T cells, cancer cells often mutate key genes of the MHC class I antigen presentation pathway. Downregulation of surface MHC class I molecules is a common feature of human cancer cells [reviewed in Ref. (72)]. Several mechanisms have been reported, including mutations in the β2-microglobulin gene, which is required for MHC class I molecule expression on the cell surface (73, 74). MHC haplotype loss in various human tumors was shown to be caused by complete or partial loss of chromosome 6, which harbor all MHC class I and class II genes (except for β2-microglobulin) (75). On the basis of its mutation pattern in cancer cells, β2-microglobulin was recently included in a list of 74 tumor suppressor genes (55). A recent study analyzed somatic point mutations in exon sequences from 4742 human cancers across 21 cancer types (76). Based on mutation frequency and pattern, 254 "cancer genes" were identified, including four genes belonging to the MHC class I antigen presentation pathway (β2-microglobulin, HLA-A, HLA-B, and TAP1), as well as the CD1D gene, which is involved in the presentation of lipid antigens to NK T cells (76). Hence, several mutations frequently observed in cancer cells are likely to result from selective pressure to evade the immune attack, in particular by cytotoxic $CD8^+$ T cells and NK T cells.

Another strategy used by cancer cells to avoid the immune response consists of secreting immunosuppressive cytokines such as transforming growth factor β (TGF-β) and interleukin 10 (IL-10). In contrast to normal cells, which produce very little, malignant cells often secrete large amounts of TGF-β and IL-10 [reviewed in Ref. (77)]. Both cytokines have various effects on non-transformed cells present in the tumor mass, most notably the inhibition of immune cell functions. For several types of cancers, elevated serum levels of TGF-β or IL-10 have been reported to be associated with worse prognosis [reviewed in Ref. (77)]. Surprisingly, TGF-β can function both as a tumor suppressor and a tumor promoter, this duality being known as the TGF-β paradox. In early stage tumors, TGF-β is a potent inducer of growth arrest. In advanced stage malignant cells, TGF-β signaling pathways are severely dysregulated, and TGF-β promotes tumor growth [reviewed in Ref. (78)]. Thus, cancer cells often produce abnormally high levels of immunosuppressive cytokines, which strongly suggests that dampening immunity is a prerequisite for tumor growth.

Experiments with immunodeficient mice have demonstrated that the immune system may exert a strong selective pressure on the cancer cells. By using the chemical carcinogen methylcholanthrene, sarcomas were induced either in wild-type mice or in RAG2-deficient mice, which lack both T and B cells (18). When transplanted into RAG2-deficient mice, all sarcomas grew progressively with equivalent kinetics. In contrast, when the tumor cells were injected into immunocompetent wild-type hosts, all sarcomas from wild-type mice grew progressively, while 8 of 20 (40%) sarcomas from RAG2-deficient mice were rejected (18). These data strongly suggest that in wild-type mice, there was selection of tumor cells that were more capable of surviving in an immunocompetent host. This provides an explanation for the apparent paradox of tumor formation in immunologically intact individuals. Based on these findings, Robert Schreiber and coworkers introduced the term "cancer immunoediting," which was further developed into a general theory, to describe the sculpting actions of the immune response on developing tumors in immunocompetent individuals (18, 79).

LYMPHOCYTES BEARING THE NKG2D RECEPTOR ARE ABLE TO RECOGNIZE AND ELIMINATE STRESSED PREMALIGNANT CELLS

NK cells are innate lymphocytes that can kill malignant or infected cells. All NK cells and some T cells express the NKG2D molecule on the cell surface. NKG2D is an activating receptor, which serves as a major recognition receptor for detection and elimination of transformed cells (80). The ligands for NKG2D are self proteins that are poorly expressed by normal resting cells but upregulated on the surface of stressed cells. NKG2D ligands in humans include MICA, MICB, and six different ULBP proteins (81). In mice, NKG2D ligands include MULT1, five isoforms of RAE-1, and three isoforms of the H60 proteins (82). In humans, cells that express NKG2D ligands may be recognized and killed by either NK cells or γδ T cells in a process called lymphoid stress surveillance (83).

NKG2D ligands were shown to be upregulated in normal cells after treatment with DNA-damaging agents like ionizing radiations and UV light (84). It was concluded that the DNA damage response, which was known to arrest the cell cycle and enhance DNA repair, may also participate in alerting the immune system to the presence of potentially dangerous cells (84). Several studies suggested that expression of NKG2D ligands on transformed cells may be directly induced by oncogenes. For example, the BCR-ABL fusion oncogene was reported to control the expression of MICA in chronic myelogenous leukemia cells at the posttranscriptional level (85). Activation of the Ras oncogene was shown to upregulate the expression of RAE-1α/β in mouse cells, and ULBP1–3 and MICA/B in human cells (86). In a recent study, surface upregulation of NKG2D ligands by human epithelial cells in response to UV irradiation, osmotic shock, or oxidative stress, was shown to depend on the activation of the epidermal growth factor receptor (EGFR) (87). The EGFR pathway is frequently dysregulated in human cancer and it was proposed that activation of EGFR may regulate the immunological visibility of stressed premalignant cells (87). Surprisingly, several isoforms of RAE-1, like RAE-1ε, were found to be expressed not only by cancer cells, but also by some normal proliferating cells such as fibroblasts (88). The E2F transcription factor, which controls cell cycle entry, was shown to regulate RAE-1ε expression. These data suggest that NKG2D-bearing lymphocytes may control the proliferation of both normal and malignant cells (88).

MICA and MICB were found to be expressed by many, but not all, freshly isolated carcinomas of the lung, breast, kidney, ovary, prostate, colon, and liver (89, 90). Moreover, *in vitro* studies revealed that MICA and MICB contributed to the lysis of hepatocellular carcinoma cells by NK cells (90). The importance of NKG2D for cancer immunosurveillance *in vivo* gained support from experiments showing that cancer cells transfected with NKG2D ligands and injected into mice were rapidly rejected by NK cells and by $CD8^+$ T cells (91, 92). Moreover, neutralization of NKG2D with blocking monoclonal antibodies rendered mice more susceptible to carcinogen-induced fibrocarcinoma (93). Gene-targeted mice deficient for NKG2D were shown to be more susceptible to the *in situ* development of prostate adenocarcinoma and B cell lymphoma (94). In humans, an association has been reported between polymorphisms of the NKG2D gene and susceptibility of developing liver and cervix cancers, supporting a protective role of NKG2D against these malignancies (95, 96). Thus, the expression of stress-induced endogenous molecules associated with cell transformation is used by the immune system to recognize and eliminate premalignant cells in mice and humans.

PROMISING NOVEL STRATEGY TO TREAT CANCER CONSISTS IN POTENTIATING THE NATURALLY OCCURRING IMMUNE RESPONSE OF THE PATIENT THROUGH BLOCKADE OF IMMUNE CHECKPOINT MOLECULES

Activation of a naïve T cell requires at least two signals: T cell receptor-mediated recognition of a cognate antigen (signal 1) and engagement of the costimulatory receptor CD28 (signal 2).

Once activated, T cells upregulate on the cell surface two co-inhibitory molecules, cytotoxic T lymphocyte-associated antigen 4 (CTLA-4) and programed death 1 (PD-1). The function of these co-inhibitory molecules is to tightly regulate the immune response by containing excessive T cell activation. For the purpose of cancer immunotherapy, monoclonal antibodies have been generated to potentiate the ongoing antitumor immune response of the patient, through "immune checkpoint blockade" of CTLA-4, PD-1, or PD-1 ligand (PD-L1). The outcome of the initial clinical trials with these new treatments is remarkable (97).

In a phase 3, randomized trial, the CTLA-4 blocking antibody ipilimumab was shown to prolong survival of patients with previously treated metastatic melanoma by ~4 months (98). This was a breakthrough in the treatment of metastatic melanoma because no other therapy had previously been shown to prolong survival in a phase 3 controlled trial. Another phase 3 trial with previously untreated metastatic melanoma patients showed that the overall survival was significantly longer in the group receiving ipilimumab combined with the chemotherapy drug dacarbazine than in the group receiving dacarbazine plus placebo (11 vs. 9 months) (99). Moreover, higher survival rates after 3 years were observed in the ipilimumab–dacarbazine group compared to controls (21 vs. 12%) (99).

Although no phase 3 trial has yet been published based on PD-1 or PD-L1 blockade, phase 1 studies showed promising results. PD-1 checkpoint blockade was tested in a phase 1 trial on patients with several types of advanced cancer. Cumulative response rates (complete or partial responses) were 18% among patients with non-small cell lung cancer (14 of 76 patients), 28% among patients with melanoma (26 of 94 patients), and 27% among patients with renal-cell cancer (9 of 33 patients). Responses were durable, 20 of 31 responses lasting 1 year or more in patients with 1 year or more of follow-up (100). In a phase 1 trial with anti-PD-L1 blocking antibodies, an objective response (complete or partial response) was observed in 9 of 52 patients with melanoma, 2 of 17 with renal-cell cancer, and 5 of 49 with non-small cell lung cancer. Responses lasted for 1 year or more in 8 of 16 patients with at least 1 year of follow-up (101). Finally, combined treatment of advanced melanoma was performed with both anti-CTLA-4 and anti-PD-1 blocking antibodies in a phase 1 trial. The objective response rate for all 53 treated patients in the concurrent-regimen group was as high as 40% (102). Thus, immune checkpoint blockade represents a promising new strategy to treat advanced cancer in humans. The success of this approach, which is based on potentiating the ongoing, naturally occurring antitumor immune response of the patient, provides another piece of evidence that fighting cancer is indeed a primary function of the immune system.

CONCLUDING REMARKS

As summarized in this review, the scientific literature over the past 50 years has provided strong support to the cancer immunosurveillance hypothesis. Thus, it appears that our immune system does not only naturally protect us against infectious non-self (pathogens) but also against malignant self (cancer). Many cell types belonging to both the innate (NK cells and macrophages) and the adaptive (T and B cells) immune systems seem to be involved in cancer control. Our current understanding on how the immune system fights cancer remains very fragmentary. There are pieces of evidence for two main strategies used by the immune system to distinguish cancer cells from normal cells. On one hand, the adaptive immune system recognizes altered (mutated) self proteins in malignant cells. On the other hand, NK cells and $\gamma\delta$ T cells recognize stress-induced self molecules (NKG2D ligands) on transformed cells. Yet, cancer cells originate from normal cells and a main challenge for successful antitumor immunity is to restrain the destruction of normal cells (autoimmunity). In fact, a recent study suggested that autoimmune disease may occur as a result of an inaccurate antitumor immune response (103). Scleroderma is an autoimmune connective tissue disease in which patients make antibodies to a limited number of autoantigens, including the RNA polymerase III subunit, encoded by the POLR3A gene. In several patients who had both scleroderma and cancer, genetic alterations of the POLR3A locus were found in the malignant cells, suggesting that POLR3A mutations triggered an adaptive antitumor immune response, which cross-reacted with normal tissue, causing autoimmune disease (103).

ACKNOWLEDGMENTS

I thank Inger Øynebråten for critical reading of the manuscript. This work was supported by grants from the Research Council of Norway, the Southern and Eastern Norway Regional Health Authority, the Norwegian Cancer Society, Anders Jahre fund, and Henrik Homans Minde fund.

REFERENCES

1. Burnet FM. The concept of immunological surveillance. *Prog Exp Tumor Res* (1970) **13**:1–27.
2. Burnet M. Cancer: a biological approach. III. Viruses associated with neoplastic conditions. IV. Practical applications. *Br Med J* (1957) **1**:841–7. doi:10.1136/bmj.1.5023.841
3. Thomas L. Discussion. In: Lawrence HS editor. *Cellular and Humoral Aspects of the Hypersensitive States.* New York: Hoeber-Harper (1959). p. 529–32.
4. Thomas L. On immunosurveillance in human cancer. *Yale J Biol Med* (1982) **55**:329–33.
5. Senovilla L, Vitale I, Martins I, Tailler M, Pailleret C, Michaud M, et al. An immunosurveillance mechanism controls cancer cell ploidy. *Science* (2012) **337**:1678–84. doi:10.1126/science.1224922
6. Smyth MJ, Godfrey DI, Trapani JA. A fresh look at tumor immunosurveillance and immunotherapy. *Nat Immunol* (2001) **2**:293–9. doi:10.1038/86297
7. Fuchs EJ, Matzinger P. Is cancer dangerous to the immune system? *Semin Immunol* (1996) **8**:271–80. doi:10.1006/smim.1996.0035
8. Willimsky G, Blankenstein T. Sporadic immunogenic tumours avoid destruction by inducing T-cell tolerance. *Nature* (2005) **437**:141–6. doi:10.1038/nature03954
9. Balkwill F, Mantovani A. Inflammation and cancer: back to Virchow? *Lancet* (2001) **357**:539–45. doi:10.1016/S0140-6736(00)04046-0
10. Mantovani A, Allavena P, Sica A, Balkwill F. Cancer-related inflammation. *Nature* (2008) **454**:436–44. doi:10.1038/nature07205
11. Gatti RA, Good RA. Occurrence of malignancy in immunodeficiency diseases. A literature review. *Cancer* (1971) **28**:89–98. doi:10.1002/1097-0142(197107)28:1<89::AID-CNCR2820280117>3.0.CO;2-Q
12. Kinlen LJ, Webster AD, Bird AG, Haile R, Peto J, Soothill JF, et al. Prospective study of cancer in patients with hypogammaglobulinemia. *Lancet* (1985) **1**:263–6. doi:10.1016/S0140-6736(85)91037-2
13. Salavoura K, Kolialexi A, Tsangaris G, Mavrou A. Development of cancer in patients with primary immunodeficiencies. *Anticancer Res* (2008) **28**:1263–9.
14. van der Meer JW, Weening RS, Schellekens PT, van Munster IP, Nagengast FM. Colorectal cancer in patients with X-linked agammaglobulinemia. *Lancet* (1993) **341**:1439–40. doi:10.1016/0140-6736(93)90883-I

15. Mueller BU, Pizzo PA. Cancer in children with primary or secondary immunodeficiencies. *J Pediatr* (1995) **126**:1–10. doi:10.1016/S0022-3476(95)70491-4
16. Hayward AR, Levy J, Facchetti F, Notarangelo L, Ochs HD, Etzioni A, et al. Cholangiopathy and tumors of the pancreas, liver, and biliary tree in boys with X-linked immunodeficiency with hyper-IgM. *J Immunol* (1997) **158**:977–83.
17. Swann JB, Smyth MJ. Immune surveillance of tumors. *J Clin Invest* (2007) **117**:1137–46. doi:10.1172/JCI31405
18. Shankaran V, Ikeda H, Bruce AT, White JM, Swanson PE, Old LJ, et al. IFN gamma and lymphocytes prevent primary tumour development and shape tumour immunogenicity. *Nature* (2001) **410**:1107–11. doi:10.1038/35074122
19. Girardi M, Oppenheim DE, Steele CR, Lewis JM, Glusac E, Filler R, et al. Regulation of cutaneous malignancy by gammadelta T cells. *Science* (2001) **294**:605–9. doi:10.1126/science.1063916
20. Dunn GP, Bruce AT, Sheehan KC, Shankaran V, Uppaluri R, Bui JD, et al. A critical function for type I interferons in cancer immunoediting. *Nat Immunol* (2005) **6**:722–9. doi:10.1038/ni1213
21. Kaplan DH, Shankaran V, Dighe AS, Stockert E, Aguet M, Old LJ, et al. Demonstration of an interferon gamma-dependent tumor surveillance system in immunocompetent mice. *Proc Natl Acad Sci U S A* (1998) **95**:7556–61. doi:10.1073/pnas.95.13.7556
22. Street SE, Trapani JA, MacGregor D, Smyth MJ. Suppression of lymphoma and epithelial malignancies effected by interferon gamma. *J Exp Med* (2002) **196**:129–34. doi:10.1084/jem.20020063
23. Smyth MJ, Thia KY, Street SE, MacGregor D, Godfrey DI, Trapani JA. Perforin-mediated cytotoxicity is critical for surveillance of spontaneous lymphoma. *J Exp Med* (2000) **192**:755–60. doi:10.1084/jem.192.5.755
24. Calne RY, White DJ, Thiru S, Evans DB, McMaster P, Dunn DC, et al. Cyclosporin A in patients receiving renal allografts from cadaver donors. *Lancet* (1978) **2**:1323–7. doi:10.1016/S0140-6736(78)91970-0
25. Hoover R, Fraumeni JF Jr. Risk of cancer in renal-transplant recipients. *Lancet* (1973) **2**:55–7. doi:10.1016/S0140-6736(73)93256-X
26. Birkeland SA, Storm HH, Lamm LU, Barlow L, Blohme I, Forsberg B, et al. Cancer risk after renal transplantation in the Nordic countries, 1964-1986. *Int J Cancer* (1995) **60**:183–9. doi:10.1002/ijc.2910600209
27. Opelz G, Dohler B. Lymphomas after solid organ transplantation: a collaborative transplant study report. *Am J Transplant* (2004) **4**:222–30. doi:10.1111/j.1600-6143.2004.00451.x
28. List AF, Greco FA, Vogler LB. Lymphoproliferative diseases in immunocompromised hosts: the role of Epstein-Barr virus. *J Clin Oncol* (1987) **5**: 1673–89.
29. Leblond V, Davi F, Charlotte F, Dorent R, Bitker MO, Sutton L, et al. Posttransplant lymphoproliferative disorders not associated with Epstein-Barr virus: a distinct entity? *J Clin Oncol* (1998) **16**:2052–9.
30. Engels EA, Pfeiffer RM, Fraumeni JF Jr, Kasiske BL, Israni AK, Snyder JJ, et al. Spectrum of cancer risk among US solid organ transplant recipients. *JAMA* (2011) **306**:1891–901. doi:10.1001/jama.2011.1592
31. Bouwes Bavinck JN, Hardie DR, Green A, Cutmore S, MacNaught A, O'Sullivan B, et al. The risk of skin cancer in renal transplant recipients in Queensland, Australia. A follow-up study. *Transplantation* (1996) **61**:715–21. doi:10.1097/00007890-199603150-00008
32. Krynitz B, Edgren G, Lindelof B, Baecklund E, Brattstrom C, Wilczek H, et al. Risk of skin cancer and other malignancies in kidney, liver, heart and lung transplant recipients 1970 to 2008 – a Swedish population-based study. *Int J Cancer* (2013) **132**:1429–38. doi:10.1002/ijc.27765
33. Ramsay HM, Fryer AA, Hawley CM, Smith AG, Harden PN. Non-melanoma skin cancer risk in the Queensland renal transplant population. *Br J Dermatol* (2002) **147**:950–6. doi:10.1046/j.1365-2133.2002.04976.x
34. Schulz TF. Cancer and viral infections in immunocompromised individuals. *Int J Cancer* (2009) **125**:1755–63. doi:10.1002/ijc.24741
35. Clifford GM, Polesel J, Rickenbach M, Dal Maso L, Keiser O, Kofler A, et al. Cancer risk in the Swiss HIV Cohort Study: associations with immunodeficiency, smoking, and highly active antiretroviral therapy. *J Natl Cancer Inst* (2005) **97**:425–32. doi:10.1093/jnci/dji072
36. Shiels MS, Cole SR, Kirk GD, Poole C. A meta-analysis of the incidence of non-AIDS cancers in HIV-infected individuals. *J Acquir Immune Defic Syndr* (2009) **52**:611–22. doi:10.1097/QAI.0b013e3181b327ca
37. Sigel K, Wisnivesky J, Gordon K, Dubrow R, Justice A, Brown ST, et al. HIV as an independent risk factor for incident lung cancer. *AIDS* (2012) **26**:1017–25. doi:10.1097/QAD.0b013e328352d1ad
38. Guiguet M, Boue F, Cadranel J, Lang JM, Rosenthal E, Costagliola D. Effect of immunodeficiency, HIV viral load, and antiretroviral therapy on the risk of individual malignancies (FHDH-ANRS CO4): a Prospective Cohort Study. *Lancet Oncol* (2009) **10**:1152–9. doi:10.1016/S1470-2045(09)70282-7
39. Fridman WH, Pages F, Sautes-Fridman C, Galon J. The immune contexture in human tumours: impact on clinical outcome. *Nat Rev Cancer* (2012) **12**:298–306. doi:10.1038/nrc3245
40. Galon J, Costes A, Sanchez-Cabo F, Kirilovsky A, Mlecnik B, Lagorce-Pages C, et al. Type, density, and location of immune cells within human colorectal tumors predict clinical outcome. *Science* (2006) **313**:1960–4. doi:10.1126/science.1129139
41. Zhang L, Conejo-Garcia JR, Katsaros D, Gimotty PA, Massobrio M, Regnani G, et al. Intratumoral T cells, recurrence, and survival in epithelial ovarian cancer. *N Engl J Med* (2003) **348**:203–13. doi:10.1056/NEJMoa020177
42. Al-Shibli KI, Donnem T, Al-Saad S, Persson M, Bremnes RM, Busund LT. Prognostic effect of epithelial and stromal lymphocyte infiltration in non-small cell lung cancer. *Clin Cancer Res* (2008) **14**:5220–7. doi:10.1158/1078-0432.CCR-08-0133
43. Kawai O, Ishii G, Kubota K, Murata Y, Naito Y, Mizuno T, et al. Predominant infiltration of macrophages and CD8(+) T Cells in cancer nests is a significant predictor of survival in stage IV nonsmall cell lung cancer. *Cancer* (2008) **113**:1387–95. doi:10.1002/cncr.23712
44. Mahmoud SM, Paish EC, Powe DG, Macmillan RD, Grainge MJ, Lee AH, et al. Tumor-infiltrating CD8+ lymphocytes predict clinical outcome in breast cancer. *J Clin Oncol* (2011) **29**:1949–55. doi:10.1200/JCO.2010.30.5037
45. Naito Y, Saito K, Shiiba K, Ohuchi A, Saigenji K, Nagura H, et al. CD8+ T cells infiltrated within cancer cell nests as a prognostic factor in human colorectal cancer. *Cancer Res* (1998) **58**:3491–4.
46. Cho Y, Miyamoto M, Kato K, Fukunaga A, Shichinohe T, Kawarada Y, et al. CD4+ and CD8+ T cells cooperate to improve prognosis of patients with esophageal squamous cell carcinoma. *Cancer Res* (2003) **63**:1555–9.
47. Hiraoka K, Miyamoto M, Cho Y, Suzuoki M, Oshikiri T, Nakakubo Y, et al. Concurrent infiltration by CD8+ T cells and CD4+ T cells is a favourable prognostic factor in non-small-cell lung carcinoma. *Br J Cancer* (2006) **94**:275–80. doi:10.1038/sj.bjc.6602934
48. Budhu A, Forgues M, Ye QH, Jia HL, He P, Zanetti KA, et al. Prediction of venous metastases, recurrence, and prognosis in hepatocellular carcinoma based on a unique immune response signature of the liver microenvironment. *Cancer Cell* (2006) **10**:99–111. doi:10.1016/j.ccr.2006.06.016
49. Kristensen VN, Vaske CJ, Ursini-Siegel J, Van Loo P, Nordgard SH, Sachidanandam R, et al. Integrated molecular profiles of invasive breast tumors and ductal carcinoma in situ (DCIS) reveal differential vascular and interleukin signaling. *Proc Natl Acad Sci U S A* (2012) **109**:2802–7. doi:10.1073/pnas.1108781108
50. Rusakiewicz S, Semeraro M, Sarabi M, Desbois M, Locher C, Mendez R, et al. Immune infiltrates are prognostic factors in localized gastrointestinal stromal tumors. *Cancer Res* (2013) **73**:3499–510. doi:10.1158/0008-5472.CAN-13-0371
51. Forssell J, Oberg A, Henriksson ML, Stenling R, Jung A, Palmqvist R. High macrophage infiltration along the tumor front correlates with improved survival in colon cancer. *Clin Cancer Res* (2007) **13**:1472–9. doi:10.1158/1078-0432.CCR-06-2073
52. Kim DW, Min HS, Lee KH, Kim YJ, Oh DY, Jeon YK, et al. High tumour islet macrophage infiltration correlates with improved patient survival but not with EGFR mutations, gene copy number or protein expression in resected non-small cell lung cancer. *Br J Cancer* (2008) **98**:1118–24. doi:10.1038/sj.bjc.6604256
53. Shimura S, Yang G, Ebara S, Wheeler TM, Frolov A, Thompson TC. Reduced infiltration of tumor-associated macrophages in human prostate cancer: association with cancer progression. *Cancer Res* (2000) **60**:5857–61.
54. Welsh TJ, Green RH, Richardson D, Waller DA, O'Byrne KJ, Bradding P. Macrophage and mast-cell invasion of tumor cell islets confers a marked survival advantage in non-small-cell lung cancer. *J Clin Oncol* (2005) **23**:8959–67. doi:10.1200/JCO.2005.01.4910
55. Vogelstein B, Papadopoulos N, Velculescu VE, Zhou S, Diaz LA Jr, Kinzler KW. Cancer genome landscapes. *Science* (2013) **339**:1546–58. doi:10.1126/science.1235122
56. Jones S, Zhang X, Parsons DW, Lin JC, Leary RJ, Angenendt P, et al. Core signaling pathways in human pancreatic cancers revealed by global genomic analyses. *Science* (2008) **321**:1801–6. doi:10.1126/science.1164368

57. Parsons DW, Jones S, Zhang X, Lin JC, Leary RJ, Angenendt P, et al. An integrated genomic analysis of human glioblastoma multiforme. *Science* (2008) **321**:1807–12. doi:10.1126/science.1164382
58. Sjoblom T, Jones S, Wood LD, Parsons DW, Lin J, Barber TD, et al. The consensus coding sequences of human breast and colorectal cancers. *Science* (2006) **314**:268–74. doi:10.1126/science.1133427
59. Wood LD, Parsons DW, Jones S, Lin J, Sjoblom T, Leary RJ, et al. The genomic landscapes of human breast and colorectal cancers. *Science* (2007) **318**:1108–13. doi:10.1126/science.1145720
60. Govindan R, Ding L, Griffith M, Subramanian J, Dees ND, Kanchi KL, et al. Genomic landscape of non-small cell lung cancer in smokers and never-smokers. *Cell* (2012) **150**:1121–34. doi:10.1016/j.cell.2012.08.024
61. Wei X, Walia V, Lin JC, Teer JK, Prickett TD, Gartner J, et al. Exome sequencing identifies GRIN2A as frequently mutated in melanoma. *Nat Genet* (2011) **43**:442–6. doi:10.1038/ng.810
62. Wang RF, Wang X, Atwood AC, Topalian SL, Rosenberg SA. Cloning genes encoding MHC class II-restricted antigens: mutated CDC27 as a tumor antigen. *Science* (1999) **284**:1351–4. doi:10.1126/science.284.5418.1351
63. Wang RF, Wang X, Rosenberg SA. Identification of a novel major histocompatibility complex class II-restricted tumor antigen resulting from a chromosomal rearrangement recognized by CD4(+) T cells. *J Exp Med* (1999) **189**:1659–68. doi:10.1084/jem.189.10.1659
64. Saeterdal I, Bjorheim J, Lislerud K, Gjertsen MK, Bukholm IK, Olsen OC, et al. Frameshift-mutation-derived peptides as tumor-specific antigens in inherited and spontaneous colorectal cancer. *Proc Natl Acad Sci U S A* (2001) **98**:13255–60. doi:10.1073/pnas.231326898
65. Wolfel T, Hauer M, Schneider J, Serrano M, Wolfel C, Klehmann-Hieb E, et al. A p16INK4a-insensitive CDK4 mutant targeted by cytolytic T lymphocytes in a human melanoma. *Science* (1995) **269**:1281–4. doi:10.1126/science.7652577
66. Echchakir H, Mami-Chouaib F, Vergnon I, Baurain JF, Karanikas V, Chouaib S, et al. A point mutation in the alpha-actinin-4 gene generates an antigenic peptide recognized by autologous cytolytic T lymphocytes on a human lung carcinoma. *Cancer Res* (2001) **61**:4078–83.
67. Hogan KT, Eisinger DP, Cupp SB III, Lekstrom KJ, Deacon DD, Shabanowitz J, et al. The peptide recognized by HLA-A68.2-restricted, squamous cell carcinoma of the lung-specific cytotoxic T lymphocytes is derived from a mutated elongation factor 2 gene. *Cancer Res* (1998) **58**:5144–50.
68. Karanikas V, Colau D, Baurain JF, Chiari R, Thonnard J, Gutierrez-Roelens I, et al. High frequency of cytolytic T lymphocytes directed against a tumor-specific mutated antigen detectable with HLA tetramers in the blood of a lung carcinoma patient with long survival. *Cancer Res* (2001) **61**: 3718–24.
69. Clark RE, Dodi IA, Hill SC, Lill JR, Aubert G, Macintyre AR, et al. Direct evidence that leukemic cells present HLA-associated immunogenic peptides derived from the BCR-ABL b3a2 fusion protein. *Blood* (2001) **98**:2887–93. doi:10.1182/blood.V98.10.2887
70. Sahin U, Tureci O, Schmitt H, Cochlovius B, Johannes T, Schmits R, et al. Human neoplasms elicit multiple specific immune responses in the autologous host. *Proc Natl Acad Sci U S A* (1995) **92**:11810–3. doi:10.1073/pnas.92.25.11810
71. Scanlan MJ, Chen YT, Williamson B, Gure AO, Stockert E, Gordan JD, et al. Characterization of human colon cancer antigens recognized by autologous antibodies. *Int J Cancer* (1998) **76**:652–8. doi:10.1002/(SICI)1097-0215(19980529)76:5<652::AID-IJC7>3.3.CO;2-9
72. Garrido F, Ruiz-Cabello F, Cabrera T, Perez-Villar JJ, Lopez-Botet M, Duggan-Keen M, et al. Implications for immunosurveillance of altered HLA class I phenotypes in human tumours. *Immunol Today* (1997) **18**:89–95. doi:10.1016/S0167-5699(96)10075-X
73. D'Urso CM, Wang ZG, Cao Y, Tatake R, Zeff RA, Ferrone S. Lack of HLA class I antigen expression by cultured melanoma cells FO-1 due to a defect in B2m gene expression. *J Clin Invest* (1991) **87**:284–92. doi:10.1172/JCI114984
74. Perez B, Benitez R, Fernandez MA, Oliva MR, Soto JL, Serrano S, et al. A new beta 2 microglobulin mutation found in a melanoma tumor cell line. *Tissue Antigens* (1999) **53**:569–72. doi:10.1034/j.1399-0039.1999.530607.x
75. Jimenez P, Canton J, Collado A, Cabrera T, Serrano A, Real LM, et al. Chromosome loss is the most frequent mechanism contributing to HLA haplotype loss in human tumors. *Int J Cancer* (1999) **83**:91–7. doi:10.1002/(SICI)1097-0215(19990924)83:1<91::AID-IJC17>3.0.CO;2-4
76. Lawrence MS, Stojanov P, Mermel CH, Robinson JT, Garraway LA, Golub TR, et al. Discovery and saturation analysis of cancer genes across 21 tumour types. *Nature* (2014) **505**:495–501. doi:10.1038/nature12912
77. Lippitz BE. Cytokine patterns in patients with cancer: a systematic review. *Lancet Oncol* (2013) **14**:e218–28. doi:10.1016/S1470-2045(12)70582-X
78. Principe DR, Doll JA, Bauer J, Jung B, Munshi HG, Bartholin L, et al. TGF-beta: duality of function between tumor prevention and carcinogenesis. *J Natl Cancer Inst* (2014) **106**:djt369. doi:10.1093/jnci/djt369
79. Dunn GP, Bruce AT, Ikeda H, Old LJ, Schreiber RD. Cancer immunoediting: from immunosurveillance to tumor escape. *Nat Immunol* (2002) **3**:991–8. doi:10.1038/ni1102-991
80. Bauer S, Groh V, Wu J, Steinle A, Phillips JH, Lanier LL, et al. Activation of NK cells and T cells by NKG2D, a receptor for stress-inducible MICA. *Science* (1999) **285**:727–9. doi:10.1126/science.285.5428.727
81. Groh V, Bahram S, Bauer S, Herman A, Beauchamp M, Spies T. Cell stress-regulated human major histocompatibility complex class I gene expressed in gastrointestinal epithelium. *Proc Natl Acad Sci U S A* (1996) **93**:12445–50. doi:10.1073/pnas.93.22.12445
82. Raulet DH, Gasser S, Gowen BG, Deng W, Jung H. Regulation of ligands for the NKG2D activating receptor. *Annu Rev Immunol* (2013) **31**:413–41. doi:10.1146/annurev-immunol-032712-095951
83. Shafi S, Vantourout P, Wallace G, Antoun A, Vaughan R, Stanford M, et al. An NKG2D-mediated human lymphoid stress surveillance response with high interindividual variation. *Sci Transl Med* (2011) **3**:113ra124. doi:10.1126/scitranslmed.3002922
84. Gasser S, Orsulic S, Brown EJ, Raulet DH. The DNA damage pathway regulates innate immune system ligands of the NKG2D receptor. *Nature* (2005) **436**:1186–90. doi:10.1038/nature03884
85. Boissel N, Rea D, Tieng V, Dulphy N, Brun M, Cayuela JM, et al. BCR/ABL oncogene directly controls MHC class I chain-related molecule A expression in chronic myelogenous leukemia. *J Immunol* (2006) **176**:5108–16. doi:10.4049/jimmunol.176.8.5108
86. Liu XV, Ho SS, Tan JJ, Kamran N, Gasser S. Ras activation induces expression of Raet1 family NK receptor ligands. *J Immunol* (2012) **189**:1826–34. doi:10.4049/jimmunol.1200965
87. Vantourout P, Willcox C, Turner A, Swanson CM, Haque Y, Sobolev O, et al. Immunological visibility: posttranscriptional regulation of human NKG2D ligands by the EGF receptor pathway. *Sci Transl Med* (2014) **6**:231ra249. doi:10.1126/scitranslmed.3007579
88. Jung H, Hsiung B, Pestal K, Procyk E, Raulet DH. RAE-1 ligands for the NKG2D receptor are regulated by E2F transcription factors, which control cell cycle entry. *J Exp Med* (2012) **209**:2409–22. doi:10.1084/jem.20120565
89. Groh V, Rhinehart R, Secrist H, Bauer S, Grabstein KH, Spies T. Broad tumor-associated expression and recognition by tumor-derived gamma delta T cells of MICA and MICB. *Proc Natl Acad Sci U S A* (1999) **96**:6879–84. doi:10.1073/pnas.96.12.6879
90. Jinushi M, Takehara T, Tatsumi T, Kanto T, Groh V, Spies T, et al. Expression and role of MICA and MICB in human hepatocellular carcinomas and their regulation by retinoic acid. *Int J Cancer* (2003) **104**:354–61. doi:10.1002/ijc.10966
91. Cerwenka A, Baron JL, Lanier LL. Ectopic expression of retinoic acid early inducible-1 gene (RAE-1) permits natural killer cell-mediated rejection of a MHC class I-bearing tumor in vivo. *Proc Natl Acad Sci U S A* (2001) **98**:11521–6. doi:10.1073/pnas.201238598
92. Diefenbach A, Jensen ER, Jamieson AM, Raulet DH. RAE1 and H60 ligands of the NKG2D receptor stimulate tumour immunity. *Nature* (2001) **413**:165–71. doi:10.1038/35093109
93. Smyth MJ, Swann J, Cretney E, Zerafa N, Yokoyama WM, Hayakawa Y. NKG2D function protects the host from tumor initiation. *J Exp Med* (2005) **202**:583–8. doi:10.1084/jem.20050994
94. Guerra N, Tan YX, Joncker NT, Choy A, Gallardo F, Xiong N, et al. NKG2D-deficient mice are defective in tumor surveillance in models of spontaneous malignancy. *Immunity* (2008) **28**:571–80. doi:10.1016/j.immuni.2008.02.016
95. Chen D, Juko-Pecirep I, Hammer J, Ivansson E, Enroth S, Gustavsson I, et al. Genome-wide association study of susceptibility loci for cervical cancer. *J Natl Cancer Inst* (2013) **105**:624–33. doi:10.1093/jnci/djt051
96. Melum E, Karlsen TH, Schrumpf E, Bergquist A, Thorsby E, Boberg KM, et al. Cholangiocarcinoma in primary sclerosing cholangitis

is associated with NKG2D polymorphisms. *Hepatology* (2008) **47**:90–6. doi:10.1002/hep.21964

97. Couzin-Frankel J. Breakthrough of the year 2013. Cancer immunotherapy. *Science* (2013) **342**:1432–3. doi:10.1126/science.342.6165.1432
98. Hodi FS, O'Day SJ, McDermott DF, Weber RW, Sosman JA, Haanen JB, et al. Improved survival with ipilimumab in patients with metastatic melanoma. *N Engl J Med* (2010) **363**:711–23. doi:10.1056/NEJMoa1003466
99. Robert C, Thomas L, Bondarenko I, O'Day S, Weber J, Garbe C, et al. Ipilimumab plus dacarbazine for previously untreated metastatic melanoma. *N Engl J Med* (2011) **364**:2517–26. doi:10.1056/NEJMoa1104621
100. Topalian SL, Hodi FS, Brahmer JR, Gettinger SN, Smith DC, McDermott DF, et al. Safety, activity, and immune correlates of anti-PD-1 antibody in cancer. *N Engl J Med* (2012) **366**:2443–54. doi:10.1056/NEJMoa1200690
101. Brahmer JR, Tykodi SS, Chow LQ, Hwu WJ, Topalian SL, Hwu P, et al. Safety and activity of anti-PD-L1 antibody in patients with advanced cancer. *N Engl J Med* (2012) **366**:2455–65. doi:10.1056/NEJMoa1200694
102. Wolchok JD, Kluger H, Callahan MK, Postow MA, Rizvi NA, Lesokhin AM, et al. Nivolumab plus ipilimumab in advanced melanoma. *N Engl J Med* (2013) **369**:122–33. doi:10.1056/NEJMoa1302369
103. Joseph CG, Darrah E, Shah AA, Skora AD, Casciola-Rosen LA, Wigley FM, et al. Association of the autoimmune disease scleroderma with an immunologic response to cancer. *Science* (2014) **343**:152–7. doi:10.1126/science.1246886

10

Mathematical model of naive T cell division and survival IL-7 thresholds

Joseph Reynolds[1], Mark Coles[2], Grant Lythe[1] and Carmen Molina-París[1]*

[1] *Department of Applied Mathematics, School of Mathematics, University of Leeds, Leeds, UK*
[2] *Centre for Immunology and Infection, University of York, York, UK*

Edited by:
Miles Davenport, University of New South Wales, Australia

Reviewed by:
Edward John Collins, The University of North Carolina at Chapel Hill, USA
Christian Schönbach, Nazarbayev University, Kazakhstan
Robin Callard, University College London, UK

****Correspondence:***
Carmen Molina-París, Department of Applied Mathematics, School of Mathematics, University of Leeds, Leeds LS2 9JT, UK
e-mail: carmen@maths.leeds.ac.uk

We develop a mathematical model of the peripheral naive T cell population to study the change in human naive T cell numbers from birth to adulthood, incorporating thymic output and the availability of interleukin-7 (IL-7). The model is formulated as three ordinary differential equations: two describe T cell numbers, in a resting state and progressing through the cell cycle. The third is introduced to describe changes in IL-7 availability. Thymic output is a decreasing function of time, representative of the thymic atrophy observed in aging humans. Each T cell is assumed to possess two interleukin-7 receptor (IL-7R) signaling thresholds: a survival threshold and a second, higher, proliferation threshold. If the IL-7R signaling strength is below its survival threshold, a cell may undergo apoptosis. When the signaling strength is above the survival threshold, but below the proliferation threshold, the cell survives but does not divide. Signaling strength above the proliferation threshold enables entry into cell cycle. Assuming that individual cell thresholds are log-normally distributed, we derive population-average rates for apoptosis and entry into cell cycle. We have analyzed the adiabatic change in homeostasis as thymic output decreases. With a parameter set representative of a healthy individual, the model predicts a unique equilibrium number of T cells. In a parameter range representative of persistent viral or bacterial infection, where naive T cell cycle progression is impaired, a decrease in thymic output may result in the collapse of the naive T cell repertoire.

Keywords: IL-7, T cell, homeostasis, threshold, IL-7R, mathematical model, thymic output

1. INTRODUCTION

The number of naive T cells in the periphery is determined by a balance between cell loss (death or differentiation) and cell renewal due to cell division and thymic export (1, 2). In humans, at least, the decline in thymic export occurs mainly in childhood, from about a year of age until 20 years of age, when the number of naive T cells is increasing (3). In adults, the decline in thymic export is much less pronounced but the number of naive T cells is, more or less, constant (4). Survival of the naive T cell population in the periphery depends on both common gamma chain cytokines and weak "tonic" signals induced by recognition of self-peptides by the T cell receptor (TCR) (5, 6). IL-7 is required for the homeostatic expansion of naive $CD8^+$ and $CD4^+$ T cells in lymphopenic hosts, while naive T cells disappear over a 1-month period upon adoptive transfer into IL-7 deficient (IL-7^-) hosts (7–9).

Signals from recognition of self-peptides bound to major histocompatibility complex (sp-MHC), and IL-7, promote cell survival. Naive T cell survival is impaired when removing access to one of these signals (10–14). Of interest are the mechanisms by which these signals are regulated, and that result in a stable number of naive T cells throughout the lifetimes of mice and humans. In this paper, we focus on IL-7 as a master regulator of naive T cell survival (15). IL-7 is produced by stromal cells in tissues, including fibroblastic reticular cells, marginal reticular cells, and lymphatic endothelial cells (16). These cells produce very small amounts of IL-7 messenger RNA, consistent with IL-7 protein levels limiting T cell expansion. IL-7 is a heparin-sulfate binding protein, and as such, it will bind extra-cellular matrix surrounding stromal cells. Thus, the interaction between naive T cells and stroma controls their homeostasis (17). Recognition of higher affinity, non-self-peptides by the T cell receptor induces naive T cells to undergo an alternative, IL-7 independent, survival program dependent on IL-2 (18). ^{1}),

Naive $CD8^+$ T cell responses depend on the amount of IL-7 cells are exposed to (19). At low IL-7 concentrations ($<10^{-2}$ ng ml^{-}) cell viability was impaired; at higher concentrations (>1 ng ml^{-} cells were observed to proliferate in response to IL-7. This difference might arise from changes in the strength of the IL-7R induced signal the cell receives. For an individual cell, IL-7R induced signaling must be greater than some threshold to prevent the accumulation of pro-apoptotic proteins. Similarly, IL-7R signaling must be greater than a second, higher, threshold to induce cell division. Heterogeneity at the single cell level in IL-7 signaling thresholds (a property reported to depend on expression of IL-7R), resulted in differential survival and division (19). Although these observations are based on two different $CD8^+$ T cell receptor transgenic mice, it is assumed that the key principles regarding T cell survival will be found in the repertoire of naive $CD4^+$ and $CD8^+$ T cells.

We introduce a deterministic mathematical model of the naive T cell population to study the change in human naive T cell numbers from birth to adulthood. We will assume cell survival depends on the availability of IL-7. We do not include availability of sp-MHC as a variable within the model, but assume sp-MHC availability is sufficient to allow cell survival and proliferation, in conjunction with sufficient IL-7 stimulus. We also make the approximation that heterogeneity is constant with changes in age. For a mathematical study of the impact sp-MHC availability has on clonal diversity, the reader is referred to Stirk et al. (20, 21). Our model is a mathematical description of the homeostasis of the naive T cell repertoire, but does not consider stimulation by foreign antigens.

2. MATERIALS AND METHODS

2.1. A MATHEMATICAL DESCRIPTION OF THE SIZE OF THE PERIPHERAL NAIVE T CELL POPULATION

Stochastic processes provide a method of treating each cell as a distinct, countable object, and permit a more realistic model than a deterministic characterization. Fluctuations in the number of cells can be considered but, in a non-linear stochastic model, approximations are often made to facilitate the analysis. In the linear noise approximation (22), for example, fluctuations are assumed to be of order $\Omega^{\frac{1}{2}}$ for a system of size Ω. The human peripheral T cell compartment is estimated to contain of the order of 10^{11} T cells (3). Letting the system size be the average number of naive T cells in humans, we find $\mathcal{O}(\Omega) = 10^{11}$ cells, and correspondingly, fluctuations are expected to be typically $10^5 - 10^6$ cells in magnitude. That is, we expect fluctuations of approximately 0.001% in the size of the human naive T cell pool due to stochasticity in the per cell division and death rates. Based on these considerations, adopting a deterministic approach to describe the total human peripheral naive T cell population is reasonable.

We assume peripheral naive T cells are either in a resting state, or proceeding through the cell cycle. The deterministic variables $R(t)$ and $C(t)$ are introduced to model the total number of T cells in the resting and cycling states, respectively. The variable $I(t)$ is introduced to model the concentration of IL-7. The deterministic approach we take does not consider any notion of space. Indeed, this approach is tantamount to assuming the resource, IL-7, is shared equally amongst all cells. Competition for the resource is introduced only so far as each cell acts to reduce the global concentration of the resource. Resting cells may receive a signal which induces them to proceed through one round of division. Upon completion of the cell cycle, a cycling cell produces two daughter cells in the resting compartment. Resting cells are assumed to die if the IL-7 induced survival signal is insufficient; cells may also die during cell cycle. The input of cells from the thymus into the resting compartment, in keeping with observations in humans, is a decreasing function of time (23, 24). Production of IL-7 is related to the size of the lymphatic system architecture, which we estimate from the body mass of an individual. In the absence of T cells, IL-7 is assumed to be degraded and/or consumed by other cell types at a constant rate. Upon signal induction through the IL-7 receptor, IL-7 is assumed to be consumed by the T cell. A diagrammatic representation of the model is given in **Figure 1**.

2.2. IL-7 SIGNALING AND HETEROGENEITY IN IL-7 THRESHOLDS

In the model, IL-7 signaling is assumed to be uniform across the population. Yet, we introduce heterogeneity in the signaling thresholds for survival and proliferation. Let $S(t)$ be the average signaling strength across the naive T cell population. Each cell experiences the same strength of signaling for a given concentration of IL-7, $I(t)$. We relate the internal signaling to the concentration of IL-7 by the equation

$$S(t) = \frac{600I(t)}{0.025 + I(t)}. \quad (1)$$

The functional form and constants of this relationship are derived from the study of IL-7 receptor dynamics summarized in the Appendix. We assume each individual cell possesses a unique pair of thresholds for survival and proliferation. Furthermore, we assume, in the continuous limit, that these thresholds are distributed log-normally across the entire population of cells. The use of log-normal distributions guarantees, first of all, that all signaling thresholds are positive real numbers. Secondly, the log-normal distribution ensures that no cell can survive or divide independently of IL-7.

Let the random variable Θ_s represent the survival threshold, and let Θ_p represent the proliferation threshold. We write

$$\Theta_s \sim \log\mathcal{N}\left(\log\theta_s, \frac{1}{2\alpha^2}\right), \quad \Theta_p \sim \log\mathcal{N}\left(\log\theta_p, \frac{1}{2\alpha^2}\right), \quad \alpha \in \mathbb{R}^+. \quad (2)$$

The respective probability density functions are

$$p_{\Theta_x}(\theta) = \frac{\alpha}{\sqrt{\pi}\theta}\exp\left[-\left(\alpha\left(\log\theta - \log\theta_x\right)\right)^2\right], \quad x = s, p. \quad (3)$$

Estimates for θ_s and θ_p are obtained from the model summarized in the Appendix. Lauffenburger et al. found a significant change in cell viability for both OT-1 and F-5 T cells at around $10^{-2.5}$ ng ml^{-1} IL-7 (19). Proliferation of OT-1 cells occurred above 1 ng ml^{-1} IL-7. We estimate the equilibrium signaling at these concentrations as 60 and 600 units, respectively, setting $\theta_s = 60$ and $\theta_p = 600$. Modeling heterogeneity in IL-7 responses by assuming heterogeneity in the IL-7 signaling thresholds, allows us to avoid modeling the naive population using either: (i) a PDE

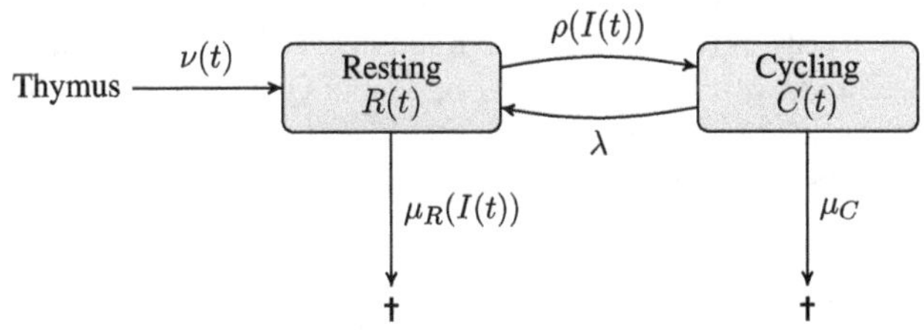

FIGURE 1 | Diagrammatic illustration of the deterministic model. T cells leaving the thymus enter the resting naive peripheral pool. Cells in either a resting or cycling state may die. The rate of death from the resting state depends on the availability of the resource (IL-7), whereas the death rate for cycling cells is constant. Resting cells enter the cell cycle at a rate that depends on the availability of the resource (IL-7). Cycling cells produce two daughter cells in the resting state upon completion of the cell cycle.

approach, where heterogeneity is continuous across the population of cells, or (ii) describing each subset of cells sharing common thresholds with its unique governing set of ODEs. However, these approaches present an obvious avenue for further research beyond the scope of this paper.

2.2.1. Death rate of resting cells

Suppose each T cell in the naive population is a distinct member possessing a unique signaling threshold for survival. As in the previous section, we assume these signaling thresholds are distributed log-normally (in the continuous limit). We suppose the death rate of an individual cell is Boolean, in the sense that if the global signaling strength is greater than the cell's individual survival threshold, then the cell can survive indefinitely. Similarly, if the signaling strength is below the survival threshold, the cell will undergo apoptosis at a rate μ_R. The death rate for cell i with survival threshold $\theta_s^{(i)}$, is given by

$$f_s\left(S(t), \theta_s^{(i)}\right) = \begin{cases} \mu_R & \text{if } S(t) < \theta_s^{(i)}, \\ 0 & \text{if } S(t) \geq \theta_s^{(i)}. \end{cases} \tag{4}$$

In the continuous limit (assuming signaling thresholds are distributed log-normally), the average death rate for the population of naive T cells is given by

$$\begin{aligned} \bar{\mu}_R(S(t)) &= \int_0^\infty f_s(S(t), \theta)\, p_{\Theta_s}(\theta)\, d\theta = \int_{S(t)}^\infty \mu_R p_{\Theta_s}(\theta)\, d\theta, \\ &= \frac{1}{2}\mu_R\left[1 - \operatorname{erf}\left(\alpha\left(\log S(t) - \log\theta_s\right)\right)\right], \end{aligned} \tag{5}$$

where $p_{\Theta_s}(\theta)$ is the probability density function of the random variable Θ_s, defined by equation (3) with $x = s$.

2.2.2. Rate of entry into cell cycle

Analogous to Section 2.2.1, we assume each T cell in the naive population is a distinct member possessing a unique signaling threshold for proliferation. We let the individual rate of entry into cell cycle be given by

$$f_p\left(S(t), \theta_p^{(i)}\right) = \begin{cases} 0 & \text{if } S(t) < \theta_p^{(i)}, \\ \rho & \text{if } S(t) \geq \theta_p^{(i)}. \end{cases} \tag{6}$$

Assume, in the continuous limit, the signaling threshold for entry into the cell cycle is represented by the random variable Θ_p, defined in equation (2), with probability density function $p_{\Theta_p}(\theta)$ (equation (3), $x = p$). The average rate of entry into cell cycle is given by

$$\begin{aligned} \bar{\rho}(S(t)) &= \int_0^\infty f_p(S(t), \theta)\, p_{\Theta_p}(\theta)\, d\theta = \int_0^{S(t)} \rho p_{\Theta_p}(\theta)\, d\theta, \\ &= \frac{1}{2}\rho\left[1 + \operatorname{erf}\left(\alpha\left(\log S(t) - \log\theta_p\right)\right)\right]. \end{aligned} \tag{7}$$

2.2.3. Cell cycle progression

Cycling cells take on average λ^{-1} days to complete the cell cycle. After a cell divides, both daughter cells are produced in the resting state and require a second signal before they can progress through another round of cell division. Cell cycle may be interrupted resulting in the death of the cell. Such death events occur at a rate μ_C.

2.2.4. Thymic export

We assume thymic output to be a decreasing function of time. In particular, we use the functional form given by Bains et al. (3). Let us introduce the thymic output function, $\nu(t)$, as follows

$$\begin{aligned} \nu(t) = {} & 2.32 \times 10^8 \exp\left(-1.1 \times 10^4 t\right) \\ & + 1.15 \times 10^8 \exp\left(-1.6 \times 10^7 t^2\right), \end{aligned} \tag{8}$$

where t corresponds to the age of the individual, measured in days. A plot of this function is shown in the left panel of **Figure 2**. The function was chosen by Bains et al. to describe the rate of thymic export of $CD4^+$ T cells. We use the same function to describe the export rate of all naive T cells ($CD4^+$ or $CD8^+$ T cells). This approximation is justified since we require the absolute cell count to roughly approximate the cell count observed in humans (indeed, such an observation is likely subject to large differences). Of interest later in the paper is the relative variation of cell numbers with different choices of parameter values. For our purposes, the important feature of $\nu(t)$ is that it is a decreasing function of time.

2.2.5. Internalization of IL-7

We use the model summarized in the Appendix to estimate the rate of IL-7 internalization. The total number of IL-7 molecules internalized by a single T cell in 1 day, exposed to IL-7 at concentration I ng ml^{-1}, is described by the function

$$\frac{6.7I(t)}{2 + I(t)}\left(3 + \frac{5}{I(t) + 3 \times 10^{-2}}\right) \times 10^3 \text{ cell}^{-1} \text{ day}^{-1}. \tag{9}$$

It is reported IL-7 has a molecular mass of 17 kDa ($\approx 2.8 \times 10^{-11}$ ng) (25). Based on this, we define the per cell rate of IL-7 internalization to be

$$\frac{2I(t)}{2 + I(t)}\left(3 + \frac{5}{I(t) + 3 \times 10^{-2}}\right) \times 10^{-7} \text{ ng day}^{-1} \text{ cell}^{-1}.$$

In order to convert the rate of change of mass to the rate of change of concentration, we must choose a volume for the system. Naive T cells are typically found in the lymph nodes, spleen, and gut of the human body. We shall make the rough estimation that the total volume is of the order of 1 l. This implies the rate of IL-7 internalization by all naive T cells in the population is given by

$$\begin{aligned} \gamma(I(t))\, R(t) = {} & \frac{2I(t)}{2 + I(t)}\left(3 + \frac{5}{I(t) + 3 \times 10^{-2}}\right) \\ & \times 10^{-10} R(t) \text{ ng ml}^{-1} \text{ day}^{-1}, \end{aligned} \tag{10}$$

where $R(t)$ is the number of resting naive T cells. The IL-7 internalization rate, $\gamma(I(t))$, is shown in the middle panel of **Figure 2**.

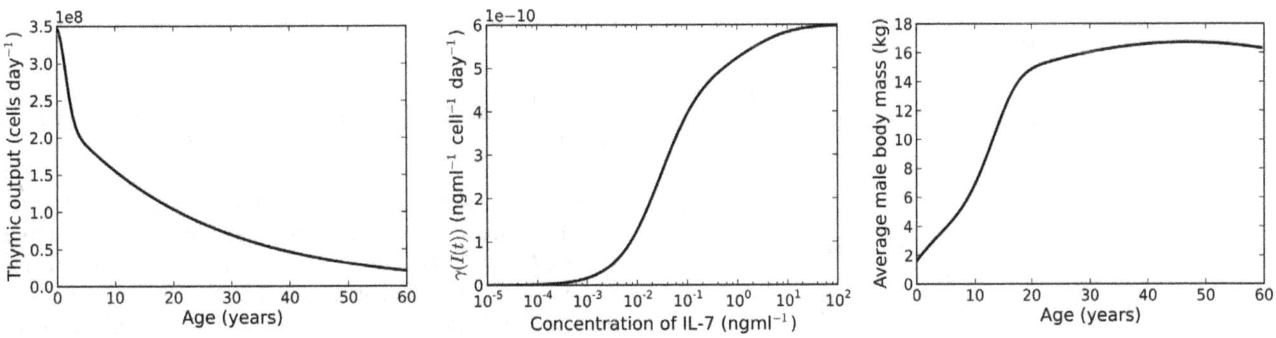

FIGURE 2 | Left panel: rate of thymic export. Plot of equation (8). Middle panel: IL-7 internalization rate. Plot of the function $\gamma(I(t))$. Right panel: plot of the function $m(s)$ (equation (11)), a model for the average body mass of male individuals.

2.2.6. *Production of IL-7*

We assume the rate of IL-7 production is proportional (with proportionality constant $\hat{\beta}$) to the body mass of an individual. To estimate average body mass we use the model given by Burmaster and Crouch (26). The explicit relationship between mass and age is given by the function $m(s)$ as follows

$$m(s) = \exp\left[4.1 + 1.4 \times 10^{-2}s - 1.5 \times 10^{-4}s^2 - 2.0\exp\left[-s\left(0.15 - 1.4 \times 10^{-2}s + 9.8 \times 10^{-4}s^2\right)\right]\right], \tag{11}$$

where s is age measured in years. A plot of this function is given in the right panel of **Figure 2**. The rate of IL-7 production is given by the function

$$\beta(t) = \hat{\beta} m(365t), \tag{12}$$

where t denotes age as measured in days.

2.2.7. *Intra-cellular degradation of IL-7*

We assume IL-7 is degraded and internalized by other cell types at a constant rate. We let the degradation rate of IL-7 be denoted by the parameter δ.

2.2.8. *Deterministic mathematical model*

From the above assumptions, the system of differential equations governing the behavior of the naive T cells (resting and cycling) and the concentration of IL-7 is given by

$$\frac{dI(t)}{dt} = \beta(t) - \gamma(I(t))R(t) - \delta I(t), \tag{13}$$

$$\frac{dR(t)}{dt} = \nu(t) - \left[\bar{\rho}(S(t)) + \bar{\mu}_R(S(t))\right]R(t) + 2\lambda C(t), \tag{14}$$

$$\frac{dC(t)}{dt} = \bar{\rho}(S(t))R(t) - (\mu_C + \lambda)C(t). \tag{15}$$

This system is subject to the initial conditions I_0, R_0, and C_0.

3. RESULTS

3.1. PARAMETER ESTIMATES

The function describing the rate of internalization of IL-7, equation (10), and the signaling relation, equation (1), were both estimated from our studies of IL-7 receptor dynamics in naive T cells (summarized in the Appendix). In the same study we have estimated the average signaling thresholds to be, respectively, $\theta_s = 60$ and $\theta_p = 600$. Our estimate for θ_p was found to be close ($\theta_p \approx 585$, which we have rounded to 600) to the limit of the signaling function equation (1), as $I(t) \to +\infty$. These estimates imply that, on average, approximately half of the naive T cell population does not proliferate in response to excess IL-7 when receptor dynamics is in equilibrium. Such a finding is consistent with the observations made by Lauffenburger et al. in the experiments described in Ref. (19). In these experiments, F-5 T cells did not proliferate (whereas OT-1 cells did proliferate), even in excess amounts of IL-7. Estimates for the IL-7 average signaling thresholds, θ_s and θ_p, have been based on OT-1 cells. However, we note that changes to these thresholds only result in quantitative differences, provided $\theta_s < \theta_p$.

We assume cycling naive T cells take 12 h to complete the cell cycle and produce two daughter cells ($\lambda^{-1} = 0.5$ day). Resting naive T cells are assumed to die after 2 days of IL-7 starvation ($\mu_R^{-1} = 2$ day). We, furthermore, set the rate of entry into cell cycle to be $\rho = 5\,\text{day}^{-1}$. Cycling cells are assumed to die at rate $\mu_C = 1\,\text{day}^{-1}$ in healthy individuals, whereas we choose $\mu_C = 3\,\text{day}^{-1}$ ($>\lambda$) to be representative of cell cycle impairment. These parameters have been estimated from the literature. We note that the model behavior we discuss in the following sections was found to be robust to changes in these parameters. Robustness was concluded since a 10-fold change in each or any combination thereof, of these four parameters did not change the qualitative behavior of the model, provided the relation $\lambda > \mu_C$ (or $\lambda < \mu_C$) was maintained. We examine the changes in model behavior arising from altering the relative values of λ and μ_C in the following sections.

We choose δ such that $\delta I(t)$ is similar in magnitude to $\gamma(I(t))R(t)$, when $R(t) \approx 10^{11}$, and $I(t) \approx 10^{-2}\,\text{ng ml}^{-1}$. The proportionality constant $\hat{\beta}$ is chosen such that we observe $\mathcal{O}(10^{11})$ naive T cells in equilibrium at 20 years of age (for $I(t) \approx 10^{-2}\,\text{ng ml}^{-1}$). We had the least inclination when choosing

Table 1 | Parameter choices for the mathematical model.

Parameter	Value	Units
θ_S	60	Signaling units
θ_P	600	Signaling units
α	2	(Log signaling units)$^{-1}$
$\hat{\beta}$	0.2	10^{-12} ml^{-1} day^{-1}
δ	500	day^{-1}
λ	2	day^{-1}
ρ	5	day^{-1}
μ_R	0.5	day^{-1}
μ_C	1	day^{-1}

the parameter α. This parameter describes the spread in the individual signaling thresholds across the naive T cell population. We choose $\alpha = 2$, however this choice has no justification from the literature. The parameter set is summarized in **Table 1**.

3.2. THERE EXISTS A UNIQUE AND STEADY STATE WHEN $\lambda > \mu_C$

Let us suppose changes in thymic output and IL-7 production occur in time scales slower than those of the changes in the number of naive T cells. Under this assumption, we look for adiabatic solutions of the system as follows:

$$0 = \beta(t) - \gamma\left(\hat{I}(t)\right)\hat{R}(t) - \delta\hat{I}(t)\,, \tag{16}$$

$$0 = \nu(t) - \left(\bar{\rho}\left(\hat{S}(t)\right) + \bar{\mu}_R\left(\hat{S}(t)\right)\right)\hat{R}(t) + 2\lambda\hat{C}(t)\,, \tag{17}$$

$$0 = \bar{\rho}\left(\hat{S}(t)\right)\hat{R}(t) - (\mu_C + \lambda)\,\hat{C}(t)\,. \tag{18}$$

For the parameter set studied, the relative error between this solution and the exact solution is within 3% for the resting naive T cell population and the concentration of IL-7, and within 14% for the cycling T cell population (see **Figure 3**).

All numerical results presented in the paper have been obtained with a Python code[1]: differential equations (13), (14), and (15) have been solved using a fourth-order Runge-Kutta scheme. Quasi-stationary solutions were found using the scipy.optimize package. Bifurcation plots were computed using a bisection scheme to search for multiple solutions of equation (21) in the interval [0,1]. Corresponding T cell numbers were calculated using equations (19) and (20).

Notice that the adiabatic solution for both cell types is uniquely defined for a given value of cytokine concentration, $\hat{I}(t)$, namely

$$\hat{R}(t) = \frac{\beta(t) - \delta\hat{I}(t)}{\gamma\left(\hat{I}(t)\right)}\,, \tag{19}$$

$$\hat{C}(t) = \frac{\bar{\rho}\left(\hat{S}(t)\right)}{\mu_C + \lambda}\,\frac{\beta(t) - \delta\hat{I}(t)}{\gamma\left(\hat{I}(t)\right)}\,. \tag{20}$$

[1] Python code available upon request.

The problem of finding adiabatic solutions can then be reduced to finding solutions, $\hat{I}(t)$, to the one-dimensional equation

$$\frac{\nu(t)\,\gamma\left(\hat{I}(t)\right)}{\beta(t) - \delta\hat{I}(t)} = \bar{\mu}_R\left(\hat{S}(t)\right) + \left(1 - \frac{2\lambda}{\lambda + \mu_C}\right)\bar{\rho}\left(\hat{S}(t)\right)\,. \tag{21}$$

By construction, $\gamma(\hat{I}(t))$ is a monotonically increasing function of $\hat{I}(t)$. Furthermore, the existence of positive adiabatic solutions requires $\beta(t) > \delta\hat{I}(t)$. Therefore, for a fixed time t, the left-hand side of equation (21) is an increasing function of $\hat{I}(t)$. For $\lambda > \mu_C$, the right-hand side of equation (21) is a monotonically decreasing function of $\hat{I}(t)$. Lastly, $\gamma(\hat{I}(t)) = 0$ for $\hat{I}(t) = 0$, and the limit as $\hat{I}(t) \to 0$ of the right-hand side is equal to μ_R. It follows that the intersection of the left and right sides must be unique and positive. We deduce that for $\lambda > \mu_C$ there exists a unique adiabatic solution to the system (see left plot of **Figure 4**). This solution is stable for the parameter set given in **Table 1**. We have also numerically explored parameter space, but have not found a parameter set for which this solution is unstable. In **Figure 5** we present numerical solutions to equations (13–15), computed with a fourth-order Runge-Kutta method implemented in Python. Initial conditions were chosen to be the adiabatic solutions of equations (16–18) at $t = 0$.

3.3. THERE EXIST TWO STEADY STATES WHEN $\lambda < \mu_C$

Let us now consider the case $\lambda < \mu_C$. The right-hand side of equation (21) is no longer a decreasing function of $\hat{I}(t)$. We find there may exist up to three solutions $\hat{I}(t)$, two of which may be stable simultaneously, whilst the third is unstable (see right plot of **Figure 4**). Further examination (by numerically finding all solutions using the bisection method) of the model reveals a saddle-node bifurcation as thymic output changes with age (see left panel, **Figure 6**). We assume that individuals with (around) 10^{11} naive T cells are healthy, in the sense that they have a sufficient number of T cells to provide protection against immune challenges. When a cell in cycle is more likely to die than to produce two daughter cells, we define cell cycle progression to be impaired. Mathematically, this corresponds to $\lambda < \mu_C$. When cell cycle progression is impaired, the model predicts an individual may possess a healthy number of T cells, thereby being immuno-competent, up until the age at which the model bifurcates. For the parameter set we have investigated, this bifurcation is inevitable given the estimated decline in thymic output established by Bains et al. (3). Indeed, for a given parameter set, from the known rate at which thymic output declines, one can estimate the age at which the model bifurcates. The bifurcation results in a decrease in the naive T cell population size of approximately two orders of magnitude, that is, following the bifurcation we expect roughly 99 out of every 100 naive T cells to be lost.

4. DISCUSSION

In a healthy individual, it is reasonable to expect that naive T cells entering the cell cycle are more likely to complete division and produce two daughter cells, than to die during the division process. Therefore, we suppose the parameter relation $\lambda < \mu_C$ represents a

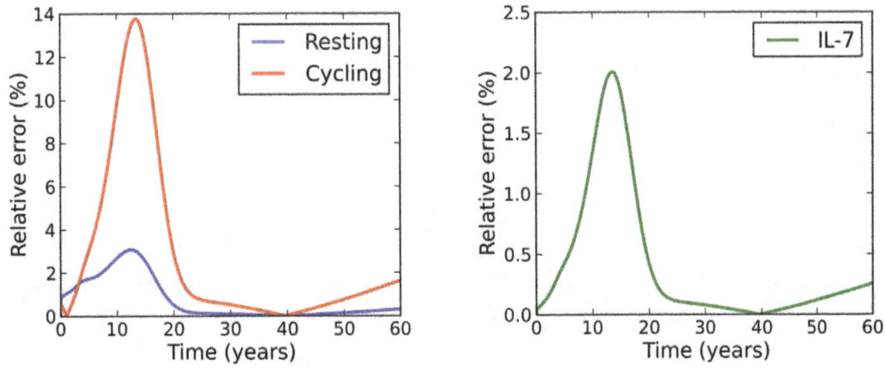

FIGURE 3 | Relative error between the adiabatic solution and the exact solution, where initial conditions were chosen to be equal to the adiabatic solution at time $t = 0$.

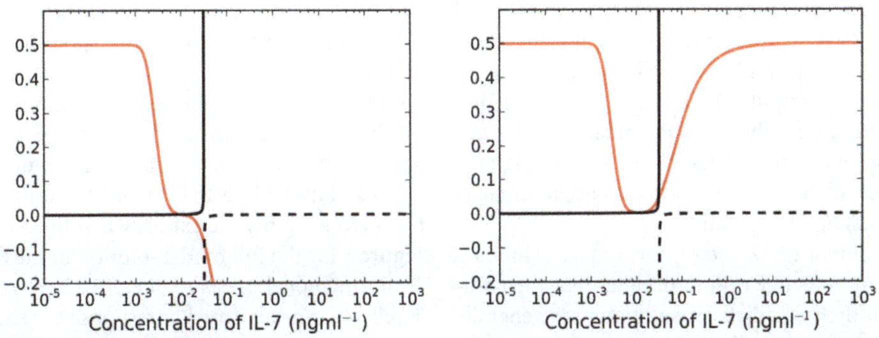

FIGURE 4 | Left panel: for $\lambda > \mu_c$ ($t = 25$ years), the right-hand side of equation (21) is a decreasing function of $I(t)$ (red line). There exists a unique, asymptotically stable solution $\hat{I}(t)$ found at the intersection of the solid black and red lines. Right panel: there exist three intersections between the red and solid black lines when $\lambda < \mu_c$ for $t = 25$ years. We require $\beta(t) > \gamma(\hat{I}(t))$ for existence of stable solutions, therefore we neglect all intersections with the dashed black line.

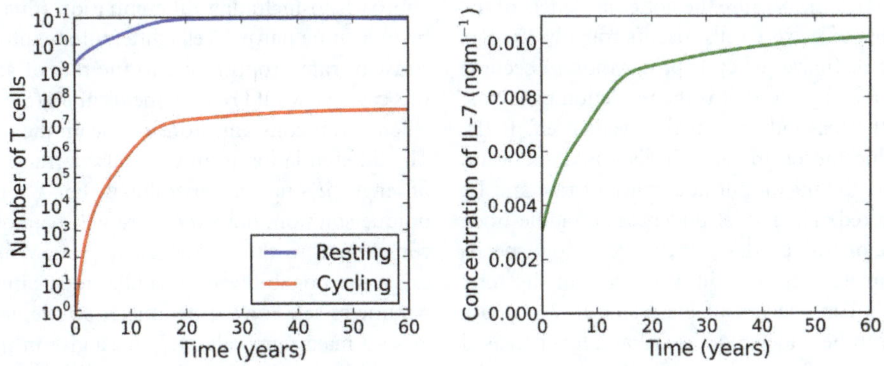

FIGURE 5 | Numerical solutions to equations (13–15) for $\lambda > \mu_c$. Initial conditions are chosen to be the adiabatic solutions of equations (16–18) at $t = 0$. We observe a large increase in the naive T cell population from birth to adulthood. During this period we see a 10^7-fold increase in the number of cycling cells, resulting from increased IL-7 availability and reduced thymic output. IL-7 availability increases continually as the individual ages.

healthy individual. We have shown, under this hypothesis, that the model allows a single asymptotically stable adiabatic solution. The total number of naive T cells per kilogram of body mass was found to increase over the first 18 years of life and decrease thereafter. The decline in this ratio for adults is seemingly a consequence of the reduction in thymic output.

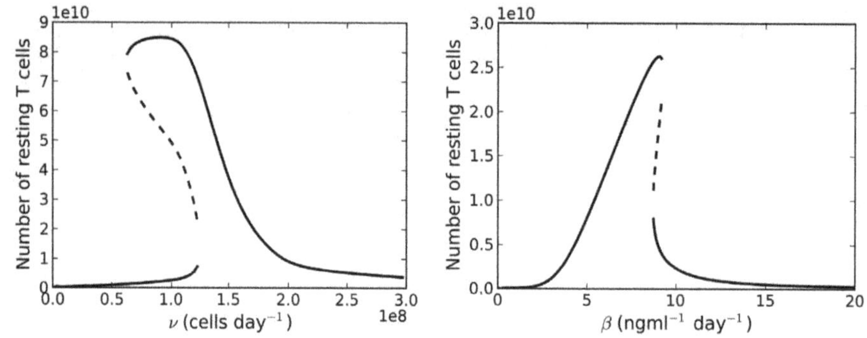

FIGURE 6 | Left panel: bifurcation diagram for varying the parameter $v(t)$ for $\lambda < \mu_C$. Right panel: bifurcation plot as a function of varying the rate of IL-7 production. Thymic export is fixed at v(60 years).

The number of cycling naive T cells in adiabatic conditions was found to increase from practically 0 (approximately 0.75 cells) cells at birth to 10^7 cells by adulthood. Whilst the number of cycling cells increased thereafter, the increase was at a markedly slower rate. The increase in the number of cycling cells is probably due to the decline in thymic output, wherein competition for IL-7 decreases. Despite the increase in the cycling population, the number of cells in cycle is several orders of magnitude smaller than the resting population. For adults, this proportion is approximately $[0.01, 0.04]$% of the total naive population.

When cell cycle is impaired ($\lambda < \mu_C$), the model exhibits a saddle-node bifurcation as thymic output declines. For the parameter set investigated, the two adiabatic solutions are generally separated by two orders of magnitude. This feature motivates the following theoretical scenario: suppose a healthy individual experiences some event which causes naive cell cycle progression to become impaired at 18 years of age. The model predicts the naive T cell repertoire will experience a dramatic reduction in cell numbers at roughly 33 years of age. See **Figure 7** for the full solution of the model illustrating this scenario. From an immunological perspective, this scenario is interesting because the noticeable effect of the event (the dramatic loss of naive T cells) occurs roughly 15 years later than the event itself (naive cell cycle progression to become impaired at 18 years of age). Indeed, it is the reduction in thymic output that triggers the loss rather than the event itself. If the thymus was not atrophic, the loss in naive T cells would not occur.

Suppose now we fix thymic output at a constant rate and let the cell cycle be impaired. The model undergoes a saddle-node bifurcation as the rate of IL-7 production changes. More specifically, the model bifurcates, resulting in a decrease in the total number of T cells, as a consequence of increasing IL-7 production. Intuitively, this can be understood as follows: for increased IL-7 production, the rate of entry into cell cycle is enhanced, however, since cells are more likely to die in cell cycle than to produce two daughter cells, the enhanced rate of entry into cell cycle actually serves to decrease the total amount of naive T cells. The bifurcation diagram for this scenario is shown in the right panel of **Figure 6.** We found the critical value of this bifurcation decreases with thymic output. In the limiting case, corresponding to thymic output at 60 years of age, we found this critical value to be approximately 9.1 ng ml^{-1}. Consider again the theoretical scenario in which a healthy individual undergoes an event resulting in cell cycle impairment at 18 years of age. Suppose now at age 25 the same individual undergoes some treatment to limit IL-7 production to 8 ng ml^{-1}, corresponding to thymic production at approximately 11 years of age. The T cell count is reduced by approximately 60%. This reduction is a significant improvement on the 99% T cell loss in the untreated individual at 33 years of age. For this theoretical scenario, the model predicts limiting IL-7 availability will partially avoid the dramatic T cell loss arising from reducing thymic export when the cell cycle is impaired. See **Figure 8** for the full model solution in the treated individual.

In the model presented here we have neglected the fact naive T cells become activated in response to recognition of ligand specific to their unique TCR. Research by Koenen et al. has shown T cell survival is IL-7 independent following T cell activation (18). Suppose now we include a term in the governing ODEs to represent differentiation of naive T cells into cells with a different phenotype, such as activated T cells. Assuming no reversion back to the naive phenotype, such a term would appear in the model as a loss term equivalent to the death rate $\hat{\mu}_R(S(t))$. The simplest approach to including differentiation (due to activation) would be to assume naive T cells differentiate into activated T cells at a constant rate proportional to the rate of antigenic challenge. In this case, we would replace the term $\hat{\mu}_R(S(t))$ by $\hat{\mu}_R(S(t)) + \mu_D$, where μ_D is constant. Consider again the red curves in **Figure 4.** The differentiation term will cause a translation in the red curve of length μ_D up the vertical axis. For $\lambda > \mu_C$, there still exists a unique solution, however there will be a quantitative change in comparison to the case when $\mu_D = 0$. When $\lambda < \mu_C$, there still exists the possibility of a saddle-node bifurcation for a general parameter set. For the parameter set we have investigated, there exists a maximum value μ_D^*, for a given time t, such that we can find more than one solution. For differentiation rates $\mu_D > \mu_D^*$, we can only find a unique solution corresponding to the stable adiabatic one, in which we have reduced T cell numbers.

In this paper we have developed and analyzed a deterministic mathematical model of a population of naive T cells, whose survival depends on the availability of the cytokine IL-7. We have shown this model predicts a stable population of cells when cell cycle progression is healthy. More interestingly, when cell cycle progression is impaired, our results indicate declining thymic

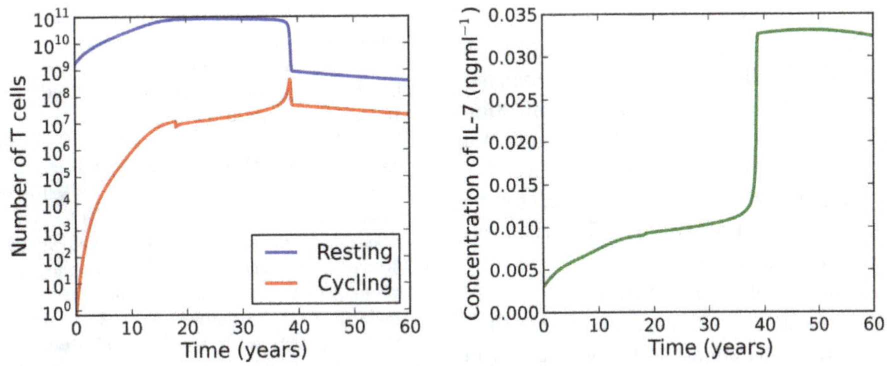

FIGURE 7 | Theoretical scenario in which we set $\mu_C = 3$ at 18 years of age. At roughly 33 years of age the model bifurcates resulting in a dramatic loss of naive T cells.

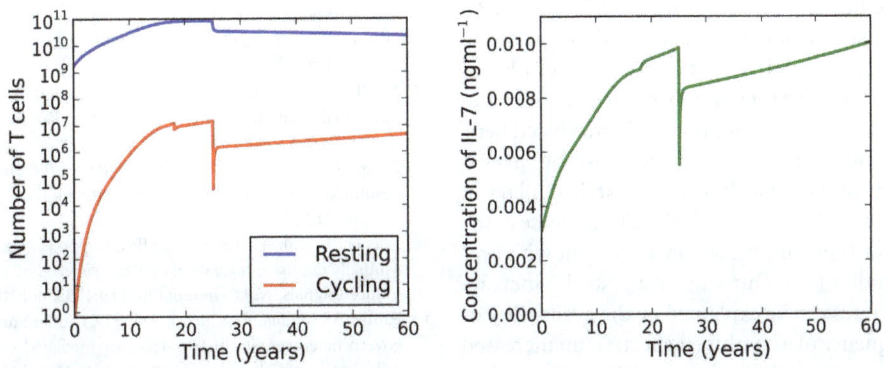

FIGURE 8 | At age 18 the individual experiences some event resulting in impaired cell cycle progression. At age 25 the individual undergoes treatment to limit IL-7 production to levels comparable to those at 11 years of age. Whilst the T cell count is reduced, this attrition is a significant improvement on the reduction observed when the individual has not received treatment (see **Figure 7**).

output may result in a dramatic loss in the number of naive T cells. Furthermore, we have been able to establish that limiting IL-7 production partially rescues this decline. However, our study has been restricted to naive T cells and we have not taken into account the accumulation of memory T cells as an individual ages. Memory T cells are generated in response to antigen or homeostatic cytokines (27), and during repeated homeostasis-driven divisions of naive T cells (28). Previous studies have shown the percentage of memory T cells increases with age, yet the percentage of naive T cells decreases with age (29). $CD4^+$ memory T cells also require IL-7 for survival and proliferation in the periphery (30). In the case of $CD8^+$ memory T cells, IL-15 is largely responsible for their peripheral survival, but IL-7 may also be required. It is, then, reasonable to assume that memory T cells compete for the IL-7 required for naive T cell survival. At least, that is, for those memory T cells which access IL-7 in the same tissues as naive T cells, such as the lymph nodes. As mentioned before, memory T cells can be derived from repeated divisions of naive T cells (31). In our model, the naive T cells that will acquire a memory-like phenotype first are those with low IL-7 survival and proliferation thresholds. We would expect, then, that over time the ratio of naive to memory T cells would decrease. Furthermore, the naive population would lose those cells with lowest survival and division thresholds. Given the distribution of signaling thresholds in our model, we would expect to see a shift to the right for the distribution of both survival and signaling thresholds. This shift, which implies that on average naive T cells require a higher concentration of IL-7 to enter cell cycle with age, together with the additional competition from an increasing memory population, is expected to cause a decrease in the total number of naive T cells and the percentage of naive T cells in cell cycle. These considerations might help explain the discrepancy between our model and data showing a reduction in the percentage of naive T cells expressing $Ki67^+$ during childhood[2]. There is support for the fact that childhood might be the phase in which most memory T cells are acquired (3). Indeed, it might be that the model presented here, better describes the total number of T cells that require IL-7, naive and memory, rather than just the naive T cell pool alone. This, however, would require a more detailed analysis, out of the scope of this paper.

[2]Our current model suggests the percentage of naive T cells in cell cycle is increasing.

Many different receptor-mediated signals are integrated by T cells in their micro-environment, such as cytokines, adhesion molecules, T cell receptors, and co-receptors (CD28, CTLA-4). However, the survival of naive T cells, the focus of this paper, has been shown to depend on IL-7 and low level TCR stimulation (8, 9, 15, 32). Other cytokines, such as IL-15, play a significant role in the homeostasis of memory $CD8^+$ T cells (33). Given the experimental support for the hypothesis that IL-7 is critical for the homeostatic proliferation and the survival of naive T cells, in this first model we have neglected other signals (7).

Previous mathematical models of naive T cell homeostasis have focused on the relative contribution of thymic export and cell division in the periphery (3, 34, 35). These models conclude that in humans, thymic export makes an important contribution to the size of the naive T cell population in early life (<20 years of age), whereas later in life the number of naive T cells is maintained by homeostatic proliferation in the periphery. Some recent studies have measured the relative contribution of thymic export by examining the average number of TRECs in naive T cells (3, 35, 36). The use of mathematical models has allowed these groups to infer the relative (young versus old) kinetics for naive T cells, based on experimental estimates of the total number of naive T cells and recent thymic emigrants (3, 34, 35). In the model introduced here, we have aimed to provide a mechanistic perspective by investigating at the molecular and cellular levels, the role IL-7 plays in regulating the homeostasis of naive T cells (37). The increase in the proportion of cycling cells in our model is in agreement with previous experimental studies (38). Our study suggests the increase in peripheral division rates can be explained by the availability of IL-7, which is a consequence of a combined effect: (i) an increased net IL-7 production as an individual ages, and (ii) a reduction of recently exported thymocytes competing for this resource.

ACKNOWLEDGMENTS

We thank Robin Callard, Megan Palmer, and Douglas Lauffenburger for sharing their advice on the approaches taken in this study. This work has been partially supported by the research grant BB/G023395/1 (BBSRC, Carmen Molina-París).

REFERENCES

1. Almeida A, Rocha B, Freitas A, Tanchot C. Homeostasis of T cell numbers: from thymus production to peripheral compartmentalization and the indexation of regulatory T cells. *Semin Immunol* (2005) **17**(3):239–49. doi:10.1016/j.smim.2005.02.002
2. Surh CD, Sprent J. Homeostasis of naive and memory T cells. *Immunity* (2008) **29**(6):848–62. doi:10.1016/j.immuni.2008.11.002
3. Bains I, Thiébaut R, Yates A, Callard R. Quantifying thymic export: combining models of naive T cell proliferation and TCR excision circle dynamics gives an explicit measure of thymic output. *J Immunol* (2009) **183**(7):4329–36. doi:10.4049/jimmunol.0900743
4. den Braber I, Mugwagwa T, Vrisekoop N, Westera L, Mögling R, Bregje de Boer A, et al. Maintenance of peripheral naive T cells is sustained by thymus output in mice but not humans. *Immunity* (2012) **36**(2):288–97. doi:10.1016/j.immuni.2012.02.006
5. Takada K, Jameson S. Naive T cell homeostasis: from awareness of space to a sense of place. *Nat Rev Immunol* (2009) **9**(12):823–32. doi:10.1038/nri2657
6. Sprent J, Surh C. Normal T cell homeostasis: the conversion of naive cells into memory-phenotype cells. *Nat Immunol* (2011) **12**(6):478–84. doi:10.1038/ni.2018
7. Tan J, Dudl E, LeRoy E, Murray R, Sprent J, Weinberg K, et al. IL-7 is critical for homeostatic proliferation and survival of naive T cells. *Proc Natl Acad Sci U S A* (2001) **98**(15):8732–7. doi:10.1073/pnas.161126098
8. Schluns K, Kieper W, Jameson S, Lefrançois L. Interleukin-7 mediates the homeostasis of naive and memory CD8 T cells in vivo. *Nat Immunol* (2000) **1**(5):426–32. doi:10.1038/80868
9. Fry T, Mackall C. The many faces of IL-7: from lymphopoiesis to peripheral T cell maintenance. *J Immunol* (2005) **174**(11):6571–6.
10. Martin B, Bécourt C, Bienvenu B, Lucas B. Self-recognition is crucial for maintaining the peripheral $CD4^+$ T-cell pool in a nonlymphopenic environment. *Blood* (2006) **108**(1):270–7. doi:10.1182/blood-2006-01-0017
11. Brocker T. Survival of mature CD4 T lymphocytes is dependent on major histocompatibility complex class II-expressing dendritic cells. *J Exp Med* (1997) **186**(8):1223–32. doi:10.1084/jem.186.8.1223
12. Markiewicz MA, Brown I, Gajewski TF. Death of peripheral $CD8^+$ T cells in the absence of MHC class I is Fas-dependent and not blocked by Bcl-xL. *Eur J Immunol* (2003) **33**(10):2917–26. doi:10.1002/eji.200324273
13. Vivien L, Benoist C, Mathis D. T lymphocytes need IL-7 but not IL-4 or IL-6 to survive in vivo. *Int Immunol* (2001) **13**(6):763–8. doi:10.1093/intimm/13.6.763
14. Kondrack R, Harbertson J, Tan J, McBreen M, Surh C, Bradley L. Interleukin 7 regulates the survival and generation of memory CD4 cells. *J Exp Med* (2003) **198**(12):1797–806. doi:10.1084/jem.20030735
15. Fry T, Mackall C. Interleukin-7: master regulator of peripheral T-cell homeostasis? *Trends Immunol* (2001) **22**(10):564–71. doi:10.1016/S1471-4906(01)02028-2
16. Mueller SN, Germain RN. Stromal cell contributions to the homeostasis and functionality of the immune system. *Nat Rev Immunol* (2009) **9**(9):618–29. doi:10.1038/nri2588
17. Kang J, Coles M. IL-7: the global builder of the innate lymphoid network and beyond, one niche at a time. *Semin Immunol* (2012) **24**(3):190–7. doi:10.1016/j.smim.2012.02.003
18. Koenen P, Heinzel S, Carrington EM, Happo L, Alexander WS, Zhang J-G, et al. Mutually exclusive regulation of T cell survival by IL-7R and antigen receptor-induced signals. *Nat Commun* (2013) **4**:1735. doi:10.1038/ncomms2719
19. Palmer M, Mahajan V, Chen J, Irvine D, Lauffenburger D. Signaling thresholds govern heterogeneity in IL-7-receptor-mediated responses of naïve $CD8^+$; T cells. *Immunol Cell Biol* (2011) **89**(5):581–94. doi:10.1038/icb.2011.5
20. Stirk ER, Lythe G, van den Berg HA, Molina-París C. Stochastic competitive exclusion in the maintenance of the naïve T cell repertoire. *J Theor Biol* (2010) **265**(3):396–410. doi:10.1016/j.jtbi.2010.05.004
21. Stirk ER, Lythe G, van den Berg HA, Hurst GA, Molina-París C. The limiting conditional probability distribution in a stochastic model of T cell repertoire maintenance. *Math Biosci* (2010) **224**(2):74–86. doi:10.1016/j.mbs.2009.12.004
22. Wallace EW. A simplified derivation of the linear noise approximation. *arXiv Preprint arXiv:1004.4280* (2010).
23. Mitchell WA, Meng I, Nicholson SA, Aspinall R. Thymic output, ageing and zinc. *Biogerontology* (2006) **7**(5–6):461–70. doi:10.1007/s10522-006-9061-7
24. Steinmann GG. Changes in the human thymus during aging. In: Müller-Hermelink HK, editor. *The Human Thymus.* Berlin: Springer (1986). p. 43–88.
25. Haugen F, Norheim F, Lian H, Wensaas AJ, Dueland S, Berg O, et al. IL-7 is expressed and secreted by human skeletal muscle cells. *Am J Physiol Cell Physiol* (2010) **298**(4):C807–16. doi:10.1152/ajpcell.00094.2009
26. Burmaster DE, Crouch EA. Lognormal distributions for body weight as a function of age for males and females in the united states, 1976–1980. *Risk Anal* (1997) **17**(4):499–505. doi:10.1111/j.1539-6924.1997.tb00890.x
27. Geginat J, Lanzavecchia A, Sallusto F. Proliferation and differentiation potential of human CD8+ memory T-cell subsets in response to antigen or homeostatic cytokines. *Blood* (2003) **101**(11):4260–6. doi:10.1182/blood-2002-11-3577
28. Goldrath AW, Bogatzki LY, Bevan MJ. Naive T cells transiently acquire a memory-like phenotype during homeostasis-driven proliferation. *J Exp Med* (2000) **192**(4):557–64. doi:10.1084/jem.192.4.557
29. Saule P, Trauet J, Dutriez V, Lekeux V, Dessaint J-P, Labalette M. Accumulation of memory T cells from childhood to old age: central and effector memory cells in CD4(+) versus effector memory and terminally differentiated memory cells in CD8(+) compartment. *Mech Ageing Dev* (2006) **127**(3):274–81. doi:10.1016/j.mad.2005.11.001

30. Seddon B, Tomlinson P, Zamoyska R. Interleukin 7 and T cell receptor signals regulate homeostasis of CD4 memory cells. *Nat Immunol* (2003) **4**(7):680–6. doi:10.1038/ni946
31. Cho B, Rao V, Ge Q, Eisen H, Chen J. Homeostasis-stimulated proliferation drives naive T cells to differentiate directly into memory T cells. *J Exp Med* (2000) **192**(4):549. doi:10.1084/jem.192.4.549
32. Fry T, Mackall C. Interleukin-7: from bench to clinic. *Blood* (2002) **99**(11):3892–904. doi:10.1182/blood.V99.11.3892
33. Tan JT, Ernst B, Kieper WC, LeRoy E, Sprent J, Surh CD. Interleukin (IL)-15 and IL-7 jointly regulate homeostatic proliferation of memory phenotype CD8+ cells but are not required for memory phenotype CD4+ cells. *J Exp Med* (2002) **195**(12):1523–32. doi:10.1084/jem.20020066
34. Thomas-Vaslin V, Altes HK, de Boer RJ, Klatzmann D. Comprehensive assessment and mathematical modeling of T cell population dynamics and homeostasis. *J Immunol* (2008) **180**(4):2240–50.
35. Murray JM, Kaufmann GR, Hodgkin PD, Lewin SR, Kelleher AD, Davenport MP, et al. Naive T cells are maintained by thymic output in early ages but by proliferation without phenotypic change after age twenty. *Immunol Cell Biol* (2003) **81**(6):487–95. doi:10.1046/j.1440-1711.2003.01191.x
36. Ribeiro RM, Perelson AS. Determining thymic output quantitatively: using models to interpret experimental T-cell receptor excision circle (TREC) data. *Immunol Rev* (2007) **216**(1):21–34. doi:10.1111/j.1600-065X.2006.00493.x
37. Fallon EM, Lauffenburger DA. Computational model for effects of ligand/receptor binding properties on interleukin-2 trafficking dynamics and T cell proliferation response. *Biotechnol Prog* (2000) **16**(5):905–16. doi:10.1021/bp000097t
38. Prelog M, Keller M, Geiger R, Brandstätter A, Würzner R, Schweigmann U, et al. Thymectomy in early childhood: significant alterations of the CD4(+)CD45RA(+)CD62L(+) T cell compartment in later life. *Clin Immunol* (2009) **130**(2):123–32. doi:10.1016/j.clim.2008.08.023
39. Park J, Yu Q, Erman B, Appelbaum J, Montoya-Durango D, Grimes H, et al. Suppression of IL7Rα transcription by IL-7 and other prosurvival cytokines: a novel mechanism for maximizing IL-7-dependent T cell survival. *Immunity* (2004) **21**(2):289–302. doi:10.1016/j.immuni.2004.07.016
40. Henriques CM, Rino J, Nibbs RJ, Graham GJ, Barata JT. IL-7 induces rapid clathrin-mediated internalization and JAK3-dependent degradation of IL-7Rα in T cells. *Blood* (2010) **115**(16):3269–77. doi:10.1182/blood-2009-10-246876
41. Palmer MJ, Mahajan VS, Trajman LC, Irvine DJ, Lauffenburger DA, Chen J, et al. Interleukin-7 receptor signaling network: an integrated systems perspective. *Cell Mol Immunol* (2008) **5**(2):79–89. doi:10.1038/cmi.2008.10

APPENDIX

A.1. A MODEL OF IL-7R DYNAMICS

In this section we present a summary of a stochastic model in which we consider the number of IL-7 receptors on the surface of naive T cells. This study is used to derive equations (1) and (9) in the main text. The model has been formulated as a continuous time Markov process. We consider the number of receptors on a single naive T cell. For our purposes, we present the mean field approximation to the model with which we estimate the parameters. We introduce the following four variables:

- $m_1(t)$ – the total number of IL-7 receptors on the surface of a naive T cell,
- $m_2(t)$ – the number of unbound internalized receptors,
- $m_3(t)$ – the number of bound internalized receptors,
- $m_4(t)$ – the quantity of IL-7 induced signal.

We assume, in equilibrium, the fraction of surface receptors bound to IL-7 is given by f_I. The system of ODEs denoting the mean field approximation to the stochastic model is given by:

$$\frac{dm_1(t)}{dt} = \phi\, e^{-m_4(t)/\kappa} + \xi_U\, m_2(t) + \xi_B\, m_3(t) - \left[\sigma_U\left(1 - f_I\right) + \sigma_B f_I\right] m_1(t)\,, \tag{A1}$$

$$\frac{dm_2(t)}{dt} = \sigma_U\left(1 - f_I\right) m_1(t) - (\xi_U + \zeta_U)\, m_2(t)\,, \tag{A2}$$

$$\frac{dm_3(t)}{dt} = \sigma_B f_I\, m_1(t) - (\xi_B + \zeta_B)\, m_3(t)\,, \tag{A3}$$

$$\frac{dm_4(t)}{dt} = \varphi\, m_3(t) - \chi\, m_4(t)\,. \tag{A4}$$

A.2. REDUCED MODEL IN THE CASE WHEN $I = 0$

Consider a T cell in an IL-7 free medium with initial conditions such that the IL-7 induced signaling vanishes and the number of IL-7:IL-7R internal complexes is zero. Then the mean field model can be reduced to the following set of ODEs:

$$\frac{dm_1(t)}{dt} = \phi + \xi_U\, m_2(t) - \sigma_U\, m_1(t)\,,$$
$$\frac{dm_2(t)}{dt} = \sigma_U\, m_1(t) - (\xi_U + \zeta_U)\, m_2(t)\,.$$

This reduced system is governed by four parameters ϕ, ξ_U, σ_U, and ζ_U, and possesses the following stable steady state:

$$m_1^* = \frac{\phi\,(\xi_U + \zeta_U)}{\sigma_U \zeta_U}\,,$$
$$m_2^* = \frac{\phi}{\zeta_U}\,.$$

We assume in the reduced model 10% of the total number of receptors are internalized in equilibrium. We set $m_1^* = 9m_2^*$. Based on the measurements of Singer et al. (39), we shall assume 4×10^4 receptors in total when the reduced model is in steady state. Therefore, we let

$$\frac{\phi\,(\xi_U + \zeta_U)}{\sigma_U \zeta_U} = 3.6 \times 10^4\,, \tag{A5}$$

$$\frac{\phi}{\zeta_U} = 4 \times 10^3\,. \tag{A6}$$

In Ref. (40), cells were cultured with the translation inhibitor cycloheximide (CHX) to prevent transcription of the IL-7 receptor. Total expression of the IL-7 receptor was measured over several time points, from which the authors estimate the half-life of the receptor in an unstimulated cell to be approximately 24 h.

In the reduced model, all receptors are guaranteed to be degraded in a finite amount of time. The expected time for a receptor, that is initially on the cell surface, to be degraded in the lysosome is given by

$$\tau_1 = \frac{\zeta_U + \sigma_U + \xi_U}{\sigma_U \zeta_U}\,.$$

Assuming exponential decay, the half-life for a receptor to undergo lysosomal degradation, starting on the cell surface, is then given by

$$t_{\frac{1}{2}} = \frac{\zeta_U + \sigma_U + \xi_U}{\sigma_U \zeta_U} \log 2\,.$$

Thus, we can write

$$\frac{\zeta_U + \sigma_U + \xi_U}{\sigma_U \zeta_U} \log 2 = 24\,\text{h}\,. \tag{A7}$$

Combining equations (A5), (A6), and (A7) we find

$$\zeta_U \approx 0.29\,\text{h}^{-1}\,,$$
$$\phi \approx 1.2 \times 10^3 \text{ receptors h}^{-1}\,,$$
$$\xi_U + 0.29\,\text{h}^{-1} \approx 9\sigma_U\,.$$

The value of ξ_U relative to ζ_U effectively dictates the ratio of receptors which are degraded to those recycled back to the cell surface. We assume the system has evolved to minimize waste of functional proteins and tentatively let $\xi_U > \zeta_U$. That is, we assume that a greater fraction of receptors are recycled back to the surface of the cell. We somewhat arbitrarily set

$$\xi_U = 1\,\text{h}^{-1} \quad \Rightarrow \quad \sigma_U \approx 0.14\,\text{h}^{-1}\,.$$

A.3. RECEPTOR-LIGAND KINETICS

Suppose the number of surface receptors is constant and denoted by R_T. Let us also assume the extra-cellular concentration of IL-7 is constant and denoted by I. Define $R_B(t)$ to be the number of IL-7 receptors bound to IL-7. Note that we assume the time to recruit the common gamma chain, γ_c, is negligible. Then, we can describe changes in the number of bound complexes by the following ODE

$$\frac{dR_B(t)}{dt} = k_+\left[R_T - R_B(t)\right] I - k_- R_B(t)\,,$$

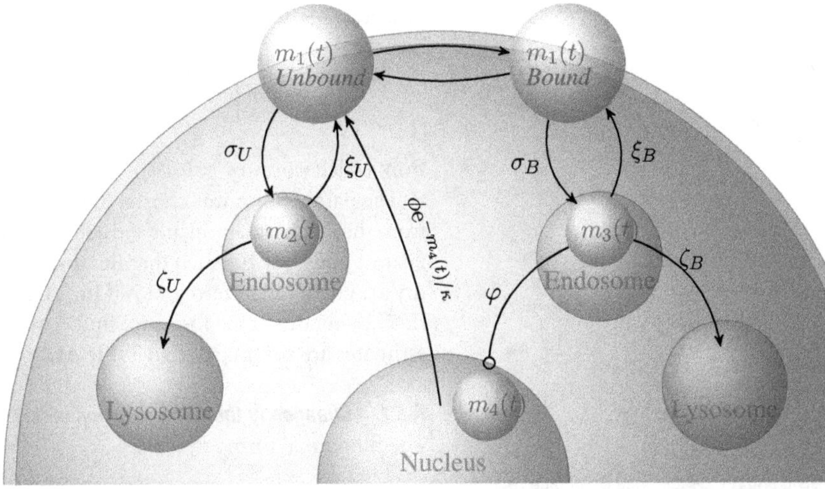

FIGURE A1 | Diagrammatic representation of the transition probabilities of the stochastic model for the IL-7 and IL-7 receptor system.

where k_+ and k_- are, respectively, the binding and unbinding rates of the IL-7:IL-7R receptor-ligand system. We assume the timescales for this reaction are faster than the timescales for changes in receptor numbers, such that we can consider these reactions to be in equilibrium. This ODE has a unique stable steady state:

$$R_B^* = \frac{R_T I}{\frac{k_-}{k_+} + I} = f_I R_T \,.$$

The Appendix for Ref. (41) provides estimates for k_+ and k_-, from which we set $k_+ = 1\,\mathrm{nM\,min^{-1}}$ and $k_- = 0.1\,\mathrm{min^{-1}}$. It is reported IL-7 has a molecular mass of around 17 kDa, from which we estimate the ratio $k_-/k_+ \approx 1.7\,\mathrm{ng\,ml^{-1}}$.

A.4. EARLY INTERNALIZATION EVENTS

In Ref. (40), surface receptor expression was assessed in human thymocytes. It is reported, cells in 50 ng ml^{-1} IL-7 culture down-regulated IL-7R expression. A 20% reduction was observed after 10 min. Using the above estimate for k_-/k_+, we find $f_I|_{I=50} \approx 0.97$. Based on this, we can neglect internalization of the unbound receptor. In the first 10 min, we shall also neglect recycling and inhibition of receptor transcription. We assume surface receptor expression loss is modeled by the ODE

$$\frac{\mathrm{d}m_1(t)}{\mathrm{d}t} = \phi - \sigma_B m_1(t) \,.$$

Given initial surface expression levels equal to $m_1(0)$, this ODE has solution

$$m_1(t) = \frac{\phi}{\sigma_B} + \left[m_1(0) - \frac{\phi}{\sigma_B}\right] \mathrm{e}^{\sigma_B t} \,. \tag{A8}$$

We assume the previous estimates obtained from the reduced model for $m_1(0)$ and ϕ. That is, we let $m_1(0) = 3.6 \times 10^4$ receptors and $\phi = 1.2 \times 10^3$ receptors h^{-1}. Then using the above expression for $m_1(t)$ equation (A8), we obtain an estimate for σ_B. We find $\sigma_B \approx 1.4\,\mathrm{h^{-1}}$. The authors of Ref. (40) estimate the half-life of the IL-7 receptor in cells treated with CHX, cultured in 50 ng ml^{-1}, to be approximately 3 h. The expected time to lysosomal degradation for a surface receptor is given by

$$\begin{aligned} \tau_2 &= \frac{\left[\sigma_U\left(1-f_I\right) + \left(\xi_U + \zeta_U\right)\right]\left(\xi_B + \zeta_B\right) + \sigma_B f_I\left(\xi_U + \zeta_U\right)}{\sigma_U\left(1-f_I\right)\zeta_U\left(\xi_B + \zeta_B\right) + \sigma_B f_I\left(\xi_U + \zeta_U\right)\zeta_B} \\ &\approx \frac{1.3\,\mathrm{h^{-1}}\left(\xi_B + \zeta_B\right) + 1.7\,\mathrm{h^{-2}}}{4.6 \times 10^3\,\mathrm{h^{-2}}\left(\xi_B + \zeta_B\right) + 1.7\,\mathrm{h^{-2}}\zeta_B} \,. \end{aligned}$$

Assuming exponential decay, with a half-life of 3 h, we find $\xi_B \approx 0.2\zeta_B + 0.3\,\mathrm{h^{-1}}$. Again, without a direct measurement, let us set $\xi_B = 1\,\mathrm{h^{-1}}$, to obtain an estimate for $\zeta_B \approx 3.5\,\mathrm{h^{-1}}$.

A.5. REMAINING PARAMETERS

Consider the observation of an approximately 98% reduction in surface receptor expression following overnight culture in 6 ng ml^{-1} IL-7 made in Ref. (39). We let $m_1^*\big|_{I=6} = 0.02\, m_1^*\big|_{I=0} = 0.02\frac{\phi(\xi_U+\zeta_U)}{\sigma_U \zeta_U} \approx 763$ receptors. We set the derivatives equal to zero in the system of ODEs equations (A1–A4), and manipulate the resulting system of equations to obtain

$$\begin{aligned} &\phi \exp\left(-\frac{\varphi \sigma_B f_I}{\chi\kappa\left(\xi_B + \zeta_B\right)} m_1^*\right) \\ &= \left[\sigma_U\left(1-f_I\right) + \sigma_B f_I - \frac{\sigma_U\left(1-f_I\right)\xi_U}{\xi_U + \zeta_U} - \frac{\sigma_B f_I \xi_B}{\xi_B + \zeta_B}\right] m_1^* \,, \end{aligned} \tag{A9}$$

$$\Rightarrow \quad \exp\left(-1.9 \times 10^2 \text{ receptors } \frac{\varphi}{\chi\kappa}\right) \approx 0.54 \,,$$

$$\Rightarrow \quad \frac{\varphi}{\chi\kappa} \approx 3.2 \times 10^{-3} \text{ receptors}^{-1}.$$

Table A1 | Parameter estimates obtained from the mean field model of IL-7 receptor dynamics.

Parameter	Value	Units
ϕ	1.2×10^3	rec h^{-1}
κ	10^3	sig
ξ_U	1	h^{-1}
ξ_B	1	h^{-1}
σ_U	0.14	h^{-1}
σ_B	1.4	h^{-1}
k_-/k_+	1.7	ng ml^{-1}
ζ_U	0.29	h^{-1}
ζ_B	3.5	h^{-1}
φ	0.61	sig rec^{-1} h^{-1}
χ	0.19	h^{-1}

We let sig be the units of the signaling and rec be the units of surface receptor numbers.

From the steady solutions of ODEs equations (A3) and (A4), we find

$$m_4^* = \frac{\phi\sigma_B f_I}{(\xi_B + \zeta_B)\,\chi} m_1^* \approx 1.9 \times 10^2 \text{ receptors } \frac{\varphi}{\chi}.$$

We use this expression to rearrange equation (A9) in terms of m_4^*. This gives

$$\exp\left(-\frac{m_4^*}{\kappa}\right) \approx 9.1\frac{m_4^*}{\kappa}.$$

Solving the above expression numerically, we find $m_4^*/\kappa \approx 0.1$. We estimate a value for χ based on the observation that following culture in 6 ng ml^{-1} IL-7, mRNA levels took approximately 12 h to return to 99% of the control levels. The transcription rate is given by $\phi\exp(-m_4(t)/\kappa)$. We again assume the IL-7 induced signal decays according to the equation $m_4(t) = m_4(0)e^{-\chi t}$, where $m_4(0) = 0.1$. Combing these assumptions with the experimental observations, we have

$$\phi \exp\left[-\frac{m_4(0)\exp(-12\chi)}{\kappa}\right] = 0.99\phi,$$

from which we find $\chi \approx 0.19\,h^{-1} \Rightarrow \varphi \approx 6.1 \times 10^{-4}$ receptors^{-1} h^{-1} κ. The parameter κ was chosen to be 1000. This choice was made from the stochastic model: $\kappa = 1000$ is the minimum value (to the nearest power of 10) such that fluctuations in the signaling quantity are greater than zero for low (10^{-2} ng ml^{-1}) concentrations of IL-7. Using this value for κ, we find $\phi \approx 0.61\,h^{-1}$. The parameter estimates are summarized in **Table A1**.

A.5.1. *Changes in the concentration of IL-7*

The functional form

$$S = \frac{aI}{b+I} \tag{A10}$$

is used to approximate the numerical solution of m_4^* as a function of the concentration of IL-7. Using this function we find $a \approx 600$ signaling units and $b \approx 0.025$ ng ml^{-1}. In a similar manner we use the functional form

$$R = c + \frac{d}{e+I} \tag{A11}$$

to approximate the numerical solution of m_1^* as a function of the concentration of IL-7. We find $c \approx 600$ receptors, $d \approx 1000$ receptors ng ml^{-1} and $e \approx 0.03$ ng ml^{-1}. The number of IL-7 molecules internalized by each T cell per day is assumed to be the same as the number of internalized IL-7:IL-7R complexes per day. We let the complex internalization rate, as a function of I, be given by

$$24\sigma_B f_I m_1^*(I) \approx \frac{6.7I}{2+I}\left(3 + \frac{5}{3 \times 10^{-2} + I}\right) \times 10^3 \text{ molecules cell}^{-1}\text{ day}^{-1}. \tag{A12}$$

Cancer vaccines in the world of immune suppressive monocytes ($CD14^{+}HLA\text{-}DR^{lo/neg}$ cells): the gateway to improved responses

Rebecca R. Laborde[1], Yi Lin[2], Michael P. Gustafson[1], Peggy A. Bulur[1] and Allan B. Dietz[1]*

[1] *Human Cellular Therapy Laboratory, Division of Transfusion Medicine, Department of Laboratory Medicine and Pathology, Mayo Clinic, Rochester, MN, USA*
[2] *Division of Hematology, Department of Medicine, Mayo Clinic, Rochester, MN, USA*

Edited by:
Lisa Helene Butterfield, University of Pittsburgh, USA

Reviewed by:
Geanncarlo Lugo-Villarino, Centre National de la Recherche Scientifique, France
Matthew Collin, Newcastle University, UK

***Correspondence:**
Allan B. Dietz, Human Cellular Therapy Laboratory, Department of Laboratory Medicine and Pathology, Division of Transfusion Medicine, Mayo Clinic, 200 First Street Southwest, Rochester, MN 55905, USA
e-mail: dietz.allan@mayo.edu

Dendritic cells are an important target in cancer immunotherapy based on their critical role in antigen presentation and response to tumor development. The capacity of dendritic cells to stimulate anti-tumor immunity has led investigators to use these cells to mediate anti-tumor responses in a number of clinical trials. However, these trials have had mixed results. The typical method for generation of *ex vivo* dendritic cells starts with the purification of $CD14^{+}$ cells. Our studies identified a deficiency in the ability to generate mature dendritic cell using $CD14^{+}$ cells from cancer patients that corresponded with an increased population of monocytes with altered surface marker expression ($CD14^{+}HLA\text{-}DR^{lo/neg}$). Further studies identified systemic immune suppression and increased concentrations of $CD14^{+}HLA\text{-}DR^{lo/neg}$ monocytes capable of inhibiting T-cell proliferation and DC maturation. Together, these findings strongly suggest that protocols aimed at immune stimulation via monocytes/dendritic cells, if optimized on normal monocytes or in systems without these suppressive monocytes, are unlikely to engender effective DC maturation *in vitro* or efficiently trigger DC maturation *in vivo*. This highlights the importance of developing optimal protocols for stimulating DCs in the context of significantly altered monocyte phenotypes often seen in cancer patients.

Keywords: $CD14^{+}HLA\text{-}DR^{lo/neg}$, MDSC, dendritic cells, immunotherapy, monocytes

DENDRITIC CELLS AS CANCER VACCINES

Dendritic cells are potent signal transducers in the immune system. These cells present antigen, are the essential bridge between the innate and adaptive arms of the immune system, and serve as regulators to modulate immune response to pathogenic invasion, tissue injury, and tumor development. As such, dendritic cells have received significant focus as a promising vehicle for the development of vaccines for cancer immunotherapy. We now have a more complete understanding of DC ontology with the realization that DCs exist in diverse subsets, all capable of activating T cells but possessing unique functions. DCs are classified into two broad categories. The first are monocyte-derived DCs resulting from stimulation due to inflammation or infection. The second category are steady-state DCs which include resident $CD8^{+}$ DCs located in the thymus, resident $CD8^{-}$ DCs in the spleen, plasmacytoid DCs (pDCs), migratory DCs, and Langerhans cells [reviewed in Ref. (1, 2)]. Each of these classes of DCs has been demonstrated to play a key role in immune surveillance and response but for the purpose of DC-based vaccines for immunotherapy in cancer, the focus has been on $CD14^{+}$ monocyte-derived DCs.

The *in vivo* pathways associated with the development of dendritic cells from monocyte precursors and the mechanisms and consequences of pathogenic activation have been described (3, 4). Briefly, DCs arise from monocyte progenitors into an immature state (iDC) responsible for immune surveillance via pathogen detection. Once activated, iDC further differentiate into mature dendritic cells (mDC) and travel to lymph nodes to activate the adaptive (typically T- and B-cell responses) and innate immune response (5). DCs also play a role in limiting the immune response against self antigen (self-tolerance) as well as limiting response to tissue damage in the absence of pathogenic signals (6). iDC can suppress immunity and have been shown to be capable of eliminating antigen-specific T cells (7). Restriction of the capacity of iDC to differentiate into mDC has been a mechanism used by viruses, parasites, and bacteria to maintain a state of self-tolerance and to enable microbial pathology (8–10). Thus, manipulation and maintenance of a state of iDC with a block on the ability to differentiate into mDC is a key mechanism of immune suppression.

To generate mDC *in vitro* for clinical use, the $CD14^{+}$ monocytes are the preferred precursor due to their abundance and ease of collection. $CD14^{+}$ monocytes are purified from mononuclear cells via adherence to plastic, antibody selection, or size centrifugation and used as source material to differentiate DC. To drive the immune response, the DCs are pulsed with tumor antigens in the form of peptides, RNA, or lysates derived from whole tumors or cell lines (11, 12). Additionally, viruses can be a potent mechanism to deliver tumor antigens (13–15). Manufacturing methods reported among clinical trials vary greatly. As a variety of methods with subtle optimizations of DC cultures have been published, there are few constants (DC activation state, tumor source, patient status, underlying disease etc.) that allow useful comparisons between the growing numbers of trials and the underlying methods and characteristics used to generate and describe the drug (in this case DC). Often, this key aspect of drug development (optimizing and describing the purity and potency of the drug) is overlooked. However, one constant regarding the majority of the trials remains; that is the use of $CD14^+$ cells as a starting material.

MONOCYTE PRECURSORS OF DC ARE OFTEN ALTERED IN CANCER PATIENTS AND ARE IMMUNE SUPPRESSIVE

In our efforts to establish a DC vaccine protocol, we worked to optimize the maturation of DCs in cancer patients. During those studies, we discovered that in many patients, $CD14^+$-isolated monocytes were incapable of differentiation into mDC using standard DC generation protocols (16–18). This result that monocytes from cancer patients were potentially altered in their capacity to differentiate into DC, led us to search for correlative markers. We identified an increased population of monocytes with an altered surface marker expression ($CD14^+HLA\text{-}DR^{lo/neg}$) in a number of malignancies (16–20) (**Figure 1A**). This phenotype has also been reported by others in melanoma (21–23), bladder cancer (24), non-small cell lung cancer (25), and hepatocellular cancer (26, 27). Our studies in glioblastoma identified evidence of systemic immune suppression and increased concentrations of $CD14^+HLA\text{-}DR^{lo/neg}$ monocytes capable of inhibiting T-cell proliferation and DC maturation that could also be re-capitulated *in vitro* co-culture systems using tumor cell lines (18). These same immunosuppressive monocytes have been characterized with increased populations in bladder carcinoma that significantly correlate with decreased T-cell proliferation and IFN-γ production (24). These cells suppress immune function in multiple ways (**Table 1**), and therefore must be considered for any approach to DC vaccine strategies.

There is also mounting evidence that correlates increased concentrations of $CD14^+HLA\text{-}DR^{lo/neg}$ monocytes in patients with poor clinical outcome. Populations of $CD14^+HLA\text{-}DR^{lo/neg}$ monocytes and TGF-β levels were significantly expanded in metastatic melanoma patients as compared to healthy donors and correlated to a lack of response to administered granulocyte–macrophage colony-stimulation factor (GM-CSF) vaccine (22). Increased $CD14^+HLA\text{-}DR^{lo/neg}$ monocytes correlated to both extrathoracic metastasis and poor response to chemotherapy in non-small lung cancer patients (25). Increased $CD14^+HLA\text{-}DR^{lo/neg}$ monocytes are associated with more aggressive disease and poorer prognosis in lymphoma (16) and hepatocellular carcinoma (40). Increased $CD14^+HLA\text{-}DR^{lo/neg}$ monocytes were associated with decreased time to progression in patients with chronic lymphocytic leukemia (CLL) (19). Increased $CD14^+HLA\text{-}DR^{lo/neg}$ monocytes and decreased $CD4^+$ T cells can predict poor overall survival across a number of malignancies (20).

The finding that $CD14^+HLA\text{-}DR^{lo/neg}$ monocytes are detectable systemically in patients with a variety of malignancies and that they are functionally immune suppressive raises important questions regarding their influence in *ex vivo* DC vaccine preparations. To address this, we have studied the effects of these altered monocytes on mDC generation across several cancer types using an *ex vivo* culture system. Briefly, $CD14^+$ mononuclear cells were isolated from buffy coats or apheresis leukoreduction system

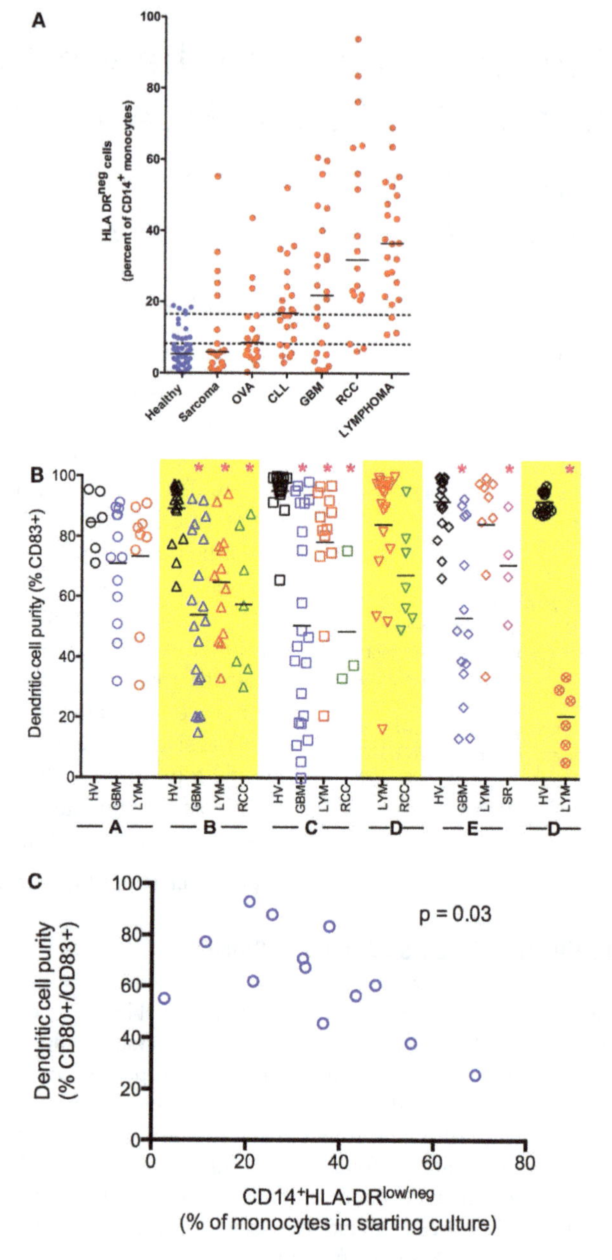

FIGURE 1 | Monocyte and dendritic cell defects in cancer. **(A)** Cancer patients have an increased percentage of $CD14^+HLA\text{-}DR^{lo/neg}$ monocytes in circulation. Peripheral blood of healthy volunteers and cancer patients was analyzed by flow cytometry for immune phenotype. **(B)** Monocytes from cancer patients have decreased capacity to differentiate to mDC ($CD83^+$) under a variety of stimulation conditions. Monocytes were selected from blood of healthy volunteers (HV) or cancer patients (GBM, glioblastoma multiforme LYM, B-cell lymphoma; RCC, renal cell carcinoma; SR, sarcoma) by $CD14^+$ immunomagnetic beads and cultured under different methods as labeled in *X* axis. Method A, fast-DC (28); B, *ex vivo* media with 5 days culture as described (29, 30); C, 5 days culture in StemLine media and GM-CSF, maturation factors TNFα and PGE2 added in the last 2 days of culture; D, method C with IL-4 added for 5 days of culture; E, method D with poly I:C added to maturation factors; F, method D with CpG used as maturation factor in place of TNF-α ($^*p < 0.05$). **(C)** Decreased generation of mDC correlates with increased percentage of $CD14^+HLA\text{-}DR^{lo/neg}$ in the monocytes selected for culture (Method B).

Table 1 | Methods of CD14$^+$HLA-DR$^{lo/neg}$ immune suppression.

CD14$^+$HLA-DR$^{lo/neg}$ functions	Targeted effect	Reference
Altered STAT signals	Resistance to cytokine/TLR signaling	(16, 24)
Increased IDO expression	Inhibits T-cell function	(31–33)
Increased arginase expression	Inhibits T-cell function	(12, 24, 34)
Prevention of DC maturation	Promotes immune tolerance	(16–18)
Altered co-stimulatory expression	Reduces T-cell stimulation	(12, 14, 15, 35)
Altered cytokine expression	Reduces T-cell stimulation	(15, 35)
Decreased antigen uptake	Reduces antigen-specific T-cell responses	(35)
Increased iNOS and NOX2 production	Reduces T-cell stimulation	(36)
Increased VEGF	Inhibits DC differentiation	(37)
Depletion of cytosine	Inhibit T-cell activation	(38, 39)

chambers of normal donors using immunomagnetic selection (41). Control DCs were cultured with 1% human AB serum, stimulated with GM-CSF and IL-4 (base media) for 3 days when one-third volume of fresh base media was added. Non-adherent cells were collected on day 6, re-suspended in base media with the addition of tumor necrosis factor alpha (TNF-α) and prostaglandin E2 (PGE2) to mature the DCs. This recipe is based on a classic method of generation of mDCs (28, 29, 41). Alternatively, the system was modified using a serum-free media and changes in cytokines to generate mDCs (**Figure 1B**).

Cancer patients showed significant deficits in the ability to generate mDCs independent of the underlying tumor. There is also substantially more variability in the efficiency of DC generation using monocytes from cancer patients (**Figure 1B**). While we primarily used CD83 up-regulation as indicative of DC maturation, we also noted a lack of CD80 expression and specific functional deficient of these cells. Increased efficiency of DC maturation can be correlated with decreased presence of CD14$^+$HLA-DR$^{lo/neg}$ monocytes in the starting culture (**Figure 1C**). However, we could consistently improve the ability to generate mDCs using serum-free methods with the addition of IL-4. Even so, it was difficult to recapitulate the efficient generation of mDCs we observed using monocytes from healthy volunteers compared to cancer patients. Knowing that CD14$^+$HLA-DR$^{lo/neg}$ monocytes have significant capacity to influence *ex vivo* DC cultures implies that these cells and the pathways to both generate and eliminate them are high-value targets to improve cancer therapies. It is striking to note that these effects occurred in the complete absence of tumors and in the continual presence (for days) with the cells in excess cytokines. This deficit likely represents a significant block in the differentiation pathway. *This strongly suggests that immune stimulation in vivo, even with precise targeting of the pathways known to convert mature DC, is unlikely to efficiently trigger mDC maturation in patients.* Further understanding of the biology of these CD14$^+$HLA-DR$^{lo/neg}$ monocytes is needed; strategies to overcome the effects of these cells can lead to better DC generation and immune reconstitution.

IMPLICATIONS OF CD14$^+$HLA-DR$^{lo/neg}$ ON DC-BASED CANCER VACCINES

Most currently active DC-based cancer immunotherapy protocols differ in either the cell source or some of the methods associated with the generation of DC. The most common approach has been the *ex vivo* generation of mature DCs from patient myeloid-derived monocyte precursors by co-culturing with GM-CSF and various cocktails of cytokines and TLR agonists to produce mature DCs. Optimizing DC culture conditions using normal healthy donors will likely not directly translate into the protocols needed for cancer patients. It will be important for those protocols that use CD14$^+$ cells to generate their DC product from primary patient samples to confirm and optimize the manufacturing method and assure that potent DCs are being generated. In our hands, a serum-free method that includes IL-4 is a good starting point. Adequate sampling size of the patient population is needed to determine the range of differentiation efficiency in each specific cancer patient population to inform the design of release criteria for vaccine manufacturing. Our data also have clear implications for other approaches attempting to mediate anti-tumor immune stimulation. *Adjuvants known to work in healthy people may not work in cancer patients if their approach is to target the DC or DC differentiation pathways.*

As we improve our understanding of the importance of CD14$^+$HLA-DR$^{lo/neg}$ monocytes in promoting immunosuppression, it is imperative that we adjust our clinical practices to ensure effective outcomes for patients using DC-based immunotherapy. This will require continued efforts to develop optimal protocols for generating *ex vivo* DC vaccine preparations and testing these protocols in individual patients. The complexity of the human immune system and individual tumor micro environments will likely require an element of individualized protocol development to achieve optimal clinical benefit.

REFERENCES

1. Moore AJ, Anderson MK. Dendritic cell development: a choose-your-own-adventure story. *Adv Hematol* (2013) **2013**:949513. doi:10.1155/2013/949513
2. Merad M, Sathe P, Helft J, Miller J, Mortha A. The dendritic cell lineage: ontogeny and function of dendritic cells and their subsets in the steady state and the inflamed setting. *Annu Rev Immunol* (2013) **31**:563–604. doi:10.1146/annurev-immunol-020711-074950
3. Chatterjee B, Smed-Sörensen A, Cohn L, Chalouni C, Vandlen R, Lee BC, et al. Internalization and endosomal degradation of receptor-bound antigens regulate the efficiency of cross presentation by human dendritic cells. *Blood* (2012) **120**(10):2011–20. doi:10.1182/blood-2012-01-402370
4. Dudek AM, Martin S, Garg AD, Agostinis P. Immature, semi-mature, and fully mature dendritic cells: toward a DC-cancer cells interface that augments anti-cancer immunity. *Front Immunol* (2013) **4**:438. doi:10.3389/fimmu.2013.00438
5. Cella M, Sallusto F, Lanzavecchia A. Origin, maturation and antigen presenting function of dendritic cells. *Curr Opin Immunol* (1997) **9**(1):10–6. doi:10.1016/S0952-7915(97)80153-7
6. Steinman RM, Hawiger D, Liu K, Bonifaz L, Bonnyay D, Mahnke K, et al. Dendritic cell function in vivo during the steady state: a role in peripheral

tolerance. *Ann N Y Acad Sci* (2003) **987**:15–25. doi:10.1111/j.1749-6632.2003.tb06029.x
7. Dhodapkar MV, Steinman RM, Krasovsky J, Munz C, Bhardwaj N. Antigen-specific inhibition of effector T cell function in humans after injection of immature dendritic cells. *J Exp Med* (2001) **193**(2):233–8. doi:10.1084/jem.193.2.233
8. De Santo C, Salio M, Masri SH, Lee LY, Dong T, Speak AO, et al. Invariant NKT cells reduce the immunosuppressive activity of influenza A virus-induced myeloid-derived suppressor cells in mice and humans. *J Clin Invest* (2008) **118**(12):4036–48. doi:10.1172/JCI36264
9. Van Ginderachter JA, Beschin A, De Baetselier P, Raes G. Myeloid-derived suppressor cells in parasitic infections. *Eur J Immunol* (2010) **40**(11):2976–85. doi:10.1002/eji.201040911
10. Martino A, Badell E, Abadie V, Balloy V, Chignard M, Mistou MY, et al. Mycobacterium bovis bacillus Calmette-Guerin vaccination mobilizes innate myeloid-derived suppressor cells restraining in vivo T cell priming via IL-1R-dependent nitric oxide production. *J Immunol* (2010) **184**(4):2038–47. doi:10.4049/jimmunol.0903348
11. Palucka K, Banchereau J. Cancer immunotherapy via dendritic cells. *Nat Rev Cancer* (2012) **12**(4):265–77. doi:10.1038/nrc3258
12. Palucka K, Banchereau J. Dendritic-cell-based therapeutic cancer vaccines. *Immunity* (2013) **39**(1):38–48. doi:10.1016/j.immuni.2013.07.004
13. Kantoff PW, Schuetz TJ, Blumenstein BA, Glode LM, Bilhartz DL, Wyand M, et al. Overall survival analysis of a phase II randomized controlled trial of a poxviral-based PSA-targeted immunotherapy in metastatic castration-resistant prostate cancer. *J Clin Oncol* (2010) **28**(7):1099–105. doi:10.1200/JCO.2009.25.0597
14. Marshall JL, Gulley JL, Arlen PM, Beetham PK, Tsang KY, Slack R, et al. Phase I study of sequential vaccinations with fowlpox-CEA(6D)-TRICOM alone and sequentially with vaccinia-CEA(6D)-TRICOM, with and without granulocyte-macrophage colony-stimulating factor, in patients with carcinoembryonic antigen-expressing carcinomas. *J Clin Oncol* (2005) **23**(4):720–31. doi:10.1200/JCO.2005.10.206
15. Blalock LT, Landsberg J, Messmer M, Shi J, Pardee AD, Haskell R, et al. Human dendritic cells adenovirally-engineered to express three defined tumor antigens promote broad adaptive and innate immunity. *Oncoimmunology* (2012) **1**(3):287–357. doi:10.4161/onci.18628
16. Lin Y, Gustafson MP, Bulur PA, Gastineau DA, Witzig TE, Dietz AB. Immunosuppressive CD14+HLA-DR(low)/- monocytes in B-cell non-Hodgkin lymphoma. *Blood* (2011) **117**(3):872–81. doi:10.1182/blood-2010-05-283820
17. Vuk-Pavlovic S, Bulur PA, Lin Y, Qin R, Szumlanski CL, Zhao X, et al. Immunosuppressive CD14+HLA-DRlow/- monocytes in prostate cancer. *Prostate* (2010) **70**(4):443–55. doi:10.1002/pros.21078
18. Gustafson MP, Lin Y, New KC, Bulur PA, O'Neill BP, Gastineau DA, et al. Systemic immune suppression in glioblastoma: the interplay between CD14+HLA-DRlo/neg monocytes, tumor factors, and dexamethasone. *Neuro Oncol* (2010) **12**(7):631–44. doi:10.1093/neuonc/noq001
19. Gustafson MP, Abraham RS, Lin Y, Wu W, Gastineau DA, Zent CS, et al. Association of an increased frequency of CD14+ HLA-DR lo/neg monocytes with decreased time to progression in chronic lymphocytic leukaemia (CLL). *Br J Haematol* (2012) **156**(5):674–6. doi:10.1111/j.1365-2141.2011.08902.x
20. Gustafson MP, Lin Y, LaPlant B, Liwski CJ, Maas ML, League SC, et al. Immune monitoring using the predictive power of immune profiles. *J Immunother Cancer* (2013) **1**(7):doi:10.1186/2051-1426-1-7
21. Meyer C, Cagnon L, Costa-Nunes CM, Baumgaertner P, Montandon N, Leyvraz L, et al. Frequencies of circulating MDSC correlate with clinical outcome of melanoma patients treated with ipilimumab. *Cancer Immunol Immunother* (2014) **63**(3):247–57. doi:10.1007/s00262-013-1508-5
22. Filipazzi P, Valenti R, Huber V, Pilla L, Canese P, Iero M, et al. Identification of a new subset of myeloid suppressor cells in peripheral blood of melanoma patients with modulation by a granulocyte-macrophage colony-stimulation factor-based antitumor vaccine. *J Clin Oncol* (2007) **25**(18):2546–53. doi:10.1200/JCO.2006.08.5829
23. Poschke I, Mougiakakos D, Hansson J, Masucci GV, Kiessling R. Immature immunosuppressive CD14+HLA-DR-/low cells in melanoma patients are Stat3hi and overexpress CD80, CD83, and DC-sign. *Cancer Res* (2010) **70**(11):4335–45. doi:10.1158/0008-5472.CAN-09-3767
24. Yuan XK, Zhao XK, Xia YC, Zhu X, Xiao P. Increased circulating immunosuppressive CD14(+)HLA-DR(-/low) cells correlate with clinical cancer stage and pathological grade in patients with bladder carcinoma. *J Int Med Res* (2011) **39**(4):1381–91. doi:10.1177/147323001103900424
25. Huang A, Zhang B, Wang B, Zhang F, Fan KX, Guo YJ. Increased CD14(+)HLA-DR (-/low) myeloid-derived suppressor cells correlate with extrathoracic metastasis and poor response to chemotherapy in non-small cell lung cancer patients. *Cancer Immunol Immunother* (2013) **62**(9):1439–51. doi:10.1007/s00262-013-1450-6
26. Arihara F, Mizukoshi E, Kitahara M, Takata Y, Arai K, Yamashita T, et al. Increase in CD14+HLA-DR -/low myeloid-derived suppressor cells in hepatocellular carcinoma patients and its impact on prognosis. *Cancer Immunol Immunother* (2013) **62**(8):1421–30. doi:10.1007/s00262-013-1447-1
27. Hoechst B, Ormandy LA, Ballmaier M, Lehner F, Krüger C, Manns MP, et al. A new population of myeloid-derived suppressor cells in hepatocellular carcinoma patients induces CD4(+)CD25(+)Foxp3(+) T cells. *Gastroenterology* (2008) **135**(1):234–43. doi:10.1053/j.gastro.2008.03.020
28. Alldawi L, Takahashi M, Narita M, Ayres F, Tsukada N, Osman Y, et al. Effect of prostaglandin E2, lipopolysaccharide, IFN-gamma and cytokines on the generation and function of fast-DC. *Cytotherapy* (2005) **7**(2):195–202. doi:10.1080/14653240510018127
29. Jonuleit H, Kühn U, Müller G, Steinbrink K, Paragnik L, Schmitt E, et al. Pro-inflammatory cytokines and prostaglandins induce maturation of potent immunostimulatory dendritic cells under fetal calf serum-free conditions. *Eur J Immunol* (1997) **27**(12):3135–42. doi:10.1002/eji.1830271209
30. Sallusto F, Lanzavecchia A. Efficient presentation of soluble antigen by cultured human dendritic cells is maintained by granulocyte/macrophage colony-stimulating factor plus interleukin 4 and downregulated by tumor necrosis factor alpha. *J Exp Med* (1994) **179**(4):1109–18. doi:10.1084/jem.179.4.1109
31. Yu J, Du W, Yan F, Wang Y, Li H, Cao S, et al. Myeloid-derived suppressor cells suppress antitumor immune responses through IDO expression and correlate with lymph node metastasis in patients with breast cancer. *J Immunol* (2013) **190**(7):3783–97. doi:10.4049/jimmunol.1201449
32. Mougiakakos D, Jitschin R, von Bahr L, Poschke I, Gary R, Sundberg B, et al. Immunosuppressive CD14+HLA-DRlow/neg IDO+ myeloid cells in patients following allogeneic hematopoietic stem cell transplantation. *Leukemia* (2013) **27**(2):377–88. doi:10.1038/leu.2012.215
33. Maeda A, Kawamura T, Ueno T, Usui N, Miyagawa S. Monocytic suppressor cells derived from human peripheral blood suppress xenogenic immune reactions. *Xenotransplantation* (2014) **21**(1):46–56. doi:10.1111/xen.12067
34. Zea AH, Rodriguez PC, Atkins MB, Hernandez C, Signoretti S, Zabaleta J, et al. Arginase-producing myeloid suppressor cells in renal cell carcinoma patients: a mechanism of tumor evasion. *Cancer Res* (2005) **65**(8):3044–8. doi:10.1158/0008-5472.CAN-045-4505
35. Poschke I, Mao Y, Adamson L, Salazar-Onfray F, Masucci G, Kiessling R. Myeloid-derived suppressor cells impair the quality of dendritic cell vaccines. *Cancer Immunol Immunother* (2012) **61**(6):827–38. doi:10.1007/s00262-011-1143-y
36. Kusmartsev S, Nefedova Y, Yoder D, Gabrilovich DI. Antigen-specific inhibition of CD8+ T cell response by immature myeloid cells in cancer is mediated by reactive oxygen species. *J Immunol* (2004) **172**(2):989–99.
37. Kusmartsev S, Eruslanov E, Kübler H, Tseng T, Sakai Y, Su Z, et al. Oxidative stress regulates expression of VEGFR1 in myeloid cells: link to tumor-induced immune suppression in renal cell carcinoma. *J Immunol* (2008) **181**(1):346–53.
38. Srivastava MK, Sinha P, Clements VK, Rodriguez P, Ostrand-Rosenberg S. Myeloid-derived suppressor cells inhibit T-cell activation by depleting cystine and cysteine. *Cancer Res* (2010) **70**(1):68–77. doi:10.1158/0008-5472.CAN-09-2587
39. Ostrand-Rosenberg S. Myeloid-derived suppressor cells: more mechanisms for inhibiting antitumor immunity. *Cancer Immunol Immunother* (2010) **59**(10):1593–600. doi:10.1007/s00262-010-0855-8
40. Shen P, Wang A, He M, Wang Q, Zheng S. Increased circulating Lin CD33 HLA-DR myeloid-derived suppressor cells in hepatocellular carcinoma patients. *Hepatol Res* (2013). doi:10.1111/hepr.12167
41. Dietz AB, Padley DJ, Butler GW, Maas ML, Greiner CW, Gastineau DA, et al. Clinical-grade manufacturing of DC from CD14+ precursors: experience from phase I clinical trials in CML and malignant melanoma. *Cytotherapy* (2004) **6**(6):563–70. doi:10.1080/14653240410005357-1

12

Estimating the diversity, completeness, and cross-reactivity of the T cell repertoire

Veronika I. Zarnitsyna[1]*, Brian D. Evavold[2], Louis N. Schoettle[3], Joseph N. Blattman[3] and Rustom Antia[1]*

[1] Department of Biology, Emory University, Atlanta, GA, USA
[2] Department of Microbiology and Immunology, Emory University, Atlanta, GA, USA
[3] Center for Infectious Diseases and Vaccinology, School of Life Sciences, Arizona State University, Tempe, AZ, USA

Edited by:
Rob J. De Boer, Utrecht University, Netherlands

Reviewed by:
Mario Castro, Comillas Pontifical University, Spain
Aridaman Pandit, Utrecht University, Netherlands

***Correspondence:**
Veronika I. Zarnitsyna and Rustom Antia, Department of Biology, Emory University, 1510 Clifton Road, Atlanta, GA 30322, USA
e-mail: veronika.i.zarnitsyna@emory.edu; rustom.antia@emory.edu

In order to recognize and combat a diverse array of pathogens the immune system has a large repertoire of T cells having unique T cell receptors (TCRs) with only a few clones specific for any given antigen. We discuss how the number of different possible TCRs encoded in the genome (the potential repertoire) and the number of different TCRs present in an individual (the realized repertoire) can be measured. One puzzle is that the potential repertoire greatly exceeds the realized diversity of naïve T cells within any individual. We show that the existing hypotheses fail to explain why the immune system has the potential to generate far more diversity than is used in an individual, and propose an alternative hypothesis of "evolutionary sloppiness." Another immunological puzzle is why mice and humans have similar repertoires even though humans have over 1000-fold more T cells. We discuss how the idea of the "protecton," the smallest unit of protection, might explain this discrepancy and estimate the size of "protecton" based on available precursor frequencies data. We then consider T cell cross-reactivity – the ability of a T cell clone to respond to more than one epitope. We extend existing calculations to estimate the extent of expected cross-reactivity between the responses to different pathogens. Our results are consistent with two observations: a low probability of observing cross-reactivity between the immune responses to two randomly chosen pathogens; and the ensemble of memory cells being sufficiently diverse to generate cross-reactive responses to new pathogens.

Keywords: $\alpha\beta$ **T cell, repertoire, precursor frequency, cross-reactivity, pathogen recognition**

1. INTRODUCTION

The clonal selection theory of adaptive immunity requires that the immune system is able to produce a large and diverse repertoire of immune cells (clones), with each cell expressing a receptor with different antigenic specificity (1, 2). Following infection, the few clones that are specific for the antigens expressed by the pathogen proliferate and differentiate into effector cells which control the infection. Subsequently, the maintenance of an increased number of these pathogen-specific cells results in long-lasting immunological memory (3–5). Accurate quantification of changes in the numbers of antigen-specific cells during infection and vaccination, together with advances in molecular and cellular biology, has allowed us to make considerable progress toward understanding the dynamics of the generation of immune responses (3, 6, 7) and the requirements for pathogen control (8, 9). Furthermore, deep sequencing technology has provided a first quantitative snapshot of the diversity of immune cells (10, 11). These technological advances set the stage for understanding the relationship between the diversity of immune cells (the repertoire) and immune protection from an extensive array of pathogens to which we are exposed.

We begin by outlining our current understanding of T cell receptor diversity and discussing problems associated with the quantification of the T cell repertoire. Next, we explore how diverse the immune system needs to be by exploring the relationship between the diversity of the T cell repertoire and its ability to provide protection from pathogens. Finally we consider how the degree of specificity of T cells (often defined by measuring how cross-reactive they are) affects the relationship between the repertoire and host response to a given pathogen. We focus on $\alpha\beta$ T cells and the term "T cell" refers to the CD8 subpopulation of T cells unless we explicitly specify a different subpopulation.

We have intentionally used simple models and calculations because, in the absence of detailed information on the terms and parameters, simpler models frequently generate more robust qualitative results than complex models (12, 13). The focus of the paper is to highlight the limitations arising from uncertainties in current estimates of parameters, and in particular to gain maximum insight from the one key parameter – the precursor frequency of T cells specific for different epitopes – that can be accurately measured. Throughout this paper we emphasize current puzzles and problems and, where possible, suggest new approaches to solving them.

2. MEASURING THE DIVERSITY OF THE T CELL REPERTOIRE

2.1. WHAT IS THE POTENTIAL REPERTOIRE?

T cells develop from progenitor cells in the thymus where the germline T cell receptor (TCR) α and β genes undergo somatic recombination of the V-J and V-D-J gene segments, respectively (14, 15). The antigenic specificity of each T cell is determined by the amino acid sequence of these rearranged TCR genes, and in particular by the hypervariable complementarity determining region 3 (CDR3) that mostly account for direct contacts with peptides presented on major histocompatibility complex (MHC) proteins, and is encoded by the junction of the V, (D), and J gene segments (16). The diversity of generated TCR genes is therefore due to: (1) selection of one from a number of possible V, D, and J gene segments, (2) semi-random cleavage of recombination hairpin intermediates, and (3) N-nucleotide addition and subtraction at the junction of V, D, and J genes (17, 18). Finally, the pairing of different α and β chains to generate a functional receptor results in additional diversity (19).

How many different T cell receptors can be generated? The first steps toward understanding the magnitude of the diversity of the T cell repertoire came from the pioneering studies that identified the molecular mechanisms involved in the recombination of V, (D), and J gene segments and N-region diversification described above for the generation of the α and β TCR chains (14, 15, 19). It was estimated that these processes together with pairing between different α and β chains could give rise to around 10^{15} possible $\alpha\beta$ TCR (19). The question of the potential number of TCR sequences has recently been revisited and significantly larger estimates for the diversity of the TCR β chain were obtained (20, 21). Murugan et al. (21) used statistical analysis of non-productive TCR β chain to conclude that the CDR3 (variable) region of the TCR β chain alone has a potential diversity of $\sim 10^{14}$ different sequences. They used empirical β chain data to show that N-nucleotide insertions at the V-D and D-J junctions are uncorrelated, their length distributions are nearly identical and their lengths could exceed six nucleotides which was assumed in previous estimates (19). We might expect that a similar analysis would result in upward revision for the potential diversity of the α chain (though the estimates of diversity would increase less than for the β chain because the α chain has only one V-J junction). This will result in a truly enormous potential repertoire of over 10^{20} for the $\alpha\beta$ TCR.

2.2. WHAT IS THE REALIZED REPERTOIRE IN AN INDIVIDUAL?

Only mature T cells that have passed thymic selection (naïve T cells) can be employed in immune responses for protection against pathogens. Thus, in order to understand the balance between diversity and protection, the most important measurement is the "realized" T cell diversity in an individual (i.e., the actual number of different TCR in the mature T cell compartment).

The diversity of the naïve T cell repertoire was initially estimated prior to the advent of deep sequencing technologies by the use of spectrotyping, which involved amplifying mRNA from particular V-J sequence combinations, separating the amplified products on the basis of size, and exhaustive conventional sequencing of a particular length CDR3 product. The diversity of TCR sequences in this sample was then extrapolated to the total T cell population.

2.2.1. *TCR diversity and clone size in humans*

Arstila et al. (22) used spectrotyping to estimate that there are 10^6 β chains in the blood each pairing on average with at least 25 different α chains, and consequently proposed a lower bound to the estimate of the T cell repertoire in humans of around 2.5×10^7 specificities. Advances in deep sequencing have confirmed that estimation of β chains is in the range of $1 - 4 \times 10^6$ (20, 23, 24).

There is however considerable uncertainty about the extent to which 2.5×10^7 specificities underestimates the diversity of T cells in humans (25, 26). A repertoire of 2.5×10^7 suggests a naïve clone size on average of over 4×10^3 cells ($>10^{11}/(2.5 \times 10^7)$). This could happen if each clone gets produced multiple times or if once produced a given clone would undergo about 12 rounds of division. The first scenario is unlikely, given the very large estimates of potential diversity (19–21). If the second scenario happens, it must occur in the periphery. Expansion of clones in the thymus would result in a much lower frequency of detectable T cell receptor excision circles (TRECs) in the naïve pool of recent thymic emigrants than is currently observed (27–29). Arstila et al. points out that naïve T cells in the periphery could divide more than 12 times during a human lifespan (26). However, as the total number of naïve T cells remains relatively stable (because division is balanced by death) changes in clone size would have to arise from stochastic drift and this seems unlikely.

2.2.2. *TCR diversity and clone size in mice*

Interestingly, it was estimated that TCR β chain diversity in mouse spleen is quite similar to the one measured in human blood. The β chain repertoire of $5 - 8 \times 10^5$ specificities with each variable domain of β chain sequence being shared by 30–40 T splenocytes have been reported using spectrotyping technology (30). Pairing with α chain was estimated to add a factor of 2.4 and resulted in total $\alpha\beta$ TCR diversity of 2×10^6. Taking into account that there are 2×10^7 splenocytes it was estimated that the clone size of $\alpha\beta$ TCR is equal to 10 cells (30). The bias in recombination and α-β TCR pairing will likely affect the T cell clone size. A recent study that enumerated the number of naïve T cells specific for different epitopes suggests that there are between 15 and 1500 unique cells in the mouse spleen specific for any given epitope, implying that the number of naïve cells with a given TCR α-β combination is very small, and indeed that most clonotypes have clone size of one (31, 32). This is in contrast with the earlier estimates that suggest an average clone size of 10 cells/clone in the spleen (30). Consequently, it brings the repertoire in the spleen toward the total number of naïve T cells in the spleen, and increases the lower bound of the total $\alpha\beta$ T cell repertoire in the mouse by an order of magnitude. In this case the estimate of 2×10^7 specificities becomes very close to a lower bound estimation for human T cell repertoire.

2.2.3. *Limitations in estimates of realized diversity*

Current estimates of the realized diversity are lower bounds. The limitations of these studies is the lack of information on the pairing of different TCR α and β chains. Bulk sequencing of a single chain, or even of both TCR α and β chains, is not sufficient to inform us of the potential diversity (33). In principle this problem could be comprehensively addressed by single cell sequencing that would obtain linked α and β chain sequences, but this remains technically and financially infeasible for the large sample sizes required to evaluate naïve repertoires with high diversity (34); the cost of single cell sequencing remains at \$1 per cell, making the analysis of T cells from a single mouse more than a \$10 million experiment! Oil emulsion lysis strategies (35) combined with micro-sequencing have increased the capacity of such single-cell studies, but these still are only able to capture <1% of the total naïve T cell repertoire in a single mouse. New techniques or methods need to be developed.

In order to have an accurate and comprehensive quantitative description of diversity, it is important to define what we mean by diversity. We can describe T cell repertoire diversity in terms of summary measures of diversity borrowed from the ecological literature. This includes enumerating the number of distinct clones or computing the Simpson diversity index (36) that takes into account the number of clones and their frequencies. However these summary approaches compress all of the diversity information into a single number. A more comprehensive statistical approach retains the frequency distribution of different clone sizes. In **Figure 1** we show a plot of the frequency distribution of β chain sequences in the mouse naïve T cells using preliminary data. We find a majority of β chain sequences are present at low frequencies and fewer sequences occurring at much higher frequencies. A key problem is that we do not know the α chain sequences pairing with each of these β chains, and this restricts our ability to infer diversity of T cells from these observations.

Several clones in **Figure 1** have very high frequencies and the exact underling mechanisms are not known. The sequences which are more common (generated more frequently) are more likely to be shared between different individuals. It was reported that inbred mice and individuals with the same MHC share some T cells with identical receptors (11, 20, 37, 38). These constitute "public" T cell clones, in contrast with the majority of the T cell clones that are unique to an individual and comprise the "private" part of a repertoire response. In general, the frequency of public TCR clonotypes exceeds what is expected if T cells were chosen at random with equal probability from the total potential repertoire, and perhaps

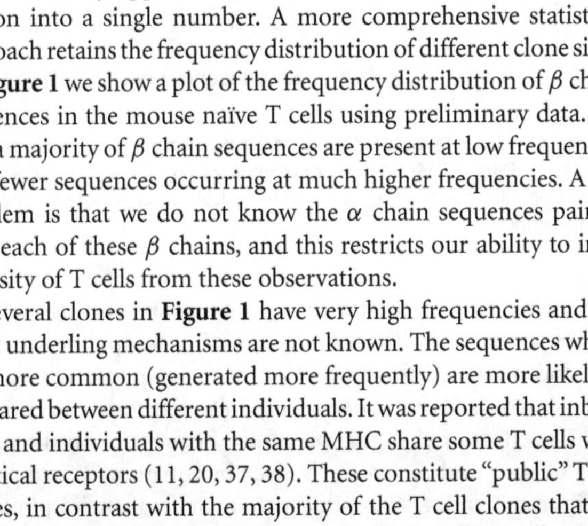

FIGURE 1 | Plot of the frequency distribution in the β chain sequences of naïve CD8 T cells. Naïve (CD44^{lo}) CD8 T cells from C57Bl/6 mice were isolated by magnetic beads and >98% purity confirmed by flow cytometry. Genomic DNA was subjected to TCRβ V-J multiplex DNA sequencing and the distribution of unique in-frame CDR3 sequences is plotted. We note that the term "clone" on the x and y axis labels refers to clones based on β chain sequences alone.

not surprisingly, the clone size of public T cells is higher than that of private T cells in the naïve T cell repertoire [(33); Blattman et al. unpublished results]. This has been suggested to arise due to MHC restriction during thymic selection, biased frequencies of recombination, as well as degeneracy in the genetic code which allows more than one nucleotide sequence to give rise to the same amino acid sequence (33, 39). The factors involved in the evolution and/or selection of public T cell clonotypes and their possible role in the control of infections remain puzzling questions.

In summary we have estimates of the potential repertoire of upward of 10^{20} TCR. The estimates of the realized repertoire suggest lower bounds of 2.5×10^7 and 2×10^6 in humans and mice. Two puzzles which we will address are: why humans and mice might have similar repertoire sizes (Section 3.2); and why the potential repertoire so greatly exceed the realized repertoire (Section 3.3).

3. UNDERSTANDING DIVERSITY, THE REPERTOIRE AND CROSS-REACTIVITY

In this section we use quantitative calculations to explore the consequences of the observations on the repertoire described in the previous section. We begin by looking at whether the diversity of the repertoire may be explained by the relationship between diversity and protection. We then address questions associated with our current understanding of repertoire diversity and cross-reactivity.

3.1. RELATIONSHIP BETWEEN DIVERSITY AND PROTECTION

Clearly a large repertoire is required to generate a T cell response to a diverse array of pathogens. However, to our knowledge, few empirical studies consider the relationship between the repertoire and protection. To some extent the paucity of experiments on this topic is because of difficulties in quantifying the repertoire (see earlier discussion). Studies on mice, expressing a single fixed transgenic TCR chain (either α or β) that measure the number of different paired endogenously recombined TCR chains, have shown that pairing is not completely random, as these mice express repertoires of reduced diversity and altered V gene usage (40–43). However, even in these mice there is still sufficient diversity to generate effective, albeit reduced, responses to control pathogen infections.

A relatively simple calculation can be made to estimate how diverse the TCR repertoire needs to be in order to provide reliable protection following infection with a pathogen. To provide protection against a pathogen there must be some number of clones present in the repertoire that are specific for that pathogen. Here, we extend the logic outlined in (44, 45). Let R be the T cell repertoire and let p_i be the probability that a randomly chosen TCR binds to i^{th} of the k epitopes derived from a given pathogen ($i = 1{:}k$). Note that p_i is also equal to the precursor frequency of T cells for i^{th} epitope. A pathogen is not detected if all R naïve T cell clones fail to recognize it, and this will happen with probability.

$$P_E = (1 - p_1)^R (1 - p_2)^R \dots (1 - p_k)^R$$

$$\approx \exp(-p_1 R)\exp(-p_2 R)\dots \exp(-p_k R) = \exp\left(-R\sum_{i=1}^{k} p_i\right) \quad (1)$$

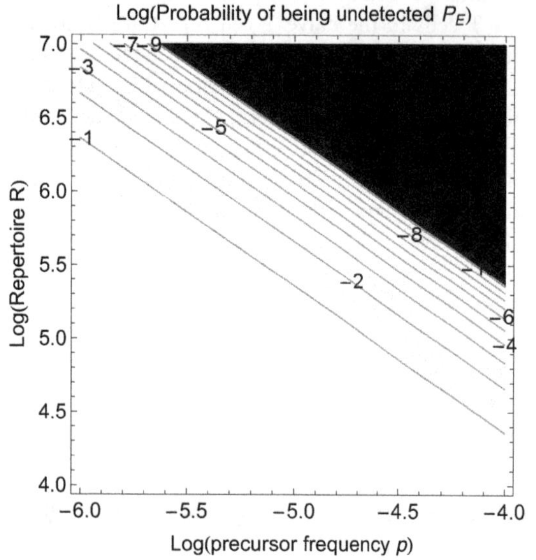

FIGURE 2 | The probability a pathogen is not detected, P_E, as a function of the log of the precursor frequency p and the log of the naïve T cell repertoire R. The numbers on the contour lines in the plot indicate log P_E values. Black color corresponds to the values of P_E below the threshold of 10^{-10}.

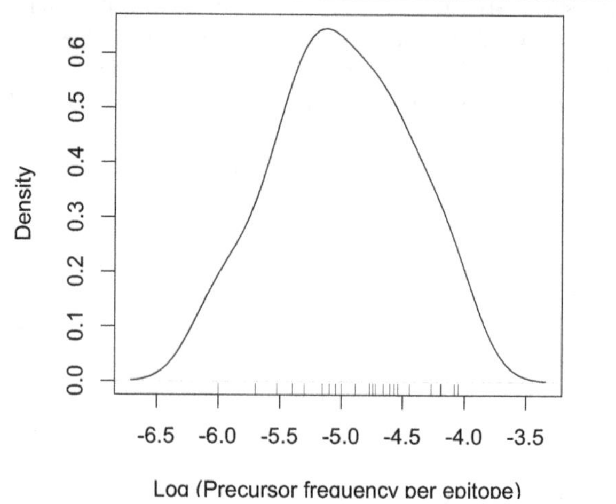

FIGURE 3 | Density distribution plotted from the precursor frequencies of naïve CD8 T cells for different epitopes reported in (31). The tick marks on the top of the x-axis indicate individual epitopes. Note the log scale on the x-axis.

which gives

$$R = \frac{-\ln(P_E)}{\sum_{i=1}^{k} p_i} \quad (2)$$

Equation (2) tells us how big the repertoire must be to detect at level P_E. **Figure 2** shows how the probability that a pathogen is not detected by the immune system depends on the repertoire size and the total precursor frequency $p = \sum p_i$. There is a very rapid decline in the probability of not being detected once the product of p and R becomes sufficiently large. We should note that P_E is often termed as the "probability of escape" but it should not be confused with the usage of the term "escape" that refers to the generation of escape mutants in T cell epitopes after recognition has already occurred following infections such as HIV.

If we know the precursor frequencies for pathogen epitopes and total number of epitopes we can relate the probability of being not detected to the repertoire R. We have much more accurate estimates for precursor frequencies against specific epitopes than for repertoire sizes (31, 46, 47). A recently developed method that combines pMHC tetramer staining with magnetic particle-based cell enrichment allows for the direct measurement of the frequency of naïve cells to different epitopes for both mice and humans (31, 48). **Figure 3** shows the density distribution of naïve T cell precursor frequencies for different CD8 T cell epitopes in mice determined by this cell enrichment method using MHC tetramers complexed with different class I-restricted peptides (31). The total number of responded cells per mouse (naïve precursor frequency multiplied by total CD8 T cell number) varied from 15 in response to the L-338:D^b epitope of LCMV to 1500 in response to an epitope from the murine cytomegalovirus (31). These estimates concur with previous *in vivo* estimates of precursor frequencies. These studies transferred different numbers of naive epitope-specific T cells and measured the proportion of the response arising from expansion of host versus donor cells following virus infection (46, 47). The effect of changing precursor frequencies on the probability of been undetected, P_E, is given by equation (2) and plotted in **Figures 2** and **4**. Note, that precursor frequencies plotted in **Figure 3** are likely biased toward immunodominant epitopes. Immunodominance is a complex issue, and the major factors that affect the magnitude of the T cell response to a particular epitope include: the processing and presentation of peptide on MHC (i.e., the amount of epitope); the number of precursor cells for this epitope; their affinities for the epitope; the extent of their recruitment and competition between the T cells for this and other pathogen epitopes (31, 49–51).

3.2. SCALING AND THE CONCEPT OF A "PROTECTON"

We now consider the scaling of the repertoire with the size of the organism. A few pathogen-specific precursors in a tadpole are likely to be able to mount a faster and more effective response than the same number of cells in an elephant (52). Langman and Cohen proposed the basic functional unit, the "protecton," capable of providing robust protection. They suggested a tadpole (smallest vertebrate) has a single "protecton," and the number of "protectons" scales with the size of an organism. Localized infections are surveyed by a draining lymph node rather than the entire immune system and thus we expect this unit should contain at least one "protecton." Clearly the calculations for P_E (how diverse the immune system needs to be to recognize pathogens) pertains to the "protecton" [see equations (1) and (2)].

Lets estimate the diversity in a "protecton." **Figure 4** shows how the probability of being undetected depends on the size of the repertoire R for different total precursor frequencies. The precursor frequency of T cells specific for a pathogen is, to a first approximation, the sum of the precursor frequencies for that

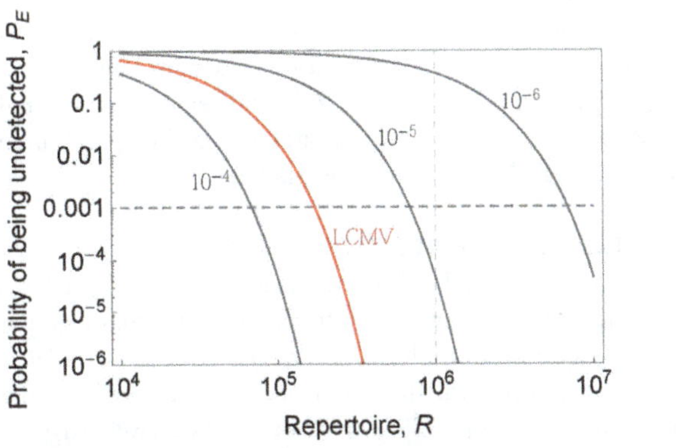

FIGURE 4 | Probability that a pathogen is not recognized P_E (y-axis) is plotted as a function of the repertoire (x-axis) for indicated pathogen-specific precursor frequencies (gray lines). LCMV case ($p = 4 \times 10^{-5}$) is shown in red color.

pathogen's different epitopes presented by MHC proteins. This can be estimated for LCMV by combining reported naïve precursor frequencies for few measured epitopes (31) and measurements of the fraction of the total LCMV specific responses which is directed against these epitopes (53). This gives us a total precursor frequency for LCMV specific T cells equal to ~4×10^{-5}, and from **Figure 4**, a level of protection $P_E = 10^{-3}$ (i.e., 1 in 1000 "protectons" will fail to recognize LCMV) requires the repertoire in the "protecton" to be about 1.7×10^5. In order to know the level of protection against diverse pathogens we need to know the distribution of precursor frequencies to pathogens. The existing data gives us lower bounds (because only cells specific for a few epitopes are measured) to the precursor frequencies of viruses such as MCMV (~1.3×10^{-4}), Influenza (~4×10^{-5}), Vaccinia (~1.1×10^{-4}), RSV (~4.5×10^{-5}), HSV (~2.9×10^{-5}), and VSV (~10^{-5}) (31). The precursor frequencies for those viruses are comparable or greater than that for LCMV with the exception of VSV and HSV for which only single epitope data were reported in (31). If this trend holds (i.e., the precursor frequency per pathogen is $>10^{-5}$) it might suggest that having a repertoire of 7×10^{-5} is sufficient to give robust protection at the level $P_E = 10^{-3}$, and thus define the size of the "protecton." For P_E one order of magnitude lower and higher, i.e., $P_E = 10^{-4} - 10^{-2}$ will require a repertoire of ~$9 \times 10^5 - 5 \times 10^5$, suggesting that our estimate is quite robust to changes in P_E (see **Figure 4**). We can expect the area of local surveillance (a small lymph node) in mice to have at least this number of different T cells.

How much bigger should the total repertoire size be so that the area corresponding to one "protecton," randomly filled with T cells from the total circulating cells, has a relatively low number of clone repeats? We estimated that if f is a fraction of clone repeats in the "protecton" area with m cells, the total repertoire size R is bounded as $(1 - f)(m - 1)/(2f) < R < (m - 1)/(2f)$. For example, for 5 or 10% of clone repeats in m we will have a multiplication factor for m for the total diversity in the ranges ~9.5 – 10 or ~4.5 – 5, respectively. To derive this formula we used two assumptions: first, the clones are equal in size and second, the size of total repertoire multiplied by clone size is much bigger than the size m. These calculations show that the total diversity doesn't need to be much higher than the diversity in a "protecton."

Several theoretical papers previously estimated that the repertoire of B and T cells scales as $ln(cM)$, where c is a constant and M is the mass of an organism (45, 54). It was also estimated that humans should have B cell repertoire 2–5 times larger than mice (45) and similar reasoning could be apply to T cell repertoire. The diversity of the repertoire is linked to clone size and it was estimated that the size of T cell clones should scale as M and, correspondingly, the total number of T cells should scale as $Mln(cM)$ (45). Wiegel and Perelson's estimate shows that the repertoire in a human need not be much higher than that in a mouse even though the number of naïve cells in these organisms differs by over 10^3 fold [mice have ~10^8 T cells (30, 46) and humans between 10^{11} and 10^{12} T cells (22, 55, 56)].

Another reason for why humans need a more diverse repertoire than mice pertains to the number of pathogens to which they are exposed. As humans live longer than mice, other factors being equal, they will be exposed to more pathogens and require a lower P_E.

3.3. EVOLUTIONARY CONSIDERATIONS: WHY ENCODE SUCH A DIVERSE POTENTIAL REPERTOIRE?

The calculations described in the previous section are consistent with the diversity of the repertoire that is observed in mice and humans (22, 30) (lower bound diversity in the range of 2×10^6 to 2.5×10^7 unique $\alpha\beta$ T cells), and the diversity is sufficient to generate a low probability that a given pathogen is not detected ($P_E < 10^{-4}$). What those estimations don't explain is why the immune system is able to generate a potential diversity of more than 10^{15} T cell specificities (19–21) that is vastly in excess of the realized repertoire?

Let's consider a number of potential explanations for why the potential repertoire needs to be much larger than the realized repertoire. One simplistic explanation takes into account the observation that most of the generated progenitor T cells are deleted during positive and negative selection in the thymus. If a fraction f of the T cells generated in the thymus gets selected (i.e., pass positive or negative selection) then the potential repertoire should be $(1/f)$ times the peripheral repertoire. Since only 3–5% of T cells pass thymic selection (57, 58), the potential repertoire need only be at most 33-fold higher than the realized repertoire, thus ruling out this explanation.

A second potential reason is the need to successfully recognize peptides in the context of the hundreds of MHC alleles in the population. The reported extent of thymic selection (see previous paragraph) allows us to reject this hypothesis – different cells may be selected in different MHC backgrounds but in all cases 3–5% of T cells pass thymic selection.

A third potential reason is the need to prevent pathogen escape mutations – mutations in an epitope that prevent it from being recognized by the immune system. To a first approximation having more than one epitope is the key factor that prevents escape – if the pathogen has k epitopes the probability of escaping all epitopes declines as μ^k, where μ is the probability of mutation leading to the loss of one epitope. The number of epitopes to which a response is generated involves many factors such as immunodominance,

MHC diversity, and T cell diversity. The relationship between these quantities is not understood and we do not know the contribution of T cell diversity to immunodominance due to problems in estimating TCR diversity described above. However from **Figure 4** we note that the repertoire is sufficiently large to enable robust detection of subdominant epitopes in a biologically reasonable range of precursor frequencies [**Figure 2**; (31)].

A fourth potential reason considers the temporal aspect and changes in the repertoire over the lifespan of an individual. Thymic emigration results in a constantly changing repertoire over time. The total number of different T cells present in the individual over its lifespan could be much greater than its repertoire at any given time. In humans, for example, if we assume that thymic emigration is of the order of $10^7 - 10^8$ cells per day (59, 60) then the realized repertoire over a lifespan might be as much as 10^{12} specificities which is much closer to the potential repertoire. There are two problems with this approach. First, it does not explain why mice have about the same potential repertoire as humans since a similar calculation for mice would result in a realized repertoire over the lifespan several orders of magnitude lower than humans. This is because both mice thymic output of the order of 10^6 cells per day (61–63) and lifespan are smaller than for humans. Second, protection is related to the repertoire at a given time point. Changing the particular clones in the repertoire over time does not help unless the relevant clones are present at the time of infection or generated during the infection and consequently able to help with clearance of the pathogen. The continual influx of cells of new specificities is thus unlikely to be of significance for acute infections which are relatively brief, but has been suggested to contribute to the maintenance of the response during persistent infections (64–66). In the case of persistent infections, however, an occasional new pathogen-specific clone is unlikely to clear the infection if the much larger number of clones at the onset were not able to do so – and the new clone is likely to be exhausted rapidly. Finally, temporal aspects could change the total repertoire if we consider the sum of both naïve and memory compartments. As naïve cells convert to memory cells each time we confront an infection, the replenishment of naïve compartment with the cells of new specificities would increase the total repertoire (naïve plus memory compartments). However, even if the memory compartment is as diverse as the naïve, the total diversity would increase at most by a factor of 2 in comparison to the naïve compartment alone. Taken together we don't expect temporal aspects to account for the differences in the sizes of the potential and realized repertoires.

We now describe a new evolutionary explanation that we call "evolutionary sloppiness." The process of generation of diversity by recombination and N nucleotide addition and deletion are sloppy processes. To reduce the amount of diversity that can be generated might require putting additional costly constraints on these processes. This would explain why organisms are able to generate far more TCR diversity (in excess of 10^{15} TCR) then is needed. Finally we note that not all aspects of biology result in perfectly optimized solutions (67).

Additionally, it has been suggested that the thymus is an energy- and resource-expensive organ (68) but these energetic costs have yet to be quantified. Energetic costs to cell production and thymic selection would favor expansion of clones after thymic selection (i.e., to have an amplifier). This amplification could take place in the thymus or periphery and would scale with the size of the organism. This would result in clone sizes in men being ~1000-fold higher than in mice, which is unlikely (see discussion on TRECs in Section 2.2.1). Accurate estimates for clone sizes in humans and mice should allow us to resolve this question.

3.4. T CELL CROSS-REACTIVITY

Cross-reactivity is related to the observation that a given T cell can respond to more than one epitope, including epitopes that show strong sequence homology or completely unrelated (69–76). As might be expected the frequency of the former is higher than that of the latter. Flexible TCR-pMHC binding sites were suggested as a possible structural explanation for known high degree of $\alpha\beta$ TCRs cross-reactivity to different pMHCs (77–80). Cross-reactivity can also arise in T cell clones with incomplete allelic exclusion at the α chain loci resulting in one β chain pairing with two different α chains. An upper bound on the frequency of such clones was estimated to be 30% (81–83).

The pioneering experiments of Selin and Welsh (69) found that the CD8 T cell responses of mice to pathogens such as the Pichinde virus (PV), Vaccinia virus (VV), and Lymphocytic choriomeningitis virus (LCMV) showed high levels of cross-reactivity. They found that prior vaccination with one of these viruses expanded a specific CD8 T cell subset that could be boosted during stimulation by the other viruses and showed an unexpectedly complex relationship between the responses to different viruses with asymmetry depending on the order of viral exposure (infection A followed by B stimulated different cross-reactivity than B followed by A) (69, 71, 84). In a very recent paper (80) the cross-reactivity studies were extended to analysis of the CD4 T cell repertoire against pathogens to which individuals had never been exposed. Surprisingly, they found that a large fraction of the CD4 T cells specific for these pathogens exhibited a memory phenotype and suggested that they had been generated by cross-reactive responses to other previously encountered pathogens including heterologous infections or environmental antigens.

The extent of cross-reactivity between the immune responses to different pathogens is of practical importance. Murine studies have not only demonstrated the presence of T cells that could cross-react between different pathogens such as PV, VV, and LCMV, but also showed that this cross-reactivity affected pathogenesis during subsequent infection (84–86). If these occurrences of cross-reactive responses are rare, then the examples above are simply interesting curiosities. If, on the other hand, cross-reactivity is common then we would need to move from our current paradigm, which looks at each infection independent of other infections, to a more complex view that incorporates the terms for the interactions between the immune responses to different pathogens. Thus a key step is to quantify the extent of cross-reactivity in the immune responses to different pathogens.

How can we predict the level of cross-reactivity between two pathogens? The current approach is based on the observation that number of possible peptide-MHC complexes is much larger than the total number of T cells, suggesting that a given T cell must be able to recognize many different peptide-MHC (i.e. have a high level of cross-reactivity) (87, 88). However it is not clear how these parameters can be measured. We propose an alternative calculation that allows estimation of the extent of cross-reactivity from the precursor frequency of T cells for pathogens – a parameter that can be reliably determined. Using slightly modified notation from (87) we first define four parameters:

R Repertoire (the number of clonotypically different naïve T cells in the repertoire)
r The number of different T cell clonotypes that will respond to the same peptide
N The total number of potentially immunogenic foreign peptides in the environment
n The number of different peptides to which a single T cell clonotype will respond

These four parameters are linked by the conservation equation (87):

$$rN = nR \tag{3}$$

Lets suggest that a given pathogen has k epitopes to which T cells can mount a response. For a given T cell, the probability to recognize at least one epitope from a given pathogen could be written as:

$$1 - \left[1 - \frac{n}{N}\right]^k \tag{4}$$

The probability that the same T cell will recognize at least one epitope on each of two pathogens with k epitopes (i.e., will be cross-reactive) will be a square of expression equation (4) and the probability to find at least one cross-reactive clone is equal to:

$$\left[1 - \left[1 - \frac{n}{N}\right]^k\right]^2 \times R \tag{5}$$

Note, that in derived equation (5) we don't know the parameters k, n, and N which makes it very difficult to apply directly. Interestingly, for one epitope ($k = 1$) and with application of cross-reactivity equation (3) the equation (5) simplifies to:

$$\left[1 - \left[1 - \frac{n}{N}\right]\right]^2 \times R = \left[1 - \left[1 - \frac{r}{R}\right]\right]^2 \times R = \left[\frac{r}{R}\right]^2 \times R \tag{6}$$

Under the assumption that all naïve T cells able to respond to a given epitope are clonotypically different, which is supported by recent data (31, 80), we can think of r/R as a precursor frequency for a given epitope. The problem of estimating cross-reactivity in this case will be similar to the problem of estimating the probability of randomly choosing a two-colored ball from an urn when the frequencies of each of two colors are known. Interestingly, the measured naïve precursor frequencies for different immunogenic epitopes are similar for mice and humans and range from 1 to 100 cells per million cells (31). According to equation (3), this similarity immediately implies that cross-reactivity of each T cell receptor, n, is in the same range for mice and humans.

For the case when $k > 1$, we could not directly use the formula (5), due to unknown parameters, but can use a simple probabilistic calculation based on sampling multiple colored balls. We can write the frequency of cross-reactive cells between two randomly chosen pathogens (A and B) in terms of the precursor frequencies of T cells to these two pathogens, p_A and p_B, and the total number of cells T:

$$\text{Expected number of cross-reactive cells} = p_A p_B \times T \tag{7}$$

and if we have clones of same size equal to T/R,

$$\text{Expected number of cross-reactive clones} = p_A p_B \times R \tag{8}$$

where R equals the repertoire (the number of different T cell clones in each individual). When the average number of cross-reactive clones is less than one, equation (8) gives us the probability of observing a cross-reactive response between two pathogens in a single individual. We can use this framework together with the data on precursor frequencies (31) described in **Figure 2** to get an estimate of the extent of cross-reactivity between the responses to unrelated pathogens. As described earlier we have an approximate precursor frequency per epitope of 10^{-5}, and a precursor frequency per pathogen, with LCMV as an example, of about 4×10^{-5}. If we assume there are about 2×10^7 naïve CD8 T cells per mouse (89) then the number of cross-reactive cells between two unrelated pathogens will be ~0.032, which suggests cross-reactivity is very rare (a single cross-reactive clone will be found <4% of the time). In order to observe cross-reactivity between two random pathogens in a mouse we would need to have a precursor frequency per pathogen of at least 2.2×10^{-4}, assuming that precursor frequencies are similar for both pathogens. There are quite a few reported examples of cross-reactive T cell responses to different pathogens. In addition to the experiments of Selin and Welsh (69), cross-reactivity has been reported between influenza virus and hepatitis C virus (72), EBV (73) or HIV (74), LCMV and vaccinia virus (75), and coronavirus and human papillomavirus (76). It remains to be seen if the observed cases of cross-reactivity arise from a reporting bias (failure to observe cross-reactivity between two pathogens is unlikely to be reported) or because some of the assumptions of our model are incorrect and need to be modified. For example, we assume all T cell clones have the same level of cross-reactivity – and introducing heterogeneity may dramatically increase the chances to observe cross-reactivity.

Even if cross-reactive T cell responses to two specific pathogens are rare, the accumulation of many successive infections could result in fairly frequent cross-reactivity between a new pathogen and sum of all the pathogens the individual has previously encountered. This is what was observed when T cell precursor frequencies were measured for novel pathogens in blood from adults (80). The precursor frequency for cells recognizing a self-antigen or an unexposed viral epitope was the same as earlier estimated in mice and humans (31) and ranged from one to ten cells per million of CD4 T cells. The surprise was that over half of the precursor cells specific for novel pathogens such as HIV (to which an individual had never been exposed) were of the memory phenotype (80), suggesting that they may have arisen as a consequence of exposure to a different previously encountered pathogen(s). Alternatively, these memory cells could be pseudo-memory cells acquired via the process known as "homeostatic proliferation" and driven by interaction with low-affinity self pMHCs that previously induced positive selection (90–94).

The Su et al. paper (80) raised an interesting question: why do memory cells invariably contribute about 50–80% of the precursors to pathogen the individual has never encountered? One possibility is that the memory repertoire is sufficiently large to be "complete." In this case if we draw the same amount of cells from either naïve or memory compartments (or mixture from both) we will have the same precursor frequency for a pathogen. Then the relative contribution of naïve and memory cells to precursors is equal to their relative frequencies, and is scaled by the stimulation threshold which is known to be lower for memory cells.

We note that our equation (7) allows an estimation of cross-reactivity for unrelated pathogens or peptides and, based on reported precursor frequencies for different epitopes, we expect cross-reactivity to be rare. Several studies allowed to estimate the rate of cross-reactivity for closely related peptides. Su et al. (80) identified potential pathogens responsible for generating T cells cross-reactive to HIV in HIV-negative individuals as follows: they generated clones from the HIV precursors and identified two epitopes to which these clones were specific. Then using a BLAST search of pathogen sequences they identified 24 sequences similar to the two HIV epitopes. About 21% of the HIV clones responded to two of the BLAST sequences corresponding to environmental pathogens. This number is comparable to result obtained in the earlier study, which showed that although the majority of 171 generated variant peptides of strongly immunodominant HLA-A2-restricted HIV gag epitope were able to bind HLA-A2, only one third were recognized by specific T cells (95). These two studies may give the rate of cross-reactivity for closely related peptides (21–33%) and could be particularly important in the context of a variable virus with an increased rate of mutations within epitopes (96).

Cross-reactive responses may be of clinical importance in the generation of pathology and autoimmunity. Several studies pointed that cross-reactivity may be the cause of increased immunopathology during successive unrelated viral infections (84–86) or as a result of application of T cell based therapy (97, 98). Expansion of cross-reactive T cell clones due to previous infections may underlie autoimmune diseases (99–101). Sometimes a pathogen epitope stimulates T cells in the context of a different MHC from the self-epitopes that react with these T cells, for example, Epstein-Barr virus EBN13-HLA-B8-specific cytotoxic T cells were shown to cross-react with a variety of self peptides presented by HLA-B35 (102). Together these observations point out that cross-reactive T cell responses might operate on different levels and much remains to be done to understand the extent of cross-reactivity and how it may differ in CD8, CD4, and regulatory populations of T cells.

4. SUMMARY

We have reviewed current estimates of the T cell repertoire and identified their key limitations. Further progress will require the development of methods to determine the pairing of TCR α and β chains and thus more accurate quantification of the T cell diversity. Current estimates raise the puzzling question of why the potential repertoire is many orders of magnitude greater than the realized repertoire. We suggest that existing hypotheses are not able to explain this puzzle and have proposed an alternative hypothesis of "evolutionary sloppiness."

One of the interesting observation that became obvious from our estimations is that precursor frequency per pathogen inherently links the TCR diversity and cross-reactivity which allows to predict the level of cross-reactivity between two random pathogens or unrelated peptides. Our estimates suggest that although cross-reactivity is a rare event for immunologically naïve individuals, probability to see the cross-reactive memory T cells becomes very high with an increase in successive infections.

Finally we note that we need to move from our current paradigm, which looks at each infection independent of other infections, to a more complex view that incorporates the terms for the interactions between the immune responses to different pathogens.

ACKNOWLEDGMENTS

Veronika I. Zarnitsyna thanks the organizers of the Multi-Scale Physics of Lymphocyte Development Summer Seminar 2012 that sparked her interest in the problem of T cell cross-reactivity. Brian D. Evavold was supported by NIH R01 NS071518 and R01 AI096879, Joseph N. Blattman was supported by a Virginia G. Piper Personalized Medicine Bridging Award, and Veronika I. Zarnitsyna and Rustom Antia were supported by an NIH MIDAS grant U01 GM070749. We also thank the Reviewers for their comments and suggestions.

REFERENCES

1. Burnet F. A modification of Jerne's theory of antibody production using the concept of clonal selection. *CA Cancer J Clin* (1957) **26**:119–21. doi:10.3322/canjclin.26.2.119
2. Talmage DW. Allergy and immunology. *Annu Rev Med* (1957) **8**:239–56. doi:10.1146/annurev.me.08.020157.001323
3. Murali-Krishna K, Altman J, Suresh M, Sourdive D, Zajac A, Miller J, et al. Counting antigen-specific CD8+ T cells: a reevaluation of bystander activation during viral infection. *Immunity* (1998) **8**:177–87. doi:10.1016/S1074-7613(00)80470-7
4. Jamieson B, Ahmed R. T cell memory: long term persistence of virus specific cytotoxic cells. *J Exp Med* (1989) **169**:1993–2005. doi:10.1084/jem.169.6.1993
5. Miller JF, Sprent J. Cell-to-cell interaction in the immune response. VI. Contribution of thymus-derived cells and antibody-forming cell precursors to immunological memory. *J Exp Med* (1971) **134**(1):66–82. doi:10.1084/jem.134.1.66
6. Perelson AS. Modeling viral and immune system dynamics. *Nat Rev Immunol* (2002) **2**(1):28–36. doi:10.1038/nri700
7. Antia R, Ganusov VV, Ahmed R. The role of models in understanding CD8+ T-cell memory. *Nat Rev Immunol* (2005) **5**(2):101–11. doi:10.1038/nri1550
8. Regoes RR, Barber DL, Ahmed R, Antia R. Estimation of the rate of killing by cytotoxic T lymphocytes in vivo. *Proc Natl Acad Sci USA* (2007) **104**(5):1599–603. doi:10.1073/pnas.0508830104
9. Yates AJ, Van Baalen M, Antia R. Virus replication strategies and the critical CTL numbers required for the control of infection. *PLoS Comp Biol* (2011) **7**(11):e1002274. doi:10.1371/journal.pcbi.1002274
10. Sherwood AM, Desmarais C, Livingston RJ, Andriesen J, Haussler M, Carlson CS, et al. Deep sequencing of the human TCRγ and TCRβ repertoires suggests that TCRβ rearranges after $\alpha\beta$ and $\gamma\delta$ T cell commitment. *Sci Transl Med* (2011) **3**(90):90ra61.
11. Venturi V, Quigley MF, Greenaway HY, Ng PC, Ende ZS, McIntosh T, et al. A mechanism for TCR sharing between T cell subsets and individuals revealed by pyrosequencing. *J Immunol* (2011) **186**(7):4285–94. doi:10.4049/jimmunol.1003898

12. Hilborn R, Mangel M. The ecological detective: confronting models with data. In: Hilborn R, Mangel M, editors. *Monographs in Population Biology*. Princeton, NJ: Princeton University Press (1997). 28 p.
13. May RM. Uses and abuses of mathematics in biology. *Science* (2004) **303**(5659):790–3. doi:10.1126/science.1094442
14. Kurosawa Y, von Boehmer H, Haas W, Sakano H, Trauneker A, Tonegawa S. Identification of d segments of immunoglobulin heavy-chain genes and their rearrangement in T lymphocytes. *Nature* (1981) **290**(5807):565–70. doi:10.1038/290565a0
15. Hayday AC, Saito H, Gillies SD, Kranz DM, Tanigawa G, Eisen HN, et al. Structure, organization, and somatic rearrangement of T cell gamma genes. *Cell* (1985) **40**(2):259–69. doi:10.1016/0092-8674(85)90140-0
16. Garboczi DN, Ghosh P, Utz U, Fan QR, Biddison WE, Wiley DC. Structure of the complex between human T-cell receptor, viral peptide and HLA-A2. *Nature* (1996) **384**(6605):134–41. doi:10.1038/384134a0
17. Oltz EM. Regulation of antigen receptor gene assembly in lymphocytes. *Immunol Res* (2001) **23**(2–3):121–33. doi:10.1385/IR:23:2-3:121
18. Jolly CJ, Cook AJL, Manis JP. Fixing DNA breaks during class switch recombination. *J Exp Med* (2008) **205**(3):509–13. doi:10.1084/jem.20080356
19. Davis MM, Bjorkman PJ. T-cell antigen receptor genes and T-cell recognition. *Nature* (1988) **334**(6181):395–402. doi:10.1038/334395a0
20. Robins HS, Srivastava SK, Campregher PV, Turtle CJ, Andriesen J, Riddell SR, et al. Overlap and effective size of the human CD8+ T cell receptor repertoire. *Sci Transl Med* (2010) **2**(47):47ra64. doi:10.1126/scitranslmed.3001442
21. Murugan A, Mora T, Walczak AM, Callan CG Jr. Statistical inference of the generation probability of T-cell receptors from sequence repertoires. *Proc Natl Acad Sci U S A* (2012) **109**(40):16161–6. doi:10.1073/pnas.1212755109
22. Arstila TP, Casrouge A, Baron V, Even J, Kanellopoulos J, Kourilsky P. A direct estimate of the human alphabeta T cell receptor diversity. *Science* (1999) **286**(5441):958–61. doi:10.1126/science.286.5441.958
23. Robins HS, Campregher PV, Srivastava SK, Wacher A, Turtle CJ, Kahsai O, et al. Comprehensive assessment of T-cell receptor beta-chain diversity in alphabeta T cells. *Blood* (2009) **114**(19):4099–107. doi:10.1182/blood-2009-04-217604
24. Warren RL, Freeman JD, Zeng T, Choe G, Munro S, Moore R, et al. Exhaustive T-cell repertoire sequencing of human peripheral blood samples reveals signatures of antigen selection and a directly measured repertoire size of at least 1 million clonotypes. *Genome Res* (2011) **21**(5):790–7. doi:10.1101/gr.115428.110
25. Kesmir C, Borghans JA, de Boer RJ. Diversity of human $\alpha\beta$ T cell receptors. *Science* (2000) **288**:1135. doi:10.1126/science.288.5469.1135a
26. Arstila TP, Casrouge A, Baron V, Even J, Kanellopoulos J, Kourilsky P. Diversity of human alpha beta T cell receptors. *Science* (2000) **288**(5469):1135. doi:10.1126/science.288.5469.1135a
27. Zhang L, Lewin SR, Markowitz M, Lin HH, Skulsky E, Karanicolas R, et al. Measuring recent thymic emigrants in blood of normal and HIV-1-infected individuals before and after effective therapy. *J Exp Med* (1999) **190**(5):725–32. doi:10.1084/jem.190.5.725
28. Bains I, Antia R, Callard R, Yates AJ. Quantifying the development of the peripheral naive CD4+ T-cell pool in humans. *Blood* (2009) **113**(22):5480–7. doi:10.1182/blood-2008-10-184184
29. McFarland RD, Douek DC, Koup RA, Picker LJ. Identification of a human recent thymic emigrant phenotype. *Proc Natl Acad Sci U S A* (2000) **97**(8):4215–20. doi:10.1073/pnas.070061597
30. Casrouge A, Beaudoing E, Dalle S, Pannetier C, Kanellopoulos J, Kourilsky P. Size estimate of the alpha beta TCR repertoire of naive mouse splenocytes. *J Immunol* (2000) **164**(11):5782–7.
31. Jenkins MK, Moon JJ. The role of naive T cell precursor frequency and recruitment in dictating immune response magnitude. *J Immunol* (2012) **188**(9):4135–40. doi:10.4049/jimmunol.1102661
32. Tubo NJ, Pagán AJ, Taylor JJ, Nelson RW, Linehan JL, Ertelt JM, et al. Single naive CD4(+) T cells from a diverse repertoire produce different effector cell types during infection. *Cell* (2013) **153**(4):785–96. doi:10.1016/j.cell.2013.04.007
33. Venturi V, Price DA, Douek DC, Davenport MP. The molecular basis for public T cell responses? *Nat Rev Immunol* (2008) **8**(3):231–8. doi:10.1038/nri2260
34. Dash P, McClaren JL, Oguin TH III, Rothwell W, Todd B, Morris MY, et al. Paired analysis of TCRα and TCRβ chains at the single-cell level in mice. *J Clin Invest* (2011) **121**(1):288–95. doi:10.1172/JCI44752
35. Turchaninova MA, Britanova OV, Bolotin DA, Shugay M, Putintseva EV, Staroverov DB, et al. Pairing of T-cell receptor chains via emulsion PCR. *Eur J Immunol* (2013) **43**(9):2507–15. doi:10.1002/eji.201343453
36. Venturi V, Kedzierska K, Turner SJ, Doherty PC, Davenport MP. Methods for comparing the diversity of samples of the T cell receptor repertoire. *J Immunol Methods* (2007) **321**(1–2):182–95. doi:10.1016/j.jim.2007.01.019
37. Bousso P, Casrouge A, Altman JD, Haury M, Kanellopoulos J, Abastado JP, et al. Individual variations in the murine T cell response to a specific peptide reflect variability in naive repertoires. *Immunity* (1998) **9**(2):169–78. doi:10.1016/S1074-7613(00)80599-3
38. Quigley MF, Greenaway HY, Venturi V, Lindsay R, Quinn KM, Seder RA, et al. Convergent recombination shapes the clonotypic landscape of the naive T-cell repertoire. *Proc Natl Acad Sci U S A* (2010) **107**(45):19414–9. doi:10.1073/pnas.1010586107
39. Livak F, Burtrum DB, Rowen L, Schatz DG, Petrie HT. Genetic modulation of T cell receptor gene segment usage during somatic recombination. *J Exp Med* (2000) **192**(8):1191–6. doi:10.1084/jem.192.8.1191
40. Brändle D, Bürki K, Wallace VA, Rohrer UH, Mak TW, Malissen B, et al. Involvement of both T cell receptor V alpha and V beta variable region domains and alpha chain junctional region in viral antigen recognition. *Eur J Immunol* (1991) **21**(9):2195–202. doi:10.1002/eji.1830210930
41. Perkins DL, Wang YS, Fruman D, Seidman JG, Rimm IJ. Immunodominance is altered in T cell receptor (beta-chain) transgenic mice without the generation of a hole in the repertoire. *J Immunol* (1991) **146**(9):2960–4.
42. Turner SJ, Cose SC, Carbone FR. TCR alpha-chain usage can determine antigen-selected TCR beta-chain repertoire diversity. *J Immunol* (1996) **157**(11):4979–85.
43. Burns RP Jr, Natarajan K, LoCascio NJ, O'Brien DP, Kobori JA, Shastri N, et al. Molecular analysis of skewed Tcra-V gene use in T-cell receptor beta-chain transgenic mice. *Immunogenetics* (1998) **47**(2):107–14. doi:10.1007/s002510050335
44. De Boer RJ, Perelson AS. How diverse should the immune system be? *Proc R Soc Lond B Biol Sci* (1993) **252**(1335):171–5. doi:10.1098/rspb.1993.0062
45. Wiegel FW, Perelson AS. Some scaling principles for the immune system. *Immunol Cell Biol* (2004) **82**(2):127–31. doi:10.1046/j.0818-9641.2004.01229.x
46. Blattman JN, Antia R, Sourdive DJ, Wang X, Kaech SM, Murali-Krishna K, et al. Estimating the precursor frequency of naive antigen-specific CD8 T cells. *J Exp Med* (2002) **195**(5):657–64. doi:10.1084/jem.20001021
47. Whitmire JK, Benning N, Whitton JL. Precursor frequency, nonlinear proliferation, and functional maturation of virus-specific CD4+ T cells. *J Immunol* (2006) **176**(5):3028–36.
48. Moon JJ, Chu HH, Pepper M, McSorley SJ, Jameson SC, Kedl RM, et al. Naive CD4(+) T cell frequency varies for different epitopes and predicts repertoire diversity and response magnitude. *Immunity* (2007) **27**(2):203–13. doi:10.1016/j.immuni.2007.07.007
49. Thomas PG, Handel A, Doherty PC, La Gruta NL. Ecological analysis of antigen-specific CTL repertoires defines the relationship between naive and immune T-cell populations. *Proc Natl Acad Sci U S A* (2013) **110**(5):1839–44. doi:10.1073/pnas.1222149110
50. La Gruta NL, Rothwell WT, Cukalac T, Swan NG, Valkenburg SA, Kedzierska K, et al. Primary CTL response magnitude in mice is determined by the extent of naive T cell recruitment and subsequent clonal expansion. *J Clin Invest* (2010) **120**(6):1885–94. doi:10.1172/JCI41538
51. Yewdell JW, Bennink JR. Immunodominance in major histocompatibility complex class I-restricted T lymphocyte responses. *Annu Rev Immunol* (1999) **17**:51–88. doi:10.1146/annurev.immunol.17.1.51
52. Langman R, Cohen M. The E-T (elephant-tadpole) paradox necessitates the concept of a unit of B-cell function: the protection. *Mol Immunol* (1987) **24**:675–97. doi:10.1016/0161-5890(87)90050-2
53. Masopust D, Murali-Krishna K, Ahmed R. Quantitating the magnitude of the lymphocytic choriomeningitis virus-specific CD8 T-cell response: it is even bigger than we thought. *J Virol* (2007) **81**(4):2002–11. doi:10.1128/JVI.01459-06
54. Perelson AS, Wiegel FW. Scaling aspects of lymphocyte trafficking. *J Theor Biol* (2009) **257**(1):9–16. doi:10.1016/j.jtbi.2008.11.007
55. Westermann J, Pabst R. Lymphocyte subsets in the blood: a diagnostic window on the lymphoid system? *Immunol Today* (1990) **11**(11):406–10. doi:10.1016/0167-5699(90)90160-B

56. Clark DR, de Boer RJ, Wolthers KC, Miedema F. T cell dynamics in HIV-1 infection. *Adv Immunol* (1999) **73**:301–27. doi:10.1016/S0065-2776(08)60789-0
57. Shortman K, Vremec D, Egerton M. The kinetics of T cell antigen receptor expression by subgroups of CD4+8+ thymocytes: delineation of CD4+8+3(2+) thymocytes as post-selection intermediates leading to mature T cells. *J Exp Med* (1991) **173**(2):323–32. doi:10.1084/jem.173.2.323
58. Huesmann M, Scott B, Kisielow P, von Boehmer H. Kinetics and efficacy of positive selection in the thymus of normal and T cell receptor transgenic mice. *Cell* (1991) **66**(3):533–40. doi:10.1016/0092-8674(81)90016-7
59. Vrisekoop N, den Braber I, de Boer AB, Ruiter AFC, Ackermans MT, van der Crabben SN, et al. Sparse production but preferential incorporation of recently produced naive T cells in the human peripheral pool. *Proc Natl Acad Sci U S A* (2008) **105**(16):6115–20. doi:10.1073/pnas.0709713105
60. Hazenberg MD, Borghans JA, de Boer RJ, Miedema F. Thymic output: a bad TREC record. *Nat Immunol* (2003) **4**(2):97–9. doi:10.1038/ni0203-97
61. Tough D, Sprent J. Turnover of naive- and memory-phenotype T cells. *J Exp Med* (1994) **179**:1127–35. doi:10.1084/jem.179.4.1127
62. Scollay RG, Butcher EC, Weissman IL. Thymus cell migration quantitative aspects of cellular traffic from the thymus to the periphery in mice. *Eur J Immunol* (1980) **10**(3):210–8. doi:10.1002/eji.1830100310
63. Gabor MJ, Scollay R, Godfrey DI. Thymic T cell export is not influenced by the peripheral T cell pool. *Eur J Immunol* (1997) **27**(11):2986–93. doi:10.1002/eji.1830271135
64. Vezys V, Masopust D, Kemball CC, Barber DL, O'Mara LA, Larsen CP, et al. Continuous recruitment of naive T cells contributes to heterogeneity of antiviral CD8 T cells during persistent infection. *J Exp Med* (2006) **203**(10):2263–9. doi:10.1084/jem.20060995
65. Yang Y, Al-Mozaini M, Buzon MJ, Beamon J, Ferrando-Martinez S, Ruiz-Mateos E, et al. CD4 T-cell regeneration in HIV-1 elite controllers. *AIDS* (2012) **26**(6):701–6. doi:10.1097/QAD.0b013e3283519b22
66. Hatzakis A, Touloumi G, Karanicolas R, Karafoulidou A, Mandalaki T, Anastassopoulou C, et al. Effect of recent thymic emigrants on progression of HIV-1 disease. *Lancet* (2000) **355**(9204):599–604. doi:10.1016/S0140-6736(99)10311-8
67. Gould S, Lewontin R. The spandrels of San Marco and the Panglossian paradigm: a critique of the adaptationist programme. *Proc R Soc Lond B Biol Sci* (1979) **205**:581–98. doi:10.1098/rspb.1979.0086
68. George A, Ritter M. Thymic involution with ageing: obsolescence or good housekeeping? *Immunol Today* (1996) **17**:267–72. doi:10.1016/0167-5699(96)80543-3
69. Selin LK, Nahill SR, Welsh RM. Cross-reactivities in memory cytotoxic T lymphocyte recognition of heterologous viruses. *J Exp Med* (1994) **179**(6):1933–43. doi:10.1084/jem.179.6.1933
70. Selin LK, Brehm MA, Naumov YN, Cornberg M, Kim S-K, Clute SC, et al. Memory of mice and men: CD8+ T-cell cross-reactivity and heterologous immunity. *Immunol Rev* (2006) **211**:164–81. doi:10.1111/j.0105-2896.2006.00394.x
71. Welsh RM, Selin LK. No one is naive: the significance of heterologous T-cell immunity. *Nat Rev Immunol* (2002) **2**(6):417–26.
72. Wedemeyer H, Mizukoshi E, Davis AR, Bennink JR, Rehermann B. Cross-reactivity between hepatitis c virus and influenza a virus determinant-specific cytotoxic T cells. *J Virol* (2001) **75**(23):11392–400. doi:10.1128/JVI.75.23.11392-11400.2001
73. Clute SC, Watkin LB, Cornberg M, Naumov YN, Sullivan JL, Luzuriaga K, et al. Cross-reactive influenza virus-specific CD8+ T cells contribute to lymphoproliferation in Epstein-Barr virus-associated infectious mononucleosis. *J Clin Invest* (2005) **115**(12):3602–12. doi:10.1172/JCI25078
74. Acierno PM, Newton DA, Brown EA, Maes LA, Baatz JE, Gattoni-Celli S. Cross-reactivity between HLA-A2-restricted FLU-M1:58-66 and HIV p17 GAG:77-85 epitopes in HIV-infected and uninfected individuals. *J Transl Med* (2003) **1**(1):3. doi:10.1186/1479-5876-1-3
75. Kim S-K, Cornberg M, Wang XZ, Chen HD, Selin LK, Welsh RM. Private specificities of CD8 T cell responses control patterns of heterologous immunity. *J Exp Med* (2005) **201**(4):523–33. doi:10.1084/jem.20041337
76. Nilges K, Höhn H, Pilch H, Neukirch C, Freitag K, Talbot PJ, et al. Human papillomavirus type 16 E7 peptide-directed CD8+ T cells from patients with cervical cancer are cross-reactive with the coronavirus NS2 protein. *J Virol* (2003) **77**(9):5464–74. doi:10.1128/JVI.77.9.5464-5474.2003
77. Reinherz EL, Tan K, Tang L, Kern P, Liu J, Xiong Y, et al. The crystal structure of a T cell receptor in complex with peptide and MHC class II. *Science* (1999) **286**(5446):1913–21. doi:10.1126/science.286.5446.1913
78. Reiser J-B, Darnault C, Grégoire C, Mosser T, Mazza G, Kearney A, et al. CDR3 loop flexibility contributes to the degeneracy of TCR recognition. *Nat Immunol* (2003) **4**(3):241–7. doi:10.1038/ni891
79. Newell EW, Ely LK, Kruse AC, Reay PA, Rodriguez SN, Lin AE, et al. Structural basis of specificity and cross-reactivity in T cell receptors specific for cytochrome c-I-E(k). *J Immunol* (2011) **186**(10):5823–32. doi:10.4049/jimmunol.1100197
80. Su LF, Kidd BA, Han A, Kotzin JJ, Davis MM. Virus-specific CD4(+) memory-phenotype T cells are abundant in unexposed adults. *Immunity* (2013) **38**(2):373–83. doi:10.1016/j.immuni.2012.10.021
81. Heath WR, Miller JF. Expression of two alpha chains on the surface of T cells in T cell receptor transgenic mice. *J Exp Med* (1993) **178**(5):1807–11. doi:10.1084/jem.178.5.1807
82. Padovan E, Casorati G, Dellabona P, Meyer S, Brockhaus M, Lanzavecchia A. Expression of two T cell receptor alpha chains: dual receptor T cells. *Science* (1993) **262**(5132):422–4. doi:10.1126/science.8211163
83. Petrie HT, Livak F, Schatz DG, Strasser A, Crispe IN, Shortman K. Multiple rearrangements in T cell receptor alpha chain genes maximize the production of useful thymocytes. *J Exp Med* (1993) **178**(2):615–22. doi:10.1084/jem.178.2.615
84. Selin LK, Varga SM, Wong IC, Welsh RM. Protective heterologous antiviral immunity and enhanced immunopathogenesis mediated by memory T cell populations. *J Exp Med* (1998) **188**(9):1705–15. doi:10.1084/jem.188.9.1705
85. Yang HY, Joris I, Majno G, Welsh RM. Necrosis of adipose tissue induced by sequential infections with unrelated viruses. *Am J Pathol* (1985) **120**(2):173–7.
86. Chen HD, Fraire AE, Joris I, Brehm MA, Welsh RM, Selin LK. Memory CD8+ T cells in heterologous antiviral immunity and immunopathology in the lung. *Nat Immunol* (2001) **2**(11):1067–76. doi:10.1038/ni727
87. Mason D. A very high level of crossreactivity is an essential feature of the T-cell receptor. *Immunol Today* (1998) **19**(9):395–404. doi:10.1016/S0167-5699(98)01299-7
88. Sewell AK. Why must T cells be cross-reactive? *Nat Rev Immunol* (2012) **12**(9):669–77. doi:10.1038/nri3279
89. Jenkins MK, Chu HH, McLachlan JB, Moon JJ. On the composition of the preimmune repertoire of T cells specific for peptide-major histocompatibility complex ligands. *Annu Rev Immunol* (2010) **28**:275–94. doi:10.1146/annurev-immunol-030409-101253
90. Murali-Krishna K, Ahmed R. Cutting edge: naive T cells masquerading as memory cells. *J Immunol* (2000) **165**(4):1733–7.
91. Ernst B, Lee DS, Chang JM, Sprent J, Surh CD. The peptide ligands mediating positive selection in the thymus control T cell survival and homeostatic proliferation in the periphery. *Immunity* (1999) **11**(2):173–81. doi:10.1016/S1074-7613(00)80092-8
92. Goldrath AW, Bevan MJ. Low-affinity ligands for the TCR drive proliferation of mature CD8+ T cells in lymphopenic hosts. *Immunity* (1999) **11**(2):183–90. doi:10.1016/S1074-7613(00)80093-X
93. Kieper WC, Jameson SC. Homeostatic expansion and phenotypic conversion of naïve T cells in response to self peptide/MHC ligands. *Proc Natl Acad Sci U S A* (1999) **96**(23):13306–11. doi:10.1073/pnas.96.23.13306
94. Muranski P, Chmielowski B, Ignatowicz L. Mature CD4+ T cells perceive a positively selecting class II MHC/peptide complex in the periphery. *J Immunol* (2000) **164**(6):3087–94.
95. Lee JK, Stewart-Jones G, Dong T, Harlos K, Di Gleria K, Dorrell L, et al. T cell cross-reactivity and conformational changes during TCR engagement. *J Exp Med* (2004) **200**(11):1455–66. doi:10.1084/jem.20041251
96. Kosmrlj A, Read EL, Qi Y, Allen TM, Altfeld M, Deeks SG, et al. Effects of thymic selection of the T-cell repertoire on HLA class I-associated control of HIV infection. *Nature* (2010) **465**(7296):350–4. doi:10.1038/nature08997
97. Cameron BJ, Gerry AB, Dukes J, Harper JV, Kannan V, Bianchi FC, et al. Identification of a titin-derived HLA-A1-presented peptide as a cross-reactive target for engineered MAGE A3-directed T cells. *Sci Transl Med* (2013) **5**(197):197ra103. doi:10.1126/scitranslmed.3006034
98. Linette GP, Stadtmauer EA, Maus MV, Rapoport AP, Levine BL, Emery L, et al. Cardiovascular toxicity and titin cross-reactivity of affinity-enhanced T cells

in myeloma and melanoma. *Blood* (2013) **122**(6):863–71. doi:10.1182/blood-2013-03-490565

99. Fujinami RS, Oldstone MB. Amino acid homology between the encephalitogenic site of myelin basic protein and virus: mechanism for autoimmunity. *Science* (1985) **230**(4729):1043–5. doi:10.1126/science.2414848
100. Oldstone MB. Molecular mimicry and immune-mediated diseases. *FASEB J* (1998) **12**(13):1255–65.
101. Wucherpfennig KW, Strominger JL. Molecular mimicry in T cell-mediated autoimmunity: viral peptides activate human T cell clones specific for myelin basic protein. *Cell* (1995) **80**(5):695–705. doi:10.1016/0092-8674(95)90348-8
102. Burrows SR, Silins SL, Khanna R, Burrows JM, Rischmueller M, McCluskey J, et al. Cross-reactive memory T cells for Epstein-Barr virus augment the alloresponse to common human leukocyte antigens: degenerate recognition of major histocompatibility complex-bound peptide by T cells and its role in alloreactivity. *Eur J Immunol* (1997) **27**(7):1726–36. doi:10.1002/eji.1830270720

13

Regulatory dendritic cells for immunotherapy in immunologic diseases

John R. Gordon*, Yanna Ma, Laura Churchman, Sara A. Gordon and Wojciech Dawicki

Department of Medicine, University of Saskatchewan, Saskatoon, SK, Canada

Edited by:
Lisa Helene Butterfield, University of Pittsburgh, USA

Reviewed by:
Theresa L. Whiteside, University of Pittsburgh, USA
Nick Giannoukakis, University of Pittsburgh, USA

***Correspondence:**
John R. Gordon, Department of Medicine, University of Saskatchewan, Room 2D30.8, 107 Wiggins Road, Saskatoon, SK S7N 5E5, Canada
e-mail: john.gordon@usask.ca

We recognize well the abilities of dendritic cells to activate effector T cell (Teff cell) responses to an array of antigens and think of these cells in this context as pre-eminent antigen-presenting cells, but dendritic cells are also critical to the induction of immunologic tolerance. Herein, we review our knowledge on the different kinds of tolerogenic or regulatory dendritic cells that are present or can be induced in experimental settings and humans, how they operate, and the diseases in which they are effective, from allergic to autoimmune diseases and transplant tolerance. The primary conclusions that arise from these cumulative studies clearly indicate that the agent(s) used to induce the tolerogenic phenotype and the status of the dendritic cell at the time of induction influence not only the phenotype of the dendritic cell, but also that of the regulatory T cell responses that they in turn mobilize. For example, while many, if not most, types of induced regulatory dendritic cells lead CD4^{+} naïve or Teff cells to adopt a CD25^{+}Foxp3^{+} Treg phenotype, exposure of Langerhans cells or dermal dendritic cells to vitamin D leads in one case to the downstream induction of CD25^{+}Foxp3^{+} regulatory T cell responses, while in the other to Foxp3^{-} type 1 regulatory T cells (Tr1) responses. Similarly, exposure of human immature versus semi-mature dendritic cells to IL-10 leads to distinct regulatory T cell outcomes. Thus, it should be possible to shape our dendritic cell immunotherapy approaches for selective induction of different types of T cell tolerance or to simultaneously induce multiple types of regulatory T cell responses. This may prove to be an important option as we target diseases in different anatomic compartments or with divergent pathologies in the clinic. Finally, we provide an overview of the use and potential use of these cells clinically, highlighting their potential as tools in an array of settings.

Keywords: dendritic cell, tolerance, regulatory T cell, immunoregulation, IL-10, retinoic acid, TGFβ, vitamin D

During the 1960s, it was thought that macrophages, with their capacity to phagocytose antigens, were required to initiate immunity to foreign substances (1). It was known that lymphocytes were mediators of immunity, but we knew little about how antigens from an invading pathogen would reach the lymph node-sequestered naïve lymphocytes (2). There was a gap in the understanding of the initiation of adaptive immunity, a gap that Ralph Steinman and Zanvil Cohn set out to fill. When Steinman began to study the spleen and lymph nodes, he observed new cells that were distinct from macrophages in appearance and function. These dendritic cells, so named because of their dendrite-like projections, had few lysosomes and only moderate phagocytic activity (3, 4), but they expressed high levels of major histocompatibility complex (MHC) molecules required for presentation of extra-cellular antigens (5). He also observed that dendritic cells were highly potent immune stimulators (6), and now we often speak of dendritic cells as the most proficient of professional antigen-presenting cells (APCs). By 1991, we had accumulated substantial knowledge on the role of the dendritic cell in the induction of immunity, but we were just beginning to recognize that extrathymic dendritic cells could also play central roles in the induction of tolerance (7), and it was not long before we began to understand more about tolerogenic dendritic cells and their potential applications (8–10). We now appreciate that there are numerous discreet populations of naturally occurring regulatory dendritic cells, but focusing on understanding the immunobiology of these cells within their individual niches has given us substantial insights on how we can generate and employ regulatory dendritic cells for immunotherapeutic applications. While dendritic cells can activate either CD4^{+} or CD8^{+}, or even CD4^{-}CD8^{-} T, B, and NK cells to become regulatory cells, this review will be confined to a discussion on tolerogenic DC in the context of CD4^{+} T cells and their responses. We will first describe

Abbreviations: AHR, airway hyperresponsiveness; APCs, antigen-presenting cells; BAL, bronchoalveolar lavage; BDCA, blood dendritic cell antigen; CTLA4, cytotoxic T lymphocyte antigen-4; DC10 or DC-10, semi-mature or immature, respectively, IL-10-differentiated dendritic cells; DC-SIGN, dendritic cell-specific intracellular adhesion molecule 3-grabbing non-integrin; Foxp3, the transcription factor forkhead box P3; ICOS and ICOS-L, inducible costimulator and inducible costimulator ligand, respectively; IDO, indoleamine-2,3-dioxygenase; ILT, immunoglobulin-like transcript; iTreg, induced CD25^{+}Foxp3^{+} regulatory T cells; MHC, major histocompatibility complex; nTreg, naturally-occurring CD25^{+}Foxp3^{+} regulatory T cells; OVA, ovalbumin; RALDH2, retinaldehyde dehydrogenase 2; Teff cell, effector T cell; TLR, toll-like receptor; Treg cell, regulatory T cell.

the populations of dendritic cells found *in vivo* and then look at the major populations of regulatory dendritic cells that have been induced *ex vivo*, as well as the effector molecules employed by these cells.

OVERVIEW OF DENDRITIC CELL BIOLOGY

In general, dendritic cells express MHCII but lack T cell (CD3), B cell (CD19), and NK cell (CD56) lineage markers (11); some subsets of dendritic cells express the monocyte/macrophage (CD14) or NK cell/neutrophil and monocyte/macrophage (CD16) lineage markers, and others the CD4 and/or CD8 T cell subset markers. Dendritic cells are formed from bone marrow progenitors that in general give rise to circulating dendritic cell precursors (12, 13) that seed the peripheral tissues as immature cells (14). As quiescent or immature cells, they express receptors for, and have an innate capacity to respond to an array of inflammatory signals, including ligands for toll-like receptor (TLR), NOD-like receptors, and scavenger receptors, as well as inflammatory mediators, cytokines, and chemokines. The various sub-populations of dendritic cells can respond in a qualitatively and quantitatively distinct fashion to such environmental triggers and differentiate extensively to become immunocompetent accessory cells, such that they provide a crucial link between the innate and adaptive immune responses (15). They upregulate cell-surface expression of their antigen-presentation machinery, including processed antigen peptide-loaded MHCII (16) and co-stimulatory molecules as well as receptors for lymph node-homing chemokines (e.g., CCR7), and they downregulate their phagocytic activities and receptors for local inflammatory signals (e.g., CCR5, CCR6) (14, 17). As dendritic cells mature, they lose their ability to process new peptides (18, 19) and migrate to their tissue-draining lymphoid organ, where they present their processed antigens to T cells in the context of cell-surface MHC (APC signal 1) together with supporting co-stimulatory molecules (e.g., CD40, CD86; APC signal 2) and T cell-polarizing cytokine signals such as IL-12 (20) (APC signal 3), inducing the T cells to differentiate into antigen-specific effector T cells (Teffs; e.g., Th1, Th2, or Th17 cells) (13). But dendritic cells can also provide a fourth APC signal of sorts to T cells, by which they direct the trafficking of the educated T cell. In the gut, retinoic acid and transforming growth factor (TGF)-β produced by dendritic cells together induce T cells to express the α4β7 and CCR9 gut-homing receptors (21), while in the skin-draining lymph nodes vitamin D metabolites released by the dendritic cell induce T cells to express CCR10, such that they become responsive to the skin-homing chemokine CCL27 (22).

Tissue-resident dendritic cells that acquire innocuous environmental or self antigens in the absence of local inflammatory responses similarly migrate to the draining lymph nodes but, as more quiescent cells, overall they express lower levels of MHCII, co-stimulatory molecules, and IL-12, and secrete instructional regulatory mediators such as IL-10 or retinoic acid (23, 24). In this way dendritic cells that are presenting innocuous environmental antigens activate one of several types of regulatory T cell (e.g., Treg, Tr1, or Th3) responses that are associated with immune tolerance (**Figure 1**).

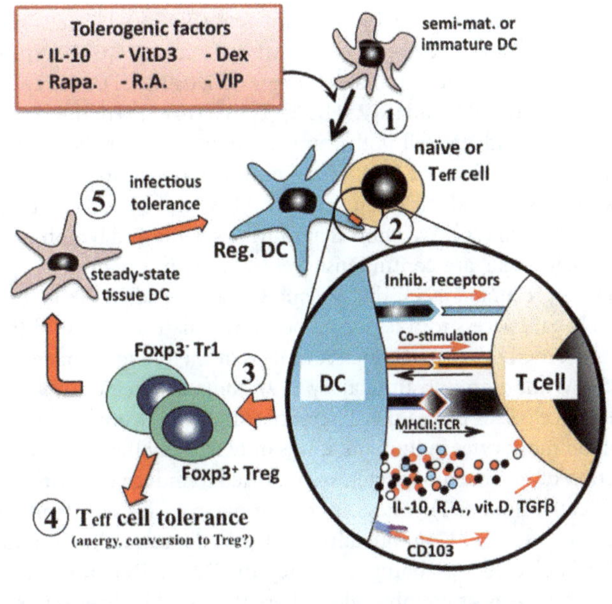

FIGURE 1 | Induction of immunologic tolerance by regulatory dendritic cells. Immature or semi-mature dendritic cells that are incubated with, or differentiated in the presence of, tolerogenic factors (e.g., IL-10, vitamin D3, corticosteroids, or retinoic acid) (1) adopt a regulatory phenotype. When these converted regulatory dendritic cells are pulsed with antigen and exposed to cognate naïve or effector T (Teff) cells (2), they present their processed antigen peptides in the context of MHCII, and also lower levels of co-stimulation (e.g., CD40, CD86) to the T cells, but at the same time many types of tolerogenic cells also provide inhibitory receptor (e.g., ILT2, ILT4) signaling to the T cell. Counter-signaling from the engaged T cell activates dendritic cell production of polarizing mediators (e.g., IL-10, TGFβ), which together instruct the T cell to adopt a regulatory phenotype. The nature of the instructional signals from the dendritic cell to the T cell determine whether it adopts an IL-10-secreting $CD25^+Foxp3^+$ Treg phenotype or an IL-10/TGFβ-secreting $Foxp3^-$ Tr1 phenotype (3). These regulatory T cells are able to suppress the responses of cognate or by-stander naïve or effector T cells in their microenvironment (4) and also to convert endogenous tissue dendritic cells to adopt a regulatory phenotype through induction of infectious tolerance (5), and thereby reinforce the tolerance phenotype.

NATURALLY OCCURRING POPULATIONS OF DENDRITIC CELLS

A large number of reports have described an array of dendritic cell types and subtypes in different organ systems and animals, and it is almost undoubtedly true that more will be described as we explore further. Many of these sub-populations are or can be tolerogenic as they are found in their steady state (e.g., pulmonary plasmacytoid or myeloid dendritic cells), but for most if not all of these there are inflammatory signals that can override this tolerogenic phenotype, converting these cells to an immunostimulatory phenotype. In some tissues (e.g., gut, liver) dominantly tolerogenic signals are constitutively expressed at high levels, while in other sites that are not routinely exposed to the external environment these signals may be much more subtle.

DENDRITIC CELLS IN THE BLOOD

Several distinct types of dendritic cells can be identified in human peripheral blood. There are two sub-populations of $MHCII^+CD11c^+CD123^{lo}$ myeloid dendritic cells, including CD1c/blood dendritic cell antigen (BDCA)-1^+ cells and CD141/BDCA-3^+ cells, as well as $MHCII^+CD1c^-CD123^{hi}$ plasmacytoid dendritic cells that also express BDCA-2/CD303, BDCA-4/CD304, IL-3RA, and ILT7 (11, 25). The $CD141^+MHCII^+CD11c^+$ myeloid dendritic cell is the human counterpart of the murine $CD8\alpha^+$ dendritic cell (25). In the mouse, the identities of circulating tissue dendritic cell precursor(s) have not been all that well documented (26). We know that murine splenic and lymph node dendritic cells are continuously replaced from a pool of blood-borne precursors (27), that splenic $CD8\alpha^+$ dendritic cells most likely gain access to this organ via the vasculature (28), and that $MHCII^{lo}CD11c^{lo}$ pDC do accumulate in the blood of mice (13, 28). While immunostimulatory (29) and tolerogenic (30) dendritic cells can be readily differentiated *ex vivo* from peripheral blood monocytes in humans, it was only recently that LPS stimulation of murine monocytes was reported to induce dendritic cell differentiation (31). These murine monocyte-derived dendritic cells express CCR7 and dendritic cell-specific intracellular adhesion molecule 3-grabbing non-integrin (DC-SIGN) and localize to T cell areas of lymph nodes, where they are highly effective in presenting and cross-presenting antigens (31).

In humans, the BDCA-1^+ and -3^+ myeloid dendritic cell populations can be mobilized from the bone marrow with Flt3 ligand alone while optimal plasmacytoid dendritic cells mobilization reportedly calls for use of Flt3 ligand and G-CSF (25). The circulating BDCA-1^+/$CD1c^+$ myeloid dendritic cell can secrete abundant IL-12 and prime cytotoxic T cell responses (32), while BDCA-3^+ myeloid dendritic cells and BDCA-2^+ plasmacytoid dendritic cells instead secrete IFNγ and IFNα, respectively, on activation (32). A minor population of tolerogenic IL-10-expressing $CD1c^-CD303^-CD14^+$ dendritic cells has recently been described in human peripheral blood, although much of the data regarding their tolerogenic activities has come from studies with an *in vitro* analog of the circulating cell (33).

INTESTINAL DENDRITIC CELLS

The intestinal immune system routinely faces the challenge of discriminating pathogens from harmless commensal organisms and other (e.g., food) antigens, as a prelude to triggering effector and regulatory T cell responses, respectively (34). The gut-associated dendritic cells include those in the mesenteric lymph nodes (MLNs), intestinal lamina propria, and the isolated lymphoid follicles (35, 36). The lamina propria contains two populations of $CD11c^+$ mononuclear cells, including $CD11c^{hi}CD103^+CD11b^+CX_3CR1^-$ cells and $CD11c^{int}CD103^-CD11b^+CX_3CR1^+$ cells; the $CD103^+$ cells are *bona fide* dendritic cells while the latter $CD103^-$ cells are now thought to be resident tissue macrophages (37). Under steady-state conditions, the $CD103^+$ dendritic cells express retinaldehyde dehydrogenase 2 (RALDH2) (23, 38), TGF-β (39), and indoleamine-2,3-dioxygenase (IDO) (40), such that targeting of antigens to these cells leads to tolerance outcomes, while gut inflammation dampens TGFβ and RALDH2 expression in these cells, such that they instead induce vigorous T and B cell responses (41, 42). CD103, the α chain of the E-cadherin ligand αEβ7 integrin (43), is expressed on almost all lamina propria dendritic cells and a subset of MLN dendritic cells (44). It has been reported that gut luminal bacteria recruit lamina propria $CD103^+$ dendritic cells into the gut epithelium, from which they extend filipodia into the lumen to sample gut antigens (37). RALDH2 is an enzyme that catalyzes the synthesis of retinoic acid, a vitamin A derivative, which plays a major role in immunologic tolerance within the gastrointestinal tract (45). Expression of CD103 and retinoic acid together induce gut T cells to express the gut-homing receptors CCR9 and α4β7 (44, 46). CCR9 and its CCL25 ligand regulate recruitment of lymphocytes to the vasculature of the small intestine (47), while α4β7 integrin expression confines extravasation of these T cells to the intestinal post-capillary venules (48). Retinoic acid and TGFβ together promote the differentiation of $Foxp3^+$ Treg from naive T cells (39), while retinoic acid further reinforces tolerance by dampening Th17 cell differentiation (49). Retinoic acid also fosters B cell isotype switching to IgA antibodies as well as their expression of CCR9 and α4β7 (50–52), and thereby contributes further to local tolerance responses.

PULMONARY DENDRITIC CELLS

Pulmonary dendritic cells can be differentially positioned in either the conducting airway or the interstitium of the lung (15, 53). In mice, $CD11c^{hi}$ myeloid cells are found in both compartments, while $CD11c^-$ cells are reportedly confined to the airway mucosa (53). The airway dendritic cells form a prototypical network of interdigitating cells positioned beneath the epithelium (54–56), with many of these cells extending dendritic processes into the airway lumen to sample airway antigens (57), just as occurs in the gut (37). In mice these airway cells express $CD11c^+$, $MHCII^+$, and $CD11b^+$, but not $CD8\alpha^-$ (15); they also express CD103 and tight junction proteins (claudin-1 and -7, and zonula occludens protein 2), which would play important roles vis-à-vis their positioning within the epithelium (43). After airway antigen sampling and processing, these cells can activate cognate T cells in their immediate environment (57, 58), but also migrate to the lung-draining lymph nodes where they present to T cells in that compartment (58). In rats the airway-associated dendritic cells are somewhat more heterogeneous (53). Bronchoalveolar lavage (59) and tissue digest (60) studies of the human lung have revealed three populations of dendritic cells, including $CD11c^+CD1c^+$ and $CD11c^+$BDCA-3^+ myeloid cells, and $CD11c^-$BDCA-2^+ plasmacytoid dendritic cells, and these are considered analogous to the $CD11b^+CD103^-$ and $CD11b^-CD103^+langerin^+$ conventional and plasmacytoid dendritic cell subsets, respectively, in mice (61). Further analysis in chronically inflamed (e.g., COPD) lung tissues have revealed langerin-positive and DC-SIGN-expressing dendritic cell sub-populations (31, 62) that were proposed to represent the human equivalent of the murine $CD11b^-CD103^+langerin^+$ and monocyte-derived inflammatory dendritic cells, respectively (31, 62). The $CD103^+$ dendritic cells that comprise the bulk of the dendritic cells found in the lung-draining lymph node migrate there from the lung mucosa under the influence of lymph node-homing chemokines that signal via the CCR7 (43). In humans, the lung plasmacytoid dendritic cells express CD123 and BDCA-2, while the mouse plasmacytoid dendritic cell is $B220^{hi}Ly6C^{hi}Gr1^{lo}CD11b^-CD11c^{lo}$ (63). Plasmacytoid dendritic cells, which contribute importantly to tolerance responses to innocuous airway antigens (64), also express CD45RA, Ly49Q, BST2/tetherin [or murine plasmacytoid dendritic cell antigen (mPDCA)], sialic acid-binding immunoglobulin-type lectin (siglec)-H, inducible costimulator ligand (ICOS-L), programed death 1 ligand (PD-L)-1, and IDO (65), but produce copious amounts of IFNα in response to viral challenge (66). Under tolerogenic conditions, the $CD103^-$ and $CD103^+$ dendritic cells reportedly are specialized in presenting antigen to $CD4^+$ versus $CD8^+$ T cells, respectively (67, 68). However, under viral challenge the $CD103^+$ dendritic cells efficiently migrate to the draining lymph nodes where they cross-present viral antigens to $CD8^+$ T cells, while the $CD103^-$ cells tend to remain within the lung parenchyma, where they present to $CD4^+$ T cells in a pro-inflammatory manner (67, 68). This separation of function is also observed in asthmatic animals, wherein the $CD103^-$ dendritic cells present allergen to parenchymal $CD4^+$ T cells, while the $CD103^+$ subset presents allergen in the draining lymph node (69).

It is clear that the pulmonary dendritic cell contributes not only to the induction of asthma, but also to allergen-tolerance. Wholesale depletion of $CD11c^+$ cells abolishes disease onset following allergen exposure in experimental animals (70), but plasmacytoid dendritic cell depletion in animals challenged with otherwise innocuous aeroallergens leads to development of allergen-specific asthmatic responses (64). Steady-state plasmacytoid dendritic cells express an immature/semi-mature phenotype, with low levels of MHCII and co-stimulatory molecules and intermediate levels of PDL-1 (15, 71), which would contribute to their tolerogenic phenotype, but IDO expression by these cells also strongly inhibits T cell proliferative responses (72). Nevertheless, $CD103^+$ dendritic cells from the lungs of allergen-tolerant mice would also affect tolerance, inasmuch as they express RALDH and secrete retinoic acid, which contributes together with TGFβ to local induction of $Foxp3^+$ regulatory T cells (73). Finally, it is important to note the contributions of other populations within the lung to tolerance. Tissue-resident (74) and alveolar (75) macrophages both express TGFβ and RALDH under steady-state conditions, such that they can also induce $CD4^+$ T cells to which they present innocuous antigens to convert into $Foxp3^+$ Treg. Alveolar macrophages can also suppress the immunostimulatory properties of steady-state lung-resident dendritic cells (76) and thereby further contribute to steady-state tolerance in the lung.

CUTANEOUS DENDRITIC CELLS

As with the intestinal tract and lungs, the skin is constantly exposed both to pathogens, which require induction of protective Teff responses, and to innocuous environmental agents for which tolerance is the desired outcome. There are at least three subsets of skin-derived dendritic cells, including the self-renewing epidermal $langerin^+CD103^-$ Langerhans cell (77), and the $langerin^+CD103^+$ (78, 79) and $langerin^-CD103^-$ (80) dermal subsets; others have reported that the dermis contains five distinct subsets of dendritic cells (81). The epidermal Langerhans cell is probably the best known dendritic cell – as in other interfaces with our environment, these superficial cells form a contiguous network of interdigitating cells that are well positioned to detect and respond to cutaneous insults (82). In general, skin dendritic cells that acquire local antigens for lymph node presentation downregulate their E-cadherin epithelial receptors and upregulate CCR7, thereby acquiring responsiveness to chemokines expressed in the T cell zones of the draining lymph nodes (e.g., CCL19, CCL21) (14). In the lymph node, the dendritic cell presents its processed antigen peptides to the T cell, along with its co-stimulatory and polarizing signals. In addition, vitamin D3 metabolites expressed by the antigen-presenting dendritic cell induces T cell upregulation of CCR10, the receptor for the skin-homing chemokine CCL27 (22).

$Langerin^+$ migratory skin dendritic cells (i.e., $CD103^+$ dermal dendritic cells and Langerhans cells) can promote T cell tolerance responses to self antigens (83). The Langerhans cell appears to be unique in some respects, however, such that exposure to potent inflammatory adjuvants by itself does not override their innate tolerogenicity (84), perhaps in part because they do not express a number of important microbial pattern recognition receptors (e.g., TLR2, TLR4, or TLR5) (85). They are also unique in that, even while in a tolerogenic mode, they strongly express APC co-stimulatory markers and express IL-12. Nevertheless they fail to effectively activate NF-κB (i.e., translocate RelB into the nucleus) following adjuvant exposure (84), which is critical to induction of the immunostimulatory phenotype in dendritic cells (86). While dermal dendritic cells can effectively induce anti-bacterial immune responses, and would need to do so in situations where microbial organisms successfully penetrate the epithelial barrier, the default function of the Langerhans cell instead leads to regulatory T cell responses, perhaps as a means of preventing the integrity of the epidermal barrier from being compromised (85). Indeed, Langerhans cell depletion (e.g., by UV-B light exposure) has long been recognized to augment pathology in multiple contact sensitivity settings (87, 88). The Langerhans cell is efficient at capture and presentation of contact irritants, but this process can culminate in anergy and/or deletion of responding $CD8^+$ T cells, with induction of $ICOS^+CD4^+Foxp3^+$ regulatory T cell responses (89). The resident $CD141^+$ dermal dendritic cell in humans can also effect tolerance through their expression of the inhibitory receptor ILT3 and of IL-10, which together upregulate $CD25^+$ regulatory T cells that protect against allograft rejection (90). Migratory $CD103^+langerin^+$ dermal dendritic cells can also induce $CD25^+Foxp3^+$ Treg outgrowth from naïve T cells, at least in part through their expression of TGFβ (91).

HEPATIC DENDRITIC AND OTHER TOLERANCE-PROMOTING CELLS

It is well recognized that operational tolerance occurs more frequently with liver transplants than with other organs, suggesting that this organ may have a unique tolerogenic capacity (92). Human liver dendritic cells comprise most prevalently $BDCA\text{-}1^+$ DC that, unlike blood dendritic cells, secrete substantial amounts of IL-10 on TLR ligation, and this contributes to their high level induction of $CD25^+Foxp3^+$ Treg (11). It has also been reported that, in the steady state, hepatic myeloid and plasmacytoid dendritic cells can both induce tolerogenic T cell responses, although by distinct mechanisms – the myeloid cells express a mature phenotype and produce high levels of regulatory factors such as IL-10, IL-27, retinoic acid, and prostaglandin E2 (93–96), whereas hepatic plasmacytoid dendritic cells express a more immature phenotype and secrete high levels of IL-10 (97, 98). The non-parenchymal hepatic stellate cell, the major storage site for retinol in the body (99), would potentially also play a role in hepatic tolerance through provision of retinoic acid and thereby by-stander contributions to hepatic regulatory T cell induction (100, 101). Another factor to consider in hepatic tolerance is the resident liver macrophage, the Kuppfer cell. Kuppfer cells are present in very large numbers in the liver and express MHCII and co-stimulatory molecules, although as quiescent cells they only poorly present antigen. Nevertheless, just as the hepatic stellate cells are a rich source of retinoic acid, Kuppfer cells constitutively express abundant prostaglandin E2 and 15d-prostaglandin J2, which strongly inhibit T cell responses to immunostimulatory dendritic cells (102). Thus, there are multiple mechanisms that may contribute to the innate tolerogenic phenotype of the liver.

EXPERIMENTAL APPLICATION OF TOLEROGENIC DENDRITIC CELLS

STEADY-STATE AND IMMATURE DENDRITIC CELLS

For practical reasons it is unlikely that steady-state dendritic cells freshly purified from donor tissues would be used clinically, but investigations into such cells have provided substantial insights into the immunobiology of tolerogenic dendritic cells. Steady-state dendritic cells from lymphoid organs (103, 104) and non-inflamed tissues (91, 104, 105) express a relatively immature phenotype – in general, such cells are tolerogenic (105, 106). For example, treatment with small numbers of antigen-pulsed steady-state CD8α^+ splenic dendritic cells can induce asthma tolerance in mouse models, reversing the asthmatic animals' bronchial hyperresponsiveness and airway eosinophil and Th2 cytokine recall responses to allergen challenge; expression of IL-10, TGFβ, and IDO, as well as direct dendritic cell–Teff cell contact each contribute to the tolerogenic activities of these cells (107). It is important to their activity that such steady-state dendritic cells remain quiescent while being purified or manipulated *ex vivo*, as even overnight exposure of CD8α^+ dendritic cells to GM-CSF, for example, converts them into potent inducers of cytotoxic CD8$^+$ T cell responses (108). Steady-state CD8α^+ dendritic cell signaling leads to attenuated IL-2 expression by T cells and increased apoptosis, at least in part through the dendritic cell's expression of FasL (109–111).

Tissue dendritic cells that acquire antigens *in situ* in such a way that they do not become activated also remain tolerogenic. Thus, as noted, steady-state airway mucosal dendritic cells routinely migrate to the draining lymph nodes and present innocuous allergens in a tolerogenic fashion – indeed, this is the default mechanism by which ≈80% of the human population remains allergen-tolerant (112). Similarly, targeting antigens to dendritic cells with anti-DEC205, for example, does not activate the cells and thus leads to antigen-specific tolerance in multiple models (113–115). And dendritic cells that phagocytose apoptotic cells remain in a largely quiescent state and thus are also tolerogenic (116, 117), at least in part via induction of TGFβ expression in the draining lymph nodes with consequent activation of Foxp3$^+$ Treg (118).

There is also a large body of data regarding the tolerogenic properties of immunologically immature dendritic cells that have been generated *in vitro* from bone marrow or blood of mice or humans. These cells tend to express low levels of MHCII and co-stimulatory markers and have thus been thought of as largely ineffective in activating T cells through the classical TCR signaling pathways (119–122), although it has also been suggested that PD-L1 and PD-L2 expression by these cells contributes to their tolerogenic activities (123). There are ≈100 genes that are differentially expressed in immature versus immunostimulatory mouse bone marrow-derived dendritic cells, including a number of cytokines (e.g., Flt3L, TNF), chemokines (e.g., MIP2, RANTES), chemokine receptors (e.g., CCR2, CCR5), and other (e.g., RP105, Axl) markers (124). Passive transfer of antigen-pulsed immature dendritic cells has been shown to induce tolerance either *in vivo* or *in vitro* in numerous experimental models and with human cells (125–132). An important caveat with use of immature dendritic cells to treat overtly inflammatory conditions is that the pro-inflammatory environment they face *in vivo* can activate these cells, such that they activate pathogenic (e.g., Th1, Th17) as opposed to regulatory T cell responses (133, 134), as discussed below.

INDUCED TOLEROGENIC DENDRITIC CELLS

Some of the first insights into the induction of a tolerogenic phenotype within dendritic cells arose from the studies of Langerhans cells that had been exposed to either ultraviolet B radiation (8) or IL-10 (8, 9). Dendritic cells from IL-10-expressing melanoma tumors (135) and IL-10-exposed immature monocyte-derived dendritic cells (136) were then also shown to be tolerogenic. This potential for using tolerogenic cells, whether dendritic cells or subsequently induced regulatory T cells, to dampen pathogenic responses has burgeoned into a field of immunology into itself. We now know that a large array of mediators can induce a tolerogenic phenotype within dendritic cell populations. These include IL-10 (9, 30, 33, 135–149) and other cytokines (150–158), corticosteroids (143, 159–162), vitamin D3 (160, 163–172), rapamycin (143, 160, 173–175), and neuropeptides (176, 177) (**Table 1**), each of which we will discuss. Although we will not discuss the following populations, it has been reported that dendritic cells can also be rendered tolerogenic by exposure to: anti-CD3 (178); *Aspergillus oryzae* protease (162); aspirin (179); atorvastatin (180); butyric or mycophenolic acids (181); the α7β0 isoform of C4b-binding protein (182); the FasL decoy receptor, decoy receptor-3 (183); galectin-1 (184, 185); growth-related oncogene (GRO)-gamma (186); intravenous immunoglobulin (IVIg) (187, 188); protein kinase C inhibitors (189); or retinoic acid (190–193), or by inhibition of miRNA let-7i (194). IL-10-, vitamin D3-, dexamethasone-, and rapamycin-induced tolerogenic dendritic cells stand out as populations that have had been particularly well-studied in mouse and/or human systems, so we will concentrate our discussions on these cells, with the interested reader referred to the cited reports for these alternate populations. Furthermore, given the potential ethical issues with use of dendritic cells transfected with viruses that express tolerogenic molecules (e.g., IL-10, CTLA4Ig) or that suppress stimulatory molecules (e.g., co-stimulatory, immunostimulatory, or pro-apoptotic molecules, such as CD80, IL-12, or TRAIL, respectively (195)), we will not devote significant discussion to these approaches at this time.

INTERLEUKIN-10-INDUCED REGULATORY DENDRITIC CELLS

As noted, IL-10 was one of the first mediators shown to induce human dendritic cells to adopt a tolerogenic phenotype (8, 9, 122,

Table 1 | Phenotypes of human tolerogenic dendritic cells differentiated using different agents.

Agent	DC	DCreg markers	Effector	Mechanisms of tolerance (outcomes)	Treg induced	Reference
Nil	Immature MDDC	↓ Co-stim, MHCII, IL-12	↓ Co-stim, MHCII	Induction of T cell anergy	N.D.	(119–122)
Apoptot. cells	Immature MDDC	↓ Co-stim, MHCII, IL-12 ↑ TGFβ	↓ Co-stim, MHCII	Induction of T cell anergy	Foxp3$^+$ Treg	(116, 118)
IL-10	Semi-mature MDDC ("DC10")	↓ Co-stim, MHCII, IL-12 ↑ IL-10, ILT-2, -3, and -4, PD-L1 and -L2, GILZ	IL-10 and contact-depend	↓ Autol. T cell prolif.	CD25$^+$Foxp3$^+$ Treg	(30, 143, 196–198)
	Immature MDDC	↓ Co-stim, MHCII ↑ ILT3, IL-10, GILZ, TLR2	N.D.	↓ Allo. T cell prolif.	N.D.	(136, 158, 164)
	Immature MDDC ("DC-10")	↓ Co-stim, MHCII ↑ ILT-2, -3, -4, HLA-G	IL-10, ILT4, HLA-G	↓ Allo. T cell prolif. ↑ Tr1	Tr1	(33)
Vit D3	Immat. MDDC	↓ Co-stim and CD83, MHCII ↑ HLA-DR	N.D.	↓ Allo. T cell prolif.	Not CD25$^+$ Foxp3$^+$ Treg	(160)
	MDDC + LPS	Intermed co-stim/MHCII ↑ IL-10, TNF, PD-L1 and ILT3	PD-L1	↓ Allo. T cell prolif., Teff > IL-10 Treg	CD25$^+$Foxp3$^+$ Treg or ND	(163, 170–172, 199)
	MDDC + TLR stim.	hMDDC, LPS maturation	LPS ≫ IL-10 med	↓ Allo. T cell prolif.	N.D.	(164)
	MDDC + LPS	↑ Surface TNF ↓ Secr. TNF	Surface TNF	↑ Treg induction	N.D.	(167)
	Dermal DC	N.D.	IL-10	↓ Allo. T cell prolif.	Tr1 cells	(200)
	Langerhans cells	N.D.	TGFβ	↓ Allo. T cell prolif.	CD25$^+$Foxp3$^+$ Treg	(200)
	CD141$^-$CD1c$^+$ blood DC	↑ CD83 ↑ CD141, CD14, ILT3, MØ mann. R	IL-10		CD25$^+$Foxp3$^+$ Treg	(90)
Dex	Immat. MDDC	↑ CD86, MHCII CD83 med	IL-10	↓ Allo. T cell prolif.	N.D.	(160)
	MDDC + LPS	Intermed co-stim/MHCII ↑ IL-10	N.D.	↓ Allo. T cell prolif., Teff > IL-10 Treg	IL-10-secreting, contact-depend. Treg	(171)
	MDDC ±TLR stim.	Intermed co-stim/MHCII ILT3$^+$, IL-10$^+$, GILZ$^+$, TLR2$^+$	N.D.	↓ Allo. T cell prolif.		(164)
	DC2.4 cells	↓ IL-12	N.D.	↓ Allo. T cell prolif.	CD25$^+$Foxp3$^+$ Treg	(201)
Steroid	MDDC	GILZ$^+$	N.D.		N.D.	(202)
VitD3 + Dex	MDDC	↓ Co-stim and CD83, MHCII > CD14, HLA-DR, CD80, CD273	IL-10	↓ Allo. T cell prolif. ↓ CD25$^+$Foxp3$^+$ Treg ↑ Tr1 and Breg	Tr1 or N.D.	(165, 203)
VIP-DC	Immature MDDC	↓ Co-stim, MHCII ↑ IL-10	N.D.	Weak naïve allo T cell activation	Tr1 and CD4$^+$ CD28$^-$CTLA4$^+$ Treg	(176, 204)
Rapamycin	Immat. MDDC	↓ Co-stim med. MHCII	IL-10?	↓ Allo. T cell prolif. ↑ Foxp3$^+$CD25$^+$ Treg	CD25$^+$Fopx3$^+$ Treg	(160, 205, 206)

135, 136, 141, 148, 150, 209–212). These reports together indicated that IL-10-differentiated monocyte-derived dendritic cells display reduced levels of MHCII and co-stimulatory markers, and can induce Teff cell anergy. Sometime later it was shown that IL-10-induced semi-mature $CD14^+$ monocyte-derived dendritic cells (DC10) from atopic asthmatic individuals suppress specific allergen-driven proliferative and Th2 cytokine responses of autologous peripheral blood $CD4^+CD25^{-/lo}Foxp3^-$ Teff cells, and convert these Teff cells into regulatory T cells (30). The maturation status of these DC10 was attributable to their exposure during differentiation to a stimulatory cocktail containing IL-1β, TNF, IL-6, and PGE2, in addition to IL-10 (30), but these cells are resistant to further, LPS-induced, maturation (209). DC10 express low levels of MHCII, co-stimulatory markers, 4-1BBL and OX40L, but they strongly express DEC205, IFNα1, CCR7, ILT2 (an inhibitory HLA-G receptor), as well as IL-10 (**Table 2**). They induce Teff cells to differentiate into IL-10-secreting $CD25^+Foxp3^+LAG\text{-}3^+CTLA4^+$ regulatory T cells, which in turn suppress allergen-driven responses of autologous Teff cells in a contact-dependent fashion (30). Others found that similar semi-mature IL-10-differentiated dendritic cells express high levels of ILT3, ILT4, PD-L1, and PD-L2, that they (but not immature cells) respond strongly to the lymph node-homing chemokine CCL19 (143), and that they induce regulatory T cells that also suppress allogeneic T cell responses in a contact, but not IL-10- or TGFβ-dependent fashion (196). These DC10 also express glucocorticoid-induced leucine zipper (GILZ), which is both necessary and sufficient for expression of IL-10, ILT3, and PD-L1 by these cells – GILZ silencing eliminates their tolerogenic activities (197, 198). IL-10-differentiated human monocyte-derived dendritic cells that have never been exposed to maturation-inducing agents are also tolerogenic (33, 148, 212). As noted above, a minor population of IL-10-producing circulating dendritic cells, called DC-10, was recently identified in humans (33), and those investigators also generated an analogous population of immature IL-10-differentiated dendritic cells (DC-10) that similarly express IL-10 (**Table 2**), as well as the inhibitory receptors ILT2, ILT3, ILT4, and HLA-G (33). Others have noted that such cells also express signaling lymphocyte activation molecule (SLAMF1, CD150) (148), which inhibits CD40-mediated signal transduction (213), and would therefore interfere with two-way dendritic cell-T cell conversations. These cells have been reported to suppress Teff cell responses in a manner that is contact-dependent, and independent of any role for secreted soluble mediators (148), although others note that IL-10 secretion and cell-surface inhibitory receptors are both important to the regulatory activities of such immature IL-10-differentiated dendritic cells (33). It is very intriguing that exposure of semi-mature human dendritic cells to IL-10 leads to their induction of classical $CD25^+Foxp3^+$ Treg (30, 196), while exposure of immature human dendritic cells to IL-10 leads to induction of $Foxp3^-$ Tr1 cells (33). It will be interesting to determine whether exposure of such immature regulatory dendritic cells to inflammatory (i.e., maturation-promoting) conditions would qualitatively or quantitatively affect their immunobiology.

Murine DC10 can prevent the onset of asthma in experimental mice, as well as reverse the asthmatic phenotype in severely affected animals (137, 138, 140, 214–216), just as do dendritic cells that have been virally transfected to express very high levels of IL-10 (146). These DC10, which are not exposed to maturational stimuli during differentiation, display low levels of cell-surface MCHII and co-stimulatory markers, are avidly phagocytic and chemotactically responsive to MIP-1α, and express elevated levels of IL-10, TGFβ (137, 138, 215), and PD-L1 (Li et al., unpublished observation). They are highly effective therapeutically in mouse models of ovalbumin (OVA) – (138, 140, 214–216) and house dust mite – (137) asthma. In both settings, DC10 abrogate airway hyperresponsiveness (AHR) within 3 weeks of treatment and dampen the allergic Th2 phenotype

Table 2 | Impact of phenotype on the levels of IL-10 secretion by regulatory dendritic cells.

Differentiating agent	DC (IL-10 levels)	Reference
NON-REGULATORY DENDRITIC CELLS		
TNF	Semi-mature MDDC (≈35 pg/ml)	(30)
Nil	semi-mature MDDC (LPS, >700 pg/ml; CD40L, >2 ng/ml)	(207)
TOLEROGENIC DENDRITIC CELLS		
Vitamin D3/dexamethasone	MDDC (9 ng/ml)	(203)
C1Q	MDDC (5 ng/ml)	(208)
Vasoactive intestinal peptide	MDDC (LPS, ≈5 ng/ml)	(176)
Galectin-1	MDDC (LPS, ≈500 pg/ml)	(185)
Vitamin D3	Dermal DC (CD40L, ≈300–700 pg/ml)	(90)
	MDDC (unstim or LPS, ≈100 pg/ml)	(160, 164)
	MDDC (LPS or CD40L, ≈2 ng/ml)	(167)
	MDDC (CD40L, 4 ng/ml)	(163)
IL-10	Immat. MDDC (unstim, 200–750 pg/ml; CD40L, 1.5 ng/ml)	(33, 143, 163, 164)
	Semi-mature MDDC (unstim, 300 pg/ml; LPS, 7 ng/ml)	(30, 158)
Dexamethasone	Immat MDDC (unstim, 25–200 pg/ml)	(143, 159, 160, 198)
	MDDC (LPS or CD40L, 0.5–3 ng/ml)	(159–161, 198)
Rapamycin	MDDC (unstim or LPS, 50–100 pg/ml)	(143, 160)
TGFβ	MDDC (unstim, 200 pg/ml; LPS, ≈2 ng/ml)	(143, 158)

in an allergen-specific fashion (137, 138, 140, 215). This suppression of allergen-induced airway eosinophil and Th2 cytokine responses and circulating allergen-specific IgE and IgG1 levels is progressive, such that at 8 months after a single DC10 treatment these parameters are at near background levels (138), although four DC10 treatments bring the asthma phenotype to near background within 2 months (138). Cell tracking studies indicate that DC10 that are delivered intraperitoneally accumulate maximally in the lungs and lung-draining lymph nodes within 1 week, but few, if any, DC10 can be detected within any anatomic compartment at 3 weeks post-treatment (214). This indicates that while tolerance induced by DC10 is long-lived, most of its impact is realized only after the treatment cells have disappeared from the body. That is consistent with the observation that DC10 treatments induce $CD4^{+}CD44^{hi}CD69^{hi}CD62L^{lo}CD25^{lo}Foxp3^{-}$ Teff cells to transdifferentiate into $CD4^{+}CD25^{+}Foxp3^{+}$ Treg, with maximal Treg activation occurring at 3 weeks after DC10 treatment (215). Human DC10-induced $CD25^{+}Foxp3^{+}$ Treg express LAG3 and CTLA3 (30), while the analogous Treg in DC10-treated asthmatic mice express LAG3, cytotoxic T lymphocyte antigen-4 (CTLA4) (137, 215), ICOS, PD-1, GITR (215), and neuropilin-1, but lower levels of Helios (217). Infectious tolerance is also evident in these animals, as the endogenous pulmonary $CD11c^{+}$ dendritic cells of DC10-treated asthmatic animals also take on a regulatory phenotype (Li et al., unpublished observation). While DC10 engage $CD4^{+}CD25^{+}Foxp3^{+}$ natural (n)Treg in a productive fashion and these T cells have a modest role in the asthma tolerance within DC10-treated animals, DC10-induced $CD25^{+}Foxp3^{+}$ (i)Treg are many-fold more effective than naturally occurring $CD25^{+}Foxp3^{+}$ regulatory T cells (nTreg) of identical TCR specificity in suppressing the asthma phenotype (217).

IL-10 expression by immature or otherwise quiescent dendritic cells has been reported numerous times to be important to tolerance induced by these cells (24, 107, 218), and DC10 (as well as DC-10) express yet higher levels of this regulatory cytokine (30, 33, 137, 138, 140, 215, 216) (**Table 2**). Indeed, expression of IL-10 by DC10 is critical (140, 214) although not sufficient for tolerance induction, inasmuch as MHCII-knock-out DC10, which expresses otherwise therapeutic levels of IL-10, do not induce tolerance (214). Moreover, combined IL-10 and MHCII expression by DC10 is still not sufficient for full expression of tolerance – allergen-presenting CD80/CD86 double knock-out (214) or CD40-knock-out (W. Dawicki, H. Huang and J.R. Gordon, unpublished observations) DC10 still do not induce tolerance at levels equivalent to wild-type DC10 (214). This underscores that conversion of Teff cells to regulatory T cells by DC10 requires not only delivery of tolerogenic signals to the T cell, but also productive feedback from the engaged T cell to the DC10.

VITAMIN D3-INDUCED REGULATORY DENDRITIC CELLS

Vitamin D and its metabolites would appear to have a significant influence within the immune system, such that there is substantial evidence of an unrealized potential for its use in an array of immunologic disorders [reviewed in Ref. (219, 220)]. It is clear that vitamin D3 can induce differentiation of tolerogenic dendritic cells (DC-VitD3) (163, 170, 221, 222). Addition of vitamin D3 to mouse bone marrow (177, 223, 224) or human monocyte-derived (164, 170, 172, 225) dendritic cell cultures induces cells that express low levels of MHC II and co-stimulatory molecules, and produce IL-10 instead of IL-12 (**Table 2**). Semi-mature monocyte-derived DC-VitD3 express augmented levels of TNF and PDL-1, and this PDL-1 is reportedly critical to their induction of IL-10-expressing contact-dependent Treg (171), as is expression of membrane-bound TNF by these dendritic cells (226). As with IL-10-differentiated dendritic cells, DC-VitD3 only respond to the lymph node-homing chemokine CCL19 if they have been exposed to maturational stimuli (143). This again raises the question of whether such chemokine-dependent lymph node homing might reasonably be expected to contribute, if not be critical, to the tolerogenic activities of regulatory dendritic cells. Addition of vitamin D3 to cultures of human skin Langerhans cells leads to expression of TGFβ by these cells and thereby downstream induction of $CD25^{hi}CD127^{lo}Foxp3^{+}$ cells (i.e., classical inducible Treg) (200). It similarly induces $CD141^{-}CD1c^{+}$ human blood dendritic cells to differentiate into IL-10-expressing dermal dendritic cell-like $CD141^{+}CD14^{+}ILT3^{+}$ cells that induce development of $CD25^{hi}CTLA4^{+}Foxp3^{+}$ Treg responses (90). In contrast, addition of vitamin D3 to cultures of human dermal dendritic cells upregulates expression of IL-10 and their induction of IL-10-expressing $Foxp3^{-}$ Tr1 cells (200). This highlights again that exposure of different dendritic cell populations to the same mediator can have very divergent outcomes in terms of the type(s) of regulatory T cells so induced. DC-VitD3 have been shown to be tolerogenic *in vivo* as well. Treatment of diabetic mice with pancreatic islet antigen-pulsed DC-VitD3 prior to pancreatic islet transplantation significantly decreases subsequent islet rejection (166), while sensitization of mice with H-Y antigen-pulsed DC-VitD3 leads to prolongation of male skin grafts in female recipients (177, 223, 224).

DEXAMETHASONE-INDUCED TOLEROGENIC DENDRITIC CELLS

The anti-inflammatory and immunosuppressive properties of corticosteroids have been known and employed clinically since their discovery some 75 years ago (227). While glucocorticoid treatments have significant clinical benefits in terms of suppressing inflammation, and it has been shown that they increase the numbers of $CD4^{+}CD25^{hi}$ cells and Foxp3 expression levels in multiple inflammatory settings, these increases are not necessarily associated with augmented Treg activity (228). Corticosteroids do induce immature dendritic cells to adopt a tolerogenic phenotype and thereby contribute to the anti-inflammatory properties of these agents (159, 229, 230), but the fact that mature dendritic cells undergo apoptosis in response to *in vitro* or *in vivo* dexamethasone treatment suggests that its effects on dendritic cells are somewhat more complex (231). Dendritic cells that are differentiated in the presence of dexamethasone (DC-Dex) express low levels of co-stimulatory markers and MHC II, produce elevated levels of IL-10 and less IL-12 (159, 161, 164, 171, 229, 230, 232), and express modestly elevated levels of ILT2 (198) and ILT3, but high levels of GILZ (164). As with semi-mature IL-10-differentiated dendritic cells, GILZ expression by DC-Dex is critical to their expression of IL-10, ILT3, and B7-H1/PDL-1 (197); both populations also maintain their immunosuppressive phenotype even after stimulation with TLR4 agonists (209, 233, 234).

The similarities between DC10 and dexamethasone-conditioned dendritic cells extends further – dexamethasone-exposed DC2.4 dendritic cells also induce Foxp3$^+$ Treg differentiation *in vitro* (201), while use of DC-Dex immunotherapy for experimental corneal allografts similarly leads to increased tissue levels of intragraft Foxp3$^+$ T cells, reduced levels of graft inflammatory cell infiltrates, and prolonged graft survival (235). And others have reported that repetitive stimulation of T cells with DC-Dex induces the T cells to adopt a contact-dependent regulatory T cell phenotype (171). DC-Dex treatment of murine recipients of MHC-mismatched heart transplants leads to delayed rejection of the allografts (234) although, oddly, DC-Dex treatments reportedly accelerate antibody-mediated graft rejection responses to transplanted MHC-mismatched pancreatic islets in rats (236). Interestingly, the contact-dependent regulatory T cells induced by DC-Dex, but not those induced by DC-VitD3, reportedly suppress T cell responses in an antigen-independent fashion (171), although others have shown that, as a general feature, activated regulatory T cells readily suppress by-stander Teff cell responses (237, 238).

VITAMIN D3 AND DEXAMETHASONE-INDUCED TOLEROGENIC DENDRITIC CELLS

While vitamin D3 and dexamethasone each can induce a tolerogenic phenotype in dendritic cells, some investigators have further assessed the regulatory activities of cells generated in the presence of both vitamin D3 and dexamethasone (DC-Dex/VitD3). DC-Dex/VitD3 produce much high levels of IL-10 (i.e., 9 ng/ml) (203) than either DC-VitD3 or DC-Dex (i.e., 0.1–4 ng/ml) (**Table 2**) (143, 159, 160, 163, 164, 167, 198), and thus display a higher IL-10/IL-12 expression ratio and poorly stimulate allogeneic T cell proliferation responses (165). They reportedly cannot effectively prime naïve CD8 T cells but, interestingly, while a single DC-Dex/VitD3 treatment drives expansion of memory CD8 T cells, any subsequent DC-Dex/VitD3 exposure leads to collapse of the CD8$^+$ T cell populations (239). DC-Dex/VitD3 have been shown to be somewhat effective in suppressing colitis pathology in a mouse model, apparently also in an antigen-independent manner (240).

NEUROPEPTIDE-INDUCED TOLEROGENIC DENDRITIC CELLS

Vasoactive intestinal peptide (VIP) is a 28-amino acid immunomodulatory neuropeptide that binds to B-class G-protein-coupled receptors such as the VPAC1 and VPAC2 (241, 242). VIP treatments induce regulatory T cell responses in experimental animals and with human Teff cells (243). For example, VIP treatment of mice with TNBS-induced colitis induces tolerance responses, dampening TLR2- and TLR4-induced inflammation and increasing expression of Foxp3 and TGFβ (244), as it does in a rat model of collagen-induced arthritis (245). But VIP can act directly on the Teff cells – culture of CD25$^-$Foxp3$^-$ Teff with VIP induces their differentiation into CD25$^+$Foxp3$^+$ Treg that express high levels of IL-10 and CTLA4 and are protective in a mouse model of graft versus host disease (GVHD) (246). Nevertheless, VIP can also induce dendritic cells to adopt a regulatory phenotype and thereby affect tolerance by this means. Differentiation of human dendritic cells in the presence of VIP (DC-VIP) or the neuropeptide pituitary adenylate cyclase-activating polypeptide (PACAP) induces the development of cells that secrete of high levels of IL-10, and strongly induce regulatory T cell responses. DC-VIP treatments dampen pathology in a number of experimental settings, including experimental allergic encephalomyelitis (EAE), rheumatoid arthritis (247), bone marrow transplant-induced GVHD (248), and colitis (249). While a number of reports indicate that DC-VIP induce Tr1 phenotype regulatory cells, as determined by secretion of IL-10/TGFβ, but not IFNγ, IL-2, IL-4, or IL-5 (204, 250–252), other reports indicate that DC-VIP instead induce CD4$^+$CD25$^+$Foxp3$^+$ Treg responses (253–255) in some of the same model systems. DC-VIP can also induce IL-10-secreting CD28$^-$CTLA4$^+$CD8$^+$ Treg (176, 252). VIP-secreting VIP-lentivirus-transfected DC are similarly tolerogenic in mouse models of acute and chronic EAE and cecal ligation-and-puncture sepsis (177). It has been speculated that DC-VIP would be more effective therapeutically when targeting Th1 rather than Th2 responses (176), ostensibly because VIP skews Th1 or Th17 T cells to a Th2 phenotype (256). This raises an important question in dendritic cell immunotherapeutics, and that is whether the specific type of regulatory cell to be employed (e.g., DC-Dex versus DC-VIP) needs to be carefully matched with, for example, the Th1, Th2, or Th17 nature of the target disease in order to ensure optimized outcomes.

RAPAMYCIN-INDUCED TOLEROGENIC DENDRITIC CELLS

Rapamycin is a macrolide immunosuppressive agent that dampens dendritic cell maturation through binding to the serine/threonine protein kinase mammalian target of rapamycin (mTOR). Signaling via mTOR has broad-ranging effects in many systems, including the nervous system, nutrition, and others, where it regulates cell growth, proliferation, motility, and survival (257). Antigen recognition by naïve CD4$^+$ and CD8$^+$ T cells activates mTOR and thereby fosters cellular progression to a committed Foxp3$^-$ Teff phenotype (205), while suppression of mTOR with rapamycin leads instead to induction of fully functional CD25$^+$Foxp3$^+$ Treg (258). Thus it was reported some time ago that rapamycin increases the regulatory activities of CD4$^+$CD25$^+$Foxp3$^+$ Treg (206). Clinically, rapamycin has been widely used to prevent allograft rejection, particularly in renal transplant patients (206), although the potential for rapamycin-related adverse cutaneous manifestations in these patients has limited its broad applicability (259). Rapamycin affects both T cells and dendritic cells, although it displays divergent effects on myeloid and monocyte-derived dendritic cells, augmenting the allostimulatory capacity of the former cells but markedly dampening the immunostimulatory phenotype of monocyte-derived dendritic cells (260). In experimental systems rapamycin treatments impair Flt3L mobilization of murine dendritic cells, their upregulation of co-stimulatory molecule and inflammatory cytokine expression, and their allostimulatory activity (261), even after exposure to activating agents such as LPS or anti-CD40 (262). Mouse dendritic cells that are differentiated in the presence of rapamycin (DC-Rap) induce naïve T cells to differentiate into CD25$^+$Foxp3$^+$ Treg (263). Moreover, such DC-Rap enhance apoptotic death among alloreactive CD8 T cells (264), further contributing to the tolerance response of transplant recipients. DC-Rap treatment of murine heart transplant recipients similarly induces outgrowth within the transplants of Foxp3$^+$ Treg and, as a consequence, long term organ survival (262), just as has been shown in numerous other studies (173, 206, 261, 262, 265, 266).

IMPACT OF DELIVERY ROUTE AND INFLAMMATION ON THERAPEUTIC OUTCOMES

SELECTING THE CORRECT DELIVERY ROUTE FOR TOLEROGENIC DENDRITIC CELLS

Not all routes for delivery of tolerogenic dendritic cells will necessarily provide the desired outcomes. For example, we reported that $CD45.2^+$ DC10 that are delivered intraperitoneally to congenic $CD45.1^+$ mice with a severe asthma phenotype appear within the lungs and airways of recipient mice within 2 days of delivery, achieve maximal numbers in this compartment by 7 days and then wane thereafter. DC10 appear in the lung-draining (mediastinal) lymph node of these animals in lower numbers, but with approximately the same kinetics, and also in the spleen but not cervical nodes, MLNs, blood, bone marrow, or liver. Within 3 weeks of delivery the treatment cells are no longer detectable in the lungs or mediastinal lymph nodes (214), suggesting that the natural lifespan of such DC10 may be 2–3 weeks. We know that DC10 treatments correct ~50% of the pathognomic bronchial hyperresponsiveness seen in asthma phenotype mice within 2 weeks of treatment and that by 3 weeks this airway response is completely normalized (138). Moreover, the time of maximal activation of regulatory T cells in the lungs of these animals is 3 weeks after DC10 delivery, but it was not determined whether the primary site within which the DC10 induce Teff cells to differentiate into regulatory T cells was *in situ* in the lungs or in the mediastinal lymph nodes (or both) (215). This remains an important, but unanswered question.

We also assessed the relative effects of intraperitoneal (i.p.), transtracheal (t.t.), subcutaneous (back skin; s.c.), or intravenous (i.v.) DC10 delivery to asthmatic animals and found that i.p. or t.t. delivery were equally effective, fully reversing bronchial hyperresponsiveness, and rapidly dampening airway eosinophil and Th2 cytokine responses to allergen challenge and circulating allergen-specific IgE and IgG1 levels (138). The s.c. DC10 treatments dampened the airway recall responses to allergen challenge, but not bronchial hyperresponsiveness, nor did they significantly reduce systemic IgE levels (138). On the other hand, multiple investigators have reported that s.c. delivery of tolerogenic dendritic cells is protective in rat models of EAE (267–271), which suggests that the anatomic site of the target pathology in immunotherapeutic applications may be important in selecting the delivery route for the treatment dendritic cells. Intravenous delivery of DC10 has no discernible impact of the disease phenotype in a mouse model of asthma (138, 272) or a rat model of EAE (271), but in mouse models of cardiomyopathy (147), experimental immune myocarditis (149, 273), and diabetes (274, 275) i.v. delivery of tolerogenic dendritic cells significantly reduces local pathology and induces tolerance. Similarly, i.v. infusion of DC-VitD/IL-10 in a rhesus macaque model of allogeneic kidney transplantation significantly prolonged survival relative to control animals (rapamycin/CTLA4Ig treatment, but no dendritic cells) (276). There has not been a sufficient number of comprehensive studies on the impact of the route of dendritic cell delivery on tolerance outcomes to generate specific guidelines at this point in time, but it does appear that the disease or compartment being targeted may be an important consideration. Certainly, we would expect that the cells should be migration-competent (i.e., express appropriate chemokine receptors), such that they are able to travel to the disease target site or its draining lymph nodes in order to best interact with the cognate Teff cells.

USE OF TOLEROGENIC DENDRITIC CELLS IN INFLAMMATORY SETTINGS

An important consideration in clinical use of tolerogenic dendritic cells, particularly when targeting inflammatory diseases (e.g., colitis, inflammatory bowel disease), is whether pre-existing adverse conditions that these cells might encounter after delivery can alter or ablate their tolerogenic activity. If so, could an inflammatory milieu convert the treatment dendritic cells into immunostimulatory populations that might exacerbate rather than ameliorate disease severity? While immature dendritic cells can have substantial tolerogenic activities, we know that exposure of these cells (133, 134) or even some populations of semi-mature dendritic cells (133, 134) to inflammatory environments can induce them to differentiate into potently immunostimulatory cells that *augment* disease severity. With this in mind, many investigators have assessed the impact of maturation-provoking (30, 90, 143, 165, 197) or otherwise inflammatory (163, 164, 167, 170, 171, 177, 222) signals on the tolerogenic phenotype of their differentiated dendritic cells. Dendritic cells express receptors for and can be activated by a number of pro-inflammatory cytokines (e.g., IL-1, TNF, IFN, TSLP) (277) and they can express numerous pattern recognition receptors [e.g., protease-activated receptors (PARs), TLR, C-type lectin receptors (78, 164, 278–281)], retinoic acid-inducible gene-1 (RIG-1) and the melanoma differentiation-associated gene-5 (MDA-5) (281), through which they interact with microbial and non-microbial agents. For example, a number of "natural" allergens (e.g., house dust mite) trigger inflammatory responses through their abilities to activate cells via PAR2 (282, 283) or C-type lectin receptors such as DC-SIGN and dectin-2 (284), while TLR signaling can potently activate expression of inflammatory signals by immature or mature dendritic cells. There have been a number of excellent reviews that address the expression of TLR by human and mouse dendritic cells [e.g., Ref. (281)], such that we will not address this issue herein.

Toll-like receptor signaling within tolerogenic dendritic cell populations does not always have a detrimental outcome. For example, BDCA-1^+ human liver dendritic cells secrete substantial amounts of IL-10 on TLR ligation, and this contributes to their high level induction of $CD25^+Foxp3^+$ Treg (11). Human DC10, DC-Dex, and DC-VitD express the same panel of TLR as monocyte-derived dendritic cells, such that all are responsive to Pam3CSK4, polyinosinic-polycytidylic acid, LPS, and flagellin (164), but the tolerogenic populations uniquely upregulate expression of TLR2 on TLR engagement (164). Moreover, TLR2 or TLR4 signaling in human DC-VitD3 and DC-Dex induces expression of the tolerance-promoting cytokines IL-10 and IL-27 (160, 285). Others have reported that human DC-Dex are refractory to challenge with an array of heat-killed gram-negative bacteria (e.g., *Escherichia coli*, *Protheus mirabillis*, *Klebsiella pneumoniae*, *Salmonella thyphimurium*) (286), while DC-Rap (160) and DC-VIP (252) are resistant to reversal of their tolerogenic phenotype by

LPS challenge. Interestingly, while isolated LPS challenge induces an IL-12 response by immature monocyte-derived dendritic cells, simultaneous exposure of these cells to LPS and IFNγ reportedly leads to a transient IL-12 response that is replaced within 24–48 h with a robust IL-10 response (287).

Finally, while we may well be able to design and generate tolerogenic dendritic cells that are resistant to reversal of phenotype by inflammatory environments, it is clear that the tolerance they induce is also dependent on transference of that phenotype to the regulatory T cells with which they interact. Moreover, infectious tolerance also involves the conversion of endogenous tissue dendritic cells into tolerogenic populations by the induced regulatory T cells (226, 288). Indeed, it has been suggested that a defect in such infectious tolerance processes may contribute to the development of an asthma phenotype in affected individuals (289). The desired outcome in dendritic cell immunotherapy is the induction of regulatory T cells that can reverse pathogenic Teff cell responses, but at least some populations of regulatory T cells can be converted into pathogenic Teff cells in the context of inflammatory environments – it has been shown that $Foxp3^+$ Treg can convert to Th17 cells in animals with colitis (290, 291), but we seem to have only scant evidence regarding the extent to which other populations of regulatory cells (e.g., Tr1 or Th3 cells) can be enticed to such reversal of phenoytpe *in vivo*. In considering whether inflammatory environments may differentially affect the phenotype of regulatory T cells (or dendritic cells), we query whether the regulatory T cells that are naturally associated with a specific compartment (e.g., Th3 cells in the gut) might be more resistant to reversal of phenotype by challenges they would routinely encounter in that compartment than other regulatory T cells (e.g., Treg, Tr1). Finally, we raise the issue of whether in some specific settings, it might be advisable to activate multiple types of regulatory T cell responses, such that the tolerance so induced might be less susceptible by reversal by subsequent coincidental inflammatory events.

CLINICAL APPLICATION OF TOLEROGENIC DENDRITIC CELLS

The first tolerogenic dendritic cell study in humans was undertaken by Ralph Steinman's lab. They demonstrated that s.c. administration of antigen-loaded immature dendritic cells (2×10^6 cells/subject) was well tolerated by the study subjects and also that the treatments could suppress antigen-specific $CD8^+$ T cell responses (128) for ≤6 months (127). More recently a clinical trial was undertaken with 10 subjects with type 1 diabetes, each of whom was given 1×10^7 autologous dendritic cells intradermally four times at 2 week intervals; the treatment cells had been transduced with anti-sense oligonucleotides to silence co-stimulatory molecules (i.e., CD40, CD80, and CD86), although efficacy data on that silencing was not reported (292). The authors had developed their silencing protocols in a mouse model of type 1 diabetes and shown that the dendritic cell treatments had had statistically significant, though quite modest, disease-sparing effects (293). As with the earlier study by Steinman (127, 128), there were no adverse events related to the dendritic cell treatments in this latter study, but there were few if any immunologically discernible tolerance outcomes attributable to the dendritic cell treatments (292).

There have been a large number of *in vitro* studies performed as proof of principle that tolerogenic dendritic cells can efficiently reduce Teff cell responses in humans. As noted above, it was shown that semi-mature IL-10-differentiated dendritic cells (i.e., DC10) generated from atopic asthmatic donors can suppress the responses of autologous T cell to specific allergen. Moreover, the DC10 induce the outgrowth of immunosuppressive $CD4^+CD25^+Foxp3^+LAG3^+CTLA4^+$ Treg from the peripheral blood Teff cell pool (30). Others have reported that DC-VitD/Dex from individuals with rheumatoid arthritis (294) or DC-VitD3 from subjects with relapsing-remitting multiple sclerosis (295) are both able to suppress autologous $CD4^+$ Teff cell responses to specific antigen-presenting mature dendritic cells.

In conclusion, it is clear that multiple mediators can induce a tolerogenic phenotype in dendritic cells, and that these substantially influence the conversations that occur between the dendritic cell and naive or Teff cells. These tolerogenic dendritic cells employ both secreted mediators (e.g., IL-10, retinoic acid) and inhibitory receptors to drive regulatory T cell induction, but can also provide additional signals (e.g., integrins) to direct these nascent Treg to the appropriate anatomic compartment (**Figure 1**). A major challenge we will face in the application of such tolerogenic dendritic cells for immunotherapy will be to carefully match or optimize the type(s) of tolerogenic dendritic cells to be employed with the clinical targets and desired endpoints.

AUTHOR CONTRIBUTIONS

Wojciech Dawicki reviewed the literature for and wrote parts of the section on naturally occurring populations of dendritic cells, Yanna Ma contributed to the section on T cell biology, Laura Churchman wrote the introduction, Sara A. Gordon collated the literature on the different types of dendritic cells that have been reported, and John R. Gordon wrote the section on the different types of experimental dendritic cells that have been reported. All authors contributed to the planning and editorial phases of the review.

ACKNOWLEDGMENTS

This work was supported by grants from the Canadian Institutes of Health Research (MOP53167) and AllerGen National Centres of Excellence (CanFAST6).

REFERENCES

1. Steinman RM. Decisions about dendritic cells: past, present, and future. *Annu Rev Immunol* (2012) **30**:1–22. doi:10.1146/annurev-immunol-100311-102839
2. Gowans JL. The role of lymphocytes in the destruction of homografts. *Br Med Bull* (1965) **21**:106–10.
3. Steinman RM, Cohn ZA. Identification of a novel cell type in peripheral lymphoid organs of mice. I. Morphology, quantitation, tissue distribution. *J Exp Med* (1973) **137**(5):1142–62. doi:10.1084/jem.137.5.1142
4. Steinman RM, Cohn ZA. Identification of a novel cell type in peripheral lymphoid organs of mice. II. Functional properties in vitro. *J Exp Med* (1974) **139**(2):380–97. doi:10.1084/jem.139.6.1431
5. Steinman RM, Kaplan G, Witmer MD, Cohn ZA. Identification of a novel cell type in peripheral lymphoid organs of mice. V. Purification of spleen dendritic cells, new surface markers, and maintenance in vitro. *J Exp Med* (1979) **149**(1):1–16. doi:10.1084/jem.149.1.1
6. Steinman RM, Witmer MD. Lymphoid dendritic cells are potent stimulators of the primary mixed leukocyte reaction in mice. *Proc Natl Acad Sci U S A* (1978) **75**(10):5132–6. doi:10.1073/pnas.75.10.5132
7. Steinman RM. The dendritic cell system and its role in immunogenicity. *Annu Rev Immunol* (1991) **9**:271–96. doi:10.1146/annurev.iy.09.040191.001415

8. Simon JC, Tigelaar RE, Bergstresser PR, Edelbaum D, Cruz PD Jr. Ultraviolet B radiation converts Langerhans cells from immunogenic to tolerogenic antigen-presenting cells. Induction of specific clonal anergy in CD4+ T helper 1 cells. *J Immunol* (1991) **146**:485–91.
9. Enk AH, Angeloni VL, Udey MC, Katz SI. Inhibition of Langerhans cell antigen-presenting function by IL-10. A role for IL-10 in induction of tolerance. *J Immunol* (1993) **151**(5):2390–8.
10. Steptoe RJ, Thomson AW. Dendritic cells and tolerance induction. *Clin Exp Immunol* (1996) **105**(3):397–402.
11. Bamboat ZM, Stableford JA, Plitas G, Burt BM, Nguyen HM, Welles AP, et al. Human liver dendritic cells promote T cell hyporesponsiveness. *J Immunol* (2009) **182**(4):1901–11. doi:10.4049/jimmunol.0803404
12. Banchereau J, Briere F, Caux C, Davoust J, Lebecque S, Liu YJ, et al. Immunobiology of dendritic cells. *Annu Rev Immunol* (2000) **18**:767–811. doi:10.1146/annurev.immunol.18.1.767
13. Merad M, Sathe P, Helft J, Miller J, Mortha A. The dendritic cell lineage: ontogeny and function of dendritic cells and their subsets in the steady state and the inflamed setting. *Annu Rev Immunol* (2013) **31**:563–604. doi:10.1146/annurev-immunol-020711-074950
14. Caux C, Ait-Yahia S, Chemin K, de Bouteiller O, Dieu-Nosjean MC, Homey B, et al. Dendritic cell biology and regulation of dendritic cell trafficking by chemokines. *Springer Semin Immunopathol* (2000) **22**(4):345–69. doi:10.1007/s002810000053
15. de Heer HJ, Hammad H, Kool M, Lambrecht BN. Dendritic cell subsets and immune regulation in the lung. *Semin Immunol* (2005) **17**(4):295–303. doi:10.1016/j.smim.2005.05.002
16. Groux H, Fournier N, Cottrez F. Role of dendritic cells in the generation of regulatory T cells. *Semin Immunol* (2004) **16**(2):99–106. doi:10.1016/j.smim.2003.12.004
17. Saeki H, Moore AM, Brown MJ, Hwang ST. Cutting edge: secondary lymphoid-tissue chemokine (SLC) and CC chemokine receptor 7 (CCR7) participate in the emigration pathway of mature dendritic cells from the skin to regional lymph nodes. *J Immunol* (1999) **162**(5):2472–5.
18. Romani N, Koide S, Crowley M, Witmer-Pack M, Livingstone AM, Fathman CG, et al. Presentation of exogenous protein antigens by dendritic cells to T cell clones. Intact protein is presented best by immature, epidermal Langerhans cells. *J Exp Med* (1989) **169**:1169–78. doi:10.1084/jem.169.3.1169
19. Hart DN. Dendritic cells: unique leukocyte populations which control the primary immune response. *Blood* (1997) **90**(9):3245–87.
20. Heufler C, Koch F, Stanzl U, Topar G, Wysocka M, Trinchieri G, et al. Interleukin-12 is produced by dendritic cells and mediates T helper 1 development as well as interferon-gamma production by T helper 1 cells. *Eur J Immunol* (1996) **26**(3):659–68. doi:10.1002/eji.1830260323
21. Weiner HL, da Cunha AP, Quintana F, Wu H. Oral tolerance. *Immunol Rev* (2011) **241**(1):241–59. doi:10.1111/j.1600-065X.2011.01017.x
22. Sigmundsdottir H, Pan J, Debes GF, Alt C, Habtezion A, Soler D, et al. DCs metabolize sunlight-induced vitamin D3 to "program" T cell attraction to the epidermal chemokine CCL27. *Nat Immunol* (2007) **8**(3):285–93. doi:10.1038/ni1433
23. Sun CM, Hall JA, Blank RB, Bouladoux N, Oukka M, Mora JR, et al. Small intestine lamina propria dendritic cells promote de novo generation of Foxp3 T reg cells via retinoic acid. *J Exp Med* (2007) **204**(8):1775–85. doi:10.1084/jem.20070602
24. Akbari O, DeKruyff RH, Umetsu DT. Pulmonary dendritic cells producing IL-10 mediate tolerance induced by respiratory exposure to antigen. *Nat Immunol* (2001) **2**(8):725–31. doi:10.1038/90667
25. Ueno H, Klechevsky E, Schmitt N, Ni L, Flamar AL, Zurawski S, et al. Targeting human dendritic cell subsets for improved vaccines. *Semin Immunol* (2011) **23**(1):21–7. doi:10.1016/j.smim.2011.01.004
26. Randolph GJ, Angeli V, Swartz MA. Dendritic-cell trafficking to lymph nodes through lymphatic vessels. *Nat Rev Immunol* (2005) **5**(8):617–28. doi:10.1038/nri1670
27. Liu K, Waskow C, Liu X, Yao K, Hoh J, Nussenzweig M. Origin of dendritic cells in peripheral lymphoid organs of mice. *Nat Immunol* (2007) **8**(6):578–83. doi:10.1038/ni1462
28. Randolph GJ, Ochando J, Partida-Sanchez S. Migration of dendritic cell subsets and their precursors. *Annu Rev Immunol* (2008) **26**:293–316. doi:10.1146/annurev.immunol.26.021607.090254
29. Sallusto F, Lanzavecchia A. Efficient presentation of soluble antigen by cultured human dendritic cells is maintained by granulocyte/macrophage colony-stimulating factor plus interleukin 4 and downregulated by tumor necrosis factor alpha. *J Exp Med* (1994) **179**(4):1109–18. doi:10.1084/jem.179.4.1109
30. Li X, Yang A, Huang H, Zhang X, Town J, Davis B, et al. Induction of type 2 T helper cell allergen tolerance by IL-10-differentiated regulatory dendritic cells. *Am J Respir Cell Mol Biol* (2010) **42**(2):190–9. doi:10.1165/rcmb.2009-0023OC
31. Cheong C, Matos I, Choi JH, Dandamudi DB, Shrestha E, Longhi MP, et al. Microbial stimulation fully differentiates monocytes to DC-SIGN/CD209(+) dendritic cells for immune T cell areas. *Cell* (2010) **143**(3):416–29. doi:10.1016/j.cell.2010.09.039
32. Nizzoli G, Krietsch J, Weick A, Steinfelder S, Facciotti F, Gruarin P, et al. Human CD1c+ dendritic cells secrete high levels of IL-12 and potently prime cytotoxic T-cell responses. *Blood* (2013) **122**(6):932–42. doi:10.1182/blood-2013-04-495424
33. Gregori S, Tomasoni D, Pacciani V, Scirpoli M, Battaglia M, Magnani CF, et al. Differentiation of type 1 T regulatory cells (Tr1) by tolerogenic DC-10 requires the IL-10-dependent ILT4/HLA-G pathway. *Blood* (2010) **116**(6):935–44. doi:10.1182/blood-2009-07-234872
34. Scott CL, Aumeunier AM, Mowat AM. Intestinal CD103+ dendritic cells: master regulators of tolerance? *Trends Immunol* (2011) **32**(9):412–9. doi:10.1016/j.it.2011.06.003
35. Medzhitov R. Recognition of microorganisms and activation of the immune response. *Nature* (2007) **449**(7164):819–26. doi:10.1038/nature06246
36. Steinman RM, Banchereau J. Taking dendritic cells into medicine. *Nature* (2007) **449**(7161):419–26. doi:10.1038/nature06175
37. Farache J, Koren I, Milo I, Gurevich I, Kim KW, Zigmond E, et al. Luminal bacteria recruit CD103+ dendritic cells into the intestinal epithelium to sample bacterial antigens for presentation. *Immunity* (2013) **38**(3):581–95. doi:10.1016/j.immuni.2013.01.009
38. Schulz O, Jaensson E, Persson EK, Liu X, Worbs T, Agace WW, et al. Intestinal CD103+, but not CX3CR1+, antigen sampling cells migrate in lymph and serve classical dendritic cell functions. *J Exp Med* (2009) **206**(13):3101–14. doi:10.1084/jem.20091925
39. Mucida D, Pino-Lagos K, Kim G, Nowak E, Benson MJ, Kronenberg M, et al. Retinoic acid can directly promote TGF-beta-mediated Foxp3(+) Treg cell conversion of naive T cells. *Immunity* (2009) **30**(4):471–2; author reply 2-3. doi:10.1016/j.immuni.2009.03.008
40. Sharma MD, Baban B, Chandler P, Hou DY, Singh N, Yagita H, et al. Plasmacytoid dendritic cells from mouse tumor-draining lymph nodes directly activate mature Tregs via indoleamine 2,3-dioxygenase. *J Clin Invest* (2007) **117**(9):2570–82. doi:10.1172/JCI31911
41. Semmrich M, Plantinga M, Svensson-Frej M, Uronen-Hansson H, Gustafsson T, Mowat AM, et al. Directed antigen targeting in vivo identifies a role for CD103+ dendritic cells in both tolerogenic and immunogenic T-cell responses. *Mucosal Immunol* (2012) **5**(2):150–60. doi:10.1038/mi.2011.61
42. Laffont S, Siddiqui KR, Powrie F. Intestinal inflammation abrogates the tolerogenic properties of MLN CD103+ dendritic cells. *Eur J Immunol* (2010) **40**(7):1877–83. doi:10.1002/eji.200939957
43. del Rio ML, Bernhardt G, Rodriguez-Barbosa JI, Forster R. Development and functional specialization of CD103+ dendritic cells. *Immunol Rev* (2010) **234**(1):268–81. doi:10.1111/j.0105-2896.2009.00874.x
44. Johansson-Lindbom B, Svensson M, Pabst O, Palmqvist C, Marquez G, Forster R, et al. Functional specialization of gut CD103+ dendritic cells in the regulation of tissue-selective T cell homing. *J Exp Med* (2005) **202**(8):1063–73. doi:10.1084/jem.20051100
45. Hall JA, Grainger JR, Spencer SP, Belkaid Y. The role of retinoic acid in tolerance and immunity. *Immunity* (2011) **35**(1):13–22. doi:10.1016/j.immuni.2011.07.002
46. den Hartog G, van Altena C, Savelkoul HF, van Neerven RJ. The mucosal factors retinoic acid and TGF-beta1 induce phenotypically and functionally distinct dendritic cell types. *Int Arch Allergy Immunol* (2013) **162**(3):225–36. doi:10.1159/000353243
47. Wurbel MA, McIntire MG, Dwyer P, Fiebiger E. CCL25/CCR9 interactions regulate large intestinal inflammation in a murine model of acute colitis. *PLoS One* (2011) **6**(1):e16442. doi:10.1371/journal.pone.0016442
48. Bowman EP, Kuklin NA, Youngman KR, Lazarus NH, Kunkel EJ, Pan J, et al. The intestinal chemokine thymus-expressed chemokine (CCL25) attracts IgA

antibody-secreting cells. *J Exp Med* (2002) **195**(2):269–75. doi:10.1084/jem.20010670
49. Mucida D, Park Y, Kim G, Turovskaya O, Scott I, Kronenberg M, et al. Reciprocal TH17 and regulatory T cell differentiation mediated by retinoic acid. *Science* (2007) **317**(5835):256–60. doi:10.1126/science.1145697
50. Cong Y, Feng T, Fujihashi K, Schoeb TR, Elson CO. A dominant, coordinated T regulatory cell-IgA response to the intestinal microbiota. *Proc Natl Acad Sci U S A* (2009) **106**(46):19256–61. doi:10.1073/pnas.0812681106
51. Uematsu S, Fujimoto K, Jang MH, Yang BG, Jung YJ, Nishiyama M, et al. Regulation of humoral and cellular gut immunity by lamina propria dendritic cells expressing Toll-like receptor 5. *Nat Immunol* (2008) **9**(7):769–76. doi:10.1038/ni.1622
52. Cerutti A, Rescigno M. The biology of intestinal immunoglobulin A responses. *Immunity* (2008) **28**(6):740–50. doi:10.1016/j.immuni.2008.05.001
53. von Garnier C, Filgueira L, Wikstrom M, Smith M, Thomas JA, Strickland DH, et al. Anatomical location determines the distribution and function of dendritic cells and other APCs in the respiratory tract. *J Immunol* (2005) **175**(3):1609–18.
54. Holt PG, Schon-Hegrad MA, Oliver J, Holt BJ, McMenamin PG. A contiguous network of dendritic antigen-presenting cells within the respiratory epithelium. *Int Arch Allergy Appl Immunol* (1990) **91**(2):155–9. doi:10.1159/000235107
55. Robays LJ, Maes T, Joos GF, Vermaelen KY. Between a cough and a wheeze: dendritic cells at the nexus of tobacco smoke-induced allergic airway sensitization. *Mucosal Immunol* (2009) **2**(3):206–19. doi:10.1038/mi.2009.7
56. Veres TZ, Rochlitzer S, Shevchenko M, Fuchs B, Prenzler F, Nassenstein C, et al. Spatial interactions between dendritic cells and sensory nerves in allergic airway inflammation. *Am J Respir Cell Mol Biol* (2007) **37**(5):553–61. doi:10.1165/rcmb.2007-0087OC
57. Holt PG, Schon-Hegrad MA. Localization of T cells, macrophages and dendritic cells in rat respiratory tract tissue: implications for immune function studies. *Immunology* (1987) **62**(3):349–56.
58. Huh JC, Strickland DH, Jahnsen FL, Turner DJ, Thomas JA, Napoli S, et al. Bidirectional interactions between antigen-bearing respiratory tract dendritic cells (DCs) and T cells precede the late phase reaction in experimental asthma: DC activation occurs in the airway mucosa but not in the lung parenchyma. *J Exp Med* (2003) **198**(1):19–30. doi:10.1084/jem.20021328
59. Plantinga M, Hammad H, Lambrecht BN. Origin and functional specializations of DC subsets in the lung. *Eur J Immunol* (2010) **40**(8):2112–8. doi:10.1002/eji.201040562
60. Demedts IK, Brusselle GG, Vermaelen KY, Pauwels RA. Identification and characterization of human pulmonary dendritic cells. *Am J Respir Cell Mol Biol* (2005) **32**(3):177–84. doi:10.1165/rcmb.2004-0279OC
61. Lambrecht BN, Hammad H. Lung dendritic cells in respiratory viral infection and asthma: from protection to immunopathology. *Annu Rev Immunol* (2012) **30**:243–70. doi:10.1146/annurev-immunol-020711-075021
62. Van Pottelberge GR, Bracke KR, Demedts IK, De Rijck K, Reinartz SM, van Drunen CM, et al. Selective accumulation of langerhans-type dendritic cells in small airways of patients with COPD. *Respir Res* (2010) **11**:35. doi:10.1186/1465-9921-11-35
63. Asselin-Paturel C, Brizard G, Pin JJ, Briere F, Trinchieri G. Mouse strain differences in plasmacytoid dendritic cell frequency and function revealed by a novel monoclonal antibody. *J Immunol* (2003) **171**(12):6466–77.
64. de Heer HJ, Hammad H, Soullie T, Hijdra D, Vos N, Willart MA, et al. Essential role of lung plasmacytoid dendritic cells in preventing asthmatic reactions to harmless inhaled antigen. *J Exp Med* (2004) **200**(1):89–98. doi:10.1084/jem.20040035
65. Gehrie E, Van der Touw W, Bromberg JS, Ochando JC. Plasmacytoid dendritic cells in tolerance. *Methods Mol Biol* (2011) **677**:127–47. doi:10.1007/978-1-60761-869-0_9
66. Wang H, Peters N, Schwarze J. Plasmacytoid dendritic cells limit viral replication, pulmonary inflammation, and airway hyperresponsiveness in respiratory syncytial virus infection. *J Immunol* (2006) **177**(9):6263–70.
67. Ho AW, Prabhu N, Betts RJ, Ge MQ, Dai X, Hutchinson PE, et al. Lung CD103+ dendritic cells efficiently transport influenza virus to the lymph node and load viral antigen onto MHC class I for presentation to CD8 T cells. *J Immunol* (2011) **187**(11):6011–21. doi:10.4049/jimmunol.1100987
68. del Rio ML, Rodriguez-Barbosa JI, Kremmer E, Forster R. CD103- and CD103+ bronchial lymph node dendritic cells are specialized in presenting and cross-presenting innocuous antigen to CD4+ and CD8+ T cells. *J Immunol* (2007) **178**(11):6861–6.
69. Plantinga M, Guilliams M, Vanheerswynghels M, Deswarte K, Branco-Madeira F, Toussaint W, et al. Conventional and monocyte-derived CD11b(+) dendritic cells initiate and maintain T helper 2 cell-mediated immunity to house dust mite allergen. *Immunity* (2013) **38**(2):322–35. doi:10.1016/j.immuni.2012.10.016
70. van Rijt LS, Jung S, Kleinjan A, Vos N, Willart M, Duez C, et al. In vivo depletion of lung CD11c+ dendritic cells during allergen challenge abrogates the characteristic features of asthma. *J Exp Med* (2005) **201**(6):981–91. doi:10.1084/jem.20042311
71. Jonuleit H, Schmitt E, Steinbrink K, Enk AH. Dendritic cells as a tool to induce anergic and regulatory T cells. *Trends Immunol* (2001) **22**(7):394–400. doi:10.1016/S1471-4906(01)01952-4
72. Fallarino F, Bianchi R, Orabona C, Vacca C, Belladonna ML, Fioretti MC, et al. CTLA-4-Ig activates forkhead transcription factors and protects dendritic cells from oxidative stress in nonobese diabetic mice. *J Exp Med* (2004) **200**(8):1051–62. doi:10.1084/jem.20040942
73. Khare A, Krishnamoorthy N, Oriss TB, Fei M, Ray P, Ray A. Cutting edge: inhaled antigen upregulates retinaldehyde dehydrogenase in lung CD103+ but not plasmacytoid dendritic cells to induce Foxp3 de novo in CD4+ T cells and promote airway tolerance. *J Immunol* (2013) **191**(1):25–9. doi:10.4049/jimmunol.1300193
74. Soroosh P, Doherty TA, Duan W, Mehta AK, Choi H, Adams YF, et al. Lung-resident tissue macrophages generate Foxp3+ regulatory T cells and promote airway tolerance. *J Exp Med* (2013) **210**(4):775–88. doi:10.1084/jem.20121849
75. Coleman MM, Ruane D, Moran B, Dunne PJ, Keane J, Mills KH. Alveolar macrophages contribute to respiratory tolerance by inducing FoxP3 expression in naive T cells. *Am J Respir Cell Mol Biol* (2013) **48**(6):773–80. doi:10.1165/rcmb.2012-0263OC
76. Holt PG, Oliver J, Bilyk N, McMenamin C, McMenamin PG, Kraal G, et al. Downregulation of the antigen presenting cell function(s) of pulmonary dendritic cells in vivo by resident alveolar macrophages. *J Exp Med* (1993) **177**(2):397–407. doi:10.1084/jem.177.2.397
77. Chorro L, Geissmann F. Development and homeostasis of "resident" myeloid cells: the case of the Langerhans cell. *Trends Immunol* (2010) **31**(12):438–45. doi:10.1016/j.it.2010.09.003
78. Merad M, Ginhoux F, Collin M. Origin, homeostasis and function of Langerhans cells and other langerin-expressing dendritic cells. *Nat Rev Immunol* (2008) **8**(12):935–47. doi:10.1038/nri2455
79. Valladeau J, Saeland S. Cutaneous dendritic cells. *Semin Immunol* (2005) **17**(4):273–83. doi:10.1016/j.smim.2005.05.009
80. Igyarto BZ, Haley K, Ortner D, Bobr A, Gerami-Nejad M, Edelson BT, et al. Skin-resident murine dendritic cell subsets promote distinct and opposing antigen-specific T helper cell responses. *Immunity* (2011) **35**(2):260–72. doi:10.1016/j.immuni.2011.06.005
81. Henri S, Poulin LF, Tamoutounour S, Ardouin L, Guilliams M, de Bovis B. CD207+ CD103+ dermal dendritic cells cross-present keratinocyte-derived antigens irrespective of the presence of Langerhans cells. *J Exp Med* (2010) **207**:189–206. doi:10.1084/jem.20091964
82. Teunissen MB, Haniffa M, Collin MP. Insight into the immunobiology of human skin and functional specialization of skin dendritic cell subsets to innovate intradermal vaccination design. *Curr Top Microbiol Immunol* (2012) **351**:25–76. doi:10.1007/82_2011_169
83. Idoyaga J, Fiorese C, Zbytnuik L, Lubkin A, Miller J, Malissen B, et al. Specialized role of migratory dendritic cells in peripheral tolerance induction. *J Clin Invest* (2013) **123**:844–54. doi:10.1172/JCI65260
84. Shklovskaya E, O'Sullivan BJ, Ng LG, Roediger B, Thomas R, Weninger W, et al. Langerhans cells are precommitted to immune tolerance induction. *Proc Natl Acad Sci U S A* (2011) **108**(44):18049–54. doi:10.1073/pnas.1110076108
85. van der Aar AM, Picavet DI, Muller FJ, de Boer L, van Capel TM, Zaat SA, et al. Langerhans cells favor skin flora tolerance through limited presentation of bacterial antigens and induction of regulatory T cells. *J Invest Dermatol* (2013) **133**(5):1240–9. doi:10.1038/jid.2012.500
86. O'Sullivan BJ, Thomas R. CD40 ligation conditions dendritic cell antigen-presenting function through sustained activation of NF-kappaB. *J Immunol* (2002) **168**(11):5491–8.

87. Kaplan DH, Jenison MC, Saeland S, Shlomchik WD, Shlomchik MJ. Epidermal langerhans cell-deficient mice develop enhanced contact hypersensitivity. *Immunity* (2005) **23**:611–20. doi:10.1016/j.immuni.2005.10.008
88. Bennett CL, van Rijn E, Jung S, Inaba K, Steinman RM, Kapsenberg ML, et al. Inducible ablation of mouse Langerhans cells diminishes but fails to abrogate contact hypersensitivity. *J Cell Biol* (2005) **169**(4):569–76. doi:10.1083/jcb.200501071
89. Gomez de Aguero M, Vocanson M, Hacini-Rachinel F, Taillardet M, Sparwasser T, Kissenpfennig A, et al. Langerhans cells protect from allergic contact dermatitis in mice by tolerizing CD8(+) T cells and activating Foxp3(+) regulatory T cells. *J Clin Invest* (2012) **122**(5):1700–11. doi:10.1172/JCI59725
90. Chu CC, Ali N, Karagiannis P, Di Meglio P, Skowera A, Napolitano L, et al. Resident CD141 (BDCA3)+ dendritic cells in human skin produce IL-10 and induce regulatory T cells that suppress skin inflammation. *J Exp Med* (2012) **209**(5):935–45. doi:10.1084/jem.20112583
91. Azukizawa H, Dohler A, Kanazawa N, Nayak A, Lipp M, Malissen B, et al. Steady state migratory RelB+ langerin+ dermal dendritic cells mediate peripheral induction of antigen-specific CD4+ CD25+ Foxp3+ regulatory T cells. *Eur J Immunol* (2011) **41**(5):1420–34. doi:10.1002/eji.201040930
92. Castellaneta A, Mazariegos GV, Nayyar N, Zeevi A, Thomson AW. HLA-G level on monocytoid dendritic cells correlates with regulatory T-cell Foxp3 expression in liver transplant tolerance. *Transplantation* (2011) **91**(10):1132–40. doi:10.1097/TP.0b013e31821414c9
93. Bamboat ZM, Ocuin LM, Balachandran VP, Obaid H, Plitas G, DeMatteo RP. Conventional DCs reduce liver ischemia/reperfusion injury in mice via IL-10 secretion. *J Clin Invest* (2010) **120**(2):559–69. doi:10.1172/JCI40008
94. Chen Y, Jiang G, Yang HR, Gu X, Wang L, Hsieh CC, et al. Distinct response of liver myeloid dendritic cells to endotoxin is mediated by IL-27. *J Hepatol* (2009) **51**(3):510–9. doi:10.1016/j.jhep.2009.04.026
95. Jinushi M, Takehara T, Tatsumi T, Yamaguchi S, Sakamori R, Hiramatsu N, et al. Natural killer cell and hepatic cell interaction via NKG2A leads to dendritic cell-mediated induction of CD4 CD25 T cells with PD-1-dependent regulatory activities. *Immunology* (2007) **120**(1):73–82. doi:10.1111/j.1365-2567.2006.02479.x
96. Xia S, Guo Z, Xu X, Yi H, Wang Q, Cao X. Hepatic microenvironment programs hematopoietic progenitor differentiation into regulatory dendritic cells, maintaining liver tolerance. *Blood* (2008) **112**(8):3175–85. doi:10.1182/blood-2008-05-159921
97. Dubois B, Joubert G, Gomez de Aguero M, Gouanvic M, Goubier A, Kaiserlian D. Sequential role of plasmacytoid dendritic cells and regulatory T cells in oral tolerance. *Gastroenterology* (2009) **137**(3):1019–28. doi:10.1053/j.gastro.2009.03.055
98. Goubier A, Dubois B, Gheit H, Joubert G, Villard-Truc F, Asselin-Paturel C, et al. Plasmacytoid dendritic cells mediate oral tolerance. *Immunity* (2008) **29**(3):464–75. doi:10.1016/j.immuni.2008.06.017
99. Friedman SL. Hepatic stellate cells: protean, multifunctional, and enigmatic cells of the liver. *Physiol Rev* (2008) **88**(1):125–72. doi:10.1152/physrev.00013.2007
100. Dunham RM, Thapa M, Velazquez VM, Elrod EJ, Denning TL, Pulendran B, et al. Hepatic stellate cells preferentially induce Foxp3+ regulatory T cells by production of retinoic acid. *J Immunol* (2013) **190**(5):2009–16. doi:10.4049/jimmunol.1201937
101. Ichikawa S, Mucida D, Tyznik AJ, Kronenberg M, Cheroutre H. Hepatic stellate cells function as regulatory bystanders. *J Immunol* (2011) **186**(10):5549–55. doi:10.4049/jimmunol.1003917
102. You Q, Cheng L, Kedl RM, Ju C. Mechanism of T cell tolerance induction by murine hepatic Kupffer cells. *Hepatology* (2008) **48**(3):978–90. doi:10.1002/hep.22395
103. Wilson NS, El-Sukkari D, Belz GT, Smith CM, Steptoe RJ, Heath WR, et al. Most lymphoid organ dendritic cell types are phenotypically and functionally immature. *Blood* (2003) **102**(6):2187–94. doi:10.1182/blood-2003-02-0513
104. Fukaya T, Takagi H, Taya H, Sato K. DCs in immune tolerance in steady-state conditions. *Methods Mol Biol* (2011) **677**:113–26. doi:10.1007/978-1-60761-869-0_8
105. Broggi A, Zanoni I, Granucci F. Migratory conventional dendritic cells in the induction of peripheral T-cell tolerance. *J Leukoc Biol* (2013) **94**(5):903–11. doi:10.1189/jlb.0413222
106. Doan T, McNally A, Thomas R, Steptoe RJ. Steady-state dendritic cells continuously inactivate T cells that escape thymic negative selection. *Immunol Cell Biol* (2009) **87**(8):615–22. doi:10.1038/icb.2009.46
107. Gordon JR, Li F, Nayyar A, Xiang J, Zhang X. CD8 alpha+, but not CD8 alpha-, dendritic cells tolerize Th2 responses via contact-dependent and -independent mechanisms, and reverse airway hyperresponsiveness, Th2, and eosinophil responses in a mouse model of asthma. *J Immunol* (2005) **175**(3):1516–22.
108. Zhang X, Huang H, Yuan J, Sun D, Hou WS, Gordon J, et al. CD4-8- dendritic cells prime CD4+ T regulatory 1 cells to suppress antitumor immunity. *J Immunol* (2005) **175**:2931–7.
109. Winkel K, Kronin V, Krummel M, Shortman K. The nature of the signals regulating CD8 T cell proliferative responses to CD8a+ or CD8a- dendritic cells. *Eur J Immunol* (1997) **27**:3350–9. doi:10.1002/eji.1830271234
110. Kronin V, Fitzmaurice CJ, Caminschi I, Shortman K, Jackson DC, Brown LE. Differential effect of CD8(+) and CD8(-) dendritic cells in the stimulation of secondary CD4(+) T cells. *Int Immunol* (2001) **13**(4):465–73. doi:10.1093/intimm/13.4.465
111. Suss G, Shortman K. A subclass of dendritic cells kills CD4 T cells via Fas/Fas-ligand-induced apoptosis. *J Exp Med* (1996) **183**(4):1789–96. doi:10.1084/jem.183.4.1789
112. Holt PG, Upham JW. The role of dendritic cells in asthma. *Curr Opin Allergy Clin Immunol* (2004) **4**(1):39–44. doi:10.1097/00130832-200402000-00009
113. Stern JN, Keskin DB, Kato Z, Waldner H, Schallenberg S, Anderson A, et al. Promoting tolerance to proteolipid protein-induced experimental autoimmune encephalomyelitis through targeting dendritic cells. *Proc Natl Acad Sci U S A* (2010) **107**(40):17280–5. doi:10.1073/pnas.1010263107
114. Ring S, Maas M, Nettelbeck DM, Enk AH, Mahnke K. Targeting of autoantigens to DEC205+ Dendritic cells in vivo suppresses experimental allergic encephalomyelitis in mice. *J Immunol* (2013) **191**(6):2938–47. doi:10.4049/jimmunol.1202592
115. Petzold C, Schallenberg S, Stern JN, Kretschmer K. Targeted antigen delivery to DEC-205(+) dendritic cells for tolerogenic vaccination. *Rev Diabet Stud* (2012) **9**(4):305–18. doi:10.1900/RDS.2012.9.305
116. Kushwah R, Wu J, Oliver JR, Jiang G, Zhang J, Siminovitch KA, et al. Uptake of apoptotic DC converts immature DC into tolerogenic DC that induce differentiation of Foxp3+ Treg. *Eur J Immunol* (2010) **40**(4):1022–35. doi:10.1002/eji.200939782
117. Gleisner MA, Rosemblatt M, Fierro JA, Bono MR. Delivery of alloantigens via apoptotic cells generates dendritic cells with an immature tolerogenic phenotype. *Transplant Proc* (2011) **43**(6):2325–33. doi:10.1016/j.transproceed.2011.06.007
118. Kushwah R, Oliver JR, Zhang J, Siminovitch KA, Hu J. Apoptotic dendritic cells induce tolerance in mice through suppression of dendritic cell maturation and induction of antigen-specific regulatory T cells. *J Immunol* (2009) **183**(11):7104–18. doi:10.4049/jimmunol.0900824
119. Jonuleit H, Schmitt E, Schuler G, Knop J, Enk AH. Induction of interleukin 10-producing, nonproliferating CD4(+) T cells with regulatory properties by repetitive stimulation with allogeneic immature human dendritic cells. *J Exp Med* (2000) **192**(9):1213–22. doi:10.1084/jem.192.9.1213
120. Mahnke K, Schmitt E, Bonifaz L, Enk AH, Jonuleit H. Immature, but not inactive: the tolerogenic function of immature dendritic cells. *Immunol Cell Biol* (2002) **80**(5):477–83. doi:10.1046/j.1440-1711.2002.01115.x
121. Bell E. Immature human dendritic cells induce regulatory T cells in vitro. *Trends Immunol* (2001) **22**(1):11. doi:10.1016/S1471-4906(00)01833-0
122. Hubo M, Trinschek B, Kryczanowsky F, Tuettenberg A, Steinbrink K, Jonuleit H. Costimulatory molecules on immunogenic versus tolerogenic human dendritic cells. *Front Immunol* (2013) **4**:82. doi:10.3389/fimmu.2013.00082
123. Chen C, Qu QX, Huang JA, Zhu YB, Ge Y, Wang Q, et al. Expression of programmed-death receptor ligands 1 and 2 may contribute to the poor stimulatory potential of murine immature dendritic cells. *Immunobiology* (2007) **212**(3):159–65. doi:10.1016/j.imbio.2007.01.004
124. Chen Z, Gordon JR, Zhang X, Xiang J. Analysis of the gene expression profiles of immature versus mature bone marrow-derived dendritic cells using DNA arrays. *Biochem Biophys Res Commun* (2002) **290**(1):66–72. doi:10.1006/bbrc.2001.6147
125. Zhou F, Ciric B, Zhang GX, Rostami A. Immune tolerance induced by intravenous transfer of immature dendritic cells via up-regulating numbers of

suppressive IL-10(+) IFN-gamma(+)-producing CD4(+) T cells. *Immunol Res* (2013) **56**(1):1–8. doi:10.1007/s12026-012-8382-7

126. Charbonnier LM, van Duivenvoorde LM, Apparailly F, Cantos C, Han WG, Noel D, et al. Immature dendritic cells suppress collagen-induced arthritis by in vivo expansion of CD49b+ regulatory T cells. *J Immunol* (2006) **177**(6):3806–13.
127. Dhodapkar MV, Steinman RM. Antigen-bearing immature dendritic cells induce peptide-specific CD8(+) regulatory T cells in vivo in humans. *Blood* (2002) **100**(1):174–7. doi:10.1182/blood.V100.1.174
128. Dhodapkar MV, Steinman RM, Krasovsky J, Munz C, Bhardwaj N. Antigen-specific inhibition of effector T cell function in humans after injection of immature dendritic cells. *J Exp Med* (2001) **193**(2):233–8. doi:10.1084/jem.193.2.233
129. Gad M, Kristensen NN, Kury E, Claesson MH. Characterization of T-regulatory cells, induced by immature dendritic cells, which inhibit enteroantigen-reactive colitis-inducing T-cell responses in vitro and in vivo. *Immunology* (2004) **113**(4):499–508. doi:10.1111/j.1365-2567.2004.01977.x
130. Jin Y, Fuller L, Ciancio G, Burke GW III, Tzakis AG, Ricordi C, et al. Antigen presentation and immune regulatory capacity of immature and mature-enriched antigen presenting (dendritic) cells derived from human bone marrow. *Hum Immunol* (2004) **65**(2):93–103. doi:10.1016/j.humimm.2003.11.002
131. Popov I, Li M, Zheng X, San H, Zhang X, Ichim TE, et al. Preventing autoimmune arthritis using antigen-specific immature dendritic cells: a novel tolerogenic vaccine. *Arthritis Res Ther* (2006) **8**(5):R141. doi:10.1186/ar2031
132. Roncarolo MG, Levings MK, Traversari C. Differentiation of T regulatory cells by immature dendritic cells. *J Exp Med* (2001) **193**(2):F5–9. doi:10.1084/jem.193.2.F5
133. Voigtlander C, Rossner S, Cierpka E, Theiner G, Wiethe C, Menges M, et al. Dendritic cells matured with TNF can be further activated in vitro and after subcutaneous injection in vivo which converts their tolerogenicity into immunogenicity. *J Immunother* (2006) **29**(4):407–15. doi:10.1097/01.cji.0000210081.60178.b4
134. Lim DS, Kang MS, Jeong JA, Bae YS. Semi-mature DC are immunogenic and not tolerogenic when inoculated at a high dose in collagen-induced arthritis mice. *Eur J Immunol* (2009) **39**(5):1334–43. doi:10.1002/eji.200838987
135. Enk AH, Jonuleit H, Saloga J, Knop J. Dendritic cells as mediators of tumor-induced tolerance in metastatic melanoma. *Int J Cancer* (1997) **73**(3):309–16. doi:10.1002/(SICI)1097-0215(19971104)73:3<309::AID-IJC1>3.3.CO;2-B
136. Steinbrink K, Wolfl M, Jonuleit H, Knop J, Enk AH. Induction of tolerance by IL-10-treated dendritic cells. *J Immunol* (1997) **159**(10):4772–80.
137. Lu M, Dawicki W, Zhang X, Huang H, Nayyar A, Gordon JR. Therapeutic induction of tolerance by IL-10-differentiated dendritic cells in a mouse model of house dust mite-asthma. *Allergy* (2011) **66**(5):612–20. doi:10.1111/j.1398-9995.2010.02526.x
138. Nayyar A, Dawicki W, Huang H, Lu M, Zhang X, Gordon JR. Induction of prolonged asthma tolerance by IL-10-differentiated dendritic cells: differential impact on airway hyperresponsiveness and the Th2 immunoinflammatory response. *J Immunol* (2012) **189**(1):72–9. doi:10.4049/jimmunol.1103286
139. Nayyar A, Gordon J. Tolerogenic bone marrow-derived dendritic cells modulate Th2 responses of pulmonary lymphocytes from mice with severe allergic lung disease. *FASEB J* (2004) **18**:A1128.
140. Koya T, Matsuda H, Takeda K, Matsubara S, Miyahara N, Balhorn A, et al. IL-10-treated dendritic cells decrease airway hyperresponsiveness and airway inflammation in mice. *J Allergy Clin Immunol* (2007) **119**(5):1241–50. doi:10.1016/j.jaci.2007.01.039
141. Bellinghausen I, Brand U, Steinbrink K, Enk AH, Knop J, Saloga J. Inhibition of human allergic T-cell responses by IL-10-treated dendritic cells: differences from hydrocortisone-treated dendritic cells. *J Allergy Clin Immunol* (2001) **108**(2):242–9. doi:10.1067/mai.2001.117177
142. Beissert S, Hosoi J, Grabbe S, Asahina A, Granstein RD. IL-10 inhibits tumor antigen presentation by epidermal antigen-presenting cells. *J Immunol* (1995) **154**(3):1280–6.
143. Boks MA, Kager-Groenland JR, Haasjes MS, Zwaginga JJ, van Ham SM, ten Brinke A. IL-10-generated tolerogenic dendritic cells are optimal for functional regulatory T cell induction – a comparative study of human clinical-applicable DC. *Clin Immunol* (2012) **142**(3):332–42. doi:10.1016/j.clim.2011.11.011
144. Chen L, Qiu M, He W, Huang A, Liu J. Functional study of immature dendritic cells co-transfected with IL-10 and TGF-beta 1 genes in vitro. *Mol Biol Rep* (2012) **39**(6):6633–9. doi:10.1007/s11033-012-1468-4
145. Figueroa-Vega N, Galindo-Rodriguez G, Bajana S, Portales-Perez D, Abud-Mendoza C, Sanchez-Torres C, et al. Phenotypic analysis of IL-10-treated, monocyte-derived dendritic cells in patients with systemic lupus erythematosus. *Scand J Immunol* (2006) **64**(6):668–76. doi:10.1111/j.1365-3083.2006.01849.x
146. Henry E, Desmet CJ, Garze V, Fievez L, Bedoret D, Heirman C, et al. Dendritic cells genetically engineered to express IL-10 induce long-lasting antigen-specific tolerance in experimental asthma. *J Immunol* (2008) **181**(10):7230–42.
147. Li WM, Liu W, Gao C, Zhou BG, Yang SS, Wang Z, et al. Antigen-specific tolerance induced by IL-10 gene modified immature dendritic cells in experimental autoimmune myocarditis in rats. *Chin Med J (Engl)* (2006) **119**(19):1646–52.
148. McBride JM, Jung T, de Vries JE, Aversa G. IL-10 alters DC function via modulation of cell surface molecules resulting in impaired T-cell responses. *Cell Immunol* (2002) **215**(2):162–72. doi:10.1016/S0008-8749(02)00007-2
149. Yang S, Li W, Liu W, Gao C, Zhou B, Li S, et al. IL-10 gene modified dendritic cells induced antigen-specific tolerance in experimental autoimmune myocarditis. *Clin Immunol* (2006) **121**(1):63–73. doi:10.1016/j.clim.2006.06.009
150. Sato K, Yamashita N, Baba M, Matsuyama T. Modified myeloid dendritic cells act as regulatory dendritic cells to induce anergic and regulatory T cells. *Blood* (2003) **101**(9):3581–9. doi:10.1182/blood-2002-09-2712
151. Menges M, Rossner S, Voigtlander C, Schindler H, Kukutsch NA, Bogdan C, et al. Repetitive injections of dendritic cells matured with tumor necrosis factor alpha induce antigen-specific protection of mice from autoimmunity. *J Exp Med* (2002) **195**(1):15–21. doi:10.1084/jem.20011341
152. Visser L, Jan de Heer H, Boven LA, van Riel D, van Meurs M, Melief MJ, et al. Proinflammatory bacterial peptidoglycan as a cofactor for the development of central nervous system autoimmune disease. *J Immunol* (2005) **174**(2):808–16.
153. Rutella S, Bonanno G, Procoli A, Mariotti A, de Ritis DG, Curti A, et al. Hepatocyte growth factor favors monocyte differentiation into regulatory interleukin (IL)-10++IL-12low/neg accessory cells with dendritic-cell features. *Blood* (2006) **108**(1):218–27. doi:10.1182/blood-2005-08-3141
154. Brandt K, Bulfone-Paus S, Foster DC, Ruckert R. Interleukin-21 inhibits dendritic cell activation and maturation. *Blood* (2003) **102**(12):4090–8. doi:10.1182/blood-2003-03-0669
155. Watanabe N, Wang YH, Lee HK, Ito T, Cao W, Liu YJ. Hassall's corpuscles instruct dendritic cells to induce CD4+CD25+ regulatory T cells in human thymus. *Nature* (2005) **436**(7054):1181–5. doi:10.1038/nature03886
156. Rutella S, Danese S, Leone G. Tolerogenic dendritic cells: cytokine modulation comes of age. *Blood* (2006) **108**(5):1435–40. doi:10.1182/blood-2006-03-006403
157. Zhang-Hoover J, Finn P, Stein-Streilein J. Modulation of ovalbumin-induced airway inflammation and hyperreactivity by tolerogenic APC. *J Immunol* (2005) **175**(11):7117–24.
158. Torres-Aguilar H, Aguilar-Ruiz SR, Gonzalez-Perez G, Munguia R, Bajana S, Meraz-Rios MA, et al. Tolerogenic dendritic cells generated with different immunosuppressive cytokines induce antigen-specific anergy and regulatory properties in memory CD4+ T cells. *J Immunol* (2010) **184**(4):1765–75. doi:10.4049/jimmunol.0902133
159. Piemonti L, Monti P, Allavena P, Sironi M, Soldini L, Leone BE, et al. Glucocorticoids affect human dendritic cell differentiation and maturation. *J Immunol* (1999) **162**(11):6473–81.
160. Naranjo-Gomez M, Raich-Regue D, Onate C, Grau-Lopez L, Ramo-Tello C, Pujol-Borrell R, et al. Comparative study of clinical grade human tolerogenic dendritic cells. *J Transl Med* (2011) **9**:89. doi:10.1186/1479-5876-9-89
161. Xia CQ, Peng R, Beato F, Clare-Salzler MJ. Dexamethasone induces IL-10-producing monocyte-derived dendritic cells with durable immaturity. *Scand J Immunol* (2005) **62**(1):45–54. doi:10.1111/j.1365-3083.2005.01640.x
162. Zimmer A, Luce S, Gaignier F, Nony E, Naveau M, Biola-Vidamment A, et al. Identification of a new phenotype of tolerogenic human dendritic cells induced by fungal proteases from *Aspergillus oryzae*. *J Immunol* (2011) **186**(7):3966–76. doi:10.4049/jimmunol.1003184
163. Penna G, Adorini L. 1 Alpha,25-dihydroxyvitamin D3 inhibits differentiation, maturation, activation, and survival of dendritic cells leading to impaired alloreactive T cell activation. *J Immunol* (2000) **164**(5):2405–11.
164. Chamorro S, Garcia-Vallejo JJ, Unger WW, Fernandes RJ, Bruijns SC, Laban S, et al. TLR triggering on tolerogenic dendritic cells results in TLR2

up-regulation and a reduced proinflammatory immune program. *J Immunol* (2009) **183**(5):2984–94. doi:10.4049/jimmunol.0801155

165. Ferreira GB, Kleijwegt FS, Waelkens E, Lage K, Nikolic T, Hansen DA, et al. Differential protein pathways in 1,25-dihydroxyvitamin d(3) and dexamethasone modulated tolerogenic human dendritic cells. *J Proteome Res* (2012) **11**(2):941–71. doi:10.1021/pr200724e
166. Ferreira GB, van Etten E, Verstuyf A, Waer M, Overbergh L, Gysemans C, et al. 1,25-Dihydroxyvitamin D3 alters murine dendritic cell behaviour in vitro and in vivo. *Diabetes Metab Res Rev* (2011) **27**(8):933–41. doi:10.1002/dmrr.1275
167. Kleijwegt FS, Laban S, Duinkerken G, Joosten AM, Zaldumbide A, Nikolic T, et al. Critical role for TNF in the induction of human antigen-specific regulatory T cells by tolerogenic dendritic cells. *J Immunol* (2010) **185**(3):1412–8. doi:10.4049/jimmunol.1000560
168. Palomares O, O'Mahony L, Akdis CA. The many routes of dendritic cells to ensure immune regulation. *J Allergy Clin Immunol* (2011) **127**(6):1541–2. doi:10.1016/j.jaci.2011.04.002
169. Penna G, Amuchastegui S, Giarratana N, Daniel KC, Vulcano M, Sozzani S, et al. 1,25-Dihydroxyvitamin D3 selectively modulates tolerogenic properties in myeloid but not plasmacytoid dendritic cells. *J Immunol* (2007) **178**(1):145–53.
170. Piemonti L, Monti P, Sironi M, Fraticelli P, Leone BE, Dal Cin E, et al. Vitamin D3 affects differentiation, maturation, and function of human monocyte-derived dendritic cells. *J Immunol* (2000) **164**(9):4443–51.
171. Unger WW, Laban S, Kleijwegt FS, van der Slik AR, Roep BO. Induction of Treg by monocyte-derived DC modulated by vitamin D3 or dexamethasone: differential role for PD-L1. *Eur J Immunol* (2009) **39**(11):3147–59. doi:10.1002/eji.200839103
172. van Halteren AG, Tysma OM, van Etten E, Mathieu C, Roep BO. 1Alpha,25-dihydroxyvitamin D3 or analogue treated dendritic cells modulate human autoreactive T cells via the selective induction of apoptosis. *J Autoimmun* (2004) **23**(3):233–9. doi:10.1016/j.jaut.2004.06.004
173. Battaglia M, Stabilini A, Roncarolo MG. Rapamycin selectively expands CD4+CD25+FoxP3+ regulatory T cells. *Blood* (2005) **105**(12):4743–8. doi:10.1182/blood-2004-10-3932
174. Macedo C, Turquist H, Metes D, Thomson AW. Immunoregulatory properties of rapamycin-conditioned monocyte-derived dendritic cells and their role in transplantation. *Transplant Res* (2012) **1**(1):16. doi:10.1186/2047-1440-1-16
175. Li X, Li JJ, Yang JY, Wang DS, Zhao W, Song WJ, et al. Tolerance induction by exosomes from immature dendritic cells and rapamycin in a mouse cardiac allograft model. *PLoS One* (2012) **7**(8):e44045. doi:10.1371/journal.pone.0044045
176. Gonzalez-Rey E, Chorny A, Fernandez-Martin A, Ganea D, Delgado M. Vasoactive intestinal peptide generates human tolerogenic dendritic cells that induce CD4 and CD8 regulatory T cells. *Blood* (2006) **107**(9):3632–8. doi:10.1182/blood-2005-11-4497
177. Toscano MG, Delgado M, Kong W, Martin F, Skarica M, Ganea D. Dendritic cells transduced with lentiviral vectors expressing VIP differentiate into VIP-secreting tolerogenic-like DCs. *Mol Ther* (2010) **18**(5):1035–45. doi:10.1038/mt.2009.293
178. Wu HY, Quintana FJ, da Cunha AP, Dake BT, Koeglsperger T, Starossom SC, et al. In vivo induction of Tr1 cells via mucosal dendritic cells and AHR signaling. *PLoS One* (2011) **6**(8):e23618. doi:10.1371/journal.pone.0023618
179. Hackstein H, Morelli AE, Larregina AT, Ganster RW, Papworth GD, Logar AJ, et al. Aspirin inhibits in vitro maturation and in vivo immunostimulatory function of murine myeloid dendritic cells. *J Immunol* (2001) **166**(12):7053–62.
180. Li XL, Liu Y, Cao LL, Li H, Yue LT, Wang S, et al. Atorvastatin-modified dendritic cells in vitro ameliorate experimental autoimmune myasthenia gravis by up-regulated Treg cells and shifted Th1/Th17 to Th2 cytokines. *Mol Cell Neurosci* (2013) **56C**:85–95. doi:10.1016/j.mcn.2013.03.005
181. Downing I, MacDonald SL, Atkinson AP, Turner ML, Kilpatrick DC. Drug modification of LPS-stimulated human monocyte-derived dendritic cells. *Br J Biomed Sci* (2012) **69**(3):126–33.
182. Olivar R, Luque A, Naranjo-Gomez M, Quer J, Garcia de Frutos P, Borras FE, et al. The alpha7beta0 isoform of the complement regulator C4b-binding protein induces a semimature, anti-inflammatory state in dendritic cells. *J Immunol* (2013) **190**(6):2857–72. doi:10.4049/jimmunol.1200503
183. Wu SF, Liu TM, Lin YC, Sytwu HK, Juan HF, Chen ST, et al. Immunomodulatory effect of decoy receptor 3 on the differentiation and function of bone marrow-derived dendritic cells in nonobese diabetic mice: from regulatory mechanism to clinical implication. *J Leukoc Biol* (2004) **75**(2):293–306. doi:10.1189/jlb.0303119
184. Cedeno-Laurent F, Opperman M, Barthel SR, Kuchroo VK, Dimitroff CJ. Galectin-1 triggers an immunoregulatory signature in Th cells functionally defined by IL-10 expression. *J Immunol* (2012) **188**(7):3127–37. doi:10.4049/jimmunol.1103433
185. Ilarregui JM, Croci DO, Bianco GA, Toscano MA, Salatino M, Vermeulen ME, et al. Tolerogenic signals delivered by dendritic cells to T cells through a galectin-1-driven immunoregulatory circuit involving interleukin 27 and interleukin 10. *Nat Immunol* (2009) **10**(9):981–91. doi:10.1038/ni.1772
186. Chen HW, Chen HY, Wang LT, Wang FH, Fang LW, Lai HY, et al. Mesenchymal stem cells tune the development of monocyte-derived dendritic cells toward a myeloid-derived suppressive phenotype through growth-regulated oncogene chemokines. *J Immunol* (2013) **190**(10):5065–77. doi:10.4049/jimmunol.1202775
187. Trinath J, Hegde P, Sharma M, Maddur MS, Rabin M, Vallat JM, et al. Intravenous immunoglobulin expands regulatory T cells via induction of cyclooxygenase-2-dependent prostaglandin E2 in human dendritic cells. *Blood* (2013) **122**(8):1419–27. doi:10.1182/blood-2012-11-468264
188. Crow AR, Brinc D, Lazarus AH. New insight into the mechanism of action of IVIg: the role of dendritic cells. *J Thromb Haemost* (2009) **7**(Suppl 1):245–8. doi:10.1111/j.1538-7836.2009.03420.x
189. Matsumoto T, Hasegawa H, Onishi S, Ishizaki J, Suemori K, Yasukawa M. Protein kinase C inhibitor generates stable human tolerogenic dendritic cells. *J Immunol* (2013) **191**(5):2247–57. doi:10.4049/jimmunol.1203053
190. Chang J, Thangamani S, Kim MH, Ulrich B, Morris SM Jr, Kim CH. Retinoic acid promotes the development of Arg1-expressing dendritic cells for the regulation of T-cell differentiation. *Eur J Immunol* (2013) **43**(4):967–78. doi:10.1002/eji.201242772
191. Cassani B, Villablanca EJ, De Calisto J, Wang S, Mora JR. Vitamin A and immune regulation: role of retinoic acid in gut-associated dendritic cell education, immune protection and tolerance. *Mol Aspects Med* (2012) **33**(1):63–76. doi:10.1016/j.mam.2011.11.001
192. Coombes JL, Siddiqui KR, Arancibia-Carcamo CV, Hall J, Sun CM, Belkaid Y, et al. A functionally specialized population of mucosal CD103+ DCs induces Foxp3+ regulatory T cells via a TGF-beta and retinoic acid-dependent mechanism. *J Exp Med* (2007) **204**(8):1757–64. doi:10.1084/jem.20070590
193. Saurer L, McCullough KC, Summerfield A. In vitro induction of mucosa-type dendritic cells by all-trans retinoic acid. *J Immunol* (2007) **179**(6):3504–14.
194. Zhang M, Liu F, Jia H, Zhang Q, Yin L, Liu W, et al. Inhibition of microRNA let-7i depresses maturation and functional state of dendritic cells in response to lipopolysaccharide stimulation via targeting suppressor of cytokine signaling 1. *J Immunol* (2011) **187**:1674–83. doi:10.4049/jimmunol.1001937
195. Hilkens CM, Isaacs JD. Tolerogenic dendritic cell therapy for rheumatoid arthritis: where are we now? *Clin Exp Immunol* (2013) **172**(2):148–57. doi:10.1111/cei.12038
196. Boks MA, Zwaginga JJ, van Ham SM, ten Brinke A. An optimized CFSE-based T-cell suppression assay to evaluate the suppressive capacity of regulatory T-cells induced by human tolerogenic dendritic cells. *Scand J Immunol* (2010) **72**(2):158–68. doi:10.1111/j.1365-3083.2010.02414.x
197. Cohen N, Mouly E, Hamdi H, Maillot MC, Pallardy M, Godot V, et al. GILZ expression in human dendritic cells redirects their maturation and prevents antigen-specific T lymphocyte response. *Blood* (2006) **107**(5):2037–44. doi:10.1182/blood-2005-07-2760
198. Zimmer A, Bouley J, Le Mignon M, Pliquet E, Horiot S, Turfkruyer M, et al. A regulatory dendritic cell signature correlates with the clinical efficacy of allergen-specific sublingual immunotherapy. *J Allergy Clin Immunol* (2012) **129**(4):1020–30. doi:10.1016/j.jaci.2012.02.014
199. Penna G, Roncari A, Amuchastegui S, Daniel KC, Berti E, Colonna M, et al. Expression of the inhibitory receptor ILT3 on dendritic cells is dispensable for induction of CD4+Foxp3+ regulatory T cells by 1,25-dihydroxyvitamin D3. *Blood* (2005) **106**(10):3490–7. doi:10.1182/blood-2005-05-2044
200. van der Aar AM, Sibiryak DS, Bakdash G, van Capel TM, van der Kleij HP, Opstelten DJ, et al. Vitamin D3 targets epidermal and dermal dendritic cells for induction of distinct regulatory T cells. *J Allergy Clin Immunol* (2011) **127**(6):1532–40.e7. doi:10.1016/j.jaci.2011.01.068

201. Gong YB, Huang YF, Li Y, Han GC, Li YR, Wang DJ, et al. Experimental study of the mechanism of tolerance induction in dexamethasone-treated dendritic cells. *Med Sci Monit* (2011) **17**(5):BR125–31. doi:10.12659/MSM.881758
202. Hontelez S, Karthaus N, Looman MW, Ansems M, Adema GJ. DC-SCRIPT regulates glucocorticoid receptor function and expression of its target GILZ in dendritic cells. *J Immunol* (2013) **190**(7):3172–9. doi:10.4049/jimmunol.1201776
203. Volchenkov R, Karlsen M, Jonsson R, Appel S. Type 1 regulatory T cells and regulatory B cells induced by tolerogenic dendritic cells. *Scand J Immunol* (2013) **77**(4):246–54. doi:10.1111/sji.12039
204. Delgado M, Gonzalez-Rey E, Ganea D. Vasoactive intestinal peptide: the dendritic cell -> regulatory T cell axis. *Ann N Y Acad Sci* (2006) **1070**:233–8. doi:10.1196/annals.1317.020
205. Chi H. Regulation and function of mTOR signalling in T cell fate decisions. *Nat Rev Immunol* (2012) **12**(5):325–38. doi:10.1038/nri3198
206. Coenen JJ, Koenen HJ, van Rijssen E, Hilbrands LB, Joosten I. Rapamycin, and not cyclosporin A, preserves the highly suppressive CD27+ subset of human CD4+CD25+ regulatory T cells. *Blood* (2006) **107**(3):1018–23. doi:10.1182/blood-2005-07-3032
207. Remes Lenicov F, Rodriguez Rodrigues C, Sabatte J, Cabrini M, Jancic C, Ostrowski M, et al. Semen promotes the differentiation of tolerogenic dendritic cells. *J Immunol* (2012) **189**(10):4777–86. doi:10.4049/jimmunol.1202089
208. Teh BK, Yeo JG, Chern LM, Lu J. C1q regulation of dendritic cell development from monocytes with distinct cytokine production and T cell stimulation. *Mol Immunol* (2011) **48**(9–10):1128–38. doi:10.1016/j.molimm.2011.02.006
209. De Smedt T, Van Mechelen M, De Becker G, Urbain J, Leo O, Moser M. Effect of interleukin-10 on dendritic cell maturation and function. *Eur J Immunol* (1997) **27**:1229–35. doi:10.1002/eji.1830270526
210. Sato K, Yamashita N, Matsuyama T. Human peripheral blood monocyte-derived interleukin-10-induced semi-mature dendritic cells induce anergic CD4(+) and CD8(+) T cells via presentation of the internalized soluble antigen and cross-presentation of the phagocytosed necrotic cellular fragments. *Cell Immunol* (2002) **215**(2):186–94. doi:10.1016/S0008-8749(02)00021-7
211. Steinbrink K, Graulich E, Kubsch S, Knop J, Enk AH. CD4(+) and CD8(+) anergic T cells induced by interleukin-10-treated human dendritic cells display antigen-specific suppressor activity. *Blood* (2002) **99**(7):2468–76. doi:10.1182/blood.V99.7.2468
212. Sato K, Nagayama H, Tadokoro K, Juji T, Takahashi TA. Extracellular signal-regulated kinase, stress-activated protein kinase/c-Jun N-terminal kinase, and p38mapk are involved in IL-10-mediated selective repression of TNF-alpha-induced activation and maturation of human peripheral blood monocyte-derived dendritic cells. *J Immunol* (1999) **162**:3865–72.
213. Rethi B, Gogolak P, Szatmari I, Veres A, Erdos E, Nagy L, et al. SLAM/SLAM interactions inhibit CD40-induced production of inflammatory cytokines in monocyte-derived dendritic cells. *Blood* (2006) **107**(7):2821–9. doi:10.1182/blood-2005-06-2265
214. Huang H, Dawicki W, Lu M, Nayyar A, Zhang X, Gordon JR. Regulatory dendritic cell expression of MHCII and IL-10 are jointly requisite for induction of tolerance in a murine model of OVA-asthma. *Allergy* (2013) **68**(9):1126–35. doi:10.1111/all.12203
215. Huang H, Dawicki W, Zhang X, Town J, Gordon JR. Tolerogenic dendritic cells induce CD4+CD25hiFoxp3+ regulatory T cell differentiation from CD4+CD25-/loFoxp3- effector T cells. *J Immunol* (2010) **185**(9):5003–10. doi:10.4049/jimmunol.0903446
216. Nayyar A. *Therapeutic Immunomodulation of Allergic Lung Disease Using Regulatory Dendritic Cells in a Mouse Model of Asthma.* Ph.D. thesis, Saskatoon, SK: University of Saskatchewan (2009).
217. Huang H, Ma Y, Dawicki W, Zhang X, Gordon JR. Comparison of induced versus natural regulatory T cells of the same TCR specificity for induction of tolerance to an environmental antigen. *J Immunol* (2013) **191**(3):1136–43. doi:10.4049/jimmunol.1201899
218. Levings MK, Gregori S, Tresoldi E, Cazzaniga S, Bonini C, Roncarolo MG. Differentiation of Tr1 cells by immature dendritic cells requires IL-10 but not CD25+CD4+ Tr cells. *Blood* (2005) **105**(3):1162–9. doi:10.1182/blood-2004-03-1211
219. Yang CY, Leung PS, Adamopoulos IE, Gershwin ME. The implication of vitamin D and autoimmunity: a comprehensive review. *Clin Rev Allergy Immunol* (2013) **45**(2):217–26. doi:10.1007/s12016-013-8361-3
220. Pludowski P, Holick MF, Pilz S, Wagner CL, Hollis BW, Grant WB, et al. Vitamin D effects on musculoskeletal health, immunity, autoimmunity, cardiovascular disease, cancer, fertility, pregnancy, dementia and mortality-A review of recent evidence. *Autoimmun Rev* (2013) **12**(10):976–89. doi:10.1016/j.autrev.2013.02.004
221. Griffin MD, Lutz WH, Phan VA, Bachman LA, McKean DJ, Kumar R. Potent inhibition of dendritic cell differentiation and maturation by vitamin D analogs. *Biochem Biophys Res Commun* (2000) **270**(3):701–8. doi:10.1006/bbrc.2000.2490
222. van Halteren AG, van Etten E, de Jong EC, Bouillon R, Roep BO, Mathieu C. Redirection of human autoreactive T-cells upon interaction with dendritic cells modulated by TX527, an analog of 1,25 dihydroxyvitamin D(3). *Diabetes* (2002) **51**(7):2119–25. doi:10.2337/diabetes.51.7.2119
223. Adorini L. Tolerogenic dendritic cells induced by vitamin D receptor ligands enhance regulatory T cells inhibiting autoimmune diabetes. *Ann N Y Acad Sci* (2003) **987**:258–61. doi:10.1111/j.1749-6632.2003.tb06057.x
224. Griffin MD, Lutz W, Phan VA, Bachman LA, McKean DJ, Kumar R. Dendritic cell modulation by 1alpha,25 dihydroxyvitamin D3 and its analogs: a vitamin D receptor-dependent pathway that promotes a persistent state of immaturity in vitro and in vivo. *Proc Natl Acad Sci U S A* (2001) **98**(12):6800–5. doi:10.1073/pnas.121172198
225. Sochorova K, Budinsky V, Rozkova D, Tobiasova Z, Dusilova-Sulkova S, Spisek R, et al. Paricalcitol (19-nor-1,25-dihydroxyvitamin D2) and calcitriol (1,25-dihydroxyvitamin D3) exert potent immunomodulatory effects on dendritic cells and inhibit induction of antigen-specific T cells. *Clin Immunol* (2009) **133**(1):69–77. doi:10.1016/j.clim.2009.06.011
226. Kleijwegt FS, Laban S, Duinkerken G, Joosten AM, Koeleman BP, Nikolic T, et al. Transfer of regulatory properties from tolerogenic to proinflammatory dendritic cells via induced autoreactive regulatory T cells. *J Immunol* (2011) **187**(12):6357–64. doi:10.4049/jimmunol.1101638
227. Coutinho AE, Chapman KE. The anti-inflammatory and immunosuppressive effects of glucocorticoids, recent developments and mechanistic insights. *Mol Cell Endocrinol* (2011) **335**(1):2–13. doi:10.1016/j.mce.2010.04.005
228. Prado C, Gomez J, Lopez P, de Paz B, Gutierrez C, Suarez A. Dexamethasone upregulates FOXP3 expression without increasing regulatory activity. *Immunobiology* (2011) **216**(3):386–92. doi:10.1016/j.imbio.2010.06.013
229. Woltman AM, de Fijter JW, Kamerling SW, Paul LC, Daha MR, van Kooten C. The effect of calcineurin inhibitors and corticosteroids on the differentiation of human dendritic cells. *Eur J Immunol* (2000) **30**(7):1807–12. doi:10.1002/1521-4141(200007)30:7<1807::AID-IMMU1807>3.0.CO;2-N
230. Matasic R, Dietz AB, Vuk-Pavlovic S. Dexamethasone inhibits dendritic cell maturation by redirecting differentiation of a subset of cells. *J Leukoc Biol* (1999) **66**(6):909–14.
231. Cao Y, Bender IK, Konstantinidis AK, Shin SC, Jewell CM, Cidlowski JA, et al. Glucocorticoid receptor translational isoforms underlie maturational stage-specific glucocorticoid sensitivities of dendritic cells in mice and humans. *Blood* (2013) **121**(9):1553–62. doi:10.1182/blood-2012-05-432336
232. Rea D, van Kooten C, van Meijgaarden KE, Ottenhoff TH, Melief CJ, Offringa R. Glucocorticoids transform CD40-triggering of dendritic cells into an alternative activation pathway resulting in antigen-presenting cells that secrete IL-10. *Blood* (2000) **95**:3162–7.
233. Bosma BM, Metselaar HJ, Nagtzaam NM, de Haan R, Mancham S, van der Laan LJ, et al. Dexamethasone transforms lipopolysaccharide-stimulated human blood myeloid dendritic cells into myeloid dendritic cells that prime interleukin-10 production in T cells. *Immunology* (2008) **125**(1):91–100. doi:10.1111/j.1365-2567.2008.02824.x
234. Emmer PM, van der Vlag J, Adema GJ, Hilbrands LB. Dendritic cells activated by lipopolysaccharide after dexamethasone treatment induce donor-specific allograft hyporesponsiveness. *Transplantation* (2006) **81**(10):1451–9. doi:10.1097/01.tp.0000208801.51222.bd
235. O'Flynn L, Treacy O, Ryan AE, Morcos M, Cregg M, Gerlach J, et al. Donor bone marrow-derived dendritic cells prolong corneal allograft survival and promote an intragraft immunoregulatory milieu. *Mol Ther* (2013) **21**(11):2102–12. doi:10.1038/mt.2013.167
236. de Kort H, Crul C, van der Wal AM, Schlagwein N, Stax AM, Bruijn JA, et al. Accelerated antibody-mediated graft loss of rodent pancreatic islets after pretreatment with dexamethasone-treated immature donor dendritic cells. *Transplantation* (2012) **94**:903–10. doi:10.1097/TP.0b013e31826acd01

237. Miller A, Lider O, Weiner HL. Antigen-driven bystander suppression after oral administration of antigens. *J Exp Med* (1991) **174**(4):791–8. doi:10.1084/jem.174.4.791
238. Derks RA, Jankowska-Gan E, Xu Q, Burlingham WJ. Dendritic cell type determines the mechanism of bystander suppression by adaptive T regulatory cells specific for the minor antigen HA-1. *J Immunol* (2007) **179**(6):3443–51.
239. Kleijwegt FS, Jansen DT, Teeler J, Joosten AM, Laban S, Nikolic T, et al. Tolerogenic dendritic cells impede priming of naive CD8(+) T cells and deplete memory CD8(+) T cells. *Eur J Immunol* (2013) **43**(1):85–92. doi:10.1002/eji.201242879
240. Pedersen AE, Schmidt EG, Gad M, Poulsen SS, Claesson MH. Dexamethasone/1alpha-25-dihydroxyvitamin D3-treated dendritic cells suppress colitis in the SCID T-cell transfer model. *Immunology* (2009) **127**(3):354–64. doi:10.1111/j.1365-2567.2008.02996.x
241. Said SI. The discovery of VIP: initially looked for in the lung, isolated from intestine, and identified as a neuropeptide. *Peptides* (2007) **28**(9):1620–1. doi:10.1016/j.peptides.2007.06.007
242. Couvineau A, Laburthe M. VPAC receptors: structure, molecular pharmacology and interaction with accessory proteins. *Br J Pharmacol* (2012) **166**(1):42–50. doi:10.1111/j.1476-5381.2011.01676.x
243. Pozo D, Anderson P, Gonzalez-Rey E. Induction of alloantigen-specific human T regulatory cells by vasoactive intestinal peptide. *J Immunol* (2009) **183**(7):4346–59. doi:10.4049/jimmunol.0900400
244. Arranz A, Juarranz Y, Leceta J, Gomariz RP, Martinez C. VIP balances innate and adaptive immune responses induced by specific stimulation of TLR2 and TLR4. *Peptides* (2008) **29**(6):948–56. doi:10.1016/j.peptides.2008.01.019
245. Chen G, Hao J, Xi Y, Wang W, Wang Z, Li N, et al. The therapeutic effect of vasoactive intestinal peptide on experimental arthritis is associated with CD4+CD25+ T regulatory cells. *Scand J Immunol* (2008) **68**(6):572–8. doi:10.1111/j.1365-3083.2008.02178.x
246. Pozo D, Gonzalez-Rey E, Chorny A, Anderson P, Varela N, Delgado M. Tuning immune tolerance with vasoactive intestinal peptide: a new therapeutic approach for immune disorders. *Peptides* (2007) **28**(9):1833–46. doi:10.1016/j.peptides.2007.04.008
247. Chorny A, Gonzalez-Rey E, Fernandez-Martin A, Pozo D, Ganea D, Delgado M. Vasoactive intestinal peptide induces regulatory dendritic cells with therapeutic effects on autoimmune disorders. *Proc Natl Acad Sci USA* (2005) **102**(38):13562–7. doi:10.1073/pnas.0504484102
248. Chorny A, Gonzalez-Rey E, Fernandez-Martin A, Ganea D, Delgado M. Vasoactive intestinal peptide induces regulatory dendritic cells that prevent acute graft-versus-host disease while maintaining the graft-versus-tumor response. *Blood* (2006) **107**(9):3787–94. doi:10.1182/blood-2005-11-4495
249. Gonzalez-Rey E, Delgado M. Therapeutic treatment of experimental colitis with regulatory dendritic cells generated with vasoactive intestinal peptide. *Gastroenterology* (2006) **131**(6):1799–811. doi:10.1053/j.gastro.2006.10.023
250. Delgado M. Generating tolerogenic dendritic cells with neuropeptides. *Hum Immunol* (2009) **70**(5):300–7. doi:10.1016/j.humimm.2009.01.020
251. Delgado M, Chorny A, Ganea D, Gonzalez-Rey E. Vasoactive intestinal polypeptide induces regulatory dendritic cells that prevent acute graft versus host disease and leukemia relapse after bone marrow transplantation. *Ann N Y Acad Sci* (2006) **1070**:226–32. doi:10.1196/annals.1317.019
252. Delgado M, Gonzalez-Rey E, Ganea D. The neuropeptide vasoactive intestinal peptide generates tolerogenic dendritic cells. *J Immunol* (2005) **175**(11):7311–24.
253. Delgado M, Chorny A, Gonzalez-Rey E, Ganea D. Vasoactive intestinal peptide generates CD4+CD25+ regulatory T cells in vivo. *J Leukoc Biol* (2005) **78**(6):1327–38. doi:10.1189/jlb.0605299
254. Fernandez-Martin A, Gonzalez-Rey E, Chorny A, Ganea D, Delgado M. Vasoactive intestinal peptide induces regulatory T cells during experimental autoimmune encephalomyelitis. *Eur J Immunol* (2006) **36**(2):318–26. doi:10.1002/eji.200535430
255. Gonzalez-Rey E, Fernandez-Martin A, Chorny A, Delgado M. Vasoactive intestinal peptide induces CD4+,CD25+ T regulatory cells with therapeutic effect in collagen-induced arthritis. *Arthritis Rheum* (2006) **54**(3):864–76. doi:10.1002/art.21652
256. Waschek JA. VIP and PACAP: neuropeptide modulators of CNS inflammation, injury, and repair. *Br J Pharmacol* (2013) **169**(3):512–23. doi:10.1111/bph.12181
257. Hay N, Sonenberg N. Upstream and downstream of mTOR. *Genes Dev* (2004) **18**(16):1926–45. doi:10.1101/gad.1212704
258. Battaglia M, Stabilini A, Migliavacca B, Horejs-Hoeck J, Kaupper T, Roncarolo MG. Rapamycin promotes expansion of functional CD4+CD25+FOXP3+ regulatory T cells of both healthy subjects and type 1 diabetic patients. *J Immunol* (2006) **177**(12):8338–47.
259. Mahe E, Morelon E, Lechaton S, Sang KH, Mansouri R, Ducasse MF, et al. Cutaneous adverse events in renal transplant recipients receiving sirolimus-based therapy. *Transplantation* (2005) **79**(4):476–82. doi:10.1097/01.TP.0000151630.25127.3A
260. Haidinger M, Poglitsch M, Geyeregger R, Kasturi S, Zeyda M, Zlabinger GJ, et al. A versatile role of mammalian target of rapamycin in human dendritic cell function and differentiation. *J Immunol* (2010) **185**(7):3919–31. doi:10.4049/jimmunol.1000296
261. Hackstein H, Taner T, Zahorchak AF, Morelli AE, Logar AJ, Gessner A, et al. Rapamycin inhibits IL-4 – induced dendritic cell maturation in vitro and dendritic cell mobilization and function in vivo. *Blood* (2003) **101**(11):4457–63. doi:10.1182/blood-2002-11-3370
262. Turnquist HR, Raimondi G, Zahorchak AF, Fischer RT, Wang Z, Thomson AW. Rapamycin-conditioned dendritic cells are poor stimulators of allogeneic CD4+ T cells, but enrich for antigen-specific Foxp3+ T regulatory cells and promote organ transplant tolerance. *J Immunol* (2007) **178**(11):7018–31.
263. Pothoven KL, Kheradmand T, Yang Q, Houlihan JL, Zhang H, Degutes M, et al. Rapamycin-conditioned donor dendritic cells differentiate CD4CD25Foxp3 T cells in vitro with TGF-beta1 for islet transplantation. *Am J Transplant* (2010) **10**(8):1774–84. doi:10.1111/j.1600-6143.2010.03199.x
264. Fischer RT, Turnquist HR, Wang Z, Beer-Stolz D, Thomson AW. Rapamycin-conditioned, alloantigen-pulsed myeloid dendritic cells present donor MHC class I/peptide via the semi-direct pathway and inhibit survival of antigen-specific CD8(+) T cells in vitro and in vivo. *Transpl Immunol* (2011) **25**(1):20–6. doi:10.1016/j.trim.2011.05.001
265. Horibe EK, Sacks J, Unadkat J, Raimondi G, Wang Z, Ikeguchi R, et al. Rapamycin-conditioned, alloantigen-pulsed dendritic cells promote indefinite survival of vascularized skin allografts in association with T regulatory cell expansion. *Transpl Immunol* (2008) **18**(4):307–18. doi:10.1016/j.trim.2007.10.007
266. Taner T, Hackstein H, Wang Z, Morelli AE, Thomson AW. Rapamycin-treated, alloantigen-pulsed host dendritic cells induce ag-specific T cell regulation and prolong graft survival. *Am J Transplant* (2005) **5**(2):228–36. doi:10.1046/j.1600-6143.2004.00673.x
267. Huang YM, Yang JS, Xu LY, Link H, Xiao BG. Autoantigen-pulsed dendritic cells induce tolerance to experimental allergic encephalomyelitis (EAE) in Lewis rats. *Clin Exp Immunol* (2000) **122**(3):437–44.
268. Pettersson A, Ciumas C, Chirsky V, Link H, Huang YM, Xiao BG. Dendritic cells exposed to estrogen in vitro exhibit therapeutic effects in ongoing experimental allergic encephalomyelitis. *J Neuroimmunol* (2004) **156**(1–2):58–65. doi:10.1016/j.jneuroim.2004.07.004
269. Xiao BG, Huang YM, Yang JS, Xu LY, Link H. Bone marrow-derived dendritic cells from experimental allergic encephalomyelitis induce immune tolerance to EAE in Lewis rats. *Clin Exp Immunol* (2001) **125**(2):300–9.
270. Yang JS, Xu LY, Huang YM, Van Der Meide PH, Link H, Xiao BG. Adherent dendritic cells expressing high levels of interleukin-10 and low levels of interleukin-12 induce antigen-specific tolerance to experimental autoimmune encephalomyelitis. *Immunology* (2000) **101**(3):397–403. doi:10.1046/j.1365-2567.2000.00115.x
271. Zhang QH, Link H, Xiao BG. Efficacy of peripheral tolerance induced by dendritic cells is dependent on route of delivery. *J Autoimmun* (2004) **23**(1):37–43. doi:10.1016/j.jaut.2004.03.010
272. Bellinghausen I, Sudowe S, Konig B, Reske-Kunz AB, Knop J, Saloga J. Interleukin-10-treated dendritic cells do not inhibit Th2 immune responses in ovalbumin/alum-sensitized mice. *Int Arch Allergy Immunol* (2006) **141**(1):61–9. doi:10.1159/000094255
273. Zimmermann O, Homann JM, Bangert A, Muller AM, Hristov G, Goeser S, et al. Successful use of mRNA-nucleofection for overexpression of interleukin-10 in murine monocytes/macrophages for anti-inflammatory therapy in a murine model of autoimmune myocarditis. *J Am Heart Assoc* (2012) **1**(6):e003293. doi:10.1161/JAHA.112.003293

274. Besin G, Gaudreau S, Menard M, Guindi C, Dupuis G, Amrani A. Thymic stromal lymphopoietin and thymic stromal lymphopoietin-conditioned dendritic cells induce regulatory T-cell differentiation and protection of NOD mice against diabetes. *Diabetes* (2008) **57**(8):2107–17. doi:10.2337/db08-0171

275. Liang X, Ma L, Thai NL, Fung JJ, Qian S, Lu L. The role of liver-derived regulatory dendritic cells in prevention of type 1 diabetes. *Immunology* (2007) **120**(2):251–60. doi:10.1111/j.1365-2567.2006.02496.x

276. Ezzelarab MB, Zahorchak AF, Lu L, Morelli AE, Chalasani G, Demetris AJ, et al. Regulatory dendritic cell infusion prolongs kidney allograft survival in nonhuman primates. *Am J Transplant* (2013) **13**(8):1989–2005. doi:10.1111/ajt.12310

277. Blanco P, Palucka AK, Pascual V, Banchereau J. Dendritic cells and cytokines in human inflammatory and autoimmune diseases. *Cytokine Growth Factor Rev* (2008) **19**(1):41–52. doi:10.1016/j.cytogfr.2007.10.004

278. Hammer GE, Ma A. Molecular control of steady-state dendritic cell maturation and immune homeostasis. *Annu Rev Immunol* (2013) **31**:743–91. doi:10.1146/annurev-immunol-020711-074929

279. Schreibelt G, Tel J, Sliepen KH, Benitez-Ribas D, Figdor CG, Adema GJ, et al. Toll-like receptor expression and function in human dendritic cell subsets: implications for dendritic cell-based anti-cancer immunotherapy. *Cancer Immunol Immunother* (2010) **59**:1573–82. doi:10.1007/s00262-010-0833-1

280. Edwards AD, Diebold SS, Slack EM, Tomizawa H, Hemmi H, Kaisho T, et al. Toll-like receptor expression in murine DC subsets: lack of TLR7 expression by CD8 alpha+ DC correlates with unresponsiveness to imidazoquinolines. *Eur J Immunol* (2003) **33**(4):827–33. doi:10.1002/eji.200323797

281. Delamarre L, Mellman I. Harnessing dendritic cells for immunotherapy. *Semin Immunol* (2011) **23**(1):2–11. doi:10.1016/j.smim.2011.02.001

282. Arizmendi NG, Abel M, Mihara K, Davidson C, Polley D, Nadeem A, et al. Mucosal allergic sensitization to cockroach allergens is dependent on proteinase activity and proteinase-activated receptor-2 activation. *J Immunol* (2011) **186**(5):3164–72. doi:10.4049/jimmunol.0903812

283. Ebeling C, Lam T, Gordon JR, Hollenberg MD, Vliagoftis H. Proteinase-activated receptor-2 promotes allergic sensitization to an inhaled antigen through a TNF-mediated pathway. *J Immunol* (2007) **179**(5):2910–7.

284. Salazar F, Sewell HF, Shakib F, Ghaemmaghami AM. The role of lectins in allergic sensitization and allergic disease. *J Allergy Clin Immunol* (2013) **132**(1):27–36. doi:10.1016/j.jaci.2013.02.001

285. Brosbol-Ravnborg A, Bundgaard B, Hollsberg P. Synergy between vitamin D(3) and toll-like receptor agonists regulates human dendritic cell response during maturation. *Clin Dev Immunol* (2013) **2013**:807971. doi:10.1155/2013/807971

286. Cabezon R, Ricart E, Espana C, Panes J, Benitez-Ribas D. Gram-negative enterobacteria induce tolerogenic maturation in dexamethasone conditioned dendritic cells. *PLoS One* (2012) **7**(12):e52456. doi:10.1371/journal.pone.0052456

287. Luger R, Valookaran S, Knapp N, Vizzardelli C, Dohnal AM, Felzmann T. Toll-like receptor 4 engagement drives differentiation of human and murine dendritic cells from a pro- into an anti-inflammatory mode. *PLoS One* (2013) **8**(2):e54879. doi:10.1371/journal.pone.0054879

288. Yates SF, Paterson AM, Nolan KF, Cobbold SP, Saunders NJ, Waldmann H, et al. Induction of regulatory T cells and dominant tolerance by dendritic cells incapable of full activation. *J Immunol* (2007) **179**(2):967–76.

289. Nguyen KD, Vanichsarn C, Nadeau KC. Impaired IL-10-dependent induction of tolerogenic dendritic cells by CD4+CD25hiCD127lo/- natural regulatory T cells in human allergic asthma. *Am J Respir Crit Care Med* (2009) **180**(9):823–33. doi:10.1164/rccm.200905-0761OC

290. Yurchenko E, Shio MT, Huang TC, Da Silva Martins M, Szyf M, Levings MK, et al. Inflammation-driven reprogramming of CD4+ Foxp3+ regulatory T cells into pathogenic Th1/Th17 T effectors is abrogated by mTOR inhibition in vivo. *PLoS One* (2012) **7**(4):e35572. doi:10.1371/journal.pone.0035572

291. Xu L, Kitani A, Fuss I, Strober W. Cutting edge: regulatory T cells induce CD4+CD25-Foxp3- T cells or are self-induced to become Th17 cells in the absence of exogenous TGF-beta. *J Immunol* (2007) **178**(11):6725–9.

292. Giannoukakis N, Phillips B, Finegold D, Harnaha J, Trucco M. Phase I (safety) study of autologous tolerogenic dendritic cells in type 1 diabetic patients. *Diabetes Care* (2011) **34**(9):2026–32. doi:10.2337/dc11-0472

293. Machen J, Harnaha J, Lakomy R, Styche A, Trucco M, Giannoukakis N. Antisense oligonucleotides down-regulating costimulation confer diabetes-preventive properties to nonobese diabetic mouse dendritic cells. *J Immunol* (2004) **173**(7):4331–41.

294. Harry R, AE A, JD I, HIlkens C. Generation and characterisation of therapeutic tolerogenic dendritic cells for rheumatoid arthritis. *Ann Rheum Dis* (2010) **69**(11):2042–50. doi:10.1136/ard.2009.126383

295. Raich-Regue D, Grau-López L, Naranjo-Gómez M, Ramo-Tello C, Pujol-Borrell R, Martínez-Cáceres E, et al. Stable antigen-specific T-cell hyporesponsiveness induced by tolerogenic dendritic cells from multiple sclerosis patients. *Eur J Immunol* (2012) **42**(3):771–82. doi:10.1002/eji.201141835

14

Germline amino acid diversity in B cell receptors is a good predictor of somatic selection pressures

Gregory W. Schwartz[1] and Uri Hershberg[1,2]*

[1] Systems Immunology Laboratory, School of Biomedical Engineering, Science, and Health Systems, Drexel University, Philadelphia, PA, USA
[2] Department of Microbiology and Immunology, College of Medicine, Drexel University, Philadelphia, PA, USA

Edited by:
Michal Or-Guil, Humboldt University Berlin, Germany

Reviewed by:
Andrew M. Collins, University of New South Wales, Australia
Nicole Wittenbrink, Humboldt University Berlin, Germany

***Correspondence:**
Uri Hershberg, Systems Immunology Laboratory, School of Biomedical Engineering, Science, and Health Systems, Drexel University, 3141 Chestnut Street, Philadelphia, PA 19104, USA
e-mail: uri.hershberg@drexel.edu

The diversity of the immune repertoire is important for the adaptive immune system's ability to detect pathogens. Much of this diversity is generated in two steps, first through the recombination of germline gene segments and second through hypermutation during an immune response. While both steps are to some extent based on the germline level repertoire of genes, the final structure and selection of specific receptors is at the somatic level. How germline diversity and selection relate to somatic diversity and selection has not been clear. To investigate how germline diversity relates to somatic diversity and selection, we considered the published repertoire of Ig heavy chain V genes taken from the blood of 12 individuals, post-vaccination against influenza, sequenced by 454 high-throughput sequencing. We here show that when we consider individual amino acid positions in the heavy chain V gene sequence, there exists a strong correlation between the diversity of the germline repertoire at a position and the number of B cell clones that change amino acids at that position. At the same time, we find that the diversity of amino acids used in the mutated positions is greater than in the germline, albeit still correlated to germline diversity. From these findings, we propose that while germline diversity and germline amino acid usage at a given position do not fully specify the amino acid mutant needed to promote survival of specific clones, germline diversity at a given position is a good indicator for the potential to survive after somatic mutation at that position. We would therefore suggest that germline diversity at each specific position is the better *a priori* model for the effects of somatic mutation and selection, than simply the division into complementarity determining and framework regions.

Keywords: B cells, somatic hypermutation, selection, diversity, evolution

1. INTRODUCTION

The adaptive immune system's ability to react to disease is based on the diversity of its immune repertoire. In the case of B cells, this diversity is generated in two rounds: the recombination of germline gene segments (V, D, and J for heavy chains, V and J for light chains) to create the B cell receptor (BCR), (1–3) as well as somatic hypermutation during an immune response (4–6). In both cases, these diversification processes are coupled with stringent somatic selection based on the binding affinity of the BCR (7). Thus, while the initial state of the BCR is at least somewhat based on an individual's germline genes, the final structure of specific BCR mutants is based on somatic selection processes related to the binding affinity of the BCR. It remains unclear how selection and diversity at the germline level relate to selection at the somatic level. In this analysis, we demonstrate a link between the diversity and selection at the germline and somatic levels for V genes.

The germline genes encoding the different regions of the BCR are themselves diverse, even before considering the diversification produced from the recombination of different gene segments. Specifically in V genes, this diversity is non-uniformly spread across the gene sequence. Some positions always utilize the same amino acid in all V genes while others can utilize many different amino acids. This differential diversity is considered an indicator of the functional role of each position in the eventual tertiary structure of the receptor. Variable regions of the V gene sequences, called complementarity determining regions (CDR), are thought to be those that encode regions which interact with antigens, while the more invariant positions, called framework regions (FR), are proposed to be involved in the backbone of the receptor (8). It has been generally thought that somatic selection segregates along these two regions. Positive selection is thought to occur in the CDR, while mutations in the FR were mostly debilitating to affinity and lethal to the cell (5). It is now clear that this segregation is not strictly true – positively selected key mutations can be found in the FR (9) and negative selection can be seen in mutations throughout the sequence (10).

Previously, the diversity measurements of the receptors were based on differing diversity indexes with varying appropriateness and on partial sets of germline and mutant sequences (8, 11). We directly measured the "true" diversity of light chain V genes and heavy chain V genes (V_H) based on the entire known BCR germline repertoire as found in the IMGT Ig gene database (12, 13). We demonstrated that the pattern of diversity in all V genes is non-uniform, with most positions showing a low level of diversity (2–5 relevant amino acids) and a few exhibiting higher levels of diversity (up to 10 relevant amino acids). If we rank all the positions in the sequence by their diversity, we can explicitly show that while the CDR is enriched for high diversity positions, many CDR positions have diversities as low as those found in FR and some FR positions have quite a high diversity (12). We previously suggested that it is the diversity of positions, not solely their association with the contiguous CDR or FR positions, which determines their functional role and the consequence of mutation.

The diversity of positions in the germline repertoire of V genes is the result of evolutionary selection of individuals and their progeny. The process of affinity maturation is based on somatic mutation and selection. It has thus far been unclear how these two processes of selection are related and if they can be connected at the V gene sequence level. To study this possible relationship, we considered a published dataset of ~17,000 recombined BCR V_H gene sequences from 12 individuals (14). We divided sequences by their clonotypes, identifying the clonal origin for each recombined sequence. In this way we could now count how many times each position was mutated in the repertoire. Comparing the number of individual times a position was mutated to its germline diversity (12), we found that while synonymous mutations were evenly spread across all positions, there was a clear positive correlation between the number of times a position had a mutated amino acid and that position's diversity in the germline repertoire. From this we conclude that the diversity at the germline level is an indication for the potential for somatic harm as a result of mutation. The diversity of each specific position is a more direct measure of the functional consequence of mutation and selection at the somatic level than a mere division into CDR and FR.

2. MATERIALS AND METHODS

2.1. SEQUENCES ANALYZED

We analyzed the amino acid and nucleotide sequences of *Homo sapiens* BCR recombined V_H genes (14). The sequences came from twelve healthy individuals post-vaccination against influenza (14). The individuals came from two age cohorts: 6 young (age range 19–45) and 6 old (age range 70–89). Sequences were acquired at days 0, 7, and 28 post-vaccination and included both IgG, IgM, and IgA class switched receptors. We divided the sequences into clones by fully aligning their nucleotide sequences to the germline V, D, and J genes from the IMGT Ig database (13). All sequences that shared the same germline source (V, J, and CDR3 length) were considered to be from the same clone. We filtered out sequences with ≥30 nt point mutations from the germline. This alignment resulted in the identification of 17,553 sequences divided into 9482 clones. Due to sequencing issues in the original dataset, we only analyzed the sequences from position 25 and on. IMGT numbering leaves gaps in order to remain consistent with all V genes. Also, the length of V genes is not always identical. Therefore, we only calculated germline diversity for amino acid positions 25 − 30, 35 − 59, 63 − 72, and 74 − 106, leaving us with 74 positions in the analysis. These positions were verified for adequate sampling by the use of rarefaction curves at each position (15). We considered a position viable if more than 99% of the curve consisted of a richness of ≥95% of the height of the curve (12). These curves rule out the possibility of having too many gaps in the germline repertoire.

We calculated the germline diversity per amino acid position using BCR V_H genes collected from IMGT as in Ref. (12). We filtered out non-functional, partial, and duplicate sequences for the analysis. All sequences were numbered according to the IMGT unique numbering system based off of the universal alignment provided by IMGT (13). We defined CDR and FR positions as in Ref. (16).

2.2. DIVERSITY MEASURES

We measured the diversity of amino acids per position as in Ref. (12) with an order of diversity equal to 1. The process of measuring diversity is dependent on the order, or "Hill number" (17), we use during calculations. While measuring the effective number of species, the order affects the influence of the sample abundances. An order of 0 does not consider abundances, thus all types are considered equally (this is equivalent to the number of different types, also called "richness"). An order gives greater weight to rare species, while an order >1 gives greater weight to common species. When the order is 1, the effective diversity is determined without any bias (18). We previously described the result of analyzing the diversity of the different amino acid positions in the V gene germline repertoire at different orders of diversity (12). We decided here to focus on the order of 1 as we found no *a priori* reason to bias toward either the more commonly used amino acids at each position or toward the rare amino acids.

At each position p, the number of amino acids at that position was N_p and the richness of the amino acids at that position was R_p.

The measure of diversity used for these positions was "true" diversity ${}^qD_p$, where

$$ {}^qD_p \equiv \left(\sum_{i=1}^{R_p} p_{i_p}^{q} \right)^{(1/1-q)} \qquad (1) $$

and q is the order of diversity and p_i is the frequency of amino acid i (17, 18). At $q = 1$, equation (1) does not exist, however the limit as q approaches 1 is

$$ {}^1D_p \equiv exp\left(-\sum_{i=1}^{R_p} p_{i_p} \ln p_{i_p} \right) \qquad (2) $$

2.3. DEFINITION OF POSITION CATEGORIES

For every amino acid position, we counted – across all clones from any time point and person – the number of times a position changed amino acids and how many times that position maintained its amino acid from the germline. If a position was found to change into several amino acids in a single clone, that position was counted once for each different amino acid. The cases where amino acids were maintained relative to the germline were in some cases further divided into non-mutated and synonymous mutations. The amino acids collected in each category (changed, maintained, or synonymous mutation) were then further analyzed for their diversity and amino acid composition tendencies.

2.4. CORRELATIONS OF DIVERSITY IN GERMLINE POSITIONS VERSUS CHANGED OR MAINTAINED AMINO ACID POSITION CATEGORIES

Using a two sided Spearman's rank correlation test, we assessed the correlation of germline diversity of human V_H genes, as calculated in Ref. (12), with the counts and diversities of the three categories (changed amino acid, maintained amino acid, and synonymous mutation) described above.

2.5. AMINO ACID USAGE ANALYSIS

We assessed if position categories were biased toward specific amino acid usage types. Following our definitions of Ig relevant amino acid categorization by hydrophobicity and tendency to be found on the surface of the receptor (16, 19), we categorized amino acids as hydrophobic (IVLFCMW), neutral (AGTSYPH), and hydrophilic (NDQEKR) (12). We then categorized a position by how biased that position was to using amino acids from only one of these categories. If a position used only amino acids from one category, that position was considered to be of that type (i.e., a hydrophobic, a neutral, or a hydrophilic position). If the position had both neutral and one other category of amino acids, that position would be considered a "weak" version of that category (i.e., weak hydrophobic or weak hydrophilic). If there were amino acids in all categories, then that position was considered indeterminate. In all instances, if a position had a single amino acid in one category, and three or more in another category, the single amino acid category was ignored (12).

3. RESULTS

3.1. CORRELATION OF GERMLINE DIVERSITY TO NUMBER OF CHANGED AMINO ACIDS PER POSITION

When comparing the germline diversity at each position – as calculated from the prototypical IMGT database (12) – and the number of unique changed amino acids at each position, we find that these two properties are highly positively correlated ($\rho = 0.710$, $p = 1.41 \times 10^{-12}$). This correlation holds true if we consider CDR ($\rho = 0.676, p = 2.18 \times 10^{-4}$) and FR ($\rho = 0.668, p = 2.17 \times 10^{-7}$) positions separately and if we consider all positions as a whole (**Figure 1**). While this correlation is monotonic, it is by no means strictly linear as the linear model explains only ~43% of variation in the extent of amino acid exchanges at the different positions

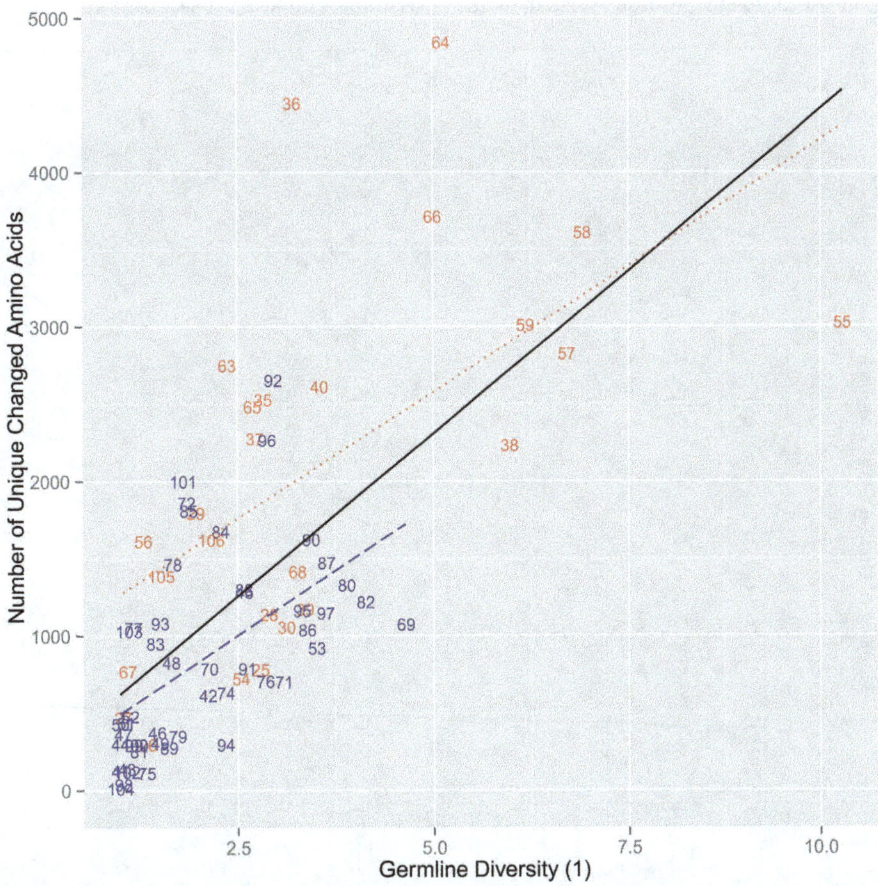

FIGURE 1 | The number of unique changed amino acids versus the diversity of order 1 of the germline sequences per position. The points are labeled by their IMGT sequence position number and if they are found in the CDR (red) or the FR (blue). The lines represent linear regressions for all positions (black, $r^2 = 0.433$), for FR positions (dashed blue, $r^2 = 0.289$), and for CDR positions (dotted red, $r^2 = 0.349$). We found a significant positive correlation for all positions ($\rho = 0.710$, $p = 1.41 \times 10^{-12}$). By correlating the positions based on FR and CDR, we found a significant positive correlation for both FR ($\rho = 0.668$, $p = 2.17 \times 10^{-7}$) and CDR ($\rho = 0.676$, $p = 2.18 \times 10^{-4}$).

($r^2 = 0.433$). Interestingly, while in general the CDR positions with similar diversity have more changed amino acids than most FR positions of similar germline diversity and the linear fits to CDR and FR are distinct, FR and CDR positions are not clearly separated in this plane (**Figure 1**).

The analysis with synonymous mutations shows no correlation ($r^2 = 1.87 \times 10^{-3}$, $\rho = 0.232$, $p = 0.0468$) and similar mutation levels across the entire range of germline position diversities and no difference between CDR ($r^2 = 0.0322, \rho = -0.223, p = 0.273$) and FR ($r^2 = 0.0127, \rho = 0.289, p = 0.0466$) positions (**Figure 2**). The results found using the diversity of the germline repertoire were at the whole repertoire level. No division into certain germlines was necessary and so the possibility for misidentification of the germlines by IMGT would have little to no impact on the diversity at the repertoire level. Moreover, when splitting up the analysis of clones by the germline they aligned with, there was no real difference in between different germlines and at the repertoire level (results now shown).

3.2. CORRELATION OF GERMLINE DIVERSITY TO CHANGED OR MAINTAINED DIVERSITY PER POSITION

We next looked to see how the actual amino acid diversity of the mutant repertoire at the different positions related to the germline diversity. We found that the maintained positions had a diversity that was essentially identical to that found in the IMGT based germline repertoire ($r^2 = 0.947, \rho = 0.961, p = 7.52 \times 10^42$) (**Figure 3A**). In the changed positions a more complex pattern emerges. While overall we find again that there is a positive correlation between germline diversity and the diversity of the changed amino acids ($r^2 = 0.284$, $\rho = 0.359$, $p = 1.70 \times 10^3$), the range of diversity is much greater in the changed positions (**Figure 3B**). This greater range of diversity is present in both CDR ($r^2 = 0.419, \rho = 0.580, p = 2.27 \times 10^3$) and FR ($r^2 = 0.0347$, $\rho = 0.132$, $p = 0.371$). However, when the FR is considered on its own this leads to a lack of significant correlation with germline diversity.

3.3. CHANGES IN AMINO ACID USAGE PATTERN

We categorized the amino acid usage patterns for each position. We found in the maintained amino acid positions the biases toward using specific amino acid types are maintained. This was especially true for the positions in the germline that had stricter categories of amino acids usage bias. 13 out of 14 hydrophobic positions, 17 out of 19 neutral positions, and 8 out of 10 hydrophilic positions retain the same bias in the maintained positions as in the germline (**Table 1**). The positions with the more intermediate

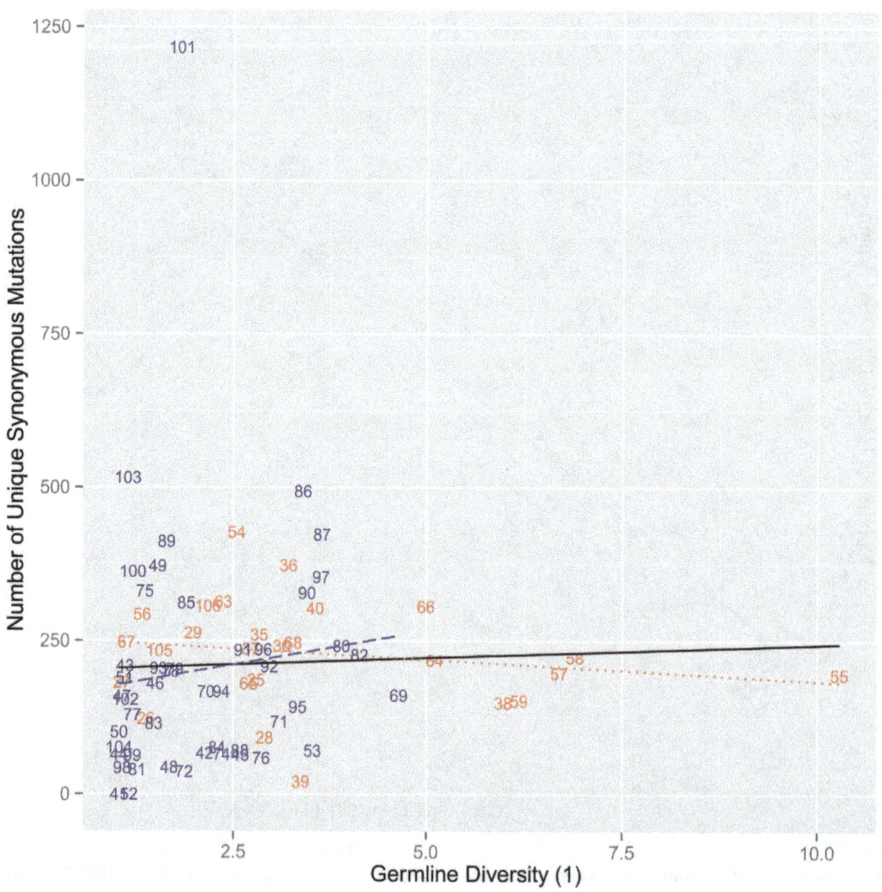

FIGURE 2 | The number of synonymous mutations versus the diversity of order 1 of the germline sequences per position. We found no positive correlation with a flat trend ($r^2 = 1.87 \times 10^{-3}$, $\rho = 0.232$, $p = 0.0468$). When splitting by region, we found no correlation for FR ($r^2 = 0.0127$, $\rho = 0.289$, $p = 0.0466$) and CDR ($r^2 = 0.0322$, $\rho = -0.223$, $p = 0.273$).

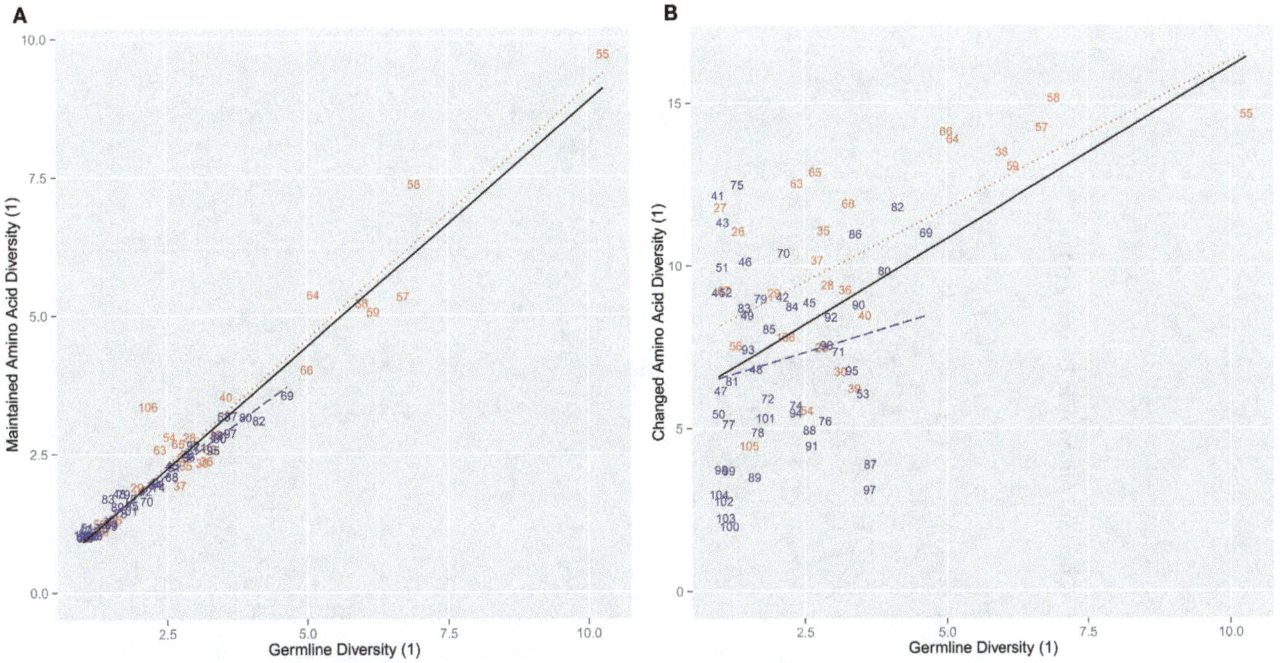

FIGURE 3 | The diversity of order 1 of the amino acids versus the diversity of order 1 for the germline sequences per position. (A) The diversity of order 1 amino acid usage in amino acids positions. We found a significant positive correlation ($r^2 = 0.947$, $\rho = 0.961$, $p = 7.52 \times 10^{-42}$). We also found positive correlations when the positions were split by region for FR ($r^2 = 0.970$, $\rho = 0.968$, $p = 3.67 \times 10^{-29}$) and CDR ($r^2 = 0.937$, $\rho = 0.880$, $p = 1.76 \times 10^{-6}$). **(B)** The diversity of order 1 amino acid usage of unique changed amino acids. We found a positive correlation ($r^2 = 0.284$, $\rho = 0.359$, $p = 1.70 \times 10^{-3}$). When splitting the positions by regions, however, FR did not correlate with the germline diversities ($r^2 = 0.0347$, $\rho = 0.132$, $p = 0.371$) while CDR did have a positive correlation ($r^2 = 0.419$, $\rho = 0.580$, $p = 2.27 \times 10^{-3}$).

Table 1 | Number of positions for each amino acid usage bias.

Category	Germline	Maintained	Changed
Hydrophobic	14	16: (13, 3, 0, 0, 0, 0)	7: (6, 1, 0, 0, 0, 0)
Weak hydrophobic	12	0: (0, 0, 0, 0, 0, 0)	8: (5, 2, 1, 0, 0, 0)
Neutral	19	27: (0, 6, 17, 4, 0, 0)	2: (0, 0, 2, 0, 0, 0)
Weak hydrophilic	13	3: (0, 0, 1, 2, 0, 0)	5: (0, 0, 1, 3, 1, 0)
Hydrophilic	11	10: (0, 0, 0, 1, 8, 1)	0: (0, 0, 0, 0, 0, 0)
Indeterminate	5	18: (1, 3, 1, 6, 3, 4)	52: (3, 9, 15, 10, 10, 5)

The numbers in parentheses after the colon signify the classifications of the respective positions in the germline repertoire: hydrophobic, weak hydrophobic, neutral, weak hydrophilic, hydrophilic, indeterminate.

biases (weak hydrophobic and weak hydrophilic) in the germline did not adhere as strictly to the same bias category but tend to have changed to one of the neighboring biases. Weak hydrophobic becomes either hydrophobic or neutral. Weak hydrophilic becomes either hydrophilic or neutral (**Table 1**). Looking now at the changed position we see that biases change much more (**Figure 4**). Most positions simply become indeterminate (i.e., have no clear bias). However, it is interesting to note that those positions that do have some bias exhibit either exactly the same bias as they have in the germline repertoire or one that is similar (**Table 1**).

4. DISCUSSION

The specificity of B cell and T cell receptors, while based on genes in the germline, is ultimately not of the germline template. Due to the imprecise nature of V(D)J recombination and, in B cells, somatic mutation, the final affinity of each immune receptor is neither inherited nor heritable. For this reason it is difficult to assess how germline diversity and its selection relate to selection during an immune response and specifically how they relate to the anticipated outcome of somatic mutation during an immune response. We have previously shown that the diversity of the germline V gene repertoire can be characterized by looking at the amino acid diversity of individual positions in the V gene sequence (12). The distribution of diversity is non-uniform with most, but not all highly diverse positions being found in the CDR. Furthermore, different positions show different biases toward the use of hydrophobic or hydrophilic amino acids (12). To contrast this picture of germline diversity with somatic changes, we have taken a published sample of the human peripheral B cell repertoire following influenza vaccination. We divided all of the sequences in this dataset into their respective clones and counted the number of times each position in the V gene sequence changed or maintained the amino acid found in the germline origin of its clone. By doing so, we could compare for each position how it contributes to repertoire diversity and its selection when changed from its germline and when it remained the same. Analyzing the maintained positions and their diversity allows us to ask to what extent clonal shift

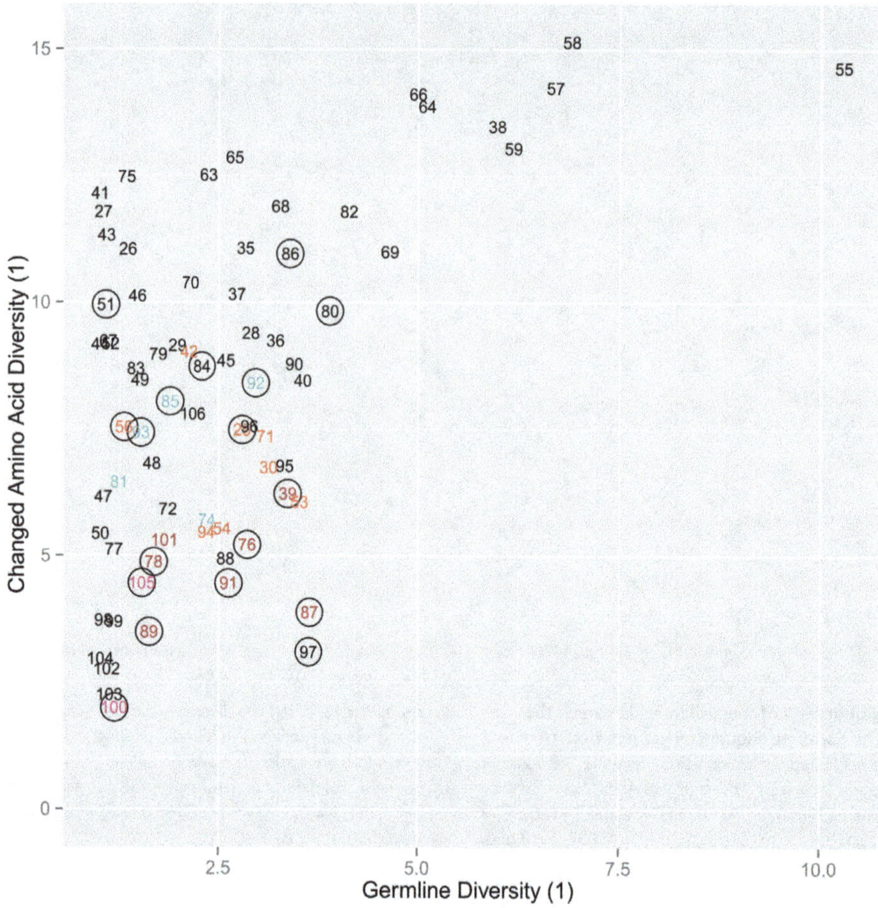

FIGURE 4 | Copy of Figure 3B annotated for amino acid usage bias. The coloring for the labels signifies whether that position is hydrophobic (red), weak hydrophobic (light red), neutral (purple), weak hydrophilic (light blue), hydrophilic (blue), or indeterminate (black), while a circle around the position indicates that the position shares the same hydrophobicity bias as the equivalent germline position. All amino acids are changed.

changes the diversity of the repertoire from the germline while analyzing the changed positions describes the effects of selection.

Starting with the maintained positions, we see that the germline diversity exhibited in the prototypic repertoire in the IMGT database, which does not assume any specific biases in V_H usage, is recapitulated in even the small and clonally shifted snapshot of the immune repertoire analyzed here. We find a significant linear correlation between germline diversity and that of positions with maintained amino acids (**Figure 3A**) and also clear conservation of amino acid usage biases (**Table 1**). Thus, despite the fact that we analyzed ~1000 clones per person (out of potentially 10^{11} clones) with a significant shift toward certain V_H genes, we still identify more or less exactly the same diversity and amino acid usage as described by the IMGT database. This suggests to us that clonal shift does not change the make up of amino acid diversity in the B cell repertoire. Furthermore, the existing IMGT database of human V genes represents this positional diversity well.

With regard to the changed positions, we find that there is a significant positive correlation between the level of diversity in the germline at a specific position and the survival of clones with changed amino acids at that position (**Figure 1**). Such a correlation suggests that there is a relationship between the tendency to diversify a position at the germline level over evolutionary time and the likelihood of mutants at those positions to survive somatic mutation and selection. We do not find any kind of correlation between germline diversity and synonymous mutation level (**Figure 2**). For this reason, while the exact observed levels of mutations and surviving mutants with specific amino acid changes may have also been influenced by biases in somatic mutation targeting or sequencing error, these explanations could not be the only reasons for our results. It would be unreasonable to think that mutation bias and sequencing error would only influence non-synonymous mutation rates and so it is thus quite clear that selection is causing this skew in mutant numbers. While assessing the exact rate of selection is beyond the scope of this paper, we can attempt to use these levels of synonymous mutations to estimate some ballpark level of expected non-synonymous mutations, which under neutral conditions we would assume to be three times as high. We can then see that all the positions with lowest germline diversity must be undergoing quite stringent negative selection and that once germline diversity gets higher (>2) there are some positions that appear to also be undergoing some positive selection. The positions with a germline diversity value >5 show rates of non-synonymous mutations 10- to 20-fold greater than synonymous mutations – a clear indicator of strong positive selection.

Another indication that specific positive selection has great influence on the final level of amino acid changed at each position is that the diversity of changed positions is much higher than the germline diversity at those positions (**Figure 3B**). Furthermore, in most cases their bias in usage is indeterminate (**Figure 4**). Thus, while the likelihood of survival is related to germline diversity, the specific change in amino acid that is needed to save the clone is also determined by the specific selection interactions in which that change was positively selected. However, it is worth noting that positions that can be classified (i.e., are not indeterminate) in the mutants all exhibit the same general amino acid bias as the germline repertoire (**Table 1**).

Taking all of these findings into account, we propose that germline diversity is a good indicator of the likelihood of survival following mutation but cannot account for the specific amino acid whose usage accounted for survival of a specific clone, although this usage can be approximated. This usage is based on the specific affinity maturation event and immune response that leads to the formation of the clone. We would further conclude that while CDR and FR do roughly segregate the sequence, a better measure of potential selection force is the specific germline diversity of each position. This is especially true for positions with <5 diversity in their germline amino acids. In such positions, while diversity indicates a range of possible levels of surviving mutants, there is no clear distinction between positions in the CDR and the FR. Indeed, the only reason one exists beyond diversity of 5 is that no FR positions have such high germline diversities.

ACKNOWLEDGMENTS

The authors would like to thank Deborah Dunn Walters for giving us access to her data from her experiments and with several interesting conversations on the meaning of its behavior. Funding: Gregory W. Schwartz is funded by the Graduate Assistance in Areas of National Need (GAANN) program.

REFERENCES

1. Alt FW, Baltimore D. Joining of immunoglobulin heavy chain gene segments: implications from a chromosome with evidence of three D-JH fusions. *Proc Natl Acad Sci U S A* (1982) **79**(13):4118–22. doi:10.1073/pnas.79.13.4118
2. Sakano H, Huppi K, Heinrich G, Tonegawa S. Sequences at the somatic recombination sites of immunoglobulin light-chain genes. *Nature* (1979) **280**(5720):288–94. doi:10.1038/280288a0
3. Weigert M, Gatmaitan L, Loh E, Schilling J, Hood L. Rearrangement of genetic information may produce immunoglobulin diversity. *Nature* (1978) **276**(5690):785–90. doi:10.1038/276785a0
4. Kim S, Davis M, Sinn E, Patten P, Hood L. Antibody diversity: somatic hypermutation of rearranged VH genes. *Cell* (1981) **27**(3):573–81. doi:10.1016/0092-8674(81)90399-8
5. Shlomchik MJ, Marshak-Rothstein A, Wolfowicz CB, Rothstein TL, Weigert MG. The role of clonal selection and somatic mutation in autoimmunity. *Nature* (1987) **328**(6133):805–11. doi:10.1038/328805a0
6. Caton AJ, Swartzentruber JR, Kuhl AL, Carding SR, Stark SE. Activation and negative selection of functionally distinct subsets of antibody-secreting cells by influenza hemagglutinin as a viral and a neo-self antigen. *J Exp Med* (1996) **183**(1):13–26. doi:10.1084/jem.183.1.13
7. Casola S, Otipoby KL, Alimzhanov M, Humme S, Uyttersprot N, Kutok JL, et al. B cell receptor signal strength determines b cell fate. *Nat Immunol* (2004) **5**(3):317–27. doi:10.1038/ni1036
8. Wu TT, Kabat EA. An analysis of the sequences of the variable regions of Bence Jones proteins and myeloma light chains and their implications for antibody complementarity. *J Exp Med* (1970) **132**(2):211–50. doi:10.1084/jem.132.2.211
9. Anderson SM, Khalil A, Uduman M, Hershberg U, Louzoun Y, Haberman AM, et al. Taking advantage: high-affinity B cells in the germinal center have lower death rates, but similar rates of division, compared to low-affinity cells. *J Immunol* (2009) **183**(11):7314–25. doi:10.4049/jimmunol.0902452
10. Hershberg U, Uduman M, Shlomchik MJ, Kleinstein SH. Improved methods for detecting selection by mutation analysis of Ig V region sequences. *Int Immunol* (2008) **20**(5):683–94. doi:10.1093/intimm/dxn045
11. Stewart JJ, Lee CY, Ibrahim S, Watts P, Shlomchik M, Weigert M, et al. A Shannon entropy analysis of immunoglobulin and t cell receptor. *Mol Immunol* (1997) **34**(15):1067–82. doi:10.1016/S0161-5890(97)00130-2
12. Schwartz GW, Hershberg U. Conserved variation: identifying patterns of stability and variability in BCR and TCR V genes with different diversity and richness metrics. *Phys Biol* (2013) **10**(3):1–10. doi:10.1088/1478-3975/10/3/035005
13. Lefranc M-P. IMGTÂ®, the international ImMunoGeneTics information systemÂ® for immunoinformatics. Methods for querying IMGTÂ® databases, tools and webresources in the context of immunoinformatics. *Mol Biotechnol* (2008) **40**(1):101–11. doi:10.1007/s12033-008-9062-7
14. Wu Y, Kipling D, Dunn-Walters DK. Age-related changes in human peripheral blood IGH repertoire following vaccination. *Front Immunol* (2012) **3**:193. doi:10.3389/fimmu.2012.00193
15. Heck LK, van Belle G, Simberloff D. Explicit calculation of the rarefaction diversity measurement and the determination of sufficient sample size. *Ecology* (1975) **56**(6):1459–61. doi:10.2307/1934716
16. Hershberg U, Shlomchik MJ. Differences in potential for amino acid change following mutation reveals distinct strategies for kappa and lambda light-chain variation. *Proc Natl Acad Sci U S A* (2006) **103**(43):15963–8. doi:10.1073/pnas.0607581103
17. Hill M. Diversity and evenness: a unifying notation and its consequences. *Ecology* (1973) **54**(2):427–32. doi:10.2307/1934352
18. Jost L. Entropy and diversity. *Oikos* (2006) **113**(2):363–75. doi:10.1111/j.2006.0030-1299.14714.x
19. Chothia C, Gelfand I, Kister A. Structural determinants in the sequences of immunoglobulin variable domain. *J Mol Biol* (1998) **278**(2):457–79. doi:10.1006/jmbi.1998.1653

15

The progression of cell death affects the rejection of allogeneic tumors in immune-competent mice – implications for cancer therapy

Ricardo A. Chaurio[1], Luis E. Muñoz[1]*, Christian Maueröder[1,2], Christina Janko[3], Thomas Harrer[1], Barbara G. Fürnrohr[4,5], Michael Niederweis[6], Rostyslav Bilyy[7], Georg Schett[1], Martin Herrmann[1†] and Christian Berens[2]*†

[1] Department of Internal Medicine 3, Friedrich-Alexander University of Erlangen-Nuremberg, Erlangen, Germany
[2] Department of Biology, Friedrich-Alexander University of Erlangen-Nuremberg, Erlangen, Germany
[3] Department of Otorhinolaryngology, Head and Neck Surgery, Section for Experimental Oncology and Nanomedicine (SEON), University Hospital Erlangen, Erlangen, Germany
[4] Division of Molecular Immunology, Department of Internal Medicine 3, Friedrich-Alexander University of Erlangen-Nuremberg, Erlangen, Germany
[5] Division of Biological Chemistry, Medical University Innsbruck, Innsbruck, Austria
[6] Department of Microbiology and Biochemistry, University of Alabama at Birmingham, Birmingham, AL, USA
[7] Institute of Cell Biology, National Academy of Sciences of Ukraine, Lviv, Ukraine

Edited by:
Fang-Ping Huang, Imperial College London, UK

Reviewed by:
Julian Pardo, Fundación Agencia Aragonesa para la Investigación y el Desarrollo, Spain
David Sancho, Centro Nacional de Investigaciones Cardiovasculares, Spain
Fang-Ping Huang, Imperial College London, UK

***Correspondence:**
Luis E. Muñoz, Department of Internal Medicine 3, Friedrich-Alexander-University Erlangen-Nuremberg, Ulmenweg 18, Erlangen 91054, Germany
e-mail: luis.munoz@uk-erlangen.de;
Christian Berens, Department of Biology, Friedrich-Alexander-University Erlangen-Nuremberg, Staudtstr. 5, Erlangen 91058 Germany
e-mail: christian.berens@fau.de

† Martin Herrmann and Christian Berens contributed equally to this work.

Large amounts of dead and dying cells are produced during cancer therapy and allograft rejection. Depending on the death pathway and stimuli involved, dying cells exhibit diverse features, resulting in defined physiological consequences for the host. It is not fully understood how dying and dead cells modulate the immune response of the host. To address this problem, different death stimuli were studied in B16F10 melanoma cells by regulated inducible transgene expression of the pro-apoptotic active forms of caspase-3 (revCasp-3), Bid (tBid), and the *Mycobacterium tuberculosis*-necrosis inducing toxin ($CpnT_{CTD}$). The immune outcome elicited for each death stimulus was assessed by evaluating the allograft rejection of melanoma tumors implanted subcutaneously in BALB/c mice immunized with dying cells. Expression of all proteins efficiently killed cells *in vitro* (>90%) and displayed distinctive morphological and physiological features as assessed by multiparametric flow cytometry analysis. BALB/c mice immunized with allogeneic dying melanoma cells expressing revCasp-3 or $CpnT_{CTD}$ showed strong rejection of the allogeneic challenge. In contrast, mice immunized with cells dying either after expression of tBid or irradiation with UVB did not, suggesting an immunologically silent cell death. Surprisingly, immunogenic cell death induced by expression of revCasp-3 or $CpnT_{CTD}$ correlated with elevated intracellular reactive oxygen species (ROS) levels at the time point of immunization. Conversely, early mitochondrial dysfunction induced by tBid expression or UVB irradiation accounted for the absence of intracellular ROS accumulation at the time point of immunization. Although ROS inhibition *in vitro* was not sufficient to abrogate the immunogenicity in our allo-immunization model, we suggest that the point of ROS generation and its intracellular accumulation may be an important factor for its role as damage associated molecular pattern in the development of allogeneic responses.

Keywords: immunogenicity, apoptosis, cancer, ROS, caspase-3, tBid, necrosis, DAMPs

INTRODUCTION

The appearance of cell death during disease therapy is a two-pronged sword. On one hand, cell death is desirable during cancer treatment in order to control malignant cell growth in the patient. On the other hand, excessive cell death should be avoided during transplantation to allow the grafted cells to survive in a foreign host. In the latter case, a considerable number of stresses are involved and several kinds of injuries may additionally compromise tissue viability, leading to progressive graft dysfunction and, eventually, also to graft loss (1, 2).

Furthermore, the mechanism and type of cell death might profoundly affect the reaction of the host toward surviving cells, making the situation more complex. Apoptosis, necrosis, autophagy, necroptosis, and other processes have been reported as common cell death mechanisms observed *in vivo* during therapies. However, how these types of cell death modulate interactions of the dying and dead cells with the immune system remains elusive. Depending on the immune response elicited, it is possible to distinguish between cases of cell death able to induce immunogenicity (immunogenic cell death) and those inducing immune tolerance or unresponsiveness (tolerogenic/silent cell death) (3, 4). Dying cells can exhibit completely different characteristics and immunological features. To understand these differences, an accurate characterization of the features, types, and phases of cell death is required.

The latter has become especially important in the context of diseases like cancer where conventional treatments (e.g., radiation and chemotherapy) are based on the massive induction of tumor cell death. In such cases, the immune system is prone to be decisive for tumor fate. Because the guidelines for drug screening in antineoplastic therapies require evaluation of human tumors xenotransplanted into immune-compromised mice (5), the role of the immune system has been neglected (6), making studies focused on the interplay between immune system and dying cells necessary. Modern anti-cancer therapies aim at inducing immunogenic cancer cell death. However, there are a plethora of factors involved in this process that have to be revisited and reassessed carefully. These include intrinsic cell immunogenicity, the nature of the initial death stimulus, the type of damage associated molecular patterns (DAMPs) released, the clearance capacity of the affected tissue for dying and dead cells, and the respective death pathway. Considering the large number of cytotoxic drugs currently used in the treatment of neoplastic diseases, much information is missing to predict the anti-tumor response of the host reliably.

In this study, we showed how different mechanisms and types of cell death, induced by different stimuli, affect the outcome of allogeneic tumor transplants in BALB/c immune-competent mice. Additionally, a morpho-physiological characterization of dying and dead cells, based on a multiparametric flow cytometry analysis, was assessed. A murine allograft model allowed evaluation of the immune response *in vivo*. The results of this work may have important implications for both cancer therapy and procedures for experimental allotransplantation.

MATERIALS AND METHODS

REAGENTS AND MOLECULAR PROBES

Dulbecco's modified eagle's medium (DMEM), fetal bovine serum (FBS), G418, penicillin–streptomycin, and glutamine were from Gibco-Invitrogen. Recombinant chicken annexin A5 (AxA5) was purchased from Responsif. The FluoroTag fluorescein isothiocyanate (FITC) conjugation kit was from Sigma-Aldrich, the 1,10,3,3,30,30-hexamethylindodicarbocyanine iodide dye [DiIC1(5)], Hoechst 33342, Lipofectamine™ 2000, and puromycin dihydrochloride were from Invitrogen. Propidium iodide (PI) was obtained from Amersham Biosciences. Doxycycline hydrochloride and trypsin–EDTA solution were purchased from Sigma-Aldrich. Ringer's solution was from Delta Select. The caspase3 inhibitor z-DEVD-fmk, the caspase-9 inhibitor Ac-LEHD-cmk, and the general caspase inhibitor z-VAD-fmk were purchased from Bachem.

CELL LINES AND CULTURE CONDITIONS

The C57BL/6 mouse-derived melanoma cell line B16F10 bearing the haplotype H2b was purchased from ATCC (#CRL-6475) and propagated in DMEM supplemented with 10% FBS and penicillin–streptomycin (D10) at 37°C in a 5% CO_2 atmosphere.

For the morpho-physiological characterization by flow cytometry, B16F10 cells were cultured in 24-well plates at 100,000 cells/2 ml D10 and harvested at the time points indicated. Harvesting was performed as follows: supernatants containing dead cells were harvested into polypropylene tubes. A trypsin–EDTA solution was added to the wells for 10–15 min at room temperature to detach the remaining adherent cells. Thus, detached cells were collected by adding D10 and combined with their corresponding supernatant fraction. Finally, cells were centrifuged at 300 g for 5 min, resuspended in 500 μl D10 medium.

GENERATION OF STABLE Tet-CONTROLLED SUICIDE CELL LINES

The cell lines B16F10-644, B16F10-tBid, and B16F10-revCasp-3 have been described (7). The parental cell line B16F10-644 was transfected with the *Ahd*I-linearized plasmid pWHE655TREtight-$CpnT_{CTD}$, carrying the C-terminal domain of the channel protein with necrosis inducing toxin ($CpnT_{CTD}$) characterized in *Mycobacterium tuberculosis* (8) (**Figures 1A–C**), and stable transfectants were selected by limited dilution in the presence of 1500 μg/ml G418. Individual subclones were cultured in 48-well plates and tested for cell death with AxA5/PI staining by FACS after 24 h of doxycycline (1 μg/ml) addition. One out of several positive clones was chosen for further experiments and named B16F10-$CpnT_{CTD}$.

MULTI-PARAMETER CLASSIFICATION OF CELL DEATH BY FLOW CYTOMETRY

The cell death characterization method analyzing size, granularity, PS exposure, plasma membrane integrity, mitochondrial membrane potential, and DNA content in a one-tube-measurement has been thoroughly described elsewhere (9). This method classifies eight different phases of cell death. Briefly, the harvested cells were incubated for 30 min at room temperature with 400 μl of freshly prepared 4-color staining solution [1.8 μg/ml AxA5-FITC, 100 ng/ml PI, 10 nM DiIC1(5), 1 ng/ml Hoechst 33342] in Ringer's solution and subsequently analyzed. Flow cytometry was performed with a Gallios cytofluorometer (Beckman Coulter, Fullerton, CA, USA). Excitation of FITC and PI was at 488 nm, the FITC fluorescence was detected with the FL1 sensor (525/38 nm BP), the PI fluorescence with the FL3 sensor (620/30 nm BP), the DiIC1(5) fluorescence was excited at 638 nm and detected with the FL6 sensor (675/20 nm BP), and the Hoechst 33342 fluorescence was excited at 405 nm and detected with the FL9 sensor (430/40 nm BP). Electronic compensation was applied to reduce bleed-through fluorescence. Data analysis was performed with Kaluza software version 2.0 (Beckman Coulter, Fullerton, CA, USA). Cells were classified according to their location in the forward scatter (FSc; size) vs. side scatter (SSc; granularity) dot plot and their staining patterns in the FL1 vs. FL3 and FL6 vs. FL9 dot plots (**Figure 2A**).

CELL DEATH INDUCTION

Cell death was induced by (1) doxycycline *in vitro* (5–10 μg/ml) for expression of the cell death inducing proteins tBid, revCasp-3, and $CpnT_{CTD}$. (2) Irradiation with ultraviolet light type B (UVB) at 1.5 mJ/cm^2/s. (3) By heat shock (56°C for 30 min).

MEASUREMENT OF INTRACELLULAR REACTIVE OXYGEN SPECIES

Intracellular reactive oxygen species (ROS) levels were assessed using the redox-sensitive dye 2,7-dichlorofluorescein diacetate (C-DCFH-DA). At the time points indicated, dying B16F10 cells were harvested, incubated for 30 min with C-DCFH-DA (10 μM) at 37°C in protein-free medium (D0) in the dark. Cells were then

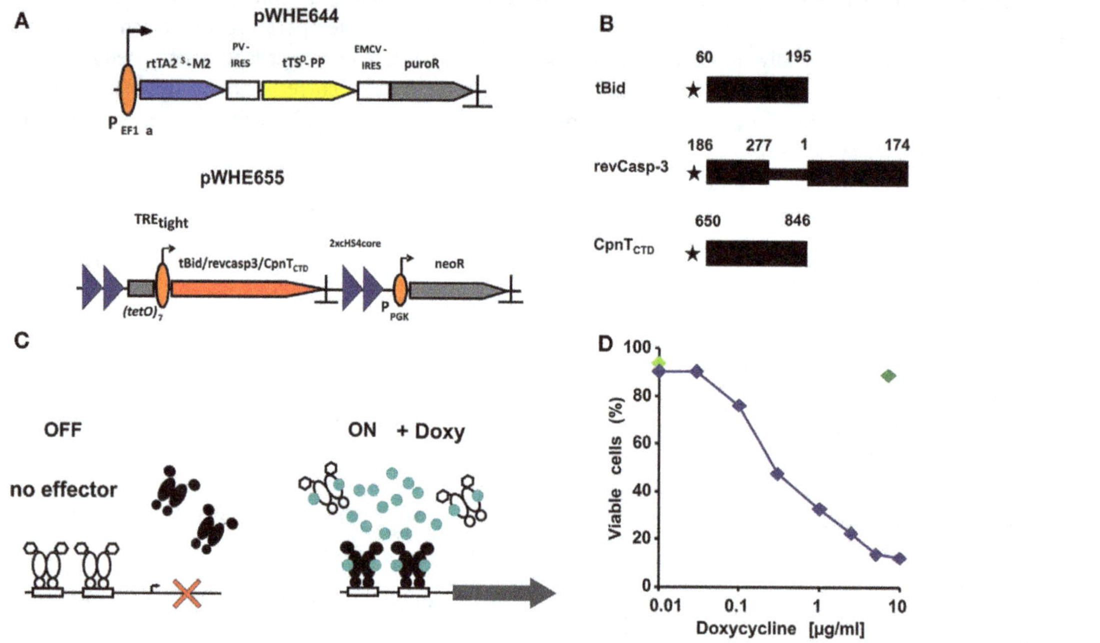

FIGURE 1 | Conditional expression of death inducing proteins. **(A)** Schematic overview of the constructs used to establish the regulatory system. The vector pWHE644 represents the regulator construct. A human EF1α promoter constitutively transcribes a tricistronic mRNA. This mRNA contains the reverse transactivator rtTA2^{S}-M2 (blue arrow), the transsilencer tTS^{D}-PP (yellow arrow), and a selection marker (puromycin resistance; gray arrow). Translation of the latter two genes is mediated by internal ribosome entry sites (IRES; open boxes) from polio-virus (PV) and encephalomyocarditis-virus (EMCV). The vector pWHE655 contains the response unit used for stable transfections. It features the target gene (red arrow) driven by the Tet-responsive promoter TRE$_{tight}$ (open box, broken arrow) and flanked by two repeats each of a 250 bp sequence from the chicken HS4 insulator (blue triangles). A murine phosphoglycerate kinase 1 promoter (PGK; broken arrow) drives expression of a gene mediating G418-resistance. PolyA sites in all vectors are marked by a "⊥." **(B)** Schematic representation of the cytotoxic test proteins. The residues that border the active domains expressed in the experiment are indicated above their respective closed box. A methionine added to allow translation is represented by a star. **(C)** Schematic overview of the regulatory system. In the OFF-State, a transsilencer (white) binds to the minimal promoter (open boxes, broken arrow) and actively suppresses transcription (cross). In the ON-State, doxycycline (blue circles) binds to both transsilencer and reverse transactivator (black). The former dissociates from, the latter binds to the minimal promoter and activates transcription (gray arrow). **(D)** Response of the regulatory system to different doxycycline concentrations. The B16F10-tBid transfected cell line was incubated for 24 h with various concentrations of doxycycline and mortality was measured, shown for one representative experiment out of three performed. Concentrations between 5 and 10 µg/ml showed the highest extent of cell death. An additional control at 10 µg/ml Doxy with the parental stably transfected cell line B16F10-644 was included to discard doxycycline toxicity at higher concentrations as cause of cell death (dark green diamond). Cell viability at time point "0" is shown as light green diamond.

washed with D10 by centrifugation, co-stained with PI, and analyzed by flow cytometry. Only PI-negative cells were analyzed and ROS levels were presented as the mean fluorescence intensity in the FL1 channel (MFI-FL1). The anti-oxidants *N*-acetylcysteine (NAC) and 2-(2,2,6,6-Tetramethylpiperidin-1-oxyl-4-ylamino)-2-oxoethyl) triphenylphosphonium chloride (mitoTEMPO) were used at 100 µM as indicated.

ALLOGENEIC TUMOR GROWTH MODEL AND IMMUNIZATIONS

The allogeneic tumor growth model consisted of the host mouse (BALB/c, MHC haplotype H2d) and B16F10 melanoma cells derived from C57BL/6 mice (MHC haplotype H2b). Specified amounts of viable cells or dead/dying cells were subcutaneously (s.c.) implanted in 500 µl Ringer's solution in the right flank using a syringe with a 25 G needle. The growth of solid melanoma tumors was registered by direct measurement of width, height, and depth of the black subcutaneous protuberance with a caliper for up to a maximum of 40 days. In accordance with the guidelines for the welfare of animals in experimental neoplasia, the animal was sacrificed if the mouse tumor volume exceeded more than 10% of the host's body weight.

In order to evaluate the immune response against implanted cells, mice were challenged s.c. with 2 million viable cells in the opposite flank, after immunization as indicated. The use of the syngeneic host (C57BL/6) as recipient of B16F10 melanoma cell lines was ruled out because of the aggressiveness of the B16F10 cells, which may cause discomfort and premature death of the animal. Mice were purchased from Charles River Laboratories International, Inc., and kept on a standard diet with drinking water available *ad libitum*. Experiments were conducted according to the European principles and local guidelines for care and use of laboratory animals at the Institute of Cell Biology, National Academy of Sciences of Ukraine, Lviv (10–12).

STATISTICAL ANALYSIS

The software package GraphPad Prism 5.0 was used for graphics and statistical tests. For comparisons between control and experimental groups, Mann–Whitney *U* test or two way ANOVA tests

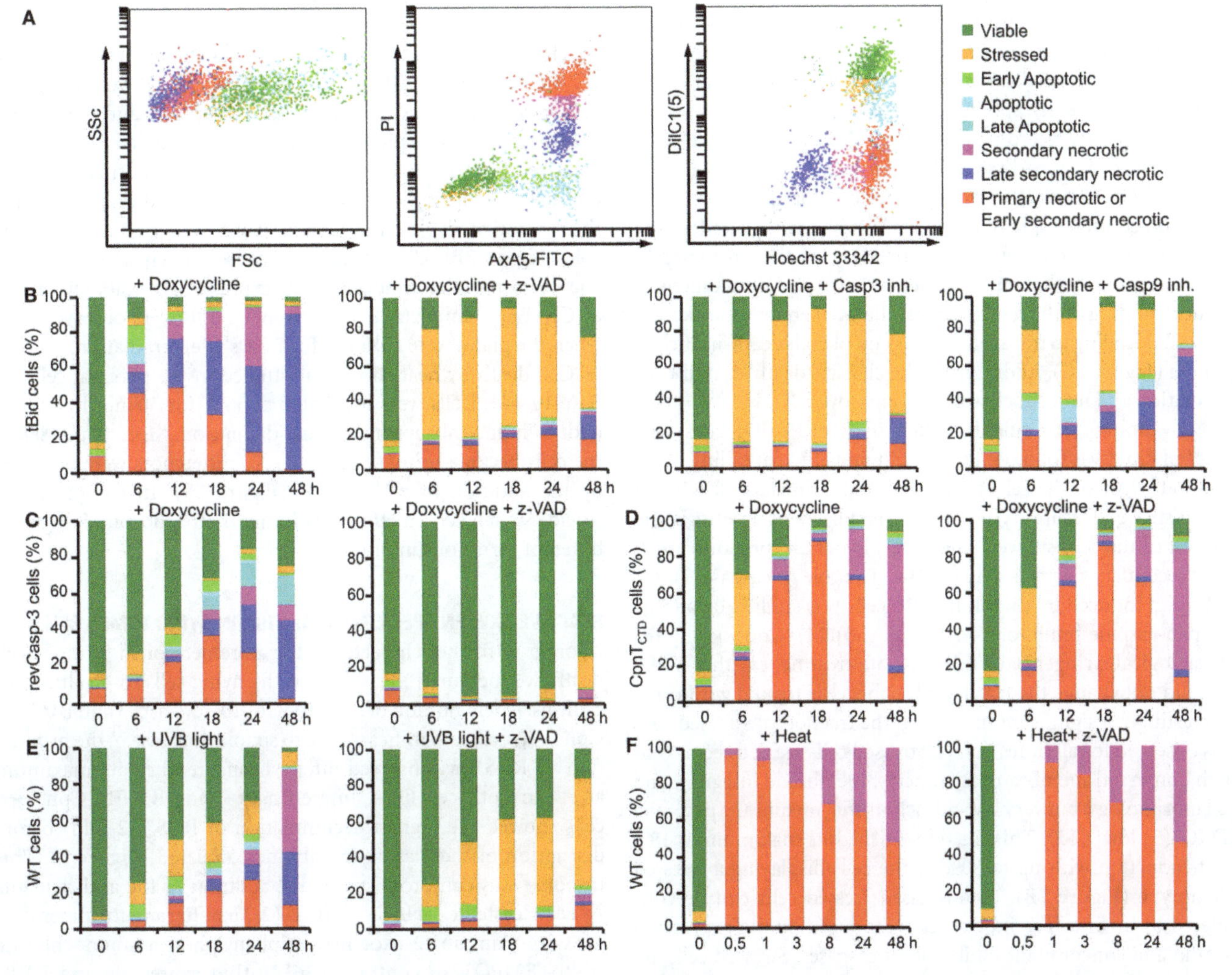

FIGURE 2 | Six parameter classification by flow cytometry of the cell death phenotype of dying and dead B16F10 cells. Cell death analysis is based on morphological features (FSc and SSc), on the exposure of PS (annexin A5-FITC) and plasma membrane ion selectivity (PI), on the mitochondrial membrane potential [DiIC1(5)] and on nuclear DNA content (Hoechst 33342) detected by flow cytometry. Note: after proper gating, up to eight physiologically different subpopulations can be recorded. Dot plots exemplarily show B16F10-revCasp-3 cells after 18 h of doxycycline (5 μg/ml) treatment **(A)**. Rapid cell death occurred after 6 h in tBid-expressing cells and more than 95% cell death was observed after 24 h. In the presence of various caspase inhibitors [z-VAD-fmk, z-DEVD-fmk (caspase-3 inhibitor) and Ac-LEHD-cmk (caspase-9 inhibitor); all 50 μM], a significant increase in the stressed cell fraction displaying low-mitochondrial potential was observed **(B)**. Expression of revCasp-3 in B16F10 cells induced cell death after 24 h in more than 80% of the cells. z-VAD-fmk (50 μM) completely inhibited doxycycline-driven apoptosis. Note: stressed cells do not arise in this type of cell death induction **(C)**. Expression of CpnT$_{CTD}$ induced cell death in more than 90% of the cells after 18 h. Note: primary necrosis was the most common type of cell death observed and death occurred independently of caspase activity (50 μM z-VAD-fmk) **(D)**. Lethal UVB irradiation (240 mJ/cm^2) of parental B16F10 cells causes a rather slow progressing kind of cell death. Note: in the presence of z-VAD-fmk (50 μM), a significant increase of the stressed cell fraction displaying low-mitochondrial potential was observed **(E)**. Heat shock (56°C, 30 min) caused immediate necrosis in 100% of cells independent of caspase activity **(F)**. Displayed are the mean values from three independent experiments of relative percentages of each cell phenotype during 48 h of culture **(B–F)**.

were employed as appropriate. Statistical significance was assumed if $p < 0.05$.

RESULTS

STABLE Tet-CONTROLLED MOUSE MELANOMA B16F10 SUICIDE CELL LINES

Subcloned transfected mouse melanoma B16F10 cell lines were tested for the response of the regulatory system to different doxycycline (doxy) concentrations after 24 h. Mortality rates were calculated by annexin A5/PI staining and flow cytometry. Concentrations around 10 μg/ml doxy showed the highest degree of cell death (**Figure 1D**).

CELL DEATH INDUCED BY EXPRESSION OF CYTOTOXIC PROTEINS IN B16F10 CELLS AND MORPHO-PHYSIOLOGICAL CLASSIFICATION OF DEAD AND DYING TUMOR CELLS BY FLOW CYTOMETRY

Since dying cells may exhibit various biological features that modulate the immune response, it is necessary to accurately characterize the phenotypes and phases of cell death. Employing a six parameter protocol to characterize the morphological and physiological features of dying and dead cells, we identified eight different states of cell death in B16F10 melanoma cells: (1) viable; (2) stressed; (3) early apoptosis; (4) apoptosis; (5) late apoptosis; (6) secondary necrosis; (7) late secondary necrosis; and (8) primary necrosis or early secondary necrosis (**Figure 2A**) (9, 13). This method allows us to closely describe biological features of death in cell lines expressing cytotoxic proteins. In our test system, doxycycline relieves active repression of the promoter by the tetracycline-dependent transsilencer (tTS) and simultaneously induces binding of the reverse tetracycline-dependent transactivator (rtTA) leading to transgene expression of each death-inducing-protein (**Figure 1C**). Additionally, the classical death stimuli UVB irradiation and heat shock were also employed.

Activation of the suicide switch in B16F10-tBid cells with 5 μg/ml doxy was followed by very fast and efficient killing. After 6 h, up to 90% of the cells were dead. Approximately 30% of the cells displayed features typical for initial phases of apoptosis and the rest of the cells showed a necrotic phenotype, predominantly early secondary necrosis (**Figure 2B**). The role of caspases in the cell death induced by tBid in B16F10 cells was studied by adding the pan-caspase inhibitor z-VAD-fmk (50 μM). Considering the physiological stringency of this method, treatment with z-VAD-fmk did not change the fraction of viable cells treated with doxy. Interestingly, a significant increase in the fraction of stressed cells was observed for all times points. Stressed cells are defined as cells with conserved membrane asymmetry, membrane integrity, and cell morphology, but very low-mitochondrial membrane potential [DiIC1(5) low] (13). This fraction reached its maximum at 18 h post-induction with up to 80% of the cells displaying a stressed phenotype (**Figure 2B**). In this case, stressed cells can be considered to be in a "pre-mortal" state, induced by the expression of tBid and concomitant inhibition of caspases. Stressed cells are detected efficiently by the six parameter method described above. tBid death kinetics in the presence of the more specific caspase-3 and caspase-9 inhibitors were similar to those observed in the presence of z-VAD-fmk, and showed comparable amounts of dead cells (**Figure 2B**).

Expression of revCasp-3 in B16F10 cells induced cell death after 24 h, albeit more slowly than tBid, with more than 80% of the cells displaying dead phenotypes (**Figure 2C**). Early stages of apoptosis were observed at 12 and 18 h, while late apoptotic and secondary necrotic stages were more predominant at 24 and 48 h. As expected, cell death by expression of revCasp-3 was completely inhibited in the presence of z-VAD-fmk (**Figure 2C**).

Expression of the necrosis inducing protein $CpnT_{CTD}$ in B16F10 cells led to cell death after 18 h with more than 80% of the cells displaying features of primary necrosis (**Figure 2D**). Early stages of apoptosis were not detected by the expression of this protein. In contrast to pro-apoptotic proteins, z-VAD-fmk did not affect the death phenotype induced by $CpnT_{CTD}$, suggesting a caspase-independent type of cell death (**Figure 2D**).

It is important to note that cell death induced by doxycycline-controlled expression of the proteins tBid, revCasp-3, and $CpnT_{CTD}$ did not kill all cells – some cells may have failed to respond to doxy. In agreement with this assumption, long-term culture of doxy-treated cells resulted in confluent growth of the surviving non-responder cells.

The parental cell line B16F10-644 was lethally irradiated with UVB (240 mJ/cm^2). After 6 h, some stressed and early apoptotic cells were observed. After 12 h, stressed, apoptotic, and some forms of necrotic cells were present. Secondary necrotic cells increasingly appeared from 24 to 48 h. The presence of z-VAD-fmk produced an important increase in the fraction of stressed cells preserving the fraction of viable cells, as was also observed for cells expressing tBid (**Figure 2E**). UVB irradiation caused much slower death in comparison to that induced by the expression of tBid, revCasp-3, or $CpnT_{CTD}$. Importantly, no surviving cells were observed even when the plates were cultured for 7 days after irradiation.

Cell death by heat shock was studied in the parental cell line B16F10-644. Cells were incubated at 56°C for 30 min in a water bath to induce abrupt membrane disruption. More than 98% of the cells became primary necrotic. No differences were observed by the addition of z-VAD-fmk (**Figure 2F**). In summary, the suicide switch system efficiently induced morpho-physiologically different forms of tumor cell death.

REACTIVE OXYGEN SPECIES PRODUCTION IN DYING TUMOR CELLS

In order to further characterize the aforementioned forms of cell death, we measured the ability of the dying cells to produce free radicals. After addition of doxy to B16F10-revCasp-3 and B16F10-$CpnT_{CTD}$ cells, a significant, five to sixfold, increase in the production of ROS was observed after 6 h and reached its maximum at 9 h in both cell lines. Interestingly, dying B16F10-$CpnT_{CTD}$ cells showed the highest accumulation of ROS (12-fold) before disruption of the plasma membranes occurred (**Figure 3**). This response was compromised by the addition of the anti-oxidants *N*-acetylcysteine (NAC) and 2-(2,2,6,6-Tetramethylpiperidin-1-oxyl-4-ylamino)-2-oxoethyl) triphenylphosphonium chloride (mitoTEMPO). In contrast, B16F10-tBid expressing and UVB-irradiated dying cells did not produce significant amounts of ROS up to 12 h after death induction.

GROWTH OF B16F10 CELLS IN THE ALLOGENEIC BALB/C HOST AND CONCOMITANT IMMUNITY

Tumor growth of the B16F10 cells was studied in BALB/c mice by implanting four million viable parental B16F10-644 cells s.c. into their right flanks (viability >90%). Five days later, black solid tumors were observed beneath the shaved skin. These tumors reached their maximum size between days 12 and 15 and spontaneously regressed thereafter (**Figure 4A**). In most cases, small tumors (5–10 mm^3) persisted subcutaneously in the animal showing no further change in size. Tumor recurrence was verified by keeping mice under observation for more than 2 months; no further tumor growth was seen during this time period. Since the tumors are growing in allogeneic hosts, we regard this as allograft rejection. Metastases were never observed in any organ.

B16F10 is a poorly immunogenic cell line, not able to generate concomitant immunity in its syngeneic host. Accordingly, C57BL/6 mice bearing a progressive tumor are not able to elicit a protective immune response (14). In order to evaluate the immunity in this allogeneic model, mice were implanted s.c. as follows:

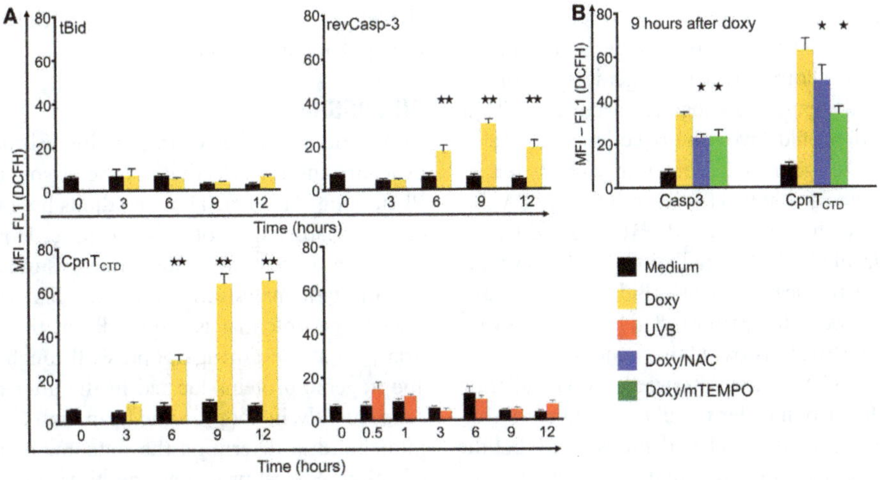

FIGURE 3 | Reactive oxygen species (ROS) production by dying B16F10 melanoma cells. Cells were induced to die by conditional expression of the death proteins tBid, revCasp-3, and $CpnT_{CTD}$ or by UVB irradiation, stained with the ROS sensor DCFH and with PI and analyzed by flow cytometry **(A)**. Inhibition of ROS production was performed by treatment with *N*-acetyl-cysteine (NAC) or mitoTEMPO, 100 μM, respectively, and recorded at 9 h after death induction **(B)**. Mean and SEM values of the mean fluorescence intensities of FL1 in viable cells (PI-negative) are displayed for different time points. At least three independent experiments were performed (Two and one stars indicate statistical significance at the $p < 0.001$ and $p < 0.05$ levels, respectively).

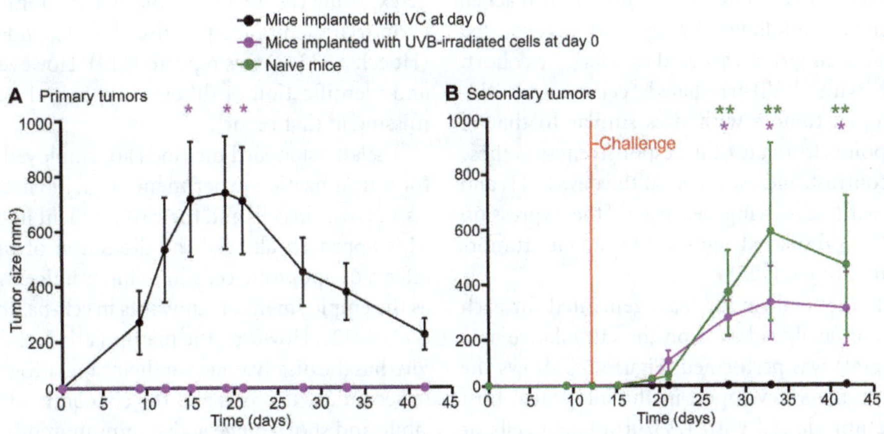

FIGURE 4 | Growth of B16F10 melanoma cells in the allogeneic host and concomitant immunity. Four million viable B16F10 cells (VC) were implanted s.c. in the right flank of BALB/c mice. Mice developed tumors reaching their maximum size after 2–3 weeks, followed by rejection [**(A)**, black line]. Mice implanted with 4 million UVB-irradiated cells did not develop primary tumors [**(A)**, purple line]. After challenge with 2 million viable cells s.c. on the left flank, those mice bearing primary tumors did not develop secondary tumors [**(B)**, black line], while mice primarily inoculated with irradiated cells developed tumors similar to those of the naïve group [**(B)**, purple and green lines, respectively]. Mean values ($n = 8$) and the SEM are displayed. Time points showing statistical significance when compared to the group of mice implanted with VC are highlighted. Two stars and one star indicate statistical significance at the $p < 0.01$ and $p < 0.05$ levels, respectively. The two way ANOVA test corrected by Bonferroni was applied in this experiment.

one group was implanted with 4 million viable cells, the second with lethally UVB-irradiated cells. A third group was injected with Ringer solution (naïve group). After 12 days, all groups were challenged s.c. with 2 million viable cells in the opposite flank. The black line in **Figure 4A** shows growth and rejection of primary tumors derived from 4 million viable cells. Mice implanted with UVB-irradiated cells showed no growth of primary tumors (**Figure 4A**, purple line $p < 0.05$ compared to the black line). After challenge, all mice carrying primary tumors rejected secondary tumors (**Figure 4B**, black line). In contrast, mice that had received UVB-irradiated cells supported the growth of secondary tumors, as the naïve group did (**Figure 4B**, purple $p < 0.05$ and green $p < 0.01$ lines compared to the black line). This observation suggests the existence of tumor related immunity in the allogeneic model. We propose to use this system for the evaluation of host immunity after immunization with dead and dying cells.

ALLOGENEIC RESPONSE ELICITED BY DYING AND DEAD CELLS

The allogeneic implantation of dead and dying tumor cells in an immune-competent host allows us to evaluate whether the mechanism of cell death induces a silent, a tolerogenic, or an immunogenic cell death by recording the response after a standardized challenge. A silent type of cell death would not affect the growth of the allotumor, a tolerogenic type of cell death would overcome the expected allograft rejection, while an immunogenic cell death would favor the rejection of the allotumor. The host response against each previously characterized form of cell death was assessed in 9–11-week-old female BALB/c (WT) mice immunized with dying/dead B16F10 cells induced to die by the following stimuli: (1) UVB irradiation; (2) doxycycline-controlled expression of the death proteins tBid, revCasp-3, and $CpnT_{CTD}$; and (3) heat shock. Stably transfected B16F10 cells were induced to die by adding 10 μg/ml doxy to the tissue culture dishes (150 cm^2) at 37°C and 5% CO_2 for 5 h. Afterward, UVB irradiation (240 mJ/cm^2) was performed in order to kill the remaining non-responsive cells. Previous experiments had demonstrated that the additional UVB irradiation at this time point neither altered the expression level of the death-inducing proteins nor the kinetics of the specific death phenotype (Figure S1 in Supplementary Material). Sixteen million dying/dead cells were injected s.c. in the right flank as single immunization dose at day 0. After 10 days, mice were challenged in the left flank with 2 million viable cells of the parental cell line B16F10-644. Tumor growth was recorded at days 5, 8, 11, 14, 20, and 30 after challenge (**Figure 5A**). Viable cells implanted in naïve BALB/c mice generated tumors that reached their maximal size after 2 weeks followed by regression, as expected (**Figure 5B**, black lines). This group was used as reference cohort.

Mice immunized with UVB-irradiated cells and tBid-expressing cells developed tumors with sizes similar to that of the naïve group. This points to a state of unresponsiveness in these mice (**Figure 5B**). In contrast, and especially at the days 8, 11, and 14, mice immunized with cells dying because of the expression of revCasp-3 or $CpnT_{CTD}$ displayed significantly smaller tumors than naïve mice (**Figure 5B**; $p < 0.05$).

In order to estimate the total tumor mass generated for each immunization cohort, an analysis based on the cumulative area under the curve (integral) was performed. **Figure 5C** shows the total amount of tumor mass developed in the allogeneic host for each cohort. Mice immunized with UVB-irradiated cells or with cells that express tBid developed similar tumor masses. Conversely, mice immunized with dying/dead cells because of revCasp-3 and $CpnT_{CTD}$ expression developed significantly smaller tumor masses (**Figure 5C**). Based on these observations, we considered UVB irradiation and over-expression of tBid as silent or tolerogenic forms of cell death. Accordingly, over-expression of revCasp-3 and $CpnT_{CTD}$ induced immunogenic cell death. At best, only a weak immunogenic response was elicited by cells treated with heat shock reflecting that the rapid induction of necrosis by heat shock has the inevitable disadvantage of diffusion of danger signals to the medium. One major advantage of doxy-controlled induction of cell death, in particular necrotic cell death, is the achievement of a necrotic phenotype without physical interaction with the cells.

Interestingly, those forms of death showing significant ROS production upon *in vitro* stimulation died in an immunogenic fashion (**Figure 5D**). To more closely address the role of ROS production in the development of allo-responses, we treated ROS-producing $CpnT_{CTD}$-expressing dead and dying cells with the anti-oxidant NAC before immunization. This treatment resulted in the amelioration of the allo-response against the challenge; however, it was not statistically significant (Figure S2 in Supplementary Material).

DISCUSSION

Conventional studies characterizing cell death are based on PS exposure and ion selectivity of the plasma membrane (AxA5 and PI staining) (15–17). These methods have traditionally classified cells as viable, apoptotic, or necrotic. However, because of the important role of the mitochondria as modulator of cell death, a concomitant analysis that monitors changes in the mitochondrial membrane potential is required. On the one hand, mitochondria play a role during apoptosis through the release of several apoptogenic proteins located in the inter-membrane space and, consequently, in apoptosome formation (18). On the other hand, mitochondria determine the outcome of many ATP-dependent cell physiological processes and, thus, are important for necrotic cell death. In this work, we used a modified staining and cytofluorometry protocol for a more detailed analysis of tumor cell death induced by various stimuli. Its major advantage is the possibility to classify at least eight different stages of cell death (viable, stressed, early/medium/late apoptosis, early/late secondary necrosis, primary necrosis) in a fast and reliable one-tube assay. A similar method employing a four-color staining for evaluation of PS exposure (AxA5-FITC), plasma membrane integrity (PI), mitochondrial membrane potential (JC-1), and nuclear DNA content (Hoechst 33342) was reported (19). However, a clear classification and identification of different types and stages of cell death was missing in that report.

Usually, standard methods are employed to generate dead cells for immunization experiments, e.g., *in vitro* induction of apoptosis/necrosis in cells and their subsequent injection into the mouse. This approach allowed the dissection of important modulatory effects of apoptotic cells in living multicellular organisms, as well as the employment of adjuvants in cell-based immunization models (20–22). However, the manipulation of dying and dead cells *ex vivo* has the disadvantage of their rapid progression from apoptosis to secondary necrosis and the concomitant decay and dilution of labile and short-range active immunomodulatory signals, respectively. In order to avoid the aforementioned limitations, we have established a conditional doxycycline-dependent expression system able to trigger various types of tumor cell death. Vectors harboring cDNAs encoding for tBid, revCasp-3, and $CpnT_{CTD}$ were stably transfected into B16F10 melanoma cells.

tBid is a major pro-apoptotic protein activated in both extrinsic and intrinsic pathways and is an important connector between these canonical apoptosis pathways. tBid translocates to the mitochondria promoting mitochondrial outer membrane permeabilization (MOMP), a process involving self-assembly of activated BAX and BAK into transmembrane pores, which can be inhibited by anti-apoptotic BCL2 family proteins (23–25). Moreover, tBid accumulation determines the timing of MOMP (26). In addition to cytochrome c, tBid induces the release of further mitochondrial death effectors that promote caspase-independent apoptosis and induce mitochondrial remodeling. All these processes result in loss of the mitochondrial membrane potential, blocking of ATP synthesis and, consequently, loss of function of ATP-dependent transporters.

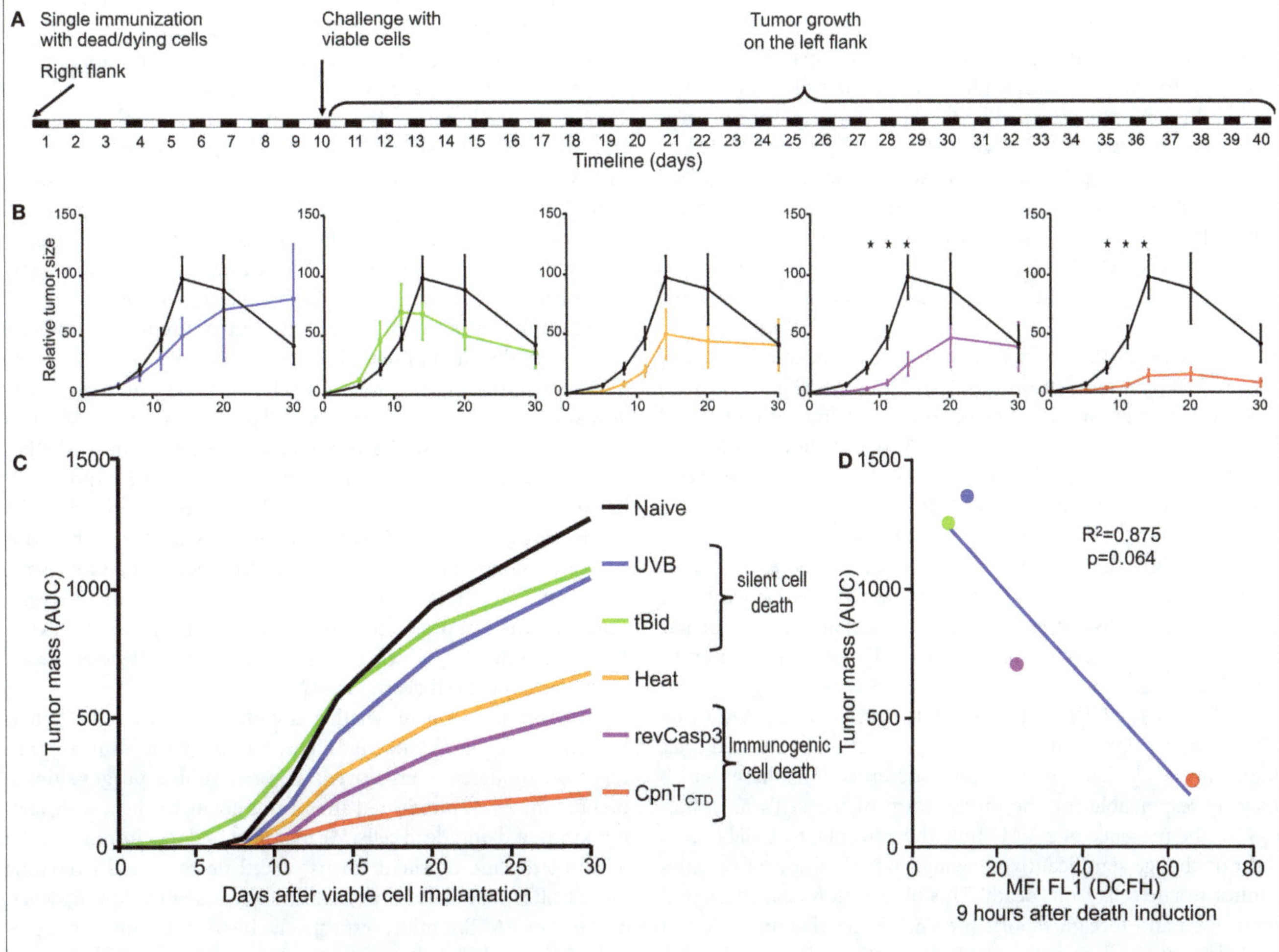

FIGURE 5 | Immune response against dead or dying allogeneic tumor cells. BALB/c mice ($n=5$) were immunized in the right flank s.c. (single dose) with B16F10 dying/dead cells. After 10 days, mice were challenged s.c. in the left flank with 2 million viable cells of the parental cell line B16F10-644. Tumor growth was monitored for 30 further days **(A)**. Cell death was induced by UVB irradiation; heat shock; doxycycline-controlled expression of death proteins tBid, revCasp-3, and $CpnT_{CTD}$. Displayed are the mean values ($n=5$) of relative tumor volumes and SEM [**(B)**, $*p < 0.05$ after Mann–Whitney U test] and the integral of tumor size [**(C)**, total tumor mass]. Inverse association between ROS production and total tumor mass developed in the allogeneic host **(D)**.

Over-expression of tBid can be considered to represent a harsh stimulus that quickly drives cells toward advanced stages of the apoptotic process with metabolic collapse leading to an early loss of plasma membrane integrity and rupture. We have defined this particular state of early loss of plasma membrane integrity as early secondary necrosis. It clearly differs from primary necrosis because of its susceptibility to inhibition by caspase inhibitors. Similar stimuli have already been reported to induce necrosis (27–29). This new cell death state may have particular relevance under clinical conditions like treatment with chemotherapy in cancer. Our cell death classification method allowed the identification of a further new stage in the process of dying, which we propose to refer to as *stressed* cells. The latter were observed especially when the over-expression of tBid was induced in the presence of z-VAD-fmk. Stressed cells show low-mitochondrial potential, suggesting the presence of MOMP and severe damage to the mitochondrial membranes in the absence of any further signs of apoptosis. The pan-caspase inhibitor z-VAD-fmk efficiently blocks certain types of apoptosis. In consequence, the common hallmarks of the execution phase of apoptosis, like PS exposure, cell shrinkage, and DNA fragmentation are inhibited. The cells appear viable although they are actually dead because of severe damage of the mitochondrial membranes after over-expression of tBid, which directly activates the mitochondrial pathway.

Compared to the expression of tBid, melanoma cells dying after the expression of revCasp-3 showed slower cell death kinetics. Twenty four hours of expression of revCasp-3 were required to reach a similar degree of cell death. Caspase-3 is the major caspase activated during the execution phase of apoptosis (30). However, expression of revCasp-3 does not directly act on the mitochondria to induce MOMP. Caspase-3 needs to cleave sufficient MOMP-inducing substrates like Bid to tBid before MOMP and cell death can occur by a feed-forward amplification loop (31). Additionally, caspase-3 can then enter the mitochondria and cleave specific substrates of the electron transfer chain, which will ultimately result in mitochondrial uncoupling and loss of membrane potential.

Addition of z-VAD-fmk to revCasp-3 expressing cells inhibited up to 95% of the cell death occurring (more than 90% viable cells). These results demonstrate that, after blocking caspases, damage to mitochondria and to cell morphology and physiology was effectively inhibited, as confirmed by the lack of appearance of large numbers of stressed cells in **Figure 2C**.

Induction of apoptosis by UVB irradiation has been recognized to be a complex process involving a variety of independent pathways. There are at least two major mechanisms involved in apoptosis induced by UVB: (1) DNA damage; UVB induces two types of lesions in chromosomal DNA, photoproducts, and cyclobutane pyrimidine dimers (CPD), the latter being the predominant ones (32). (2) Cell death receptor activation; UVB is able to directly activate cell surface receptors (i.e., CD95/Fas and TNF receptor-1) by inducing receptor trimerization and clustering without ligand interaction (33–35). In our study, B16F10 melanoma cells were lethally irradiated with 240 mJ/cm^2 UVB applied as a single dose. Lower doses failed to completely kill the cells (data not shown). In the 24 h period following irradiation, we observed slow cell death kinetics mainly characterized by the presence of stressed (mitochondrial damage) and early secondary necrotic cells (membrane disruption and DNA preservation). Substantial amounts of late apoptotic and late secondary necrotic cells were only observed after 48 h.

Cells dying by UVB irradiation in the presence of z-VAD-fmk also showed a significant increase in the fraction of stressed cells, indicating a blockade of the apoptotic execution phase, which may be responsible for the preservation of the cell's morphology. In the presence of z-VAD-fmk, the percentage of viable cells did not change significantly, showing that inhibition of caspases cannot rescue cells from death. This observation challenges previous own and foreign reports presenting effective inhibition of UVB-induced apoptosis by z-VAD-fmk (36–38). Employing our multiparametric analysis, we here put forward a more detailed characterization of cell death phenotypes induced by several stimuli. We conclude that UVB mainly acts in B16F10 cells by triggering the intrinsic mitochondrial death pathway.

Necrosis is a cellular state that follows acute injuries, sudden anoxia, or extreme stimuli (heat, irradiation, toxins, mechanical, or oxidative stress) and, according to that, it can be viewed as a violent kind of cell death. Conventional methods used to induce necrosis in immunological studies applied heat shock at 56°C or alternating cycles of freeze–thawing. In this work, we present an alternative approach expressing a necrosis inducing protein (CpnT$_{CTD}$) via a doxy-dependent inducible expression system. CpnT is a novel outer membrane protein of *M. tuberculosis* containing a C-terminal domain that is cytotoxic when expressed in eukaryotic cells (8). It has been suggested to be required for the escape of *M. tuberculosis* from macrophages allowing subsequent bacterial dissemination. However, how CpnT$_{CTD}$ induces necrosis is still mechanistically elusive. Six hours after the addition of doxy, a significant fraction of stressed cells was observed. This suggests loss of the mitochondrial membrane potential and mitochondrial damage. Twelve and 18 h after the addition of doxy, more than 50 and 80% of the cells were primary necrotic, respectively. Only after 48 h post-doxy addition, was DNA degradation observed. The decreased DNA content of the latter mimics some features of secondary necrotic death. However, DNA degradation occurred in cells that had already lost their membrane integrity. The cells should, therefore, be referred to as post-necrotic and not as post-apoptotic. The passive influx of DNA degrading enzymes and/or Ca^{2+} most likely causes the chromatin degradation observed in necrotic cells. Expression of the CpnT$_{CTD}$ protein in the presence of z-VAD-fmk showed the same phenotype as those not treated with the inhibitor, arguing for a caspase-independent type of cell death. A classical method to induce necrosis is a heat shock at 56°C for 30 min. As expected, cells became necrotic immediately after heating. This process was also not affected by the presence of z-VAD-fmk, suggesting that caspases were not required for death induced by this kind of heat shock.

Most anti-cancer therapies, like chemotherapy and radiotherapy, aim to induce cancer cell death. However, a central problem is to understand how the immune system determines whether cell death elicits immunogenic, tolerogenic, or silent responses. It has been reported that type and/or phase of cell death affect the immune response (3, 39). For example, cells treated with antracyclines, oxaliplatin, or UVC light develop a kind of endoplasmic reticulum (ER) stress response that involves recruitment of several actors of the apoptotic pathway and contributes to the exposure of calreticulin, which represents an important determinant of immunogenic cell death (40–42).

In order to evaluate whether a certain type of cell death is immunogenic or tolerogenic/silent, an allogeneic murine graft rejection model was employed. The s.c. tumor progression in BALB/c mice was monitored after immunizing the host with various kinds of dying/dead cells. We hypothesized that immunization with tolerogenic or silent forms of cell death would overcome or not affect the natural host immunity allowing tumor development in BALB/c mice, respectively. In contrast, immunogenic cell death would result in faster and more efficient rejection and persistent immunity (3, 43–47). Syngeneic implantation of viable B16F10 cells in C57/Bl6 mice reportedly resulted in high mortality because of the potent carcinogenicity making it difficult to evaluate the immune response against various kinds of cell death (48, 49). The allogeneic model, instead, allows us to compare the immune modulatory effects of cell death forms without compromising the welfare of the host (10–12).

Immune responses elicited by dying/dead cells in BALB/c mice were dependent on the death stimulus applied to the vaccine. Mice implanted with viable melanoma cells transiently produced primary tumors, but never developed secondary tumors after rechallenge (100% rejection). In contrast, mice immunized with irradiated cells supported the growth of secondary tumors similar to the naïve cohort. In order to explore this effect thoroughly, mice were challenged after having been immunized with dying/dead cells killed by various mechanisms.

Expression of the necrosis inducing protein domain CpnT$_{CTD}$ in a B16F10 cell-based vaccine resulted in the most immunogenic type of cell death. Unexpectedly, expression of the pro-apoptotic constitutively active form of caspase-3 (revCasp-3) also induced a strongly immunogenic type of cell death. Massive apoptosis induced by the regulated expression of revCasp-3 in already implanted syngeneic tumors has been reported to be immunogenic (50). Expression of caspase-3 induced a high percentage of necrotic cell death (early and late secondary necrosis). Heat-necrotized cells, which display membrane disruption already before injection, exhibited poor immunogenicity. This points to short-lived necrotic cell-derived signaling molecules, which would not be active anymore in the vaccine that had been necrotized before injection. Summarizing, in our model the time of appearance of membrane disruption in B16F10 cells did not correlate with the type of immune response the cells elicited. Noteworthy, UVB-irradiated cells showed the lowest percentage of necrotic cells and failed to trigger immunity. tBid-expressing cells and UVB-irradiated cells used for immunization clearly behaved silently and allowed the growth of allogeneic tumors, despite the presence of high levels of necrotic cells, as in naïve animals.

The unresponsiveness observed in our system cannot be explained solely by the exposure of PS. Similarly, DAMPs released or expressed after disruption of the plasma membrane are also not sufficient to explain the immunogenicity observed in our model. Therefore, we looked for common features of the two "silent" types of cell death, over-expression of tBid and UVB irradiation, and of the two immunogenic types of cell death, over-expression of revCasp-3 and $CpnT_{CTD}$. The common denominator in both cases is the prominent role of the mitochondria in the execution of death (39).

In our system, activation of the intrinsic pathway either by the recombinant expression of cleaved active Bid or by UVB irradiation may have caused death without relevant ROS production during the time frame the cells were employed for immunization (3–9 h after doxy treatment). Although some caspase-3 activity is to be expected in both tBid- and UVB-induced death, this was not enough to secondarily generate ROS. In contrast, downstream expression of revCasp-3 and $CpnT_{CTD}$ may have caused death by activation of terminal effector mechanisms excluding the involvement of mitochondria. Therefore, we assume that in the revCasp-3 and $CpnT_{CTD}$ cases, execution of cell death starts before mitochondrial function is severely compromised. After over-expression of revCasp-3, MOMP formation is induced allowing access of caspase-3 to the mitochondrial inter-membrane space, cleaving specific substrates in the complex I of the electron transport chain (like p75 NDUSF1) (51, 52). As a consequence, the electron transport is disrupted, and ROS is generated. In contrast, tBid expression causes severe damage to the mitochondria measured as a fast loss of the mitochondrial potential, suggesting fast MOMP formation thereby destroying electron transport abruptly. We propose that ROS can be produced in cells overexpressing revCasp-3 and possibly $CpnT_{CTD}$ because mitochondrial activity is not severely affected by an intrinsic death stimulus. Ongoing cell death in the presence of functioning mitochondria would be important for intracellular ROS accumulation. Free radicals generated in this context may induce considerable stress in the ER, which has been associated with immunogenicity of the dying cells (3).

We suggest that intracellular accumulation of ROS intermediates may play a critical role in the generation of DAMPs affecting the ongoing allogeneic immune response. For example, oxidative damage to DNA enhances its immune-stimulatory capabilities once processed by the immune system (53). Avoiding intracellular accumulation of ROS by a selective manipulation of mitochondrial functionality before killing cells is a possible option to down-regulate the subsequent immune response. Reversely, conserving mitochondrial function as long as possible during cancer cell killing may increase the immunogenicity, if this is wanted.

Although NAC significantly inhibited ROS production in $CpnT_{CTD}$-expressing cells *in vitro* (**Figure 3**), the employment of this anti-oxidant during cell death induced by the expression of $CpnT_{CTD}$ was not sufficient to abrogate their immunogenicity in our allo-immunization model. Interestingly, the addition of the specific mitochondrial ROS scavenger mitoTEMPO induced significant inhibition of ROS production in B16F10-revCasp-3 and B16F10-$CpnT_{CTD}$ dying cells *in vitro* arguing for an important role of the mitochondria in ROS production. Since inhibition *in vitro* by NAC or mitoTEMPO was partial, ROS may be additionally produced in other cellular compartments like the ER. Noteworthy, it was demonstrated in yeasts that mitochondrial dysfunction indirectly induces ROS production in the ER by a novel mechanism mediated by suppression of the endoplasmic reticulum-associated degradation (ERAD) pathway (54, 55). In line with this, ER stress may result in increased cytoplasmic Ca^{2+} concentrations and immunogenic cell death (56). Further investigation addressing the source and localization of ROS in these cells is needed to elucidate the exact role of ROS production during cell death and its immunological consequences, especially in *in vivo* models.

We speculate that some of the mechanisms observed in this manuscript might also work in patients with tumors, during tumor therapy and in some syngeneic tumor models. However, the application of tumor vaccines in human beings has, so far, been less successful. The association between intracellular ROS accumulation in dying cells and allogeneic tumor rejection may have the potential to intentionally shape anti-tumor immunity.

ACKNOWLEDGMENTS

This project was supported by the German Research Foundation (SPP1468-IMMUNOBONE, collaborative research center 643 TP-B5, GA 1507/1-1, and DFG-Graduiertenkolleg 1660: key signals of the adaptive immune response), by the Emerging Fields Initiative (EFI) of the FAU Erlangen-Nuremberg, by the German Federal Ministry of Education and Research (BMBF; m4 Cluster, 01EX1021R) and the K. und R. Wucherpfennig-Stiftung. The authors acknowledge support by the Deutsche Forschungsgemeinschaft and the Friedrich-Alexander-Universität within the open access publishing funding program. The authors alone are responsible for the content and writing of the paper.

SUPPLEMENTARY MATERIAL

Figure S1 | UVB irradiation of B16F10 cells after doxycycline treatment. In order to rule out that an additional irradiation step interferes with the type of cell death induced by specific expression of the respective cytotoxic protein in the cell lines B16F10-tBid, B16F10-revCasp-3, and B16F10-$CpnT_{CTD}$, cells were induced to die with doxycyline (5 μg/ml) and irradiated with a single dose of 240 mJ/cm² UVB at different time points ($t = 4$ h, $t = 5$ h, $t = 6$ h, and $t = 7$ h). Eighteen hours after doxycycline addition (t_0), the cells were harvested by trypsinization and analyzed by FACS for PI staining. Cells killed solely by UVB or doxycycline were used as controls. Blue bars show death induced by irradiation alone. Red bars show death by doxycycline-regulated expression of each cytotoxic protein alone. Green bars show the combined effect of cytotoxic protein expression plus irradiation at different time points. Note that cells irradiated 4, 5, 6, and 7 h after doxycycline addition (green bars) died to the same extent as cells killed by doxycycline alone (red bars).These results suggest that after 4 h of incubation with doxy, the additional irradiation step did not significantly affect the degree of doxycycline-induced cell death despite of the additional damage caused by the irradiation. We, therefore, assumed that after 4 h the cytotoxic protein expression is sufficient to induce cell death as it would happen without irradiation. Irradiation at earlier time points significantly impaired doxycycline-regulated cell death (data not shown). This procedure ensured killing of the doxycycline-resistant cells in primary grafts in order to consequently avoid complications caused by proliferative signals emitted from the dying cells acting on the surviving tumor cells.

Figure S2 | Immune response against allogeneic dead and dying cells in the presence of the ROS inhibitor NAC. BALB/c mice were immunized in the right flank s.c. (single dose) with dying B16F10 cells expressing $CpnT_{CTD}$ (red lines/bars) or dying B16F10 cells expressing $CpnT_{CTD}$ in the presence of the ROS inhibitor *n*-Acetylcysteine (NAC, green lines/bars). Displayed are the mean values ($n = 7$) of the relative tumor volumes and their SEMs and the respective integral of tumor size (total tumor mass) that was obtained in mice challenged s.c. in the left flank with 2 million VC of the parental cell line B16F10-644 10 days after immunization. The Mann–Whitney *U* test was applied to compare groups.

REFERENCES

1. Matzinger P. The danger model: a renewed sense of self. *Science* (2002) **296**(5566):301–5. doi:10.1126/science.1071059
2. Schroppel B, Legendre C. Delayed kidney graft function: from mechanism to translation. *Kidney Int* (2014) **86**:251–8. doi:10.1038/ki.2014.18
3. Green DR, Ferguson T, Zitvogel L, Kroemer G. Immunogenic and tolerogenic cell death. *Nat Rev Immunol* (2009) **9**(5):353–63. doi:10.1038/nri2545
4. Kepp O, Senovilla L, Kroemer G. Immunogenic cell death inducers as anticancer agents. *Oncotarget* (2014) **5**(14):5190–1.
5. Kelland LR. Of mice and men: values and liabilities of the athymic nude mouse model in anticancer drug development. *Eur J Cancer* (2004) **40**(6):827–36. doi:10.1016/j.ejca.2003.11.028
6. Kepp O, Galluzzi L, Martins I, Schlemmer F, Adjemian S, Michaud M, et al. Molecular determinants of immunogenic cell death elicited by anticancer chemotherapy. *Cancer Metastasis Rev* (2011) **30**(1):61–9. doi:10.1007/s10555-011-9273-4
7. Maueroder C, Chaurio RA, Platzer S, Munoz LE, Berens C. Model systems for rapid and slow induction of apoptosis obtained by inducible expression of pro-apoptotic proteins. *Autoimmunity* (2013) **46**(5):329–35. doi:10.3109/08916934.2012.752463
8. Danilchanka O, Sun J, Pavlenok M, Maueröder C, Speer A, Siroy A, et al. An outer membrane channel protein of *Mycobacterium tuberculosis* with exotoxin activity. *Proc Natl Acad Sci U S A* (2014) **111**:6750–5. doi:10.1073/pnas.1400136111
9. Munoz LE, Maueroder C, Chaurio R, Berens C, Herrmann M, Janko C. Colourful death: six-parameter classification of cell death by flow cytometry – dead cells tell tales. *Autoimmunity* (2013) **46**(5):336–41. doi:10.3109/08916934.2012.755960
10. United Kingdom Co-ordinating Committee on Cancer Research (UKCCCR) guidelines for the welfare of animals in experimental neoplasia (second edition). *Br J Cancer* (1998) **77**(1):1–10. doi:10.1038/bjc.1998.1
11. Jones-Bolin S. Guidelines for the care and use of laboratory animals in biomedical research. *Curr Protoc Pharmacol* (2012) **59**:4B:A.4B.1–9. doi:10.1002/0471141755.pha04bs59
12. Vale C, Stewart L, Tierney J. Trends in UK cancer trials: results from the UK coordinating committee for cancer research national register of cancer trials. *Br J Cancer* (2005) **92**(5):811–4. doi:10.1038/sj.bjc.6602425
13. Janko C, Munoz L, Chaurio R, Maueroder C, Berens C, Lauber K, et al. Navigation to the graveyard-induction of various pathways of necrosis and their classification by flow cytometry. *Methods Mol Biol* (2013) **1004**:3–15. doi:10.1007/978-1-62703-383-1_1
14. Turk MJ, Guevara-Patino JA, Rizzuto GA, Engelhorn ME, Sakaguchi S, Houghton AN. Concomitant tumor immunity to a poorly immunogenic melanoma is prevented by regulatory T cells. *J Exp Med* (2004) **200**(6):771–82. doi:10.1084/jem.20041130
15. Appelt U, Sheriff A, Gaipl US, Kalden JR, Voll RE, Herrmann M. Viable, apoptotic and necrotic monocytes expose phosphatidylserine: cooperative binding of the ligand annexin V to dying but not viable cells and implications for PS-dependent clearance. *Cell Death Differ* (2005) **12**(2):194–6. doi:10.1038/sj.cdd.4401527
16. Franz S, Frey B, Sheriff A, Gaipl US, Beer A, Voll RE, et al. Lectins detect changes of the glycosylation status of plasma membrane constituents during late apoptosis. *Cytometry A* (2006) **69**(4):230–9. doi:10.1002/cyto.a.20206
17. Zhang G, Gurtu V, Kain SR, Yan G. Early detection of apoptosis using a fluorescent conjugate of annexin V. *Biotechniques* (1997) **23**(3):525–31.
18. Saelens X, Festjens N, Vande Walle L, van Gurp M, van Loo G, Vandenabeele P. Toxic proteins released from mitochondria in cell death. *Oncogene* (2004) **23**(16):2861–74. doi:10.1038/sj.onc.1207523
19. Troiano L, Ferraresi R, Lugli E, Nemes E, Roat E, Nasi M, et al. Multiparametric analysis of cells with different mitochondrial membrane potential during apoptosis by polychromatic flow cytometry. *Nat Protoc* (2007) **2**(11):2719–27. doi:10.1038/nprot.2007.405
20. Frey B, Schildkopf P, Rodel F, Weiss EM, Munoz LE, Herrmann M, et al. AnnexinA5 renders dead tumor cells immunogenic – implications for multimodal cancer therapies. *J Immunotoxicol* (2009) **6**(4):209–16. doi:10.3109/15476910903204058
21. Gaipl US, Munoz LE, Rodel F, Pausch F, Frey B, Brachvogel B, et al. Modulation of the immune system by dying cells and the phosphatidylserine-ligand annexin A5. *Autoimmunity* (2007) **40**(4):254–9. doi:10.1080/08916930701357331
22. Munoz LE, Frey B, Pausch F, Baum W, Mueller RB, Brachvogel B, et al. The role of annexin A5 in the modulation of the immune response against dying and dead cells. *Curr Med Chem* (2007) **14**(3):271–7. doi:10.2174/092986707779941131
23. Li H, Zhu H, Xu CJ, Yuan J. Cleavage of BID by caspase 8 mediates the mitochondrial damage in the Fas pathway of apoptosis. *Cell* (1998) **94**(4):491–501. doi:10.1016/S0092-8674(00)81590-1
24. Luo X, Budihardjo I, Zou H, Slaughter C, Wang X. Bid, a Bcl2 interacting protein, mediates cytochrome c release from mitochondria in response to activation of cell surface death receptors. *Cell* (1998) **94**(4):481–90. doi:10.1016/S0092-8674(00)81589-5
25. Youle RJ, Strasser A. The BCL-2 protein family: opposing activities that mediate cell death. *Nat Rev Mol cell Biol* (2008) **9**(1):47–59. doi:10.1038/nrm2308
26. Spencer SL, Gaudet S, Albeck JG, Burke JM, Sorger PK. Non-genetic origins of cell-to-cell variability in TRAIL-induced apoptosis. *Nature* (2009) **459**(7245):428–32. doi:10.1038/nature08012
27. Eastman A. Apoptosis: a product of programmed and unprogrammed cell death. *Toxicol Appl Pharmacol* (1993) **121**(1):160–4. doi:10.1006/taap.1993.1141
28. Lieberthal W, Triaca V, Levine J. Mechanisms of death induced by cisplatin in proximal tubular epithelial cells: apoptosis vs. necrosis. *Am J Physiol* (1996) **270**(4 Pt 2):F700–8.
29. Martin SJ, Green DR. Protease activation during apoptosis: death by a thousand cuts? *Cell* (1995) **82**(3):349–52. doi:10.1016/0092-8674(95)90422-0
30. Elmore S. Apoptosis: a review of programmed cell death. *Toxicol Pathol* (2007) **35**(4):495–516. doi:10.1080/01926230701320337
31. Shelton SN, Shawgo ME, Robertson JD. Cleavage of Bid by executioner caspases mediates feed forward amplification of mitochondrial outer membrane permeabilization during genotoxic stress-induced apoptosis in Jurkat cells. *J Biol Chem* (2009) **284**(17):11247–55. doi:10.1074/jbc.M809392200
32. Patrick MH. Studies on thymine-derived UV photoproducts in DNA – I. Formation and biological role of pyrimidine adducts in DNA. *Photochem Photobiol* (1977) **25**(4):357–72. doi:10.1111/j.1751-1097.1977.tb07355.x
33. Aragane Y, Kulms D, Metze D, Wilkes G, Poppelmann B, Luger TA, et al. Ultraviolet light induces apoptosis via direct activation of CD95 (Fas/APO-1) independently of its ligand CD95L. *J Cell Biol* (1998) **140**(1):171–82. doi:10.1083/jcb.140.1.171
34. Rehemtulla A, Hamilton CA, Chinnaiyan AM, Dixit VM. Ultraviolet radiation-induced apoptosis is mediated by activation of CD-95 (Fas/APO-1). *J Biol Chem* (1997) **272**(41):25783–6. doi:10.1074/jbc.272.41.25783
35. Rosette C, Karin M. Ultraviolet light and osmotic stress: activation of the JNK cascade through multiple growth factor and cytokine receptors. *Science* (1996) **274**(5290):1194–7. doi:10.1126/science.274.5290.1194
36. Garcia-Calvo M, Peterson EP, Leiting B, Ruel R, Nicholson DW, Thornberry NA. Inhibition of human caspases by peptide-based and macromolecular inhibitors. *J Biol Chem* (1998) **273**(49):32608–13. doi:10.1074/jbc.273.49.32608
37. Kulms D, Zeise E, Poppelmann B, Schwarz T. DNA damage, death receptor activation and reactive oxygen species contribute to ultraviolet

radiation-induced apoptosis in an essential and independent way. *Oncogene* (2002) **21**(38):5844–51. doi:10.1038/sj.onc.1205743
38. Schiller M, Blank N, Heyder P, Herrmann M, Gaipl US, Kalden JR, et al. Induction of apoptosis by spermine-metabolites in primary human blood cells and various tumor cell lines. *Apoptosis* (2005) **10**(5):1151–62. doi:10.1007/s10495-005-1188-5
39. Galluzzi L, Vitale I, Abrams JM, Alnemri ES, Baehrecke EH, Blagosklonny MV, et al. Molecular definitions of cell death subroutines: recommendations of the nomenclature committee on cell death 2012. *Cell Death Differ* (2012) **19**(1):107–20. doi:10.1038/cdd.2011.96
40. Casares N, Pequignot MO, Tesniere A, Ghiringhelli F, Roux S, Chaput N, et al. Caspase-dependent immunogenicity of doxorubicin-induced tumor cell death. *J Exp Med* (2005) **202**(12):1691–701. doi:10.1084/jem.20050915
41. Panaretakis T, Kepp O, Brockmeier U, Tesniere A, Bjorklund AC, Chapman DC, et al. Mechanisms of pre-apoptotic calreticulin exposure in immunogenic cell death. *EMBO J* (2009) **28**(5):578–90. doi:10.1038/emboj.2009.1
42. Zitvogel L, Kepp O, Senovilla L, Menger L, Chaput N, Kroemer G. Immunogenic tumor cell death for optimal anticancer therapy: the calreticulin exposure pathway. *Clin Cancer Res* (2010) **16**(12):3100–4. doi:10.1158/1078-0432.CCR-09-2891
43. Kepp O, Tesniere A, Schlemmer F, Michaud M, Senovilla L, Zitvogel L, et al. Immunogenic cell death modalities and their impact on cancer treatment. *Apoptosis* (2009) **14**(4):364–75. doi:10.1007/s10495-008-0303-9
44. Kepp O, Tesniere A, Zitvogel L, Kroemer G. The immunogenicity of tumor cell death. *Curr Opin Oncol* (2009) **21**(1):71–6. doi:10.1097/CCO.0b013e32831bc375
45. Kono H, Rock KL. How dying cells alert the immune system to danger. *Nat Rev Immunol* (2008) **8**(4):279–89. doi:10.1038/nri2215
46. Krysko DV, Garg AD, Kaczmarek A, Krysko O, Agostinis P, Vandenabeele P. Immunogenic cell death and DAMPs in cancer therapy. *Nat Rev Cancer* (2012) **12**(12):860–75. doi:10.1038/nrc3380
47. LaLadoire S, Hannani D, Vetizou M, Locher C, Aymeric L, Apetoh L, et al. Cell-death-associated molecular patterns as determinants of cancer immunogenicity. *Antioxid Redox Signal* (2013) **20**(7):1098–116. doi:10.1089/ars.2012.5133
48. Briles EB, Kornfeld S. Isolation and metastatic properties of detachment variants of B16 melanoma cells. *J Natl Cancer Inst* (1978) **60**(6):1217–22.
49. Fidler IJ. Biological behavior of malignant melanoma cells correlated to their survival in vivo. *Cancer Res* (1975) **35**(1):218–24.
50. Melis MH, Simpson KL, Dovedi SJ, Welman A, MacFarlane M, Dive C, et al. Sustained tumour eradication after induced caspase-3 activation and synchronous tumour apoptosis requires an intact host immune response. *Cell Death Differ* (2013) **20**(5):765–73. doi:10.1038/cdd.2013.8
51. Ricci JE, Gottlieb RA, Green DR. Caspase-mediated loss of mitochondrial function and generation of reactive oxygen species during apoptosis. *J Cell Biol* (2003) **160**(1):65–75. doi:10.1083/jcb.200208089
52. Ricci JE, Munoz-Pinedo C, Fitzgerald P, Bailly-Maitre B, Perkins GA, Yadava N, et al. Disruption of mitochondrial function during apoptosis is mediated by caspase cleavage of the p75 subunit of complex I of the electron transport chain. *Cell* (2004) **117**(6):773–86. doi:10.1016/j.cell.2004.05.008
53. Gehrke N, Mertens C, Zillinger T, Wenzel J, Bald T, Zahn S, et al. Oxidative damage of DNA confers resistance to cytosolic nuclease TREX1 degradation and potentiates STING-dependent immune sensing. *Immunity* (2013) **39**(3):482–95. doi:10.1016/j.immuni.2013.08.004
54. Leadsham JE, Sanders G, Giannaki S, Bastow EL, Hutton R, Naeimi WR, et al. Loss of cytochrome c oxidase promotes RAS-dependent ROS production from the ER resident NADPH oxidase, Yno1p, in yeast. *Cell Metab* (2013) **18**(2):279–86. doi:10.1016/j.cmet.2013.07.005
55. Murphy MP. Mitochondrial dysfunction indirectly elevates ROS production by the endoplasmic reticulum. *Cell Metab* (2013) **18**(2):145–6. doi:10.1016/j.cmet.2013.07.006
56. Kepp O, Menger L, Vacchelli E, Locher C, Adjemian S, Yamazaki T, et al. Crosstalk between ER stress and immunogenic cell death. *Cytokine Growth Factor Rev* (2013) **24**(4):311–8. doi:10.1016/j.cytogfr.2013.05.001

16

Quantifying the protection of activating and inhibiting NK cell receptors during infection with a CMV-like virus

Paola Carrillo-Bustamante*, Can Keşmir and Rob J. de Boer

Theoretical Biology and Bioinformatics, Department of Biology, Utrecht University, Utrecht, Netherlands

Edited by:
Ramit Mehr, Bar-Ilan University, Israel

Reviewed by:
Ramit Mehr, Bar-Ilan University, Israel
Becca Asquith, Imperial College London, UK
Jayajit Das, The Ohio State University, USA

***Correspondence:**
Paola Carrillo-Bustamante, Theoretical Biology and Bioinformatics, Department of Biology, Utrecht University, Padualaan 8, Utrecht 3584 CH, Netherlands
e-mail: p.carrillobustamante@uu.nl

The responsiveness of natural killer (NK) cells is controlled by balancing signals from activating and inhibitory receptors. The most important ligands of inhibitory NK cell receptors are the highly polymorphic major histocompatibility complex (MHC) class I molecules, which allow NK cells to screen the cellular health of target cells. Although these inhibitory receptor–ligand interactions have been well characterized, the ligands for most activating receptors are still unknown. The mouse cytomegalovirus (MCMV) represents a helpful model to study NK cell-driven immune responses. Many studies have demonstrated that CMV infection can be controlled by NK cells via their activating receptors, but the exact contribution of the different signaling potential (i.e., activating vs. inhibiting) remains puzzling. In this study, we have developed a probabilistic model, which predicts the optimal specificity of inhibitory and activating NK cell receptors needed to offer the best protection against a CMV-like virus. We confirm our analytical predictions with an agent-based model of an evolving host population. Our analysis quantifies the degree of protection of each receptor type, revealing that mixed haplotypes (i.e., haplotypes composed of activating and inhibiting receptors) are most protective against CMV-like viruses, and that the protective effect depends on the number of MHC loci per individual.

Keywords: NK cell receptors, evolution, CMV infection, models, theoretical, agent-based modeling

INTRODUCTION

Natural killer (NK) cells contribute to the host immune response by recognizing and killing viral-infected and tumor cells (1). Their activity is controlled by balancing signals from a vast repertoire of activating and inhibiting receptors enabling them to distinguish healthy from unhealthy cells (2). The most important ligands for inhibitory NK cell receptors (iNKR) are MHC class I molecules on other cells. An infected cell may have lower MHC expression, altering the binding with inhibitory receptors, disrupting the balance of signals, and allowing for NK cell activation. The mechanism by which NK cells attack MHC class I deficient cells was coined by Kärre et al. as "missing-self" detection (3).

There are several NKRs that contribute to missing-self detection. In humans, for example, the inhibitory receptor CD96/NKG2A binds to complexes of the human leukocyte antigen-E (HLA-E), which presents peptides derived from the leader sequences of HLA-A, -B, and -C molecules (4, 5). Both the receptor and the ligand are highly conserved in these inhibitory interactions, and the down-stream effects are remarkably similar across individuals (6). The killer immunoglobulin-like receptors (KIRs) also contribute to monitor abnormalities in MHC class I expression on cell surfaces. In contrast to the CD96/NKG2 superfamily, KIRs are highly polygenic and polymorphic, exhibit both inhibitory and activating potential, and bind to the highly polymorphic HLA-A, -B, and -C molecules (7–9). Consequently, the interactions between KIRs and classical HLA-class I molecules are very diverse (10). Thus, humans have two types of NKRs, one conserved and one highly diverse, performing seemingly the same function.

Humans are not the only species that have an expanded and polymorphic NKR gene complex. During mammalian radiation, many different species have diversified alternative NKR gene families recognizing MHC class I. This example of convergent evolution includes three gene families from two structurally unrelated superfamilies: KIRs, the CD94/NKG2, and the Ly49 (11). Higher primates have expanded their KIR genes (12); a group of lower primates have expanded NKG2 (13), whereas rodents and equids have expanded Ly49 (14, 15). These alternative genetic strategies illustrate the evolutionary complexity of these systems, and suggest that an expanded NKR gene complex is beneficial for survival. But, if conserved inhibitory receptor–ligand interactions (such as NKG2A–HLA-E in humans) are capable to successfully detect missing-self, why have several NKR families evolved to become polygenic and polymorphic? Even more intriguing, why have they evolved receptors with activating potential?

In humans, some activating NKRs (aNKRs) are associated with the disease outcome of viral infections and malignancies (16). For example, in combination with HLA–Bw4, the activating KIR3DS1 has been associated with a delayed progression to AIDS in HIV-1 infected individuals (17, 18). KIR3DS1 has also been linked to an increased rate of spontaneous recovery after hepatitis B infections (19), a reduced risk of developing hepatocellular carcinoma in patients infected with HCV (20), and a reduced risk of Hodgkin's lymphoma (21). Moreover, maternal activating KIRs are related to protection against several pregnancy disorders (22). But because only a few ligands for activating KIRs have been identified so far, the exact mechanisms underlying the provided protection in humans remain puzzling.

Studies in mice have revealed important insights into the role of aNKR during viral infections (23, 24). Viruses like the mouse cytomegalovirus (MCMV) down-regulate the expression of MHC class I molecules from the cell surface to escape T cell response, and may additionally code decoy MHC molecules (m157) that can inhibit NK cell activation (23). Mouse strains that are resistant to MCMV carry the activating Ly49H gene, which binds with high affinity to the MHC-like viral protein m157. In contrast, mice susceptible to MCMV lack the activating gene but carry the inhibiting receptor Ly49I, which also binds strongly to the m157 protein. The activating Ly49H emerged from an inhibitory counterpart (25), suggesting that the evolution of an aNKR was due to the immune pressure induced by the "MHC decoy" m157 during CMV infection (26, 27).

Although these studies shed light into the importance of NKR in general, the specific contribution of activating and inhibitory receptors to the NK cell response is still unknown. We previously studied the evolution of KIR diversity in a human population infected with CMV-like viruses by using a computational agent-based model (28). We showed that iNKRs require sufficient specificity to protect populations against viruses evolving MHC-like molecules, and that diversity in the NK cell genetic complex evolves as a result of the required discrimination between self-MHC molecules and viral decoy molecules. Here, we also consider aNKRs, and develop a probabilistic model to quantify the optimal specificity of inhibitory and activating NKRs needed to render maximal protection against CMV-like viruses. We also analyze the effect of mixed haplotypes (i.e., composed of aNKR and iNKR) on protection, and confirm the expectations of the probabilistic model with an agent-based computational model. Our studies reveal that mixed haplotypes composed of specific activating and inhibitory NKRs render high protection against CMV-like viruses encoding for decoy molecules, and that the protective effect depends on the number of MHC loci per individual.

RESULTS

We analyze the effect of the specificity of activating and inhibitory NKRs on the detection of a virus presenting MHC-like molecules with a simple probabilistic model. Our model estimates the chance of protection P, i.e., the probability of a host detecting an infection by NK cells, as a function of the haplotype size, specificity (i.e., the probability p of recognizing any random MHC molecule), and number of MHC loci.

The responsiveness of NK cells (i.e., their ability to discriminate cells with normal MHC expression from those lacking MHC) is regulated by a process called "education" or "licensing" taking place during NK cell development (29). During this process, the interactions of iNKRs with their MHC ligands render the NK cells with functional competence (13, 29, 30). To prevent NK cell-related autoimmunity, activating receptors also participate in the education process, where the chronic exposure of aNKR ligands during development results in hyporesponsive NK cells (31, 32).

For simplicity, we do not model individual NK cells, each expressing a random set of tuned receptors. We rather consider for each individual a global repertoire of receptors, which have the potential to license NK cells. Henceforth, we will refer to these receptors as "licensed" receptors. We mimic the MHC-dependent education process during NK cell development by creating a repertoire of NKRs composed of iNKRs that recognize at least one of the MHC molecules of the host, and of aNKRs that recognize none of the MHC molecules of the host (**Figure 1**). By considering a global repertoire, we assume that there will be at least one subset of NK cells expressing at least one of the "licensed" NKRs. Upon infection, we consider only those NK cell subsets having licensed receptors. If these can successfully detect the virus, they will become activated, expand, and protect (see Appendix for a full discussion). Therefore, only the licensed repertoire of NKRs is allowed to participate in the immune response.

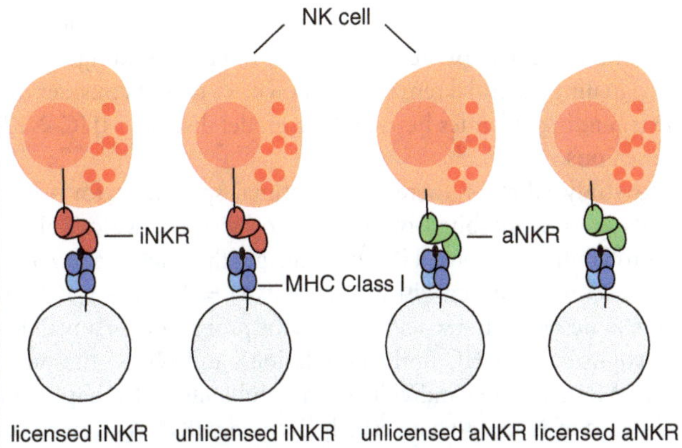

FIGURE 1 | Cartoon of NK cell education. iNKRs (represented in red) recognizing at least one of the MHC molecules per individual will become licensed. In contrast, aNKRs (depicted in green), which do not recognize *any* of the host's MHC molecules will become licensed.

Whether a decoy protein allows a virus to successfully escape the NK response, i.e., whether that individual is protected against the infection, depends on the receptor type and on the receptor specificity. iNKRs that bind the decoy molecule cannot detect missing-self and are "fooled" by the decoy. Conversely, aNKRs binding the foreign decoy protein can specifically recognize the infection and therefore protect the host. With this model, we quantify the contribution of each receptor type and its specificity to the detection of CMV-like viruses.

INHIBITORY AND ACTIVATING NK CELL RECEPTORS DIFFER IN THE PROTECTION LEVEL THEY PROVIDE

There are two crucial processes for a single iNKR to detect virus evolving MHC-like molecules. First, iNKRs have to be licensed during the NK cell education to become fully functional during an immune response. Second, iNKRs should not bind decoy molecules upon infection. Because, in our model, iNKRs are only licensed if they recognize at least one of the MHC molecules in their host, and decoy molecules are similar to self-MHC molecules, iNKRs face the challenge of distinguishing self-MHC molecules from foreign decoy molecules. We previously demonstrated that this challenge can be solved by evolving sufficiently specific iNKRs (28). In that study, we defined specificity as the probability (p) of any NKR to recognize a random MHC molecule in the population. Herewith, degenerate receptors (i.e., with $p = 1$) are able to recognize all MHC molecules in the population, whereas specific receptors (i.e., with $p \sim 0$) recognize only a small fraction of them. Since the exact relation between ligand–receptor binding affinity and signaling potential remains unknown, we do not consider different binding affinities here, and we model discrete MHC–NKR interactions.

To study whether there is an optimal specificity for which iNKRs are not inhibited by such "decoy viruses," we calculated the probability of licensed iNKRs detecting the infection. A single iNKR becomes licensed with a probability $q_I = 1-(1-p_I)^{2N_{MHC}}$, where p_I describes the specificity (i.e., the probability of any iNKR to recognize any MHC in the population), and N_{MHC} the number of MHC loci per individual. The probability of a haplotype composed of N_{iNKR} to have exactly licensed iNKRs is given by the binomial distribution as follows:

$$P(\text{iNKR}_{\text{licensed}} = \ell) = \binom{N_{\text{iNKR}}}{\ell}(1-q_I)^{N_{\text{iNKR}}-\ell}q_I^{\ell}. \quad (1)$$

To successfully detect a decoy virus, none of the licensed iNKRs should bind the decoy molecule. Thus, the overall probability of detecting the infection is determined by the chance that none of the licensed iNKRs recognizes a decoy molecule, and can be calculated by:

$$P_I(\text{detection}) = \sum_{\ell=1}^{N_{\text{iNKR}}}\binom{N_{\text{iNKR}}}{\ell}(1-p_I)^{\ell}(1-q_I)^{N_{\text{iNKR}}-\ell}q_I^{\ell}. \quad (2)$$

Our analysis confirms that for any haplotype size, there is an optimal specificity. For $N_{iNKR} \leq 25$, our model predicts a maximal level of protection (i.e., $P_I = 0.85$), which can only be obtained with high specificity values ($p_I \leq 0.2$) and a large number of genes per haplotype ($N_{iNKR} \geq 20$) (**Figure 2A**).

A host with degenerate iNKRs (e.g., $p_I \geq 0.8$) has a large repertoire of licensed iNKRs. But because of the low specificity, the iNKRs within that individual are expected to also recognize any foreign decoy molecule as self, offering no protection. In contrast, when iNKRs are specific (e.g., $p_I \leq 0.2$) the repertoire of licensed iNKRs per individual is lower, but if there are several genes per haplotype, the chance of having at least one licensed specific iNKR increases. Due to their high specificity, it is unlikely for a licensed iNKR to also recognize a foreign decoy molecule, impeding the virus to escape the NK immune response. Therefore, an infection with a decoy virus can be controlled with a probability of at least 70% in a haplotype composed of more than 10 iNKRs when $p_I \leq 0.25$. Thus, the probability of detecting the virus increases with both a higher specificity and a larger number of genes per haplotype (i.e., N_{iNKR}). This confirms our previous results, suggesting that large haplotypes composed of non-overlapping specific iNKRs are most protective (28).

We next developed a model considering only aNKRs. Similar to the iNKRs, the two crucial processes for an aNKR to detect the virus depends on the probability of becoming licensed and recognizing the decoy molecule as a foreign antigen. However, the licensing process is almost opposite between aNKRs and iNKRs. An aNKR becomes licensed if it does not recognize any MHC molecule within an individual. The probability of a single aNKR to become licensed is therefore described by $q_A = (1-p_A)^{2N_{MHC}}$, where p_A is the specificity of an aNKR. Opposite to an iNKR, an aNKR detects a "decoy virus" if it binds the MHC decoy. Thus, the overall probability of protection in this case is determined by the chance of at least one licensed aNKR binding the decoy molecule, and is given by:

$$P_A(\text{detection}) = \sum_{\ell=1}^{N_{\text{aNKR}}}\binom{N_{\text{aNKR}}}{\ell}\left(1-(1-p_A)^{\ell}\right) \times (1-q_A)^{N_{\text{aNKR}}-\ell}q_A^{\ell}, \quad (3)$$

where N_{aNKR} is the number of aNKRs per haplotype.

This model reveals that there is again an optimal specificity, and the protection range for aNKR is much broader than that for iNKR, covering also less specific receptors (i.e., $0.1 \leq p_A \leq 0.7$) (**Figure 2B**). In these cases, the optimal protection (i.e., $P_A = 1$) is obtained with haplotypes composed of 12 genes, having intermediate specificity values ($0.2 \leq p_A \leq 0.65$). To avoid self-reactivity, aNKRs become licensed only if they fail to recognize all self-MHC molecules. Additionally, an aNKR must recognize foreign MHC-like molecules to detect the infection. Therefore, the challenge for an aNKR is opposite to that of an iNKR, since it must recognize foreign antigens but not self-MHC molecules. A degenerate aNKR will recognize every decoy in the population but it will never become licensed. As a result, the optimal protection is reached in large haplotypes composed of aNKRs with intermediate specificity.

Note that we consider individuals to be heterozygous for all MHC loci. Allowing individuals to be homozygous in some MHC loci does not qualitatively change our results on specificity and protection, since MHC homozygosity has only a mild effect on the number of licensed receptors, ℓ (results not shown).

THE PROTECTION LEVEL DEPENDS ON THE NUMBER OF MHC LOCI

Above, we considered only one MHC locus per individual as a representation of HLA-C as the main identified ligand for inhibitory KIRs. However, HLA-A and -B molecules have also been identified as KIR ligands, and HLA-E is the ligand for CD94/NKG2A. Therefore, we expanded our model to consider two MHC loci per individual. The distribution of protection levels is similar to the model with one MHC locus, showing a small protective area for individuals carrying only iNKRs (**Figure 2C**), whereas individuals carrying aNKRs have a broader protective range (**Figure 2D**). However, the area of maximal protection is skewed in both cases. Because iNKRs have to recognize at least one self-MHC molecule to become licensed, the chance of having several licensed NKRs per haplotype increases by having 2 MHC loci (and thus 4 MHC molecules per heterozygous individual). Therefore, a high protection (e.g., $P_I \geq 0.85$) can be reached already with a smaller haplotype, e.g., one composed of at least 11 iNKRs.

In contrast, the probability of an aNKR to become licensed decreases with 2 MHC loci because aNKRs should not recognize *any* of the MHC molecules within an individual. Consequently, the protection with aNKRs reaches high values (i.e., $P_A \geq 0.85$) only with large haplotypes composed of at least 20 genes and the optimal protection level ($P_A = 1$) is never obtained. Thus, the

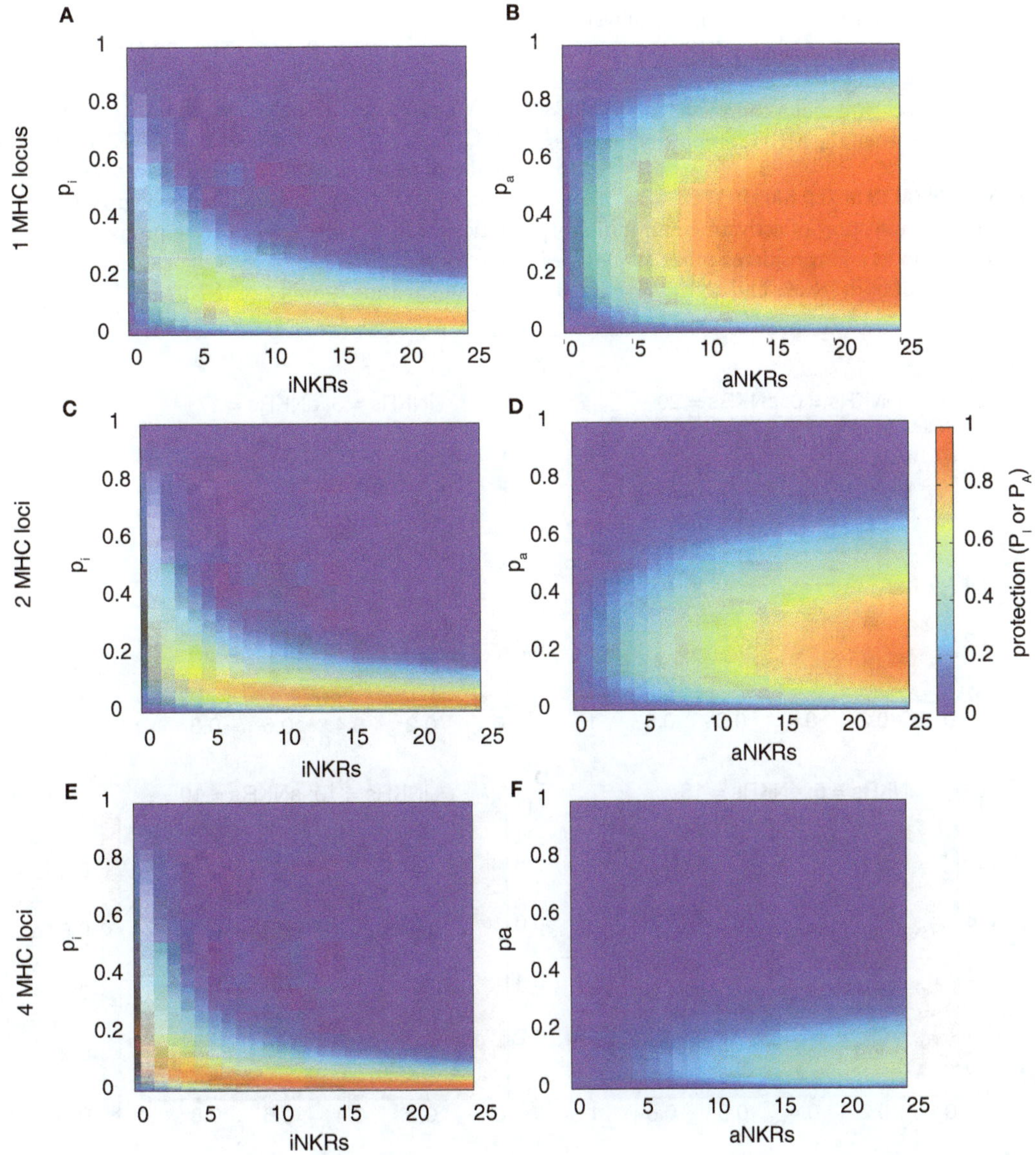

FIGURE 2 | Range of protection differs between iNKRs and aNKRs. The heatmaps show the protection level as the probability of detecting the infection with a virus expressing a decoy molecule to mask MHC down-regulation. In the left column, the protection for individuals carrying only iNKRs [calculated by equation (2)] is shown, whereas in the right column, the protection for individuals carrying only aNKRs [calculated by equation (3)] is depicted. The protection level is shown in the color bar from highest (red) to lowest (blue). p_i and p_a correspond to the specificity of iNKR and aNKR, respectively. **(A,B)** The protective range for iNKRs is small and skewed toward a large haplotype size and high specific values. In contrast, aNKRs offer a broad range of protection for intermediate specificity values and a smaller haplotype size. Calculations were done with 1 MHC locus **(A,B)**, 2 MHC loci **(C,D)**, and 4 MHC loci **(E,F)**.

protection of aNKRs is highly dependent on the number of MHC molecules per individual.

With even higher MHC complexity, i.e., by increasing the number of MHC loci per individual to 4, fewer iNKRs are sufficient to successfully clear the infection (**Figures 2E,F**). Because of the education process in our model, hosts with 4 MHC loci have a much larger licensed iNKR repertoire compared to individuals having 1 MHC locus. These hosts reach the maximal protection already with a haplotype size of 4 receptors. Even for lower haplotype sizes, a good protection level (i.e., $0.3 \leq P_I \leq 0.7$) can be reached at lower specificity values ($p_I \leq 0.35$) (**Figure 2E**). This effect was further increased when considering 8 MHC loci per individual, where the maximal protection was reached with only one specific iKIR (results not shown).

However, an expanded MHC haplotype is disadvantageous for individuals having only aNKRs. Because in our model the licensing process is more difficult with a higher number of MHC molecules, little protection can be provided. The infection can be controlled with a maximal probability of 50 and 35% in individuals with 4 (**Figure 2F**) and 8 MHC loci (results not shown), respectively.

Taken together, these results show that aNKRs provide little protection against a virus evolving MHC decoy proteins in individuals having several MHC loci, and that a contracted haplotype of iNKRs is already protective when the MHC complexity increases.

VIRAL DETECTION IS MAXIMAL IN MIXED HAPLOTYPES

To predict the combined protection of activating and inhibitory NKRs, we expanded our model and considered mixed haplotypes, i.e., haplotypes composed of both iNKRs and aNKRs. We predict the combined probability of detecting the virus as follows:

$$P = 1 - (1 - P_{\mathrm{I}})(1 - P_{\mathrm{A}}). \quad (4)$$

We computed the protection in hosts carrying two MHC and 20 NKR loci, and varied the fraction of aNKRs in the NKR haplotype, while keeping the total number of loci constant. The best protection is reached in mixed haplotypes (**Figure 3**). As seen above, haplotypes with aNKRs only provide protection (i.e., $0.5 \leq P \leq 0.8$) for intermediate specificity values $0.15 \leq p_{\mathrm{A}} \leq 0.4$ (**Figure 3A**). With increasing number of iNKRs per haplotype, the protection

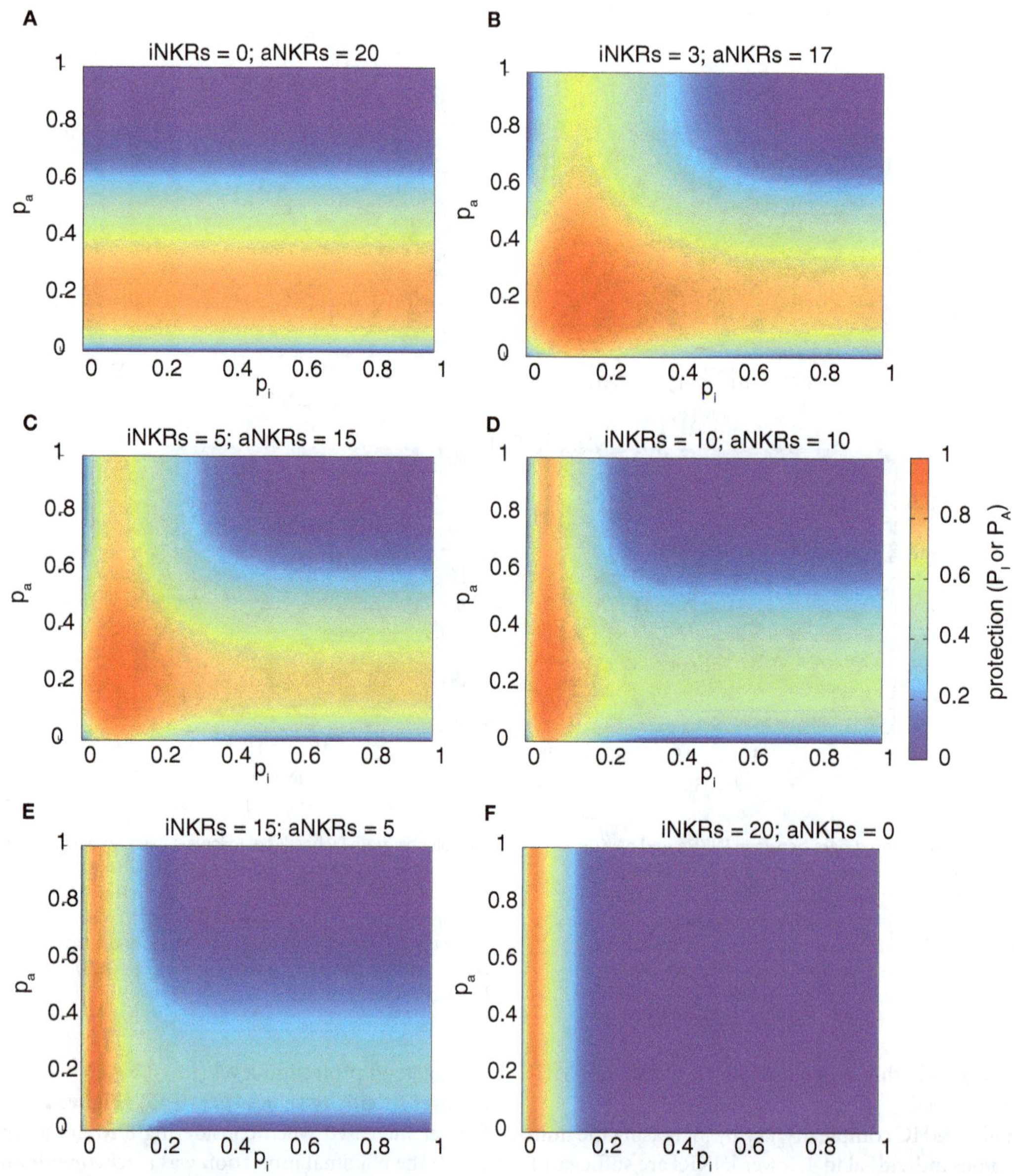

FIGURE 3 | Mixed haplotypes render highest protection. The heatmaps show the protection level as the probability of detecting the infection for haplotypes composed of iNKRs and aNKRs [as calculated by equation (4)]. The protection level is shown in the color bar from highest (red) to lowest (blue). **(A–F)** Show the NKR haplotype composition for different fractions of iNKR and aNKR. Considering a haplotype size of $N_{\mathrm{NKR}} = 20$, we first modeled haplotypes composed of aNKRs only **(A)**, and reduced their number, while increasing the number of iNKRs **(B–E)**, until we obtained a haplotype composed only of iNKRs **(F)**. We here consider 2 MHC loci (i.e., $N_{\mathrm{MHC}} = 2$).

reaches higher values (approaching $P = 1$) (**Figures 3B,C**), covering a larger range of specificity values and having a skewed distribution toward more specific inhibitory and activating receptors. A large number of iNKRs per haplotype reduces the contribution of aNKRs, and therefore the latter can have low specificity values without affecting the protection level (**Figures 3D,E**). Note that the area of high protection shrinks when the fraction of aNKRs is decreased, where maximal protection can only be achieved for extremely high specificities (i.e., $p_I \leq 0.1$) (**Figure 3F**).

These results depend on a similar manner on the number of MHC loci per individual as those shown in **Figure 2**, with aNKRs having a lower protective effect with increasing MHC loci number (results not shown). Therefore, we conclude that the maximal protection against CMV-like viruses is easier to achieve in mixed haplotypes.

AGENT-BASED MODEL OF ACTIVATING AND INHIBITORY NKRs

Our probabilistic model allows us to quantify the expected protection, given a certain number of aNKRs and iNKRs. However, it is not clear whether a population with evolving NKRs would find the same basin of attraction for the specificity (i.e., p) when infected with a CMV-like virus.

To study the evolution of NKR specificity in populations infected with a CMV-like virus, we developed an agent-based model similar to the one published in Ref. (28) (for a detailed description of the model, see Materials and Methods). Briefly, our model considers a human population infected with a non-lethal herpes-like virus causing chronic infections. The hosts carry a diploid genome with one or two MHC loci and ten NKR loci. We consider 15 MHC alleles per locus (mimicking the common HLA-B and -C alleles in the European populations) and this polymorphism is kept constant throughout the entire simulation (i.e., we do not allow for mutation of the MHC genes). The initial NKR haplotype consists of ten different genes, and all individuals are homozygous for the same NKR haplotype.

Upon birth, novel receptors can be created, allowing for evolution within the NKR gene complex. Each new receptor comes with a randomly chosen receptor type (i.e., either inhibitory or activating) and a randomly chosen specificity value (corresponding to $0 \leq p \leq 1$, see Materials and Methods). Receptors are so specific that they are unable to recognize any MHC in the population will never be functional, and are considered to be pseudogenes. Thus, haplotypes expand by acquiring receptors with novel p values and signaling potential, but can also contract due to the accumulation of pseudogenes.

In this agent-based model, we also mimic the MHC-dependent NK cell education process (**Figure 1**). We remove iNKRs which fail to recognize any MHC molecule within an individual from the licensed repertoire. Similarly, those aNKRs capable of recognizing self-MHC molecules are deleted from the licensed repertoire. Only the licensed NKRs are able to participate during the immune response.

Infection of a host starts with a short acute phase, after which the individual either recovers or becomes chronically infected. We consider one wild-type virus and several decoy viruses (1 decoy per MHC molecule in the population). We do not allow for super-infection nor co-infection, thus hosts can be infected with only one of the viruses. A decoy virus down-regulates the expression of all MHC molecules within an individual, and expresses an MHC-like molecule. Thus, every virus expressing a decoy molecule has the potential to escape the immune response of both T and NK cells. The evolution of decoy proteins is modeled by allowing the virus to adopt a randomly selected MHC molecule from its host. Therefore, each decoy protein is actually an MHC molecule.

The population is first inoculated with the wild-type virus, which can be typically cleared after the acute phase because of the implicit response of both T and NK cells. We model the immune response with one parameter describing the probability of clearing the infection. For the wild-type virus, this is set to $p_{wt} = 0.85$ (**Table 1**), resulting in approximately 85% of the wild-type infections being cleared. Individuals clearing the infection become immune for a period t_i of 10 years. At steady state, approximately 20% of the population becomes chronically infected (**Figures 4A,B**; green solid lines), 65% become immune (**Figures 4A,B**; green dashed lines), and 5% are susceptible for infection. The immune escape of the decoy viruses is modeled by decreasing the clearance probability to zero ($p_{dec,1} = 0$, **Table 1**), which occurs if at least one of the licensed iNKRs or none of the aNKRs binds to the decoy molecule (**Table 2**). With this agent-based model, we can study the evolution of NKR specificity, and quantify the protection provided by activating and inhibitory receptors.

INHIBITORY RECEPTORS EVOLVE HIGHER SPECIFICITY THAN ACTIVATING RECEPTORS AFTER A CMV-LIKE INFECTION

We first study the protection provided by iNKRs against a CMV-like virus. After 5000 years of infection with the wild-type virus, we allow for the emergence of decoy viruses. The initial specificity of the iNKRs is set to $p \approx 0.4$ (see Materials and Methods). The decoy viruses spread easily among individuals carrying only iNKRs, resulting in a high fraction of chronically infected individuals (**Figure 4A**; red solid lines). Moreover, almost none of the hosts is able to control the infection (**Figure 4A**; red dashed lines), and the total population size decreases dramatically to 50% of the carrying capacity (i.e., maximal population size), confirming the results from the probabilistic model. However, after centuries of infection, the fraction of recovered individuals increases, and with it the total population size, indicating a recovery of the population. This observation is consistent in all ten simulations we performed for iNKRs (**Figures 4A,C**).

To study how these individuals evolve to control an infection with a virus having an MHC-like molecule, we analyze the average specificity of the NKRs over time. We determine how many MHC molecules in the population can be recognized by each receptor, and normalize it by the number of total MHC molecules in the population (**Figure 4E**; red line). We observe that the specificity increases after the emergence of the decoy viruses. At the end of the simulations, each iNKR recognize <20% of the MHC molecules in the population, indicating that evolution selects for specific iNKRs.

We perform the same simulations and analysis for populations having only aNKRs. Compared to populations having iNKRs, the initial spread of the virus is somewhat impaired (**Figure 4B**; red solid lines). Already at the beginning of the infection, some

Table 1 | Parameters of the agent-based model.

Parameter	Value
Time step	1 week
Simulation time	2 Million years
HOST PARAMETERS[a]	
Maximal population size, N_{max}	5000 Individuals
MHC diversity	1–2 Loci, each with 15 alleles
Number of NKR loci	5–10
Bit string length	16 Bits[b]
Host mutation rate, μ	0.00005 Per gene per birth event
INFECTION[c]	
Infection state, i	1 (Acute), 2 (chronic)
Effect of viral load on the death rate, VL_i	0.1 (For $i=1$), 0.06 (for $i=2$) per year
Probability of viral transmission during acute phase, p_{ac}	0.85 Per contact
Probability of viral transmission during chronic phase, p_{ch}	0.15 Per contact
Probability of clearing the wild-type virus, p_{wt}	0.85
Success state of the decoy virus, s	0 (Successful), 1 (unsuccessful)
Probability of clearing the virus evolving decoy molecules, $p_{dec,s}$	0 (For $s=0$), 0.5 (for $s=1$)
Immunity time, t_i	10 years
Acute infection time, t_{inf}	4 weeks
VIRUS PARAMETERS	
Virus mutation rate, μ_v[d]	0.0001 Per week
INITIAL CONDITIONS	
Initial population size, N_{init}	4500 Individuals
KIR initial diversity (SRI)	5–10 (1 Allele per locus)

[a]*The death and birth rate parameters are age-dependent and have been chosen according to a human population (33). For a full description of the age-dependency of birth and death rate, see Ref. (28).*

[b]*The choice to use 16-bit strings represents a large enough theoretical repertoire of 65,536 sequences.*

[c]*The parameters used for the infection are chosen to maintain the epidemic. Changing the length of the acute phase or the probabilities of clearance do not affect our results on the evolution of the NKRs qualitatively (results not shown).*

[d]*We manually switch on the mutation of the viruses at specific points in time, and after that the mutation rate determines the waiting time for the mutant to arrive. The mutant viruses appear in a short time scale and once the virus has spread in the population, mutation does not occur anymore. Since we analyze the genetic diversity long after the arrival of the virus, changes in mutation rate should not affect the outcome.*

individuals are able to control the virus (**Figure 4B**; red dashed lines). The population size decreases to 60% of the carrying capacity, and is therefore fitter than in those simulations considering only iNKRs (**Figures 4A–C**). Thus, aNKRs provide a better initial protection than iNKRs. Accordingly, the number of recovered individuals and thereby the total population increases rapidly, reflecting their fast recovery against viruses evolving decoy proteins.

The higher protection of aNKRs compared to iNKRs can be explained by the initial specificity. Because we initialize all populations with intermediate specificity, individuals carrying only aNKR are initially better protected (**Figure 2**). Nevertheless, aNKRs also evolve to be more specific (**Figure 4E**; black lines). At the end of the simulation, aNKRs recognize on average approximately 35% of all MHC molecules, and hence decoys in the population. Taken together, our agent-based model reveals that iNKRs need to be more specific than aNKRs to protect during an infection with a CMV-like virus, confirming the results from our probabilistic model.

Note that we do not explore all possible loci number in the agent-based model. To save computational time, we test the evolution of the specificity given a fixed loci number of NKRs. Populations carrying 10 NKR loci correspond to 20 NKRs in the probabilistic model, where the protection is maximal at very high specificity values for iNKR, and intermediate values for aNKR. These values correspond indeed to the specificity values that the populations evolve in our simulations. We carried out additional simulations for 5 and 15 NKR loci, the results of which confirmed the predictions of the mathematical model (results not shown).

POPULATIONS HAVING ONLY aNKRs EVOLVE A LARGER NKR POLYMORPHISM THAN POPULATIONS WITH ONLY iNKRs

Our probabilistic model predicts that the protection by iNKRs and aNKRs increases with the number of receptors per individual (**Figure 2**), because a large receptor number increases the chance of a host carrying very specific NKRs to have licensed receptors. This observation suggests that heterozygous hosts should have an advantage over homozygotes. We therefore hypothesized that heterozygous advantage must be selecting novel NKRs in our agent-based model, driving polymorphism of NKRs in the population.

To measure the polymorphism at population level, we use the Simpson's reciprocal index (SRI, see Materials and Methods). The SRI is a diversity measure that is equal to the total number of NKRs if they are equally distributed in the population, whereas the SRI is lower than that in a population where some alleles dominate (34).

The initial polymorphism of aNKRs (i.e., SRI = 10) increases over time (**Figure 4G**; black line), reflecting that a high number of aNKRs provides indeed an advantage. But surprisingly, this is not the case for iNKRs, where the diversity decreases to SRI = 7. Because the agent-based model considers a limited number of MHC molecules in the population, the specificity that the iNKRs evolve in the simulations is lower than that observed in the analytical model (i.e., $p_{i,\text{simulations}} \approx 0.18$ compared to $p_{i,\text{analytical}} = 0.10$) (see **Figure 2**). With this specificity value that is slightly lower than expected, all haplotypes tend to cover the entire (finite) MHC space, making it possible to have at least one licensed receptor. As a result, these populations can be well protected with a lower number of receptors. Therefore, there is little heterozygous advantage in populations having only iNKRs, resulting in a low level of polymorphism. Thus, the agent-based model finds a different solution for an optimal protection: it evolves contracted haplotypes (i.e., composed only of seven receptors) with slightly less specific iNKRs than expected.

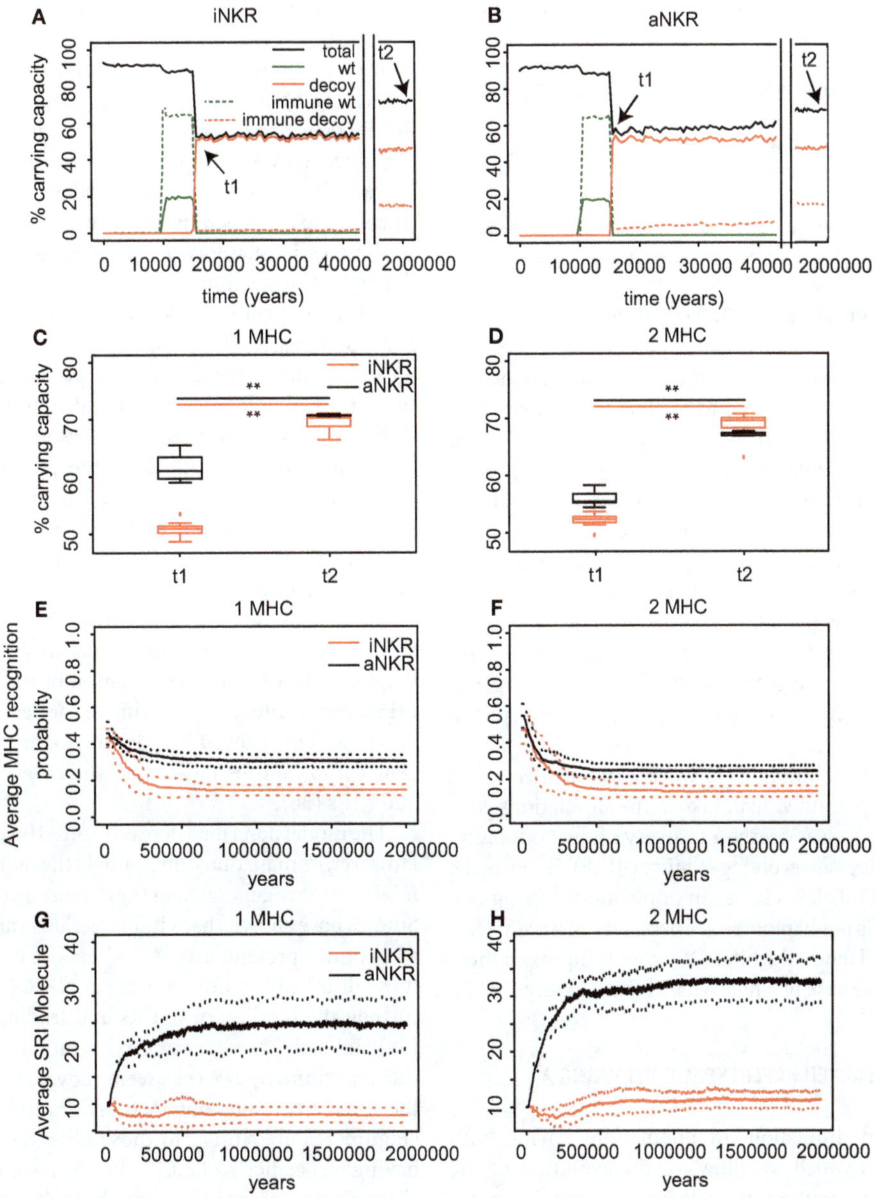

FIGURE 4 | Agent-based model confirms probabilistic model. (A) A host population having only iNKRs was inoculated with a wild-type virus (green lines) after a period of $t = 5000$ years (green solid lines show the chronically infected individuals and the dashed lines the immune individuals). Ten thousand years after the initial epidemic (i.e., t_1), we allowed for the evolution of decoy viruses (red lines). During the wild-type infection, most individuals recover (dashed green line). In contrast, almost none of the individuals are initially capable of clearing a CMV-like infection (red dashed line), resulting in a large decrease of the total population size (black line). **(B)** A host population having only aNKRs is initially better protected against decoy viruses, resulting in a higher fraction of the population clearing the infection, and a lower decrease of the total population size. **(A,B)** Show single representative simulations. **(C)** The average population size during the initial spread of decoy viruses (t_1) is lower than that at the end of the simulations (i.e., $t_2 = 3$ million years), indicating that over time, the populations learn to cope with the viral infection. Individuals in simulations considering only aNKRs (black) are initially better protected than those in simulations considering only iNKRs (red). In these simulations, all hosts carry only one MHC locus. **(D)** The initial advantage that aNKRs have over iNKRs receptors decreases in simulations considering two MHC loci per individual. **(E)** The probability of iNKRs recognizing any random MHC molecule in the population decreases over time (red line), indicating that more specific receptors are being selected for. In contrast, aNKRs (black line) do not evolve such high degree of specificity. **(F)** aNKRs evolve to become more specific in simulations where individuals have two MHC loci. **(G)** The degree of NKR polymorphism (expressed as the SRI score) increases in time, as a result of the evolved higher specificity. **(H)** SRI score in simulations considering two MHC loci. In **(C,D)**, the boxes represent the interquartile range, and the thick horizontal lines the median out of ten simulations (**represent p values < 0.005 and were calculated using the Mann–Whitney U test). In **(E–H)**, the solid lines represent the average out of ten simulations, and the dashed lines are the standard deviation.

Table 2 | Levels of protection against a decoy virus in the agent-based model.

	No. of $aNKR_{binding} = 0$	No. of $aNKR_{binding} > 0$
No. of $iNKR_{binding} = 0$	$p_{dec,1}$	$p_{dec,1}$
No. of $iNKR_{binding} > 0$	$p_{dec,0}$	$p_{dec,1}$

$aNKR_{binding}$ and $iNKR_{binding}$ refer to the number of iNKRs and aNKRs binding the decoy molecule, respectively. The receptors here are considered to be licensed.

PROTECTION DEPENDS ON THE NUMBER OF MHC LOCI

To confirm our results concerning the dependency on MHC loci number, we also perform simulations with individuals having two MHC loci. An increasing number of MHC loci has a large effect on the protection provided by aNKRs. Although these populations are initialized with intermediate specific NKRs, the initial protection is lower than in the population carrying only one MHC locus (**Figure 4D**). For better protection, a higher specificity is required, and the selection for more specific aNKRs is stronger in these simulations (**Figure 4F**). As a result of the higher specificity, a larger number of receptors per haplotype are necessary to become licensed and to recognize the foreign decoy molecules. Therefore, the advantage of heterozygotes over homozygotes is larger in these populations, resulting in a higher degree of polymorphism (**Figure 4H**).

The protection and evolution of iNKRs is less sensitive to the number of MHC loci per individual. Like in the simulations considering one MHC locus, we observe a recovery of the population as more specific receptors are evolving (**Figures 4D,F**). Because the total number of MHC alleles is larger in populations having two MHC loci, more iNKRs per haplotype are necessary to have at least one licensed receptor. Hence, the total SRI score is higher in these simulations, than in the case of single MHC locus (**Figures 4G,H**; red line).

BASIN OF ATTRACTION: MIXED HAPLOTYPES CONTAINING A MAJORITY OF aNKRs

Finally, we performed simulations of populations having both iNKRs and aNKRs, in which we allow for the evolution of the specificity and also the receptor type. The initial specificity values for both receptor types was intermediate (i.e., $p \approx 0.4$) and we initialized the genotypes with a random number of activating and inhibitory receptors.

After the appearance of decoy viruses, the populations suffered similar effects to those having only iNKRs and aNKRs. The population size decreases dramatically at first, and with time it recovers. The final population size is higher than in the simulations considering only one type of receptor, approaching 70% of the carrying capacity (**Figure 5A**) because mixed haplotypes protect better than only one type of receptors. At the end of the simulations, we observe more aNKRs than iNKRs per haplotype (**Figure 5B**), i.e., the final haplotypes are composed on average of 6 aNKRs and 4 iNKRs. In agreement with the predictions of the analytical model, both receptor types evolve high specificity (i.e., $p \leq 0.35$), and a high polymorphism (**Figures 5C,D**). Summarizing, the agent-based model confirms the prediction of the probabilistic model.

CONCLUSION AND DISCUSSION

Our mathematical model predicts the optimal protection level provided by inhibiting and activating NKRs against viruses expressing MHC-like molecules. Haplotypes composed only of iNKRs detect the viral infection within a small range, requiring high specificity and large haplotype size. In contrast, the maximal protection is reached for intermediate specificity values and at a smaller haplotype size in individuals having only aNKRs. Mixed haplotypes, i.e., haplotypes carrying both iNKRs and aNKRs offer the highest protection.

All these results are dependent on the number of MHC loci per individual. With increasing MHC loci, aNKRs lose their ability to become licensed and thus provide little or no protection. In contrast, haplotypes composed only of iNKR have a higher chance of having licensed receptors when the number of MHC loci is increased. In this case, the protection level is maximal already with a contracted NKR haplotype. Thus, there seem to be several combinations of MHC–NKR genotypes that provide maximal protection. A high protection is reached with a simple MHC complex and a high number of NKR genes. With increasing complexity of the MHC, a contracted NK complex is sufficient to render protection. These last results are particularly interesting, as they provide a possible explanation of the differences in KIR and MHC gene content across primate species (35), and the expansion of new KIR lineages corresponding to the contraction of the MHC gene complex, thus illustrating the co-evolution of MHC class I and KIRs (36).

The model described here is inspired by viruses evolving decoys. However, its main outcome, namely the requirement for specificity, might be more general than the defense against such decoy viruses. Studies have shown that viral infections can change the repertoire of peptides presented by MHC class I molecules (37), and that these different peptides affect the NKR–MHC interactions, perturbing the binding of iNKRs and leading to NK cell activation (38). In such cases, specific recognition of the changes in peptide repertoire by NK cells seems advantageous for the host. Also, the specificity ranges obtained in our model for mixed haplotypes (**Figure 3E**) are similar to those observed in reality, with iNKRs having a specificity of 0.2. This corresponds to the four mutually exclusive epitopes that have been detected so far for inhibitory KIRs in humans: HLA-A11, -Bw4, -C1, and -C2.

The exact role of aNKRs remains intriguing. Since only a few aNKRs tend to recognize MHC class I molecules (39), we speculate that aNKRs could specifically recognize new ligands expressed upon viral infection (e.g., decoy molecules or stress ligands). Our model predicts that to face the challenge of not recognizing self but specifically recognize foreign antigens, aNKRs do not need to be so specific. Indeed, the haplotype providing the highest protection is a combined haplotype composed of more aNKRs than iNKRs, which disagrees with the most primate KIR haplotypes (36). Most primate NKRs are inhibitory, and activating receptors have been linked to selection pressure induced by reproduction (36). Our model predicts that aNKRs should evolve to an intermediate specificity upon CMV-like infections. However, not many activating ligands have been identified yet, and it remains puzzling what other roles aNKRs might play.

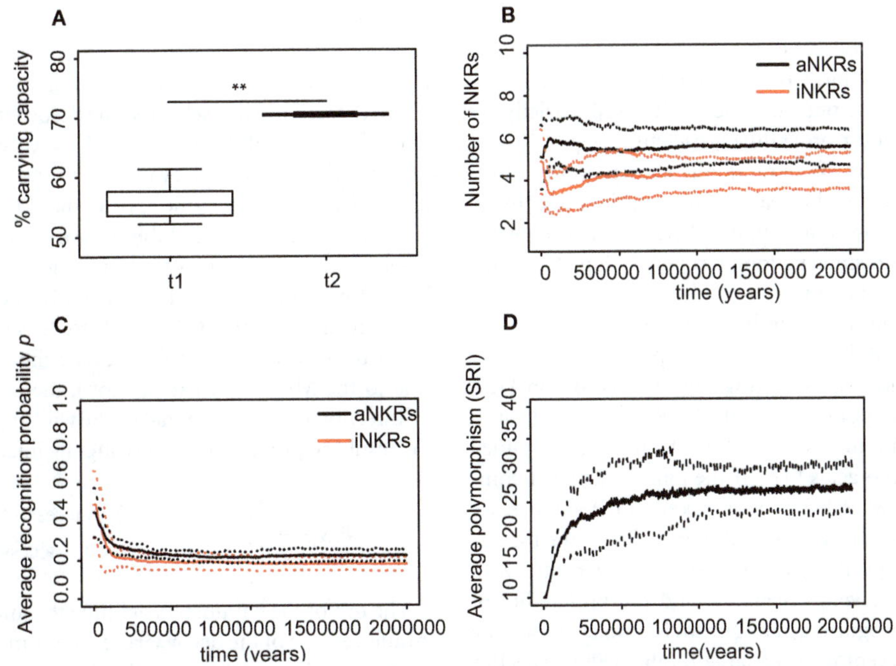

FIGURE 5 | Mixed haplotypes offer the highest protection. A host population having iNKRs and aNKRs was inoculated with a wild-type virus after a period of $t = 5000$ years; we allowed for the evolution of decoy viruses 10,000 years after the initial epidemic (i.e., t_1). **(A)** The population size during the initial spread of decoy viruses (t_1) is lower than that at the end of the simulations (i.e., $t_2 = 3$ million years), indicating that over time, the population recovers from the viral infection. **(B)** The number initial haplotype is composed of five iNKRs and five aNKRs. The number of aNKRs and iNKRs per haplotype varies over time, resulting in a selection for haplotypes with a larger activating potential. **(C)** The probability of NKRs recognizing any random MHC molecule in the population, decreases over time, indicating that more specific receptors are being selected for. **(D)** The degree of NKR polymorphism (expressed as the SRI score) increases in time, as a result of the heterozygote advantage due to the evolved higher specificity. Averages are taken out of ten different simulations. In **(A)**, the boxes represent the interquartile range, and the thick horizontal lines the median (** represent p values <0.005, and were calculated using the Mann–Whitney U test). In **(B–D)**, the solid lines represent the average out of ten simulations, and the dashed lines are the standard deviation.

The expansion of NKR superfamilies, presumably in order to gain resistance against pathogens, illustrates the high evolutionary complexity of NKRs. We aimed to fully understand the effects of a single possible driving force of this evolutionary process, namely that of a viral encoded MHC-like molecule. Therefore, we focused on modeling only the evolution of NKRs in a simple model, which requires simplifying assumptions. For instance, we fixed MHC polymorphism despite the evidence of the co-evolution between MHC class I and KIRs (35, 36). Given their different evolutionary timescales, i.e., that MHC molecules are older than both Ly49 and KIRs, we chose to model the expansion and contraction of NKR systems within an already existing MHC diversity. Additionally, we assumed that decoy viruses down-regulate the expression of all MHC molecules in the host. Even though we do not expect selective MHC down-regulation to affect the evolution of aNKRs (since activating receptors cannot detect missing-self), the evolution of iNKRs might be affected because more licensed iNKRs will be necessary to recognize a virus that down-regulates only one of the host's MHC-I molecules. Note that if the licensed repertoire of iNKRs is larger, these receptors should be even more specific to avoid being "fooled" by the decoy molecule. The exact effect of selective MHC down-regulation on the specificity of iNKRs is an open interesting question, which we are currently working on.

Other simplifying assumptions were also necessary, such as considering a global NKR repertoire and ignoring the synergy between NKRs or the direct interaction between immune cells. Additionally, we ignored mutational operators that conserve similarity between pre- and post-mutation receptors (e.g., point mutations), as we only model mutations that significantly change receptor functionality. Including point mutations, did not affect the results qualitatively (results not shown), however a longer evolutionary time was necessary to approach the same solution of specificity. Overall, since our main results are of a qualitative nature, it seems unlikely that relaxing any of these assumptions would affect our main results. Note also that our agent-based model is inspired on humans and KIRs, with the advantage of having realistic parameters for processes like birth and death. However, the model can be generalized to other species, and qualitatively it represents a model of the evolution of the expansion of the NKR complex.

All our analytical results were consistent with the agent-based model and our analysis allowed us to quantify the protection against an infection for both receptor types. It confirmed our previous results that iNKRs should become specific enough (28). Our new approach has shed light into the possible contribution that each receptor type confers upon infection, and allowed us to conclude that mixed haplotypes render the best protection.

MATERIALS AND METHODS

AGENT-BASED MODEL

The agent-based model consists of two types of actors (hosts and viruses) and three events (birth, death, and infection). This model is virtually identical to the one published in Ref. (28). Briefly, we screen all hosts in a random order during each time step of 1 week, and confront them to one of the randomly chosen events. Hosts age over time and at the end of each time step, their age, infection state, and type of infection is updated. This cycle is repeated for two million years to simulate long term evolution. All model parameters are given in **Table 1**.

We model simplified diploid individuals, carrying gene complexes for NKR and MHC class I. For simplicity, we consider 15 MHC alleles per locus, resembling the most common HLA alleles in the European population (40). NKRs and their ligands are modeled with randomly generated bit strings as a simplified representation of amino acids (41). If the longest adjacent complementary match between two strings exceeds a threshold L, we allow for the receptor to interact with its ligand. Thus, the threshold L determines the specificity of each receptor: a receptor with a small L value will be very degenerate and the probability of a random NKR to recognize a random MHC molecule will be $p \approx 1$. In contrast, a receptor with a large L value will be specific, and accordingly, the probability of this receptor binding any MHC molecule in the population will be $p \sim 0$ [for a detailed description, see Ref. (28)].

RECEPTOR TYPES

In the present model, we allow for the evolution of aNKRs. When a novel NKR is generated, a random L value between 1 and 16 is assigned to it, and its type (i.e., whether it is activating or inhibitory) is also randomly chosen. Thus, each receptor has its particular specificity and functionality. Receptors with L values larger than 13 will usually not recognize any MHC molecules in the population, and are typically not functional. Genes encoding such non-functional NKRs are considered to be pseudogenes. Haplotypes containing pseudogenes are effectively shorter than haplotypes composed of fully functional NKRs. Thus, we can model the contraction and expansion of the NKR gene complex.

VIRAL INFECTIONS

In our simulations, we consider one wild-type virus and several "decoy viruses," i.e., viruses expressing MHC decoys. Each virus comes with a viral load, which is implemented as an increase of the host's death rate, VL_i depending on the infection state i (see **Table 1**), and a probability of clearing the infection p_{wt} and $p_{dec,s}$ for the wild-type and the decoy viruses, respectively. A decoy virus down-regulates the expression of all MHC molecules in that host, and encodes one MHC-like molecule. The evolution of decoy molecules is modeled by allowing the virus to adopt a randomly selected MHC molecule from its host with a rate μ_v. The virus keeps this decoy for the rest of the simulation. Because we fix the MHC polymorphism to 15 alleles per locus, the maximal number of decoy proteins that can evolve in the population is 15 for the simulations considering 1 MHC locus, and 30 for those considering two MHC loci.

We consider different levels of protection against a decoy virus, depending on the success of the virus to escape the NK cell response, s. If at least one of the licensed iNKR binds to the decoy molecule, there will be an inhibitory signal, the host will not be able to detect "missing-self," and the decoy virus will be successful. Similarly, if none of the licensed aNKRs recognizes the decoy molecule, the decoy virus will evade the NK cell response. Thus, none of the iNKRs or at least one aNKRs should bind the decoy molecule to render protection (**Table 2**). We model the immune escape by setting the probability of clearing the infection to zero, letting the host become chronically infected. In the case that a decoy is not successful, the host will be able to detect "missing-self." Since this virus is nevertheless able to evade the response from T cells (due to the MHC down-regulation), the probability of clearing the infection is lower than that of the wild-type virus ($p_{wt} = 0.85$). The resulting probability of clearing the infection is described by:

$$p_{dec,s} = \begin{cases} 0, & \text{if } s = 0 \text{ (successful decoy)} \\ 0.5, & \text{if } s = 1 \text{ (unsuccessful decoy)}. \end{cases} \quad (5)$$

The rest of the parameters defining the infection dynamics and immune escape of the decoy viruses (i.e., time of infection, immunity time, and transmission probabilities) were set like in Ref. (28) and are described in **Table 1**.

MUTATION

During each birth event, NKRs undergo mutation with a probability, μ. To decrease computation time, we model mutation by randomly creating a new receptor with its particular specificity and signaling type. We do not consider other mutational operators, e.g., point mutations, recombination, deletion, or duplication.

We first perform simulations where only the specificity can evolve (i.e., a random value L is assigned to each new receptor), while the receptor type remains fixed. Hereby, we are able to compare what the basin of attraction for the specificity will be, if a population has only aNKRs or only iNKRs. We also simulate populations with mixed haplotypes, by allowing the receptor type to mutate.

NK CELL EDUCATION

During the birth event, an NK cell education process takes place. Like in our probabilistic model explained above, iNKRs which recognize *at least one* of the MHC molecules within one individual, and aNKRs that fail to recognize *all* of the MHC molecules within the host, are set to be licensed. In our model, only the licensed repertoire of NKRs will participate in an NK cell response (**Figure 1**).

MODEL INITIALIZATION

The model is initialized with a host population of 4500 hosts, with random ages between 1 and 70 years corresponding to a uniform age distribution. After approximately 10 host generations, this age distribution corresponds to more modern age distributions with the majority of individuals having an age between 15 and 60.

At the start of every simulation, a gene pool for MHC alleles is generated, the size of which depends on the number of MHC loci per individual. It consists of 15 alleles in simulations considering one MHC locus per individual, and of 30 alleles in those simulations considering two MHC loci per individual. To create the initial genome of each individual, MHC genes were randomly drawn from the pool, while ten NKRs with intermediate specificity ($2 \leq L \leq 4$, i.e., $p \approx 0.4$) were generated. Thus, the initial haplotypes did not contain any pseudogenes. In the simulations considering mixed NKR haplotypes, the initial genes can be both activating and inhibitory. The type of each receptor was randomly chosen as explained above, resulting in approximately 50% of the receptors being activating. All individuals were initialized with the same NKR haplotype, but with different MHC genes.

GENETIC DIVERSITY

The Simpson's Index is a measurement of diversity that can be interpreted as the probability that two randomly chosen receptors from two random hosts in the population are identical (34). The reciprocal of the Simpson's Index defines a "weighted" diversity. The SRI was calculated as follows: $\mathrm{SRI} = \frac{1}{\sum_{i=1}^{N} f_i^2}$, where f_i is the frequency of the receptor i over all NKRs in the population, and N is the total number of unique NKRs.

IMPLEMENTATION

The model was implemented in the C++ programing language. We considered populations with haplotypes composed of only aNKRs, only iNKRs, or both. In every scenario, we compared the effects of one or two MHC loci per individual. For each of these settings, we performed ten simulations for 2 million years. The code is available upon request.

ACKNOWLEDGMENTS

We thank Chris van Dorp, Leïla Perie, and Hanneke van Deutekom for helpful discussions and carefully reading the manuscript. We also thank Oussama Jarrousse and Johannes Textor for their technical support during the development of the code. This work was financially supported by the CLS program of the Netherlands Organization for Scientific Research (NWO), grant 635.100.025. This study was also supported by the "Virgo consortium," funded by the Dutch government (project number FES0908) and by the "Netherlands Genomics Initiative (NGI)" (project number 050-060-452). The funders had no role in study design, data collection and analysis, decision to publish, or preparation of the manuscript.

REFERENCES

1. Lanier LL. Evolutionary struggles between NK cells and viruses. *Nat Rev Immunol* (2008) **8**(4):259–68. doi:10.1038/nri2276
2. Lanier LL. NK cell recognition. *Annu Rev Immunol* (2005) **23**:225–74. doi:10.1146/annurev.immunol.23.021704.115526
3. Ljunggren HG, Kärre K. In search of the "missing self": MHC molecules and NK cell recognition. *Immunol Today* (1990) **11**(7):237–44. doi:10.1016/0167-5699(90)90097-S
4. O'Callaghan CA. Molecular basis of human natural killer cell recognition of HLA-E (human leukocyte antigen-E) and its relevance to clearance of pathogen-infected and tumour cells. *Clin Sci (Lond)* (2000) **99**(1):9–17. doi:10.1042/CS19990334
5. Braud VM, Allan DS, O'Callaghan CA, Söderström K, D'Andrea A, Ogg GS, et al. HLA-E binds to natural killer cell receptors CD94/NKG2A, B and C. *Nature* (1998) **391**(6669):795–9. doi:10.1038/35869
6. Shum BP, Flodin LR, Muir DG, Rajalingam R, Khakoo SI, Cleland S, et al. Conservation and variation in human and common chimpanzee CD94 and NKG2 genes. *J Immunol* (2002) **168**(1):240–52.
7. Trowsdale J, Barten R, Haude A, Stewart CA, Beck S, Wilson MJ. The genomic context of natural killer receptor extended gene families. *Immunol Rev* (2001) **181**:20–38. doi:10.1034/j.1600-065X.2001.1810102.x
8. Moesta AK, Parham P. Diverse functionality among human NK cell receptors for the C1 epitope of HLA-C: KIR2DS2, KIR2DL2, and KIR2DL3. *Front Immunol* (2012) **3**:336. doi:10.3389/fimmu.2012.00336
9. Jiang W, Johnson C, Jayaraman J, Simecek N, Noble J, Moffatt MF, et al. Copy number variation leads to considerable diversity for B but not A haplotypes of the human KIR genes encoding NK cell receptors. *Genome Res* (2012) **22**(10):1845–54. doi:10.1101/gr.137976.112
10. Vilches C, Parham P. KIR: diverse, rapidly evolving receptors of innate and adaptive immunity. *Annu Rev Immunol* (2002) **20**:217–51. doi:10.1146/annurev.immunol.20.092501.134942
11. Kelley J, Walter L, Trowsdale J. Comparative genomics of natural killer cell receptor gene clusters. *PLoS Genet* (2005) **1**(2):e27. doi:10.1371/journal.pgen.0010027
12. Guethlein LA, Older Aguilar AM, Abi-Rached L, Parham P. Evolution of killer cell Ig-like receptor (KIR) genes: definition of an orangutan KIR haplotype reveals expansion of lineage III KIR associated with the emergence of MHC-C. *J Immunol* (2007) **179**(1):491–504.
13. Anfossi N, André P, Guia S, Falk CS, Roetynck S, Stewart CA, et al. Human NK cell education by inhibitory receptors for MHC class I. *Immunity* (2006) **25**(2):331–42. doi:10.1016/j.immuni.2006.06.013
14. Wilhelm BT, Gagnier L, Mager DL. Sequence analysis of the ly49 cluster in C57BL/6 mice: a rapidly evolving multigene family in the immune system. *Genomics* (2002) **80**(6):646–61. doi:10.1006/geno.2002.7004
15. Wilhelm BT, Mager DL. Rapid expansion of the Ly49 gene cluster in rat. *Genomics* (2004) **84**(1):218–21. doi:10.1016/j.ygeno.2004.01.010
16. Körner C, Altfeld M. Role of KIR3DS1 in human diseases. *Front Immunol* (2012) **3**:326. doi:10.3389/fimmu.2012.00326
17. Pelak K, Need AC, Fellay J, Shianna KV, Feng S, Urban TJ, et al. Copy number variation of KIR genes influences HIV-1 control. *PLoS Biol* (2011) **9**(11):e1001208. doi:10.1371/journal.pbio.1001208
18. Martin MP, Gao X, Lee J-H, Nelson GW, Detels R, Goedert JJ, et al. Epistatic interaction between KIR3DS1 and HLA-B delays the progression to AIDS. *Nat Genet* (2002) **31**(4):429–34. doi:10.1038/ng934
19. Zhi-Ming L, Yu-lian J, Zhao-lei F, Chun-xiao W, Zhen-fang D, Bing-chang Z, et al. Polymorphisms of killer cell immunoglobulin-like receptor gene: possible association with susceptibility to or clearance of hepatitis B virus infection in Chinese Han population. *Croat Med J* (2007) **48**(6):800–6. doi:10.3325/cmj.2007.6.800
20. López-Vázquez A, Rodrigo L, Martínez-Borra J, Pérez R, Rodríguez M, Fdez-Morera JL, et al. Protective effect of the HLA-Bw4I80 epitope and the killer cell immunoglobulin-like receptor 3DS1 gene against the development of hepatocellular carcinoma in patients with hepatitis C virus infection. *J Infect Dis* (2005) **192**(1):162–5. doi:10.1086/430351
21. Besson C, Roetynck S, Williams F, Orsi L, Amiel C, Lependeven C, et al. Association of killer cell immunoglobulin-like receptor genes with Hodgkin's lymphoma in a familial study. *PLoS One* (2007) **2**(5):e406. doi:10.1371/journal.pone.0000406
22. Hiby SE, Apps R, Sharkey AM, Farrell LE, Gardner L, Mulder A, et al. Maternal activating KIRs protect against human reproductive failure mediated by fetal HLA-C2. *J Clin Invest* (2010) **120**(11):4102–10. doi:10.1172/JCI43998
23. Smith HR, Heusel JW, Mehta IK, Kim S, Dorner BG, Naidenko OV, et al. Recognition of a virus-encoded ligand by a natural killer cell activation receptor. *Proc Natl Acad Sci U S A* (2002) **99**(13):8826–31. doi:10.1073/pnas.092258599
24. Arase H, Mocarski ES, Campbell AE, Hill AB, Lanier LL. Direct recognition of cytomegalovirus by activating and inhibitory NK cell receptors. *Science* (2002) **296**(5571):1323–6. doi:10.1126/science.1070884
25. Abi-Rached L, Parham P. Natural selection drives recurrent formation of activating killer cell immunoglobulin-like receptor and Ly49 from inhibitory homologues. *J Exp Med* (2005) **201**(8):1319–32. doi:10.1084/jem.20042558
26. Arase H, Lanier LL. Virus-driven evolution of natural killer cell receptors. *Microbes Infect* (2002) **4**(15):1505–12. doi:10.1016/S1286-4579(02)00033-3
27. Sun JC, Lanier LL. The natural selection of herpesviruses and virus-specific NK cell receptors. *Viruses* (2009) **1**(3):362. doi:10.3390/v1030362
28. Carrillo-Bustamante P, Kesmir C, de Boer RJ. Virus encoded MHC-like decoys diversify the inhibitory KIR repertoire. *PLoS Comput Biol* (2013) **9**(10):e1003264. doi:10.1371/journal.pcbi.1003264

29. Elliott JM, Yokoyama WM. Unifying concepts of MHC-dependent natural killer cell education. *Trends Immunol* (2011) **32**(8):364–72. doi:10.1016/j.it.2011.06.001
30. Chalifour A, Scarpellino L, Back J, Brodin P, Devèvre E, Gros F, et al. A role for cis interaction between the inhibitory Ly49A receptor and MHC class I for natural killer cell education. *Immunity* (2009) **30**(3):337–47. doi:10.1016/j.immuni.2008.12.019
31. Sun JC, Lanier LL. Tolerance of NK cells encountering their viral ligand during development. *J Exp Med* (2008) **205**(8):1819–28. doi:10.1084/jem.20072448
32. Fauriat C, Ivarsson MA, Ljunggren HG, Malmberg KJ, Michaëlsson J. Education of human natural killer cells by activating killer cell immunoglobulin-like receptors. *Blood* (2010) **115**(6):1166–74. doi:10.1182/blood-2009-09-245746
33. Carnes BA, Holden LR, Olshansky SJ, Witten MT, Siegel JS. Mortality partitions and their relevance to research on senescence. *Biogerontology* (2006) **7**(4):183–98. doi:10.1007/s10522-006-9020-3
34. Simpson E. Measurement of diversity. *Nature* (1949) **163**:688. doi:10.1038/163688a0
35. Sambrook JG, Bashirova A, Palmer S, Sims S, Trowsdale J, Abi-Rached L, et al. Single haplotype analysis demonstrates rapid evolution of the killer immunoglobulin-like receptor (KIR) loci in primates. *Genome Res* (2005) **15**(1):25–35. doi:10.1101/gr.2381205
36. Parham P, Moffett A. Variable NK cell receptors and their MHC class I ligands in immunity, reproduction and human evolution. *Nat Rev Immunol* (2013) **13**(2):133–44. doi:10.1038/nri3370
37. Hickman HD, Luis AD, Bardet W, Buchli R, Battson CL, Shearer MH, et al. Cutting edge: class I presentation of host peptides following HIV infection. *J Immunol* (2003) **171**(1):22–6.
38. Fadda L, O'Connor GM, Kumar S, Piechocka-Trocha A, Gardiner CM, Carrington M, et al. Common HIV-1 peptide variants mediate differential binding of KIR3DL1 to HLA-Bw4 molecules. *J Virol* (2011) **85**(12):5970–4. doi:10.1128/JVI.00412-11
39. Moesta AK, Graef T, Abi-Rached L, Older Aguilar AM, Guethlein LA, Parham P. Humans differ from other hominids in lacking an activating NK cell receptor that recognizes the C1 epitope of MHC class I. *J Immunol* (2010) **185**(7):4233–7. doi:10.4049/jimmunol.1001951
40. Meyer D, Singe R, Mack S, Lancaster A, Nelson M, Erlich H, et al. Single locus polymorphism of classical HLA genes. In: Hansen JA, editor. *Immunobiology of the Human MHC: Proceedings of the 13th International Histocompatibility Workshop and Conference.* (Vol. 1), Seattle, WA: IHWG Press (2007). p. 653–704.
41. Farmer JD, Packard NH, Perelson AS. The immune system, adaptation, and machine learning. *Physica D* (1986) **22**:187–204. doi:10.1016/0167-2789(86)90240-X

APPENDIX

GLOBAL REPERTOIRE OF LICENSED NKRs

Instead of considering individual NK cells expressing a tuned set of NKRs, we model a global repertoire of "licensed" NKRs in each host. Hereby, we assume that the expression of at least one "licensed" receptor is sufficient to educate NK cells, and that those functional NK cells can become activated upon viral infection. This assumption needs further explanation.

If an aNKR recognizes some self-molecule (or self-MHC), all developing NK cells expressing that receptor should additionally express at least one iNKR recognizing self to prevent self-reactivity. As a consequence, all NK cells expressing that aNKR should never become activated, even if a virus encodes a ligand which engages that aNKR. Therefore, we call such an aNKR "unlicensed": it will never contribute to detect a viral infection. In contrast, if an aNKR that does not recognize any self-molecule, all developing NK cells expressing that receptor will not be influenced by it, and these cells will express other iNKRs and aNKRs that balance their self-reactivity. NK cells expressing that aNKR will become activated when a virus expressing its ligand engages that aNKR. Therefore we call such an aNKR "licensed." Any NK cell expressing this aNKR should breach its activation threshold, expand, and protect, when the ligand is present.

Now consider an iNKR that recognizes some self-MHC. All developing NK cells expressing that receptor will be tuned to balance its self-reactivity. As a consequence, all NK cells expressing that iNKR should become activated when a virus down-regulates this particular MHC. Therefore, we call such an iNKR "licensed": it detects MHC down-regulation. However, for an iNKR that does not recognize any self-MHC, the developing NK cells expressing that receptor will not be influenced by that iNKR. Consequently, these cells will express other iNKRs and other aNKRs in order to balance their self-reactivity. Therefore, NK cells expressing that iNKR will not become activated by this iNKR when a virus down-regulates self-MHC. Therefore, we call such an iNKR "unlicensed": it would never contribute to the detection of virus infected cells.

What happens with the NK cells expressing such an unlicensed iNKR if it happens to recognize something else on virus infected cells, e.g., a decoy? Then the iNKR should deliver an extra inhibitory signal to those cells. Consequently, these NK cells cannot expand and protect, even if their other iNKR detect MHC down-regulation, or if their other aNKR detect a new ligand. Hence, such an unlicensed iNKR will not protect, and can be considered to be non-functional at the repertoire level.

17

Gut microbiota and the paradox of cancer immunotherapy

Theofilos Poutahidis[1,2], Markus Kleinewietfeld[3,4,5] and Susan E. Erdman[1]*

[1] Division of Comparative Medicine, Massachusetts Institute of Technology, Cambridge, MA, USA
[2] Laboratory of Pathology, Faculty of Veterinary Medicine, Aristotle University of Thessaloniki, Thessaloniki, Greece
[3] Departments of Neurology and Immunobiology, Yale School of Medicine, New Haven, CT, USA
[4] Broad Institute, Massachusetts Institute of Technology and Harvard University, Cambridge, MA, USA
[5] Faculty of Medicine, Dresden University of Technology (TUD), Dresden, Germany

Edited by:
Fang-Ping Huang, Imperial College London, UK

Reviewed by:
Graham Robert Leggatt, University of Queensland, Australia
Yong Lu, Cleveland Clinic Foundation, USA

***Correspondence:**
Susan E. Erdman, Massachusetts Institute of Technology, 77 Mass Avenue, Cambridge, MA 02139, USA
e-mail: serdman@mit.edu

It is recently shown that beneficial environmental microbes stimulate integrated immune and neuroendocrine factors throughout the body, consequently modulating regulatory T-lymphocyte phenotypes, maintaining systemic immune balance, and determining the fate of preneoplastic lesions toward regression while sustaining whole body good health. Stimulated by a gut microbiota-centric systemic homeostasis hypothesis, we set out to explore the influence of the gut microbiome to explain the paradoxical roles of regulatory T-lymphocytes in cancer development and growth. This paradigm shift places cancer prevention and treatment into a new broader context of holobiont engineering to cultivate a tumor-suppressive macroenvironment.

Keywords: tumor macroenvironment, regulatory T-cells, cancer immunotherapy, inflammation and cancer, probiotic bacteria

INTRODUCTION

The neoplastic process is characterized by overwhelming complexity. Cancer is comprised of a genetically unstable population of cells that proliferate at an extraordinarily high rate. Millions of cancer deaths each year make it obvious that the battle against cancer is asymmetric, with humankind often being the weaker element (1). To date, cancer research efforts directly confront malignancy by targeting properties of individual cancer cells. In 2000, Hanahan and Weinberg described that most of the research on origins and treatment of cancer had just contributed toward "adding further layers of complexity to a scientific literature that is already complex almost beyond measure" (2).

In the same landmark paper, however, the authors were optimistic enough to predict groundbreaking upcoming advances in the conceptual rather than the technical level (2). They were proven right. One such advancement was the increased awareness for the importance of the tumor microenvironment in the etiopathogenesis of neoplasia (3, 4). We now know that initially transformed cells are much less autonomous in their growth than previously thought (5, 6). Among the microenvironment elements, immune cells and factors have emerged as fundamental players (4–6). Accumulating evidence suggests that tumor-associated inflammatory cell accumulation, whether overt or smoldering, could be viewed as a tumor-promoting event (7–9). These inflammatory responses enhance mutagenesis by oxidative DNA damage and shape the tumor stroma in favor of cancer cell survival and expansion (6, 10, 11).

Will this knowledge base in the field of inflammation, immunity, and cancer lead to new, highly effective, and biologically safe cancer immunotherapy modalities? We assert that the outcome will depend upon the philosophy and the strategic goals that will dominate the bench-to-bedside research. We propose that research in this field should focus upon stimulating systemic innate immune balance and adaptive immune resiliency, making the mammalian host more powerful to resist its cancer challenger. One possible approach utilizes gut microbiota or microbial antigens to stimulate beneficial immune cells. On the other hand, existing immunotherapy aims to selectively interrupt immune factors to better recognize and exterminate cancer cells (12–17), an approach that may ultimately lead to host instability. To further explain this point of view, we will refer to the recently discovered paradoxical roles of regulatory T-cells (T_{REG}) in cancer (10, 14).

T_{REG} ARE CENTRAL IN PRESERVING SYSTEMIC IMMUNE HOMEOSTASIS AND GOOD HEALTH

$FOXP3^+$ $CD4^+$ $CD25^{+/high}$ T_{REG} are dominant cellular elements of the professional suppressor arm of the immune system and are important for orchestrating the control of peripheral immunological tolerance (18). The transcription factor FOXP3 is a fundamental regulator of T_{REG} function in rodents and humans, and so far the most reliable phenotypic indicator of their identity. Recent studies on human T_{REG} subpopulations, however, revealed that low but discernible levels of FOXP3 expression could be detected in non-suppressive T_{REG} or even in activated effector T-cells. It is probable that this finding reflects the inherent plasticity of T_{REG}; $FOXP3^+$ cells co-expressing effector T-cell phenotypic markers or cytokines may be in stages of a progressive, epigenetically regulated, phenotypical, and functional shift process (14, 16, 19–22), ultimately favorable for healthful recovery of the host after environmental challenges. The role of T_{REG} is central in preserving immune system homeostasis for health and the balance of beneficial inflammatory responses during infections while minimizing collateral tissue damage. In cancer, however, roles of T_{REG} are traditionally considered to be negative (14–16, 23).

T_{REG} GATHER NEAR TUMORS AND FAVOR CANCER SURVIVAL

A large body of data suggest that T_{REG} gather near tumors and suppress the anti-tumor inflammatory response, thus favoring cancer cell survival. To this end, tumor-associated T_{REG} are thought as a major impediment of anti-tumor vaccines (13–16, 23). Clinical and experimental data suggest that tumor-associated T_{REG} recognize both self and neoantigens expressed by tumor cells, counteracting antigen-specific effector T-cell responses. Consequently, immunotherapy strategies based on the vaccination with tumor-associated antigens fail to evoke an effective response against cancer cells due to the activation and expansion of tumor antigen-specific T_{REG} (14–16). This potential interplay of T_{REG} within tumors has been reviewed in detail elsewhere (12–16), and has led to the proposal of several anti-T_{REG} regimens for cancer immunotherapy. These regimens aim to deplete T_{REG}, inhibit their suppressive function, prevent their homing into tumor sites, or block their differentiation/proliferation (12–16).

Several of these T_{REG}-targeting modalities have already been tested in the clinic, with mixed results (13, 16). Blocking T_{REG} function by depleting the cytotoxic T-lymphocyte-associated antigen 4 (CTLA-4) appears promising (24), due to the depletion of T_{REG} from tumor tissues (25, 26). However, a similar regimen could lead to an opposite effect with the accumulation of T_{REG} and $CD8^+$ T-cells in tumors (27, 28). A phase III study of melanoma patients using a gp100 peptide vaccine with interleukin (IL)-2 administration led to equally promising results with discovery of T_{REG} expansion in responding patients (29).

GUT MICROBIOTA INDUCE POTENT T_{REG} WITH SYSTEMIC ANTI-NEOPLASTIC PROPERTIES

As the results of these trials are anticipated, the literature reveals contradictory evidence. Indeed, the studies associating high densities of tumor-associated cells expressing T_{REG} markers including FOXP3 with a poor prognosis in several types of human cancers are now challenged by similar studies on the very same types of cancer showing the opposite outcome (30–34). The different $CD8^+$:T_{REG} ratios and the presence of $FOXP3^+$ cell subsets of undetermined identity in the tumor microenvironment have been proposed as probable explanations (16). Indeed, data from animal models show under certain conditions of microbial priming that T_{REG} not only protect but also alter the tumor microenvironment to induce remission of already established intestinal, mammary, and prostate cancers (35–41). The hypothesis that the composition of the different subsets of $FOXP3^+$, which may include effector $Foxp3^+$ cells, is intriguing (16). Indeed, it was previously shown that IFN-γ levels were increased during T_{REG}-mediated tumor regression in mice (37). Further, feeding of probiotic microbes to mice induces systemic oxytocin secretion that shifts immunity toward IFN-γ and CD25 for improved wound healing capacity and systemic good health (42). A question subsequently arising is whether gut microbiota may be engineered to harness an anti-neoplastic $FOXP3^+$ cell milieu (5, 10, 41).

GUT-CENTRIC HYPOTHESIS: PRIOR EXPOSURES TO MICROBES EXPLAIN BENEFICIAL ROLES OF T_{REG}

Stimulated by a gut-centric systemic homeostasis hypothesis, we set out to explore and explain the paradoxical roles of T_{REG} in cancer using several different mouse models of cancer and adoptive cell transfer methodologies (10). We found that T_{REG} may suppress, promote, or have no effect in carcinogenesis depending upon their timing and prior exposure to gut bacterial antigens and presence of IL-10 (35–39, 41, 43, 44). Under some conditions, adoptive transfer of T_{REG} rapidly led to apoptosis of emerging tumor cells (37, 45). Using as a model organism an opportunistic pathogen, *Helicobacter hepaticus*, commonly residing in the lower bowel of mice, we have shown in Rag2-deficient mice (otherwise lacking lymphocytes) that gut microbiota modulate inflammatory bowel disease and inflammation-associated colon cancer, a cancer process inhibited by properly functioning IL-10-dependent T_{REG} (35, 36). Subsequently, by introducing *H. hepaticus* into the large bowel flora of mice lacking the APC tumor suppressor gene ($Apc^{Min/+}$), we found that intestinal polypogenesis was greatly enhanced by bacteria and subsequently suppressed by immune-competent T_{REG}. Furthermore, adenomas of infected $Apc^{Min/+}$ mice progressed into adenocarcinoma, a transition atypical of polyps of aged-matched uninfected controls (38, 41). Interestingly, $Apc^{Min/+}$ mice having *H. hepaticus* in their gut flora were prone to develop cancer in tissues distant from intestine, such as prostate and the mammary glands (40, 41, 43, 46, 47). *H. hepaticus*-induced tumorigenic events were inhibited by supplementation with T_{REG} from immune-competent wild type donor mice.

A potent treatment to counteract these local and systemic *H. hepaticus*-induced tumorigenic events was supplementation with T_{REG} in an IL-10-dependent manner (10, 36, 38–40, 44, 46, 48). Purified T_{REG} exhibited greatest anti-cancer potency when taken from donor mice previously colonized with *H. hepaticus*. By contrast, T_{REG} taken from donor mice without prior *H. hepaticus* exposure were ineffective, and in some cases actually enhanced tumorigenesis (10). Based on these results, we theorize that the tumor microenvironment is subject to systemic inflammatory events arising from environmental exposures in the gastrointestinal tract (**Figure 1**). This microbe-inducible pro-inflammatory condition contributes to tumor trophic signaling. Interestingly, bacterial antigen triggered IL-10-dependent activities in the GI-tract impart sustained protection from the aforementioned events, resulting in immune cell recruitment, including T_{REG}, which, by being more potent in their anti-inflammatory roles, work locally and systemically to suppress sepsis, myeloid precursor mobilization, and inflammatory signaling important in extra-intestinal cancer evolution (10, 43). These systemic events comprise the tumor macroenvironment.

The roles of intestinal microflora in promoting cancer development within the bowel have been well established (35, 49–52). Linking gut microbial flora and local and systemic effects that promote (38) or suppress (45) tumors throughout the body, expands this paradigm in a challenging manner. Recent findings show that gut flora imbalances considerably undermine the response to both immune (53, 54) and non-immune chemotherapeutic regimens, such as cisplatin and oxaliplatin (53).

A WEAKENED T_{REG} FEEDBACK LOOP UNIFIES AUTOIMMUNE DISEASES AND CANCER

These gut microbe-centric findings in mice are consistent with the "hygiene hypothesis," according to which insufficient microbial exposures earlier in life predispose to allergies, autoimmune disorders, and uncontrollable inflammation-associated pathologies later in life. We have shown that the basic principles of this

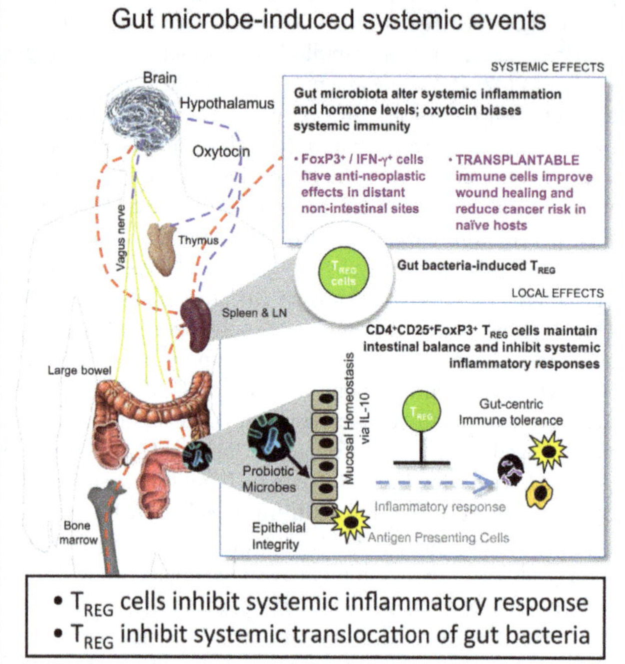

FIGURE 1 | Gut bacteria–host crosstalk is continuous and reciprocal in the cancer macroenvironment. Beneficial microbes trigger IL-10-mediated GI-tract immune and neuronal networks that lower systemic inflammatory tone and up-regulate hypothalamic–hypophyseal targets, including oxytocin, constituting a gut–systemic immunity-endocrine-axis. In this way, microbiota stimulate $CD4^+$ lymphocytes including regulatory T cells (T_{REG}) that suppress, promote, or have no effect in carcinogenesis depending upon their timing and prior exposure to gut bacterial antigens and presence of interleukin (IL)-10. This places neoplastic development and growth into a new broader context of the holobiont (comprised of the mammalian host plus resident microbes) and the cancer macroenvironment, highlighting microbes that may be engineered for sustained good health.

hypothesis may apply not only to auto-immunity, but also to neoplastic disease as well, and that T_{REG} play a central role in this phenomenon (10, 41, 55). The ability of T_{REG} to decrease risk for cancer and counteract established tumors depends upon microbe-triggered IL-10, which works to maintain immune system homeostasis and reinforce a protective anti-inflammatory, anti-neoplastic T_{REG} phenotype (41). T_{REG} display inherent phenotypic plasticity (10). Hygienic individuals with a weakened IL-10 and T_{REG} feedback loop are prone to a re-direction of unstable resting peripheral T_{REG} toward a T helper (Th)-17 pro-inflammatory process. As a result "hygienic" subjects are at higher risk to develop auto-immune diseases and cancer (10). It is tempting to postulate that this may explain why only a few people go on to develop cancer, while nearly everyone bears dysplastic and early neoplastic lesions throughout their body (56).

Depending on composition of gut microbiota, the immune system of mice may acquire different subclinical characteristics, even in the absence of overt inflammatory processes. The clinically silent immune system status may determine the risk of developing sporadic cancer in epithelia throughout the body. Further, we found that consuming beneficial probiotic bacteria led to the expansion of a $Foxp3^+$ cell population in the periphery (42, 45, 57) conferring protection to diet-related and genetic predisposition to mammary cancer (45). Targeted oral challenge with such probiotic bacteria resulted in the activation of interrelated systemic inflammatory and metabolic pathways, either through blood circulation or via the vagus nerve (**Figure 1**). Consequently, there was an upregulation of systemic hormone levels, such as oxytocin, testosterone, and thyroxin. Oxytocin serves to sustain immune and integumentary homeostasis, biasing the immune system toward IL-10 and IFN-γ, without anergy, subsequently minimizing the deleterious systemic effects of IL-17 (57). This altered immune system and metabolic profile of mice imparted healthful phenotypes including shiny fur and youthful hair follicle cycling, accelerated skin wound healing capacity, and resistance to diet-induced obesity and senility (42, 47, 57, 58). Through tightly regulated immune activities, competent T_{REG} permit brief beneficial host inflammatory responses to eliminate invading pathogens, and later inhibit chronic deleterious inflammatory tissue damage (43). The results of our wound healing assays further suggest that the probiotic microbe-induced enhancement of the T_{REG}-dominated arm of the immune system did not compromise the ability of mice to respond to invading pathogens (42).

BENEFICIAL SYSTEMIC EFFECTS OF GUT MICROBES ARE TRANSPLANTABLE VIA FOXP3+ T_{REG} INTO NAÏVE HOSTS

Adoptive cell transfer models offer mechanistic insight as these beneficial effects were isolated to bacteria-primed T_{REG} (42, 47, 57–59). In fact, healthful phenotypes were entirely reproducible in naive recipient mice by the adoptive transfer of highly purified T_{REG} derived from probiotic-fed cell donors (42, 57, 59). These results suggest gut microbe-induced crosstalk with the host in a continuous and reciprocal manner. The fate of preneoplastic and neoplastic lesions arising in epithelia throughout the body depends upon this macroenvironment at the whole organism level. Consequently, the tumor macroenvironment is defined as the "holobiont," i.e., the mammalian organism plus the microbial symbionts it bears. The T_{REG} population is a central player of the tumor macroenvironment connecting gut bacteria with reproductive fitness, youthful phenotypes, and anti-neoplastic properties.

MICROBIAL ENGINEERING OFFERS NEW STRATEGIES FOR PUBLIC HEALTH

Taken together, microbial engineering strategies using food-grade bacteria highlight alternative directions in cancer immunotherapy. Modulating beneficial T_{REG} via diet is a biologically safe and efficient approach, originating from genetic programs that have been shaped during the millions of years of co-evolution of mammals with their gut bacteria symbionts. These attributes remain largely inactive in individuals with a modern lifestyle, Westernized dietary habits, and stringent hygiene practices. Awakening these latent T_{REG}-mediated capabilities may provide an alternative avenue to reduce cancer risk at a population level for public health. The perspectives presented here should be considered as an alternative paradigm – not only for fighting cancer – but also for promoting overall good health and longevity.

AUTHOR CONTRIBUTIONS

Theofilos Poutahidis, Markus Kleinewietfeld, and Susan E. Erdman wrote the paper.

ACKNOWLEDGMENTS

This work was supported by National Institutes of Health grants P30-ES002109 (pilot project award to Susan E. Erdman), U01 CA164337 (to Susan E. Erdman), and RO1CA108854 (to Susan E. Erdman).

REFERENCES

1. Stewart BW, Wild CP editors. *World Cancer Report 2014*. Lyon: Cedex (2014).
2. Hanahan D, Weinberg RA. The hallmarks of cancer. *Cell* (2000) **100**:57–70. doi:10.1016/S0092-8674(00)81683-9
3. Bissell MJ, Radisky D. Putting tumours in context. *Nat Rev Cancer* (2001) **1**:46–54. doi:10.1038/35094059
4. Hanahan D, Weinberg RA. Hallmarks of cancer: the next generation. *Cell* (2011) **144**:646–74. doi:10.1016/j.cell.2011.02.013
5. Erdman S, Poutahidis T. Roles for inflammation and regulatory T cells in colon cancer. *Toxicol Pathol* (2010) **38**:76–87. doi:10.1177/0192623309354110
6. Hanahan D, Coussens LM. Accessories to the crime: functions of cells recruited to the tumor microenvironment. *Cancer Cell* (2012) **21**:309–22. doi:10.1016/j.ccr.2012.02.022
7. Balkwill F, Mantovani A. Inflammation and cancer: back to Virchow? *Lancet* (2001) **357**:539–45. doi:10.1016/S0140-6736(00)04046-0
8. Balkwill F, Coussens LM. Cancer: an inflammatory link. *Nature* (2004) **431**:405–6. doi:10.1038/431405a
9. Balkwill F. Cancer and the chemokine network. *Nat Rev Cancer* (2004) **4**:540–50. doi:10.1038/nrc1388
10. Erdman SE, Poutahidis T. Cancer inflammation and regulatory T cells. *Int J Cancer* (2010) **127**:768–79. doi:10.1002/ijc.25430
11. Colotta F, Allavena P, Sica A, Garlanda C, Mantovani A. Cancer-related inflammation, the seventh hallmark of cancer: links to genetic instability. *Carcinogenesis* (2009) **30**:1073–81. doi:10.1093/carcin/bgp127
12. Curiel TJ. Regulatory T cells and treatment of cancer. *Curr Opin Immunol* (2008) **20**:241–6. doi:10.1016/j.coi.2008.04.008
13. Whiteside TL. What are regulatory T cells (Treg) regulating in cancer and why? *Semin Cancer Biol* (2012) **22**:327–34. doi:10.1016/j.semcancer.2012.03.004
14. Mougiakakos D, Choudhury A, Lladser A, Kiessling R, Johansson CC. Regulatory T cells in cancer. *Adv Cancer Res* (2010) **107**:57–117. doi:10.1016/S0065-230X(10)07003-X
15. Colombo MP, Piconese S. Regulatory-T-cell inhibition versus depletion: the right choice in cancer immunotherapy. *Nat Rev Cancer* (2007) **7**:880–7. doi:10.1038/nrc2250
16. Nishikawa H, Sakaguchi S. Regulatory T cells in cancer immunotherapy. *Curr Opin Immunol* (2014) **27C**:1–7. doi:10.1016/j.coi.2013.12.005
17. Gajewski TF, Fuertes MB, Woo SR. Innate immune sensing of cancer: clues from an identified role for type I IFNs. *Cancer Immunol Immunother* (2012) **61**:1343–7. doi:10.1007/s00262-012-1305-6
18. Sakaguchi S, Yamaguchi T, Nomura T, Ono M. Regulatory T cells and immune tolerance. *Cell* (2008) **133**:775–87. doi:10.1016/j.cell.2008.05.009
19. Roncador G, Brown PJ, Maestre L, Hue S, Martinez-Torrecuadrada JL, Ling KL, et al. Analysis of FOXP3 protein expression in human CD4+CD25+ regulatory T cells at the single-cell level. *Eur J Immunol* (2005) **35**:1681–91. doi:10.1002/eji.200526189
20. Gavin MA, Torgerson TR, Houston E, Deroos P, Ho WY, Stray-Pedersen A, et al. Single-cell analysis of normal and FOXP3-mutant human T cells: FOXP3 expression without regulatory T cell development. *Proc Natl Acad Sci U S A* (2006) **103**:6659–64. doi:10.1073/pnas.0509484103
21. Miyara M, Yoshioka Y, Kitoh A, Shima T, Wing K, Niwa A, et al. Functional delineation and differentiation dynamics of human CD4+ T cells expressing the FoxP3 transcription factor. *Immunity* (2009) **30**:899–911. doi:10.1016/j.immuni.2009.03.019
22. Kleinewietfeld M, Hafler DA. The plasticity of human Treg and Th17 cells and its role in autoimmunity. *Semin Immunol* (2013) **25**:305–12. doi:10.1016/j.smim.2013.10.009
23. Curiel TJ, Coukos G, Zou L, Alvarez X, Cheng P, Mottram P, et al. Specific recruitment of regulatory T cells in ovarian carcinoma fosters immune privilege and predicts reduced survival. *Nat Med* (2004) **10**:942–9. doi:10.1038/nm1093
24. Hodi FS. Overcoming immunological tolerance to melanoma: targeting CTLA-4. *Asia Pac J Clin Oncol* (2010) **6**(Suppl 1):S16–23. doi:10.1111/j.1743-7563.2010.01271.x
25. Hodi FS, Butler M, Oble DA, Seiden MV, Haluska FG, Kruse A, et al. Immunologic and clinical effects of antibody blockade of cytotoxic T lymphocyte-associated antigen 4 in previously vaccinated cancer patients. *Proc Natl Acad Sci U S A* (2008) **105**:3005–10. doi:10.1073/pnas.0712237105
26. Liakou CI, Kamat A, Tang DN, Chen H, Sun J, Troncoso P, et al. CTLA-4 blockade increases IFNgamma-producing CD4+ICOShi cells to shift the ratio of effector to regulatory T cells in cancer patients. *Proc Natl Acad Sci U S A* (2008) **105**:14987–92. doi:10.1073/pnas.0806075105
27. Quezada SA, Peggs KS, Curran MA, Allison JP. CTLA4 blockade and Gm-Csf combination immunotherapy alters the intratumor balance of effector and regulatory T cells. *J Clin Invest* (2006) **116**:1935–45. doi:10.1172/JCI27745
28. Kavanagh B, O'Brien S, Lee D, Hou Y, Weinberg V, Rini B, et al. CTLA4 blockade expands FoxP3+ regulatory and activated effector CD4+ T cells in a dose-dependent fashion. *Blood* (2008) **112**:1175–83. doi:10.1182/blood-2007-11-125435
29. Schwartzentruber DJ, Lawson DH, Richards JM, Conry RM, Miller DM, Treisman J, et al. gp100 peptide vaccine and interleukin-2 in patients with advanced melanoma. *N Engl J Med* (2011) **364**:2119–27. doi:10.1056/NEJMoa1012863
30. Salama P, Phillips M, Grieu F, Morris M, Zeps N, Joseph D, et al. Tumor-infiltrating FOXP3+ T regulatory cells show strong prognostic significance in colorectal cancer. *J Clin Oncol* (2009) **27**:186–92. doi:10.1200/JCO.2008.18.7229
31. Badoual C, Hans S, Fridman WH, Brasnu D, Erdman S, Tartour E. Revisiting the prognostic value of regulatory T cells in patients with cancer. *J Clin Oncol* (2009) **27**:e5–6. Author reply e7.
32. Whiteside TL. Disarming suppressor cells to improve immunotherapy. *Cancer Immunol Immunother* (2012) **61**:283–8. doi:10.1007/s00262-011-1171-7
33. Leffers N, Gooden MJ, De Jong RA, Hoogeboom BN, Ten Hoor KA, Hollema H, et al. Prognostic significance of tumor-infiltrating T-lymphocytes in primary and metastatic lesions of advanced stage ovarian cancer. *Cancer Immunol Immunother* (2009) **58**:449–59. doi:10.1007/s00262-008-0583-5
34. Wilke CM, Wu K, Zhao E, Wang G, Zou W. Prognostic significance of regulatory T cells in tumor. *Int J Cancer* (2010) **127**:748–58. doi:10.1002/ijc.25464
35. Erdman SE, Poutahidis T, Tomczak M, Rogers AB, Cormier K, Plank B, et al. CD4+ CD25+ regulatory T lymphocytes inhibit microbially induced colon cancer in Rag2-deficient mice. *Am J Pathol* (2003) **162**:691–702. doi:10.1016/S0002-9440(10)63863-1
36. Erdman SE, Rao VP, Poutahidis T, Ihrig MM, Ge Z, Feng Y, et al. CD4(+)CD25(+) regulatory lymphocytes require interleukin 10 to interrupt colon carcinogenesis in mice. *Cancer Res* (2003) **63**:6042–50.
37. Erdman SE, Sohn JJ, Rao VP, Nambiar PR, Ge Z, Fox JG, et al. CD4+CD25+ regulatory lymphocytes induce regression of intestinal tumors in ApcMin/+ mice. *Cancer Res* (2005) **65**:3998–4004. doi:10.1158/0008-5472.CAN-04-3104
38. Rao VP, Poutahidis T, Ge Z, Nambiar PR, Boussahmain C, Wang YY, et al. Innate immune inflammatory response against enteric bacteria *Helicobacter hepaticus* induces mammary adenocarcinoma in mice. *Cancer Res* (2006) **66**:7395–400. doi:10.1158/0008-5472.CAN-06-0558
39. Poutahidis T, Haigis KM, Rao VP, Nambiar PR, Taylor CL, Ge Z, et al. Rapid reversal of interleukin-6-dependent epithelial invasion in a mouse model of microbially induced colon carcinoma. *Carcinogenesis* (2007) **28**:2614–23. doi:10.1093/carcin/bgm180
40. Poutahidis T, Rao VP, Olipitz W, Taylor CL, Jackson EA, Levkovich T, et al. CD4+ lymphocytes modulate prostate cancer progression in mice. *Int J Cancer* (2009) **125**:868–78. doi:10.1002/ijc.24452
41. Erdman SE, Rao VP, Olipitz W, Taylor CL, Jackson EA, Levkovich T, et al. Unifying roles for regulatory T cells and inflammation in cancer. *Int J Cancer* (2010) **126**:1651–65. doi:10.1002/ijc.24923
42. Poutahidis T, Kleinewietfeld M, Smillie C, Levkovich T, Perrotta A, Bhela S, et al. Microbial reprogramming inhibits western diet-associated obesity. *PLoS One* (2013) **8**:e68596. doi:10.1371/journal.pone.0068596
43. Rao VP, Poutahidis T, Fox JG, Erdman SE. Breast cancer: should gastrointestinal bacteria be on our radar screen? *Cancer Res* (2007) **67**:847–50. doi:10.1158/0008-5472.CAN-06-3468

44. Erdman SE, Rao VP, Poutahidis T, Rogers AB, Taylor CL, Jackson EA, et al. Nitric oxide and TNF-alpha trigger colonic inflammation and carcinogenesis in *Helicobacter hepaticus*-infected, Rag2-deficient mice. *Proc Natl Acad Sci U S A* (2009) **106**:1027–32. doi:10.1073/pnas.0812347106
45. Lakritz JR, Poutahidis T, Levkovich T, Varian BJ, Ibrahim YM, Chatzigiagkos A, et al. Beneficial bacteria stimulate host immune cells to counteract dietary and genetic predisposition to mammary cancer in mice. *Int J Cancer* (2013). doi:10.1002/ijc.28702
46. Rao VP, Poutahidis T, Ge Z, Nambiar PR, Horwitz BH, Fox JG, et al. Proinflammatory CD4+ CD45RB(hi) lymphocytes promote mammary and intestinal carcinogenesis in Apc(Min/+) mice. *Cancer Res* (2006) **66**:57–61. doi:10.1158/0008-5472.CAN-05-3445
47. Poutahidis T, Cappelle K, Levkovich T, Lee CW, Doulberis M, Ge Z, et al. Pathogenic intestinal bacteria enhance prostate cancer development via systemic activation of immune cells in mice. *PLoS One* (2013) **8**:e73933. doi:10.1371/journal.pone.0073933
48. Houghton J, Li H, Fan X, Liu Y, Liu JH, Rao VP, et al. Mutations in bone marrow-derived stromal stem cells unmask latent malignancy. *Stem Cells Dev* (2010) **19**:1153–66. doi:10.1089/scd.2009.0439
49. Terzic J, Grivennikov S, Karin E, Karin M. Inflammation and colon cancer. *Gastroenterology* (2010) **138**(2101–2114):e5. doi:10.1053/j.gastro.2010.01.058
50. Zhu Y, Michelle Luo T, Jobin C, Young HA. Gut microbiota and probiotics in colon tumorigenesis. *Cancer Lett* (2011) **309**:119–27. doi:10.1016/j.canlet.2011.06.004
51. Arthur JC, Perez-Chanona E, Muhlbauer M, Tomkovich S, Uronis JM, Fan TJ, et al. Intestinal inflammation targets cancer-inducing activity of the microbiota. *Science* (2012) **338**:120–3. doi:10.1126/science.1224820
52. Song X, Gao H, Lin Y, Yao Y, Zhu S, Wang J, et al. Alterations in the microbiota drive interleukin-17C production from intestinal epithelial cells to promote tumorigenesis. *Immunity* (2014) **40**:140–52. doi:10.1016/j.immuni.2013.11.018
53. Iida N, Dzutsev A, Stewart CA, Smith L, Bouladoux N, Weingarten RA, et al. Commensal bacteria control cancer response to therapy by modulating the tumor microenvironment. *Science* (2013) **342**:967–70. doi:10.1126/science.1240527
54. Viaud S, Saccheri F, Mignot G, Yamazaki T, Daillere R, Hannani D, et al. The intestinal microbiota modulates the anticancer immune effects of cyclophosphamide. *Science* (2013) **342**:971–6. doi:10.1126/science.1240537
55. Rook GA, Dalgleish A. Infection, immunoregulation, and cancer. *Immunol Rev* (2011) **240**:141–59. doi:10.1111/j.1600-065X.2010.00987.x
56. Folkman J, Kalluri R. Cancer without disease. *Nature* (2004) **427**:787. doi:10.1038/427787a
57. Poutahidis T, Kearney SM, Levkovich T, Qi P, Varian BJ, Lakritz JR, et al. Microbial symbionts accelerate wound healing via the neuropeptide hormone oxytocin. *PLoS One* (2013) **8**:e78898. doi:10.1371/journal.pone.0078898
58. Levkovich T, Poutahidis T, Smillie C, Varian BJ, Ibrahim YM, Lakritz JR, et al. Probiotic bacteria induce a 'glow of health.' *PLoS One* (2013) **8**:e53867. doi:10.1371/journal.pone.0053867
59. Poutahidis T, Erdman S. Probiotic "glow of health": more than skin deep. *Benef Microbes* (2014) **5**:109–19. doi:10.3920/BM2013.0042

18

Mathematical models of the impact of IL2 modulation therapies on T cell dynamics

Kalet León*, Karina García-Martínez and Tania Carmenate

Systems Biology Department, Center of Molecular Immunology, Habana, Cuba

Edited by:
Carmen Molina-Paris, University of Leeds, UK

Reviewed by:
Tomasz Zal, University of Texas MD Anderson Cancer Center, USA
Joseph Reynolds, University of Leeds, UK

***Correspondence:**
Kalet León, Systems Biology Department, Center of Molecular Immunology, 216 Street, PO Box 16040, Atabey, Habana 11600, Cuba
e-mail: kalet@cim.sld.cu

Several reports in the literature have drawn a complex picture of the effect of treatments aiming to modulate IL2 activity *in vivo*. They seem to promote either immunity or tolerance, probably depending on the specific context, dose, and timing of their application. Such complexity might derive from the pleiotropic role of IL2 in T cell dynamics. To theoretically address the latter possibility, our group has developed several mathematical models for Helper, Regulatory, and Memory T cell population dynamics, which account for most well-known facts concerning their relationship with IL2. We have simulated the effect of several types of therapies, including the injection of: IL2; antibodies anti-IL2; IL2/anti-IL2 immune-complexes; and mutant variants of IL2. We studied the qualitative and quantitative conditions of dose and timing for these treatments which allow them to potentiate either immunity or tolerance. Our results provide reasonable explanations for the existent pre-clinical and clinical data, predict some novel treatments, and further provide interesting practical guidelines to optimize the future application of these types of treatments.

Keywords: mathematical model, T cell dynamics, interleukin 2, interleukin 2 mutants, regulatory T cells

INTRODUCTION

Several reports in the literature have drawn a complex picture of the effect of treatments aiming to modulate IL2 activity *in vivo*. These treatments seem to promote either immunity or tolerance, probably depending on the specific context, dose, and timing of their application.

Treatments that increase IL2 activity, simply by injecting it, have been shown to potentiate the immune response to vaccines (1–4) and are a current medical practice to enhance the natural anti-tumor immunity in patients with melanoma. However, several reports in the literature have shown that HIV (5–8) and melanoma (9) patients treated with IL2, experience an increase in $CD4^+$ $CD25^+$ $FoxP3^+$ regulatory T cells, which typically mediate natural immune tolerance. Moreover, several pre-clinical studies have further documented a tolerogenic effect of IL2. Injections of IL2 have been shown to prevent or ameliorate autoimmune responses in mice (10–12). Treatments which reduce natural IL2 activity, by sequestering it with anti-IL2 monoclonal antibodies, have been shown to induce autoimmune responses (13). And treatments intending to block IL2 activity, with non-depleting anti-IL2-receptor antibodies, are showed to have anti-tumoral effects (14). Nevertheless, in the clinical practice non-depleting anti-IL2-receptor antibodies are used to ameliorate the autoimmune reaction in patients with neoplasia, autoimmune diseases, and organ allograft rejection (15).

Further complexity to the latter picture has been recently added with the pre-clinical assessment of treatments based on immune-complexes formed by IL2 and monoclonal antibodies anti-IL2. This treatment shows a much more potent *in vivo* effect than IL2 alone, appears again to potentiate either immunity (16, 17) or tolerance (18), depending on the specific antibody used to form the immune-complexes. In particular, the specific epitope in the IL2 recognized by the antibody has been postulated as critical for this phenomenon (19, 20).

IL2 interacts with many different cells types, which express the three known chains of the IL2 receptor. Particularly relevant and complex is its relationship with the population dynamics of the CD4 T lymphocytes. IL2 was originally described as a potent $CD4^+$ T cell growth factor (21), which should in consequence enhance overall T cell immunity. However, several experiments have shown lately a critical role for this cytokine in the survival and proliferation of the $CD4^+CD25^+FoxP3^+$ T cells (regulatory T cells) (22, 23), which mediate the maintenance of natural and induced tolerance. The $CD4^+CD25^-FoxP3^-$ T cells (helper T cells) have been identified as the principal source of IL2 *in vivo* (24), suggesting that the regulatory T cells have to sequester the IL2 produced by these cells in order to proliferate and survive (25). Moreover, *in vitro and in vivo* experiments have shown that regulatory T cells inhibit the production of IL2 by the helper T cells (26), limiting in this way their own source of this essential cytokine. Thus, overall, it seems that IL2 has a dual role on its circuit of interactions with $CD4^+$ T cells. It could promote the proliferation of the helper T cells, which may drive effective immunity and foster IL2 production. But, it could also promote the expansion of regulatory T cells, which may turn off the immune reaction, as well as the IL2 production on its own. The dynamic balance between these opposite forces might explain the complexity observed in the effect of treatments that modulate IL2 activity, either sequestering it or further increasing it.

To theoretically address the latter hypothesis, our group has developed mathematical models for Helper, Regulatory, and Memory T cells dynamics, which account for most well-known facts relative to their relationship with IL2. We have simulated the effect of several types of therapies including the injection of: IL2; antibodies anti-IL2; IL2/anti-IL2 immune-complexes, and mutants variants of IL2. We studied the qualitative and quantitative conditions of dose and timing for these treatments which allow them to potentiate either immunity or tolerance. Our results provide reasonable explanations for the existent pre-clinical and clinical data, predict some novel treatments, and further provide interesting practical guidelines to optimize the future application of these types of treatments.

MATERIALS AND METHODS

INTRODUCTION TO THE MATHEMATICAL MODEL

The mathematical model used in this paper is based on the one developed in Ref. (27) to describe the interaction between IL2 and helper (E) and regulatory (R) $CD4^+$ T cells and memory $CD8^+$ T cells inside a lymph node. The model includes several physical compartments, which minimally capture the bio-distribution of T cells, IL2, and antibodies in the immune system (see **Figure 1**). It includes several compartments, which represent different lymph nodes, where T cells are confined interacting with each other's, with the antigen presenting cells (APCs) and available soluble molecules. It includes also a compartment representing the blood (i.e., the circulatory system), which contains only soluble molecules, IL2, mutant variants of IL2 or anti-IL2 antibodies. Each lymph node in the system is connected to the blood compartment, allowing the free exchange of these soluble molecules.

DYNAMICS IN THE BLOOD COMPARTMENT

The concentration of soluble molecules in the blood compartment is assumed to decay with a constant characteristic rate, which represent renal elimination in the kidney. An external source term for these molecules is added in this compartment to simulate particular treatment applications. Interaction between free IL2 and anti-IL2 antibodies are modeled in this and other compartments as a dynamic equilibrium characterized by a given biding affinity. Equations for the dynamics in this compartment are presented in "Dynamics in the Blood Compartment" in Appendix A.

DYNAMICS FOR T CELLS INSIDE LYMPH NODES

The model includes, inside the lymph nodes, the dynamics of Helper (E), and Regulatory (R) T cells on three different functional states of their life cycle: resting, activated, and cycling cells. All the interactions involving these T cells occur in the presence of a constant amount of their cognate APCs and relevant homeostatic cytokines. The basic processes and interactions included in the model dynamics for these T cells are (see **Figure 2** and (27, 28) for a more detailed biological explanation, including references to experiments that sustained their validity):

i. Resting E and R cells are produced at constant rate by the thymus; they die with a constant decay rate; they get activated (becoming an activated cell) following conjugation to their cognate APCs. The activation of E cells can be inhibited by the presence of co-localized R cells on the APCs.
ii. The activated E and R cells could become cycling cells following a dose-dependent response to cytokine derived signals. The activated R cells get this signal from the interaction with available IL2 while the E cells could additionally use other homeostatic cytokines[1], which are referred in the model as

[1] Note that, although other cytokines are able to stimulate Tregs *in vitro*, several reports in the literature have indicated IL2 as the key cytokine for the proliferation

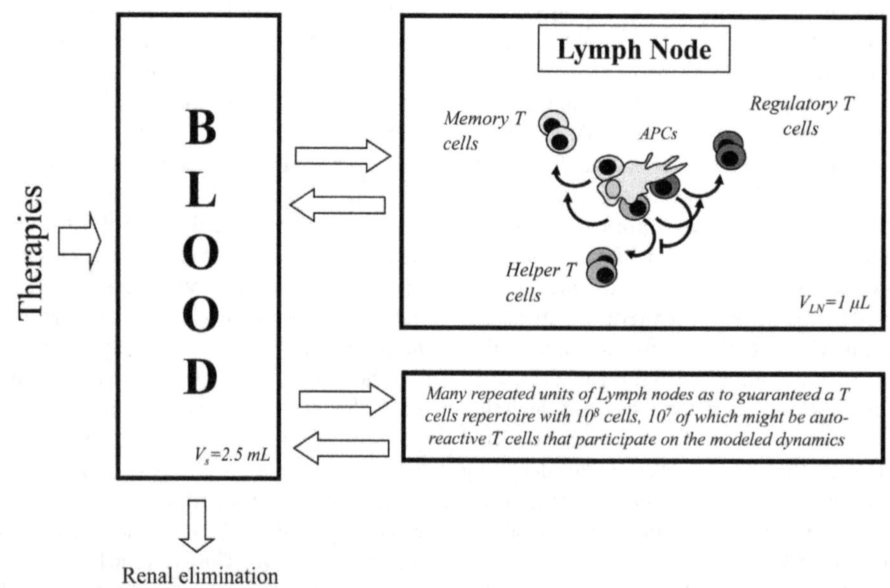

FIGURE 1 | Diagram of the processes occurring in the two compartments considered in the model. At the left side of the diagram the blood compartment is shown, where soluble molecules related with IL2 modulatory therapies are introduced and eliminated. This compartment is in constant molecular exchange with the lymph nodes (right side of the diagram). In this last class of compartment, occur the processes related with the dynamics of T cells and their interaction with the IL2 and other soluble molecules.

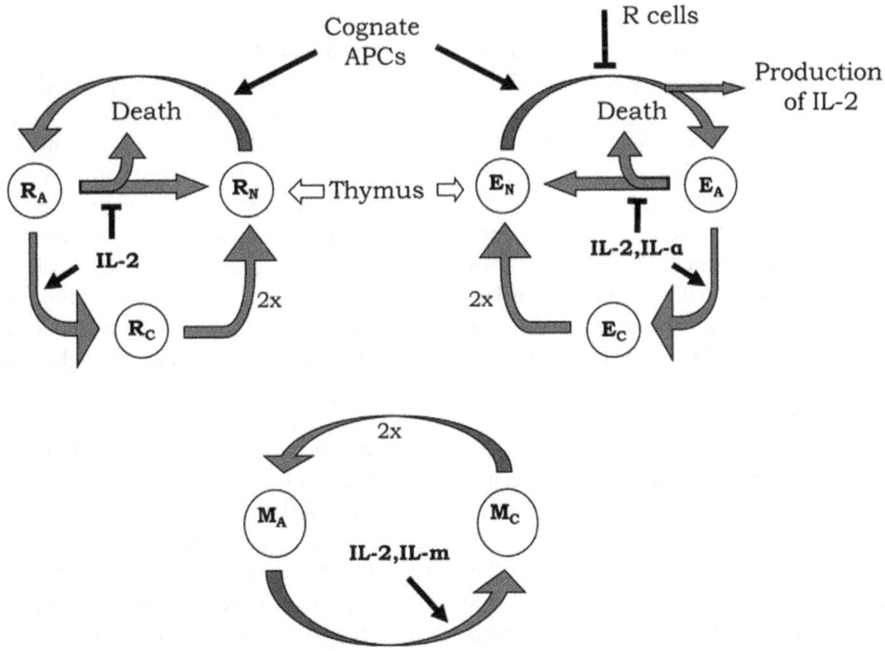

FIGURE 2 | Diagrams of helper (E), regulatory (R), and memory (M) T-cell life cycle considered in the model. New resting E (E_N) and R (R_N) cells are constantly generated by the thymus. These resting T cells become activated by interaction with their cognate APCs. During activation, E cells produce IL2, although the whole process can be inhibited by the presence of co-localized R cells. Activated E (E_A) and R (R_A) enter the cell cycle (becoming cycling cells) when receiving enough signal from IL2 or another external cytokine (IL-α) in the case of E cells. In the absence of enough cytokines, activated T cells become inactivated, where a fraction of cells simply returns back to the resting state and the other dies. Cycling E (E_C) and R (R_C) cells divide with a constant rate generating two new resting E or R cells, respectively. Memory T cells are assumed as being always in a sort of naturally activated state (even without any strong cognate interaction with APCs). Activated M (M_A) cells enter the cell cycle when receiving enough signals from IL2 or another external cytokine (IL-m). Cycling M cells (M_C) divide generating two new activated M cells.

ILa and are available inside the lymph node in a constant but limited amount. In the absence of enough cytokine derived signal, a fraction of the activated E or R cells revert to the resting state and the remaining fraction just die.

iii. The cycling E and R cells are fully committed to divide, producing two new resting cells. Thus, they are presumed to do so with a constant rate.

The model includes also the dynamics of a generic population of non-CD4 T cells, which binds weakly to the existent APCs, but proliferates in response to IL2 signal, with similar sensitivity than the activated helper $CD4^+$ T cells. This cells (referred as M cells) represent, the memory $CD8^+CD44^+$ T cells, which can proliferate in response to IL2 without any requirements of activation by cognate APCs (see **Figure 2**).

The dynamics of the number of T cells in the lymph node compartment, following the process described above, are modeled with the set of equations presented in "Dynamics of T Cells in the Lymph Node Compartment" in Appendix B.

DYNAMICS IL2 AND ANTIBODIES ANTI-IL2 INSIDE THE LYMPH NODE

The dynamics of IL2 molecules inside the lymph node takes into account the role of T cells in the production and degradation of this cytokine. The following processes are considered in the model [see **Figure 2** and Ref. (27) for a more detailed biological explanation, including references to experiments that sustained their validity]:

iv. IL2 is produced by E cells upon activation. It is produced as a burst whenever a resting E cell becomes an activated E cell. Such production of IL2 is inhibited, together with the E cell activation, by the presence of co-localized R cells on the APCs.

v. IL2 is degraded in the lymph nodes, after being internalized by the T cells in the form of complexes with the IL2 receptor at their cell surface.

Interactions of IL2 and T cells in the model are based on the expression by these cells, either in the resting, activated or cycling state, of different levels of the IL2 receptor. These receptors mediate the binding of IL2, which provide a stimulatory signal in a dose-dependent fashion to the T cell. In this model the three known chains of the IL2 receptor, alpha, beta, and gamma (29) are included. These three chains are

and survival of Treg cells *in vivo*. The group of Freitas (24) have shown that the absence of $CD4^+$ T cells capable of producing IL2, leads to the absence of Treg cells and to the development of autoimmunity. Moreover, mice knockouts of IL2 or IL2 receptor components have been shown to lack the accumulation of Tregs *in vivo*, exhibiting once more an autoimmune phenotype (48, 49). Interestingly in these latter scenarios of autoimmune mice, other cytokines besides IL2 are capable to maintain and expand the auto-reactive helper $CD4^+$ T cells (perhaps IL7, IL15, or IL21).

combined dynamically at the cell surface, upon IL2 binding, to conform the two known signaling forms of the IL2 receptors. The following processes and known facts are considered in the model regarding this interaction [see **Figure 3** and Ref. (27)]:

vi. IL2/IL2Receptor complexes formation is modeled as a multi-step process: free, soluble, IL2 binds initially to the available free alpha or free beta chains of the receptor, and only then can form dimers or trimers with the remaining IL2 receptor chains at the cell membrane. The gamma chain is assumed to be always in excess compared with the amount of beta chain bound to IL2, either alone or together with alpha chain. Therefore gamma chain joins immediately to these membrane complexes, forming the well known intermediate (beta-gamma-IL2) or high affinity (alpha-beta-gamma-IL2) IL2–IL2 receptor complexes.

vii. IL2/IL2Receptor configurations, which include the beta and gamma chains (high-affinity alpha-beta-gamma, and intermediate affinity beta-gamma receptor), trigger a signal into the T cells (19). Therefore, in the model, the mean number of such signaling receptors per activated E cell, R cell, and M cell are counted. Then, the probability of getting enough signal as to become a cycling cell, for any particular activated E, R, or M cell, is computed with a sigmoid dose response curve, of the mean signaling level. The use of a sigmoid dose response curve is based on direct experimental observations on *in vitro* culture of $CD4^+$ T cells (30) stimulated with recombinant IL2.

viii. Beta and gamma chain of the IL2 receptor are similarly expressed by E and R cells in all functional states, but the expression of the alpha chain is modulated with T cell activation (31). R cells constitutively express the alpha chain in the resting state, but further increase its expression level with activation. E cells do not express the alpha chain in the resting state, but gain a significant expression level with activation.

ix. The M cells are assumed to express a negligible amount of the alpha chain of IL2 receptor, but have levels of the beta and gamma chain which are higher than those of helper and regulatory T cells (32).

Antibodies anti-IL2 are modeled as molecules that can form complexes with the IL2, blocking or not its binding to the different chains of the IL2 receptor at the T cell surface. IL-2 mutants are modeled as a molecule bearing similar properties than wild-type IL-2, but differing in some specific parameter value on each case. In particular, we simulate the effects of IL2 mutants with an either reduced or increased Kon for the alpha or beta chains of the IL2R.

The equations in the model describing the dynamics of the number of molecules circulating in the Lymph Node (IL2, anti-IL2

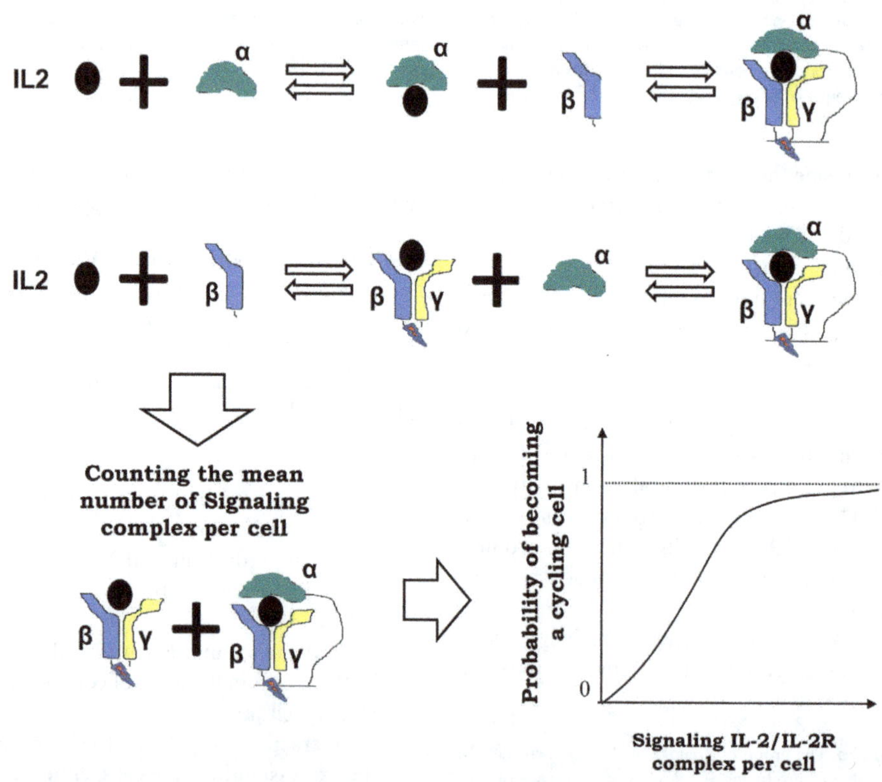

FIGURE 3 | Interactions between IL2 and T cells in the model are mediated by the IL2 receptor (IL2R), which is formed by three chains: alpha, beta, and gamma chain. These chains are combined dynamically in multi-step process at the cell surface, upon IL2 binding, to conform the two known signaling forms of the IL2 receptors: high affinity alpha-beta-gamma and intermediate affinity beta-gamma receptor. In the model, the mean number of such signaling IL2-IL2R complexes per activated T cell are counted, and the probability of becoming a cycling cell is computed with a sigmoid function of the mean number of bound cytokines signaling receptors per cell (as shown at the right side of the arrow).

antibodies, and immune-complexes) and the number of complexes IL2-IL2R and IL2-mAb-IL2R formed in a single cell membrane are described in "Dynamics of Molecules in the Lymph Node" in Appendix C.

SIMULATION OF DIFFERENT THERAPIES

Four types of treatments are simulated in the model: injections of IL2; injections of anti-IL2 monoclonal antibodies; injections of immune complex composed of a mixture of IL2 and anti-IL2 antibodies with a specified constant proportion of them; and injection of mutant variants of IL2.

Treatments are simulated to represent a continuous infusion of the involved molecules for a defined period of time. This is implemented by setting on, transiently, the external source term of the molecules involved in a specific treatment (i.e., IL2; IL2m; and/or anti-IL2 antibody). Two parameters always control treatment application: the "dose," which set up the total amount per day of IL2, IL2m, and/or anti-IL2 antibody infused; and the "treatment duration," which set the time period for which continuous infusion is maintained. In all cases, we explore how the dose and treatment duration determine the outcome of the system simulation. We study whether or not different treatments can condition a significant preferential expansion (dominance) of helper T cells or regulatory T cells or M cells in the system.

PARAMETER AND VARIABLE VALUES IN MODEL SIMULATIONS

Model parameters were previously calibrated in Ref. (27). The actual values of parameter used in our simulations are provided in **Tables 1–3**. The majority of the model parameters are fixed to values directly taken or derived from available independent experimental data; just a few parameters remain unknown, and their influence in result was explored inside a range of biologically reasonable values. Given the realistic values and units of the most model parameters used in the simulations, we report in this paper the values of treatments doses in milligrams and the values of treatment duration in weeks. However, the reader should note that our model is only roughly calibrated, thus one should believe on the order of magnitude and general qualitative trends of the predicted effects. But, the exact values of dose and treatment duration reported here to cause a given effect in the simulations should not be taken as a solid prediction.

The simulations of the model dynamics was implemented using the program Mathematica v.4.0.

RESULTS AND DISCUSSION

BASIC MODEL AND SIMULATIONS SETUP

The model is setup to study the basic homeostasis of the immune system of a mouse (27). Therefore the APCs in the model are interpreted as those APCs, which present self-antigens to T cells in the absence of infections. In consequence, the $CD4^+$ T cells in the model are taken to represent the populations of auto-reactive E and R cells, which significantly recognizes the existent self-antigens and thus interact with the available APCs.

Two main problems are then studied in the model simulations. (a) The basic dynamics states of the system in the absence of treatments; and (b) The effect of perturbations which represent specific IL2 modulation treatments on the stability of these dynamics states.

TOLERANCE AND IMMUNITY AS THE BASIC MODEL STEADY STATES (IN THE ABSENCE OF TREATMENT)

The model has two stable steady states which can be interpreted as natural tolerance and autoimmunity in the system. The steady state, which is interpreted as an autoimmune state (**Figure 4A**), is one where auto-reactive helper cells are significantly expanded while the auto-reactive Regulatory T cells are outcompeted from their cognate APCs. This steady state is also characterized by the existence of high levels of free IL2 and some subsequence expansion of the memory $CD8^+$ T cells population (M cells) in the lymph nodes. The steady state, which is interpreted as natural tolerance in the model, is one where the auto-reactive E and R cells co-exist in a dynamic equilibrium (**Figure 4B**). In this steady state the expansion of the auto-reactive helper cells is actively controlled by their interaction with the auto-reactive Regulatory T cells, the amount of free IL2 remains very low and the size of M cell population remains close to its basal homeostatic level.

A key dynamical property of the model is the existence of a parameter regime where these steady states of tolerance and autoimmunity can co-exist. This is a regime of bistable behavior (**Figure 4C**), where the model could evolve dynamically into either to the autoimmune or the tolerant steady state, but depending on the initial conditions used to seed the simulation without any change of parameter values (i.e., changing the initial proportion of auto-reactive E to R cells). The model is set to operate inside this bistable parameter regime. Thus in equilibrium, in the absence of treatments, the system will be either in the tolerant or the autoimmune steady state referred above. Such parameter choice is required to explain properly with the model the results of adoptive transfer experiments in mice, where transferring different proportions of $CD4^+CD25^-$ (helper) and $CD4^+CD25^+$ (regulatory) T cells into immune deficient mice (those lacking T cells, $Rag^{-/-}$ or $nu^{-/-}$), they either reconstitute a normal (tolerant to self-antigens) immune system or develop an autoimmune disease mediated by the uncontrolled expansion of the transferred auto-reactive $CD4^+$ T cells (28).

Moreover, it is important to note that the model reviewed here is an extension of the cross-regulation model of immunity, which studies the interaction of helper and regulatory $CD4^+$ T cells in the lymph node of the normal mice (33). Interestingly, despite of substantial increase on the number of variable and parameters, the new model conserves the three main dynamical properties of the original one reviewed in Ref. (34). In Ref. (28), three parameter conditions were presented as necessary in the extended model to behave as the original model and therefore to explain the same phenomenology. These conditions are:

(1) Regulatory T cells have to be more efficient using IL-2 at low concentrations than helper and memory T cells.
(2) The existence of a cytokine alternative to IL-2 that promote helper T cell proliferation and survival.
(3) The helper cells must become activated and proliferate more rapidly than Regulatory T cells in conditions of IL-2 excess.

A detailed discussion of the validity of these constrains, from an experimental point of view, is provided in Ref. (28).

Table 1 | Variables and parameters appearing in the equations that model the dynamics in the blood compartment.

Variables	Definitions	
$IL2_S$	Total number of IL2 molecules in the blood	
$IL2m_S$	Total number of IL2m molecules in the blood	
Ab_S	Total number of anti-IL2 mAb in the blood	
$IL2_S^{Ab}$	Total number of IL2-mAb complexes in the blood	
IL2	Total number of free IL2 molecules (non-conjugated to IL2R at the cell membrane) in the lymph node	
IL2m	Total number of free IL2m molecules (non-conjugated to IL2R at the cell membrane) in the lymph node	
Ab	Total number of free anti-IL2 mAb (non-conjugated to IL2-IL2R complex at the cell membrane) in the lymph node	
$IL2^{Ab}$	Total number of free IL2-mAb complexes (non-conjugated to IL2R at the cell membrane) in the lymph node	
Symbolic labels	**Definitions**	
j	Symbolic label that denotes the different IL2R chains: $j = \alpha$ (alpha chain) and $j = \beta$ (beta chain)	
l	Symbolic label that denotes the possible functional states of the T cells: $l = N$ resting state, $l = A$ activated state and $l = C$ cycling state	
Parameters	**Definitions**	**Values used in simulations**
Γ_i	External influx of IL2, typically used to simulate IL2 addition treatment	–
K_{pi}	Rate of IL2 production by helper CD4+ T cells upon activation	10^3 M/h
K_{di}	Elimination rate of IL2 in the blood	Ln(2)/10 min
N_{LN}	Total number of equivalent lymph nodes considered in the system	10
D_{il}, D_{ab}	Diffusion rate for the exchange of IL2 and mAbs, between the blood and peripheral lymph nodes	10^{-7} L × Ln(2)/10 min
V_S, V_{LN}	Volume of the blood and lymph node compartments, respectively	2.5×10^{-3} L, 10^{-6} L
fve	Fraction of the lymph node volume, in which molecules and mAbs can diffuse	0.1
K_{on}^{Ab}, K_{off}^{Ab}	Association and dissociation constants of IL2-mAb complexes	Face alpha mAb: 1.5×10^5 $M^{-1}s^{-1}$, 1.4×10^{-4} s^{-1}; face beta mAb: 2.3×10^4 $M^{-1}s^{-1}$, $6.6 \times 10^{-5} s^{-1}$
Γ_{mi}	External influx of IL2m, typically used to simulate IL2 addition treatment	–
Γ_{ab}	External influx of mAb, typically used to simulate anti-IL2 mAbs addition treatment	–
K_{da}	Elimination rate of mAbs and IL2-mAbs complexes in the blood	Ln(2)/3 days
N_A	Avogadro's number	6,02 × 10^{23} mol^{-1}

RESPONSE TO TREATMENTS THAT MODULATE IL2 CONCENTRATION

In following sections, the effects of different treatments, which aim to modulate IL2 activity, are studied. Treatments simulate a continuous infusion for a defined period of time of the involved molecules (IL2, IL2m, and/or anti-IL2 antibody). Two parameters control their application: the "dose," which set up the total amount per day of IL2, IL2m, and/or anti-IL2 antibody infused; and the "treatment duration," which set the time period of sustained infusion. Treatments are always applied in a system which is initially set to a dynamic equilibrium (i.e., either into the tolerant or the autoimmune steady state). We systematically study, whether a given treatment induces a significant change in the initial proportion of Regulatory (R) versus Helper (E + M) T cells, both transiently or permanently. We interpret that a treatment promotes immunity when it induces a transition from the tolerant steady state (dominated by R cells) to the autoimmune steady state (dominated by E cells). We interpret that a treatment promotes tolerance when it induces a transition from the autoimmune state to the tolerant steady state.

Simulating the injection of IL2

Simulations of IL2 injections show that, when this treatment is applied to a system initialized into the autoimmune steady state, it is unable to take the system into the tolerant steady state, irrespectively of the dose and treatment duration chosen. Moreover, it further promotes the expansion of the auto-reactive E cells and the M cells (**Figure 5**) reinforcing transiently the ongoing autoimmune response. However, when this treatment is applied

Table 2 | Variables and parameters appearing in the equations that model the T cells dynamics.

Variables	**Definitions**	
E_N, E_A, E_C	Total number (conjugated plus non-conjugated) of resting, activated, and cycling E cells	
R_N, R_A, R_C	Total number (conjugated plus non-conjugated) of resting, activated, and cycling R cells	
M_A, M_C	Total number (conjugated plus non-conjugated) of activated and cycling M cells	
Intermediate variables	**Definitions**	
E_N^B, E_A^B, E_C^B	Number of resting, activated, and cycling E cells conjugated to APCs	
E_T^B	Total number of conjugated E cells: $E_T^B = E_N^B + E_A^B + E_C^B$	
E_N^F, E_A^F, E_C^F	Number of resting, activated, and cycling E cells non-conjugated to APCs: $E_l^F = E_l - E_l^B, \ \forall l \in \{N, A, C\}$	
R_N^B, R_A^B, R_C^B	Number of resting, activated, and cycling R cells conjugated to APCs	
R_T^B	Total number of conjugated R cells: $R_T^B = R_N^B + R_A^B + R_C^B$	
R_N^F, R_A^F, R_C^F	Number of resting, activated and cycling R cells non-conjugated to APCs: $R_l^F = R_l - R_l^B, \ \forall l \in \{N, A, C\}$	
M_A^B, M_C^B	Number of activated and cycling M cells conjugated to APCs	
M_T^B	Total number of conjugated M cells: $M_T^B = M_A^B + M_C^B$	
M_A^F, M_C^F	Number of activated and cycling M cells non-conjugated to APCs: $M_l^F = M_l = M_l^B, \ \forall l \in \{A, C\}$	
F	Total number of APC conjugation sites that remain free in the system	
SigE, SigR, SigM	Number of bound cytokines signaling receptors at the surface of an activated *E*, *R*, and *M* cells	
Symbolic labels	**Definitions**	
l	Symbolic label that denotes the possible functional states of the T cells: $l = N$ resting state, $l = A$ activated state, and $l = C$ cycling state	
Parameters	**Definitions**	**Values used in simulations**
Γ_e, Γ_r	Input rate of new resting self-reactive E and R cells from the thymus	2.5×10^4 cells/day
K_A^E, K_A^R	Activation rate for resting E and R cells conjugated to APCs	Ln(2)/2 h, Ln(2)/6 h
K_P^E, K_P^R, K_P^M	Division rate for cycling E, R, and M cells	Ln(2)/4 h
K_S^E, K_S^R	IL2 signaling-waiting rate for activated E and R cells	Ln(2)/2 h
K_S^M	IL2 signaling-waiting rate for activated M cells	Ln(2)/4 h
K_d^E, K_d^R, K_d^M	Death rate for free resting E and R cells, and free activated M cells	Ln(2)/1 week
A	Number of total APCs	2×10^5
s	Total number of conjugations site per APC	5
K^E, K^R	Equilibrium conjugation constants (K_{on}/K_{off}) for E and R cells to the APC conjugation sites	$K_{on} = 10^{-13}\ \mathrm{L\,s^{-1}\,cell^{-1}}$, $K_{off} = 6 \times 10^{-4}\ \mathrm{s^{-1}}$
K^M	Equilibrium conjugation constants (K_{on}/K_{off}) for M cells to the APC conjugation sites	$K_{on} = 10^{-13}\ \mathrm{L\,s^{-1}\,cell^{-1}}$, $K_{off} = 6 \times 10^{-3}\ \mathrm{s^{-1}}$
α_E, α_R	Fraction of activated E and R cells reverting to the resting state in the absence of cytokine related signal	0.95
h	Hill coefficient at the sigmoid response curve	4
S_E, S_R, S_M	Sensitivities thresholds for E, R, and M cells to cytokines signal	500

Table 3 | Variables and parameters related to dynamics of IL2, IL2R, and mAb complexes fomation.

Variables	Definitions	
$C_j^{E_I}$, $C_j^{R_I}$, $C_j^{M_I}$	Number of IL2 molecules bound to *j* chain of IL2R, at the surface of the indicated T cell type	
$Cm_j^{E_I}$, $Cm_j^{R_I}$, $Cm_j^{M_I}$	Number of IL2m molecules bound to *j* chain of IL2R, at the surface of the indicated T cell type	
$CAb_j^{E_I}$, $CAb_j^{R_I}$, $CAb_j^{M_I}$	Number of IL2/mAb complexes bound to the *j* chain of IL2R, at the surface of the indicated T cell type	
T^{E_I}, T^{R_I}, T^{M_I}	Number of IL2 molecules bound to high affinity IL2R (alpha + beta), at the surface of the indicated T cell type	
Tm^{E_I}, Tm^{R_I}, Tm^{M_I}	Number of IL2m molecules bound to high affinity IL2R (alpha + beta), at the surface of the indicated T cell type	
Intermediate variables	**Definitions**	
$P_j^{E_I}$, $P_j^{R_I}$, $P_j^{M_I}$	Number of IL2R of *j* chain free (not bound to IL2), at the surface of the indicated T cell type	
SigE, SigR, SigM	Number of cytokines signaling receptors at the surface of an activated *E*, *R*, and *M* cells	
Parameters	**Definitions**	**Values used in simulations**
K_{off}^{j}, K_{on}^{j}	Dissociation and association constant of IL2 to the *j* chain of the IL2R	$K_{off}^{\alpha} = 0.6\ s^{-1}$, $K_{on}^{\alpha} = 10^7 M^{-1}s^{-1}$, $K_{off}^{\beta} = 3 \times 10^{-3}s^{-1}$, $K_{on}^{\beta} = 3.4 \times 10^6 M^{-1}s^{-1}$
f_j	Parameter that control the properties of different IL2m	10^{-3}, 10^3
N_j	Switch parameter setting if the mAb blocks (=1) or not (=0) the interaction of IL2 with the *j* chain of the IL2R	0, 1
ila_{E_A}, ila_{M_A}	Number of cytokine signaling receptors, at the surface of an activated *E* and *M* cells, bounds to an alternative cytokine (not IL2)	10^8, 10^7
Ra^{E_I}, Rb^{E_I}	Total number of alpha and beta chains of IL2R per E cells in the state *I*	$Ra^{E_N} = 10$, $Ra^{E_A} = 10^4$, $Ra^{E_C} = 10^3$, $Rb^{E_I} = 10^3$
Ra^{R_I}, Rb^{R_I}	Total number of alpha and beta chains of IL2R per R cells in the state *I*	$Ra^{R_N} = 10^4$, $Ra^{R_A}=10^5$, $Ra^{R_C}=10^4$, $Rb^{R_I}=10^3$
Ra^{M_I}, Rb^{M_I}	Total number of alpha and beta chains of IL2R per M cells in the state *I*	$Ra^{M_I}=10$, $Rb^{M_I}=10^4$
$K_{on}^{\alpha\beta}$, $K_{off}^{\alpha\beta}$	Association and dissociation rates for the interaction of free beta chain to preformed IL2/alpha chain complexes, at the T cell membrane	$K_{on}^{\alpha\beta}=2.2 \times 10^{-3}s^{-1}$, $K_{off}^{\alpha\beta}= 3 \times 10^{-3}s^{-1}$
$K_{on}^{\beta\alpha}$, $K_{off}^{\beta\alpha}$	Association and dissociation rates for the interaction of free alpha chain to preformed IL2/beta chain complexes, at the T cell membrane	$K_{on}^{\beta\alpha} = 0.6 \times 10^{-2}s^{-1}$, $K_{off}^{\beta\alpha} = 0.6\ s^{-1}$
K_{in}	Internalization (degradation) rate of signaling IL2/IL2R complex by T cells	$K_{in} = 0.04\ min^{-1}$

to a system initialized in the tolerant steady state it reinforces the preexistent tolerance, by further expanding the regulatory populations (**Figure 5**). Interestingly, increasing the IL2 dose applied to a preexistent tolerant state could induce immunity by expanding the M cells; although, this effect is obtained for significantly high (unrealistic) values of the IL2 dose.

Thus overall in the model, IL2 injections appear to reinforce the preexistent steady state, this is expanding transiently either the R or the E cells respectively for a preexistent tolerant or autoimmune situation. A closer look to the model behavior qualitatively explains these results. Briefly: in a preexistent autoimmune steady state there is an excess of IL2 in the lymph node, thus is not lack of IL2 what limits regulatory T cell expansion, is their competition with auto-reactive E cells for the cognate APCs. In consequence injecting IL2 would never reestablish tolerance. In a preexistent tolerant steady state, there is a small amount of IL2 in the lymph node, which is almost exclusively used by the regulatory T cells, limiting their expansion. The helper T cells do not expand as result of the direct suppression of their activation exerted by the R cells. In this situation the injection of IL2, naturally leads to the enhanced expansion of R cells reinforcing the suppression over the E cells. Only when the IL2 concentration is extremely high at the lymph nodes it triggers a significant expansion of the Memory T cells, signaling through the intermediate affinity IL2 receptor beta-gamma. The excessive expansion of the M cells in the system affects the suppressive interaction between E and R cells at the APCs, since these cells, although much weakly, also interact with and compete for the available APCs.

Interestingly the latter model predictions are indeed compatible with existent experimental observations and further provide a guideline for its future practical application. On the one hand, the reinforcement of ongoing immune reactions by IL2 injections, predicted by the model, explains classical observations on *in vivo* animal models, where IL2 have been shown to potentiate immune reactions to viral infection (35) and to well-adjuvated vaccines (1–3). In these systems the immune response induced to

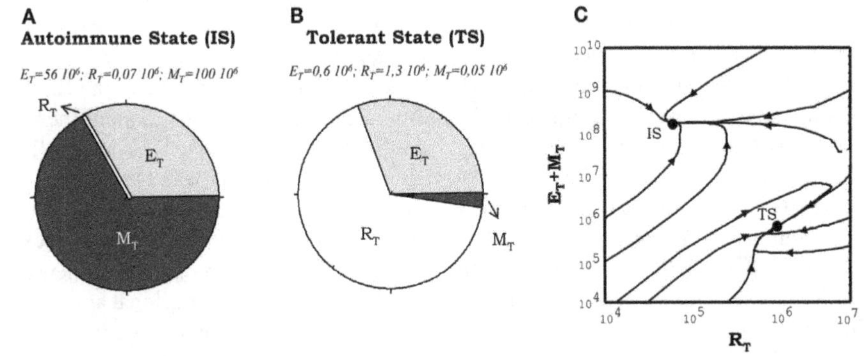

FIGURE 4 | Illustration of the steady states obtained from numerical simulations of the model. (A,B) shows the proportion of the total T cell number corresponding to helper (E), regulatory (R), and memory (M) T cells. The situation showed in **(A)**, corresponds to the autoimmune steady state (IS) where the memory and helper T cells dominate the system. The situation depicted in **(B)**, correspond to the tolerant steady state (TS) where the regulatory T cells dominate the dynamics. The graph in **(C)** illustrates how these two types of steady state of the system co-exist in the same region of parameter values (the region of bistability). It is shown how different initial conditions, changing just the proportion of E, R, and M cells at time $t=0$, leads to trajectories taking the system either in the tolerant (TS) or the autoimmune (IS) steady state.

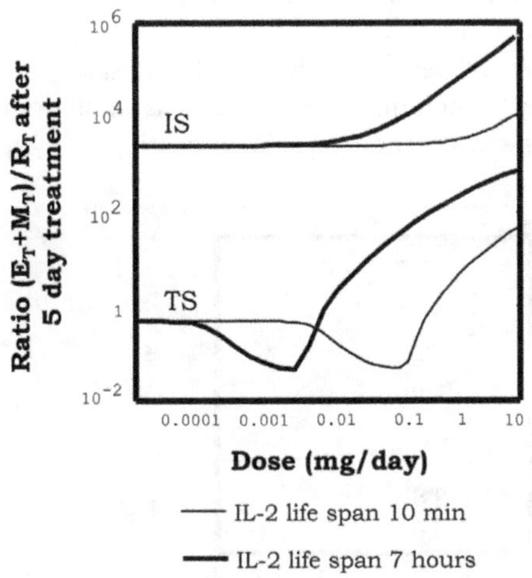

FIGURE 5 | Effect of injections of IL2, on the proportion of helper + memory T cells versus regulatory T cells [ratio (E + M)/R], in a system initialized either in tolerant (TS) or the autoimmune (IS) steady state. The graph shows the ratio (E + M)/R attained in the system right after 5 days of continuous injections of the indicated dose (*x* axis of the graph) of an IL2 with either 10 min (thin curves) or 7 h (thick curves) life span in solution. It can be seen how when the simulations start with a system at the TS, the ratio (E + M)/R reduce its values for intermediate dose of the treatment. This is a direct consequence of a preferential expansion of the R cells in the system. However, if the dose is further increased then the ratio (E + M)/R is significantly increased. This is a direct consequence of the expansion of helper and memory T cells, by the treatment application. When the treatment start on a system at the IS, then increasing the dose always leads to an increase of the ratio (E + M)/R. This is, it further increments the number of E and R cells in the system. Interestingly increasing the life span of the injected IL2 moves to lower values the dose ranges where treatment is effective, but does not change the qualitative pattern of response observed.

the involved foreign antigens, which are most probably loosely or just not controlled by regulatory T cell activity, is further promoted by the injected IL2. Furthermore, the observed enhancement of immunity, in these experimental systems, might not relay just on the model predicted expansion of helper $CD4^+$ T cells. It might also involve important direct effects of IL2 on memory $CD8^+$ T cell and/or NK cells, which are known to be relevant in many of these particular systems. In any case the model here, will further predict that optimal application of IL2 for the purpose of enhancing immunity, will be obtained when providing IL2 after the immune reaction have already started and never before, because some reminiscent of immune regulation might still exist and could be potentiated by the added IL2.

On the other hand, the capacity of IL2 addition to reinforce natural tolerance mediated by regulatory T cells, predicted by the model, explains as well several experimental observations. Particularly, it explains clinical data stating that regulatory T cells populations are significantly expanded, both in cancer (9, 36) and HIV (37) patients, treated with IL2. Such effect might be related to the poor efficacy observed in these clinical applications of IL2. Particularly, in the case of cancer, less than 20% of the treated patients show some anti-tumor effect, perhaps, according to the model here, because just an small fraction of the patients, happen to have a naturally preexistent immune response against tumor antigens, which could be further enhanced by the injected IL2. In the case HIV patients, IL2 based therapy have led to the recovery of $CD4^+$ T cells counts, but the patients do not seem to recover their capacity to fight general infections, perhaps, according to the model here, because this treatment is just reinforcing tolerance mediated by regulatory T cell activity.

Furthermore, this second model prediction also explains many results in pre-clinical animal models. It explains, for instance, that IL2 injections can prevents allograft rejection (10); or attenuate the induction of Experimental Autoimmune Encephalomyelitis (EAE) (10); or fully prevent the development of diabetes in the NOD mice (11). Interestingly, in the EAE and allograft reaction models the latter effects are observed for scheme of IL2 applications where this cytokine is injected in the system before implanting the allogeneic tissue or before inducing the EAE. This is before the immune/autoimmune reaction has been expanded; i.e., when there is a preexistent natural tolerance, mediated by regulatory T cells, which could be reinforced by the applied treatment. However, in the NOD mice model, recent data (12) have shown that IL2 treatment at the onset of diabetes could revert disease development. Interestingly, in this "therapeutically relevant scenario" treatment efficacy is much lower than in the preventive settings. Only 40–60% of the NOD mice appear to be cured, while 100% of the NOD mice are diabetes free when treating in the preventive settings. Whether or not at the onset of NOD mice diabetes the balance between regulatory T cells and helpers T cells have been fully disrupted in favor of immunity, just as considered in our model simulations of an autoimmune disease therapeutic scenario, is a matter of discussion. Actually Grinberg-Bleyer et al. have shown that at the onset of NOD diabetes a significant amount of regulatory T cells can still be found in the pancreas and its draining lymph node. Unfortunately in the NOD mice, the acute nature of diabetes development (with a full irreversible destruction beta islet) invalidates any displacement of the treatment application toward a more advanced stage of the disease, to better compare with our model predictions.

Simulating the injections of different anti-IL2 mAbs

Anti-IL2 antibodies are molecules that form complexes with the IL2, blocking or not its binding to the different chains of the IL2 receptor at the T cell surface and therefore interfering with the associated signaling process. Three classes of antibodies are systematically explored in our simulations following its documented existence in the literature (20, 38): (1) The anti-IL2 mAbs, which bind and thus block the site in the IL2 surface implicated on the interaction with the alpha chain of the IL2 receptor (referred here as the face alpha mAbs); (2) The anti-IL2 mAbs, which bind and thus block the site in the IL2 surface implicated on the interaction with the beta chain of the IL2 receptor (referred here as face beta mAbs); and (3) the anti-IL2, which block the binding of IL2 to all chains of the IL2 receptor (referred here as a fully blocking mAbs).

The injection of monoclonal antibodies anti-IL2, in the model simulations, when applied to a previously tolerant system could induce a breakdown of tolerance (**Figure 6A**), with the consequent transition of the system to the autoimmune steady state. Such effect can be obtained with the three classes of anti-IL2 mAbs studied, but it requires a minimal effective dose of the anti-IL2 mAb and treatment duration (**Figure 6A**) which varies significantly with the type of mAbs used. Face alpha mAbs are significantly more efficient than fully blocking or face beta mAbs (**Figure 6A**) in this simulation. Moreover, for the three classes of mAbs studied the higher the affinity for the IL2 the higher their efficacy in these simulation (27).

The effect of treatment with anti-IL2 mAbs in a system with a preexistent autoimmune reaction is also quite significant. In this case, the treatment is capable of resetting the system into the

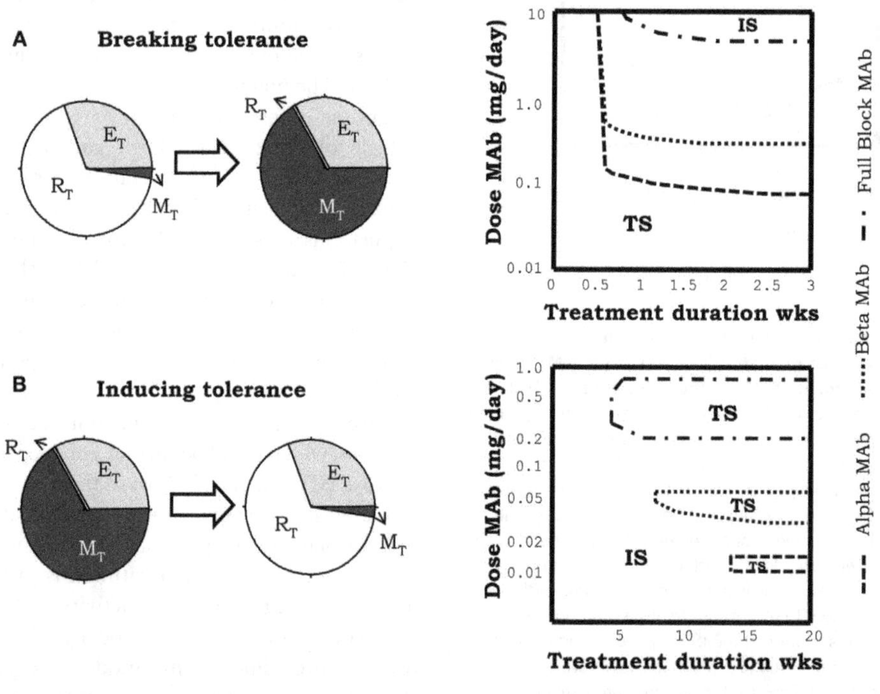

FIGURE 6 | Effect of the simulation of treatments of IL2 depletion, using different anti-IL2 antibodies. mAbs in the simulation, can block the interaction of IL2 with the alpha (face alpha mAb), or with the beta (face beta mAb) or with both (fully blocking mAb) chains of the IL2R. The graphs in **(A)** corresponds to the case in which the treatment induces a breakdown of the preexistent tolerant steady state, i.e., a transition to the autoimmune steady state. The graphs in **(B)** corresponds to the case in which treatment induces tolerance, taking into the tolerant steady state, a system initially set in the autoimmune steady state. Breakdown of a preexistent tolerant state requires a minimal effective dose of mAb and treatment duration [graph in the right side of **(A)**]. In this scenario, face alpha mAbs are more efficient than face beta or fully blocking mAb. This means that the latter need higher doses of mAb to achieve a similar effect. Induction of tolerance requires minimum treatment duration with a mAb dose inside an intermediate window of values [graph in the right side of **(B)**]. This effect is obtained when face alpha, face beta, or fully blocking mAbs are used.

tolerant steady state (i.e., inducing tolerance) (**Figure 6B**). This effect occur under quite restrictive treatment conditions: there is a minimal treatment duration required and the dose of the anti-IL2 mAbs used has to be set inside some particular intermediate range of values (**Figure 6B**). The tolerogenic effect of the anti-IL2 mAbs is obtained with all type of mAbs (**Figure 6B**). Differences in the mAbs affinity and mAbs class strongly change the dose range where this effect is observed[2].

Overall the simulations of IL2 depletion treatments using anti-IL2 antibodies predict that this type of therapy is able to break a preexistent tolerant state, inducing an autoimmune response, or to render tolerant a preexistent autoimmune system. A closer look to the model behavior qualitatively explains these results as follows. The injected mAbs appear to sequester the IL2, limiting its availability to provide signal to the T cells. When the treatment is applied into an initially tolerant steady state, the initial effective concentration of IL2 is low and it is further reduced to insignificant levels, where this cytokine is incapable to signal neither to E, R, or M cells. Therefore, if the treatment is sustained long enough, the number of R cells fall down to a minimum determined by the size of the thymic output, because the proliferation and survival of R cells is strictly dependent on IL2. But the number of E cells, on the other hand, set back to a value determined by the availability of the homeostatic cytokine of ILα, which they could use as alternative to IL2 signal. Therefore once the injected mAbs are cleared, the auto-reactive E cells could have some initial advantage in respect to the R cells, leading the T cell expansion, which drive the system into the autoimmune steady state. However, when the treatment is applied to an initially autoimmune system, the effective concentration of IL2 is quite large and it is reduced by the presence of the antibody. The efficacy of the mAbs to affect IL2 signaling in the different T cell population is strongly dependent on its affinity for the IL2 and the side of the IL2 recognized. For a very high antibody dose, the effective IL2 concentration falls to negligible values, which as before are unable to signal neither to E, R, or M cells. Thus the size of the auto-reactive E cell population is reduced to the value set by the availability of ILα and the number of R cell remains low in a value determined by the size of thymic output. When the injected antibody is cleared the system could return back to the autoimmune equilibrium. However, for some intermediate doses of the antibody, the effective IL2 concentration is reduced to values where it is unable to signal on the E and M cells, but it is still significant for the R cells, which are more sensitive due to their higher expression of the alpha chain of the IL2 receptor. Therefore, for these mAbs doses the E cell population is reduced to the minimal size, which can be sustained by the available ILα. But the R cells are stimulated to grow forcing the system to switch into the tolerant steady state.

The model prediction of a higher efficacy of treatments with face alpha mAbs, to break a preexistent tolerant steady state, relates to the impact of this type of mAbs on the dynamics of the M cells. Face alpha mAbs bind the available IL2 forming immune-complexes that can still signal through the intermediate affinity IL2 receptor (beta + gamma chain). This form of the receptor is prevalent in the M cells, thus face alpha mAbs partially redirect IL2 signaling into the M cells expanding this population. The growth of the M cells interferes with the dynamics of CD4$^+$ T cells, i.e., M cells consume the available IL2 and reduce the capacity of CD4$^+$ T cells to interact with the APCs. The combination of the latter effects explains the advantage of the face alpha mAb to break a preexistent tolerant steady state. On the other hand, the differences observed between fully blocking and face beta mAbs in the model simulations (compare dose dependencies in **Figure 6**), must rely on the fact that face beta mAbs do not block the interaction with the alpha chain of the IL2 receptor, conditioning the attachment of the immune-complexes formed to cells that express this molecule at the cells surface. These interactions significantly alter the bio-distribution of both the IL2 and the antibody.

Interestingly, the latter model predictions are indeed compatible with existent experimental observations. On the one hand, the predicted capacity of treatments blocking IL2 activity to promote autoimmunity/immunity, explains observations where monoclonal antibodies against IL2 have been shown to promote effective immune responses to tumors (16) and to induce autoimmune disease in naïve mice (13). In both cases, the model explains the observed effects as being associated to the treatment capacity to weaken regulatory cell activity, just as argued by their original authors. It must be also noted that in these reports the S4B6 anti-IL2 mAbs was used, a mAb which has been recently proven to block only the interaction of IL2 with the alpha chain of the IL2 receptor (38).

On the other hand, the model predicted capacity of IL2 blocking therapies to reestablish tolerance in the context of ongoing immune/autoimmune reactions, is not documented in the literature. This model prediction is very interesting from the practical perspectives for the treatment of autoimmune diseases. However, the fact that the predicted treatment effect just occurs for a particular intermediate range of antibody doses, applied during a relatively long period of time, makes difficult the practical implementation of the treatment. To overcome the latter problem we suggested, based on model simulations, an alternative/simpler strategy to capitalize this therapeutic effect. A large initial dose of the mAb could be used, reducing it periodically with a fixed rate. With this alternative strategy the model predict a much simpler dose dependency (see **Figure 7**) of treatment efficacy, i.e., the applied initial dose used must be large enough (as to induce significant initial immunosuppression), and the reduction rate used should be sufficiently slow.

Simulating the injection of IL2/mAb immune-complexes

Immune-complexes of IL2 plus anti-IL2 mAbs (in a 1:2 mAb:IL2 molar proportion), has been recently highlighted as a novel therapeutic strategy (18, 20, 39) which could significantly potentiate the activity of the IL2 *in vivo*. Intuitively it should be expected that the therapy with immune-complexes share properties with

[2]Treatment using the face alpha mAbs is the best option (it work for lower MAb dose windows, example shown in **Figure 6B**) when the mAb used has an affinity for IL2 lower than 10^{10} M^{-1}. But the capacity of this mAb to revert an autoimmune state is completely lost if the mAb affinity for IL2 is assumed to be higher. The face beta mAbs seems to work well for a larger range of mAbs affinities. Its effect is lost only for unrealistically high affinities (larger than 10^{11} M^{-1}) and it is always better than the one obtained with a fully blocking mAb. In Ref. (27), **Figure 7**, we presented results considering a mAb affinity higher than 10^{10} M^{-1}, where the face alpha mAb is not effective in reverting an autoimmune state.

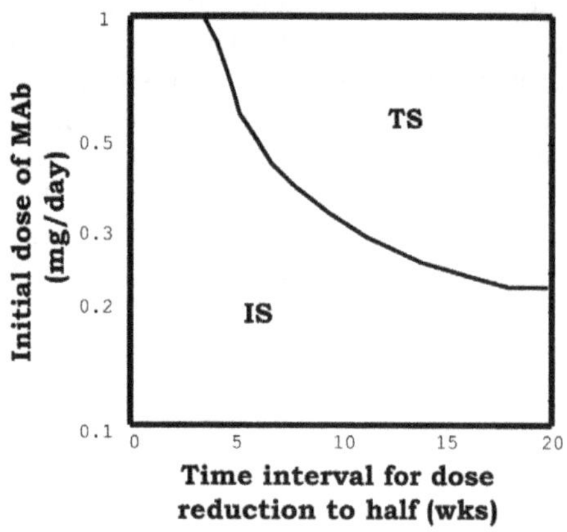

FIGURE 7 | The graph summarizes the results of simulations of a model system set initially to the IS and then perturbed with, an initial dose of the face beta mAb, which is periodically reduced to the half at the indicated time (*x* axis). The curve indicates the minimal value of the initial mAb dose required to induce tolerance (taking the system into the tolerant steady state) with the applied treatment.

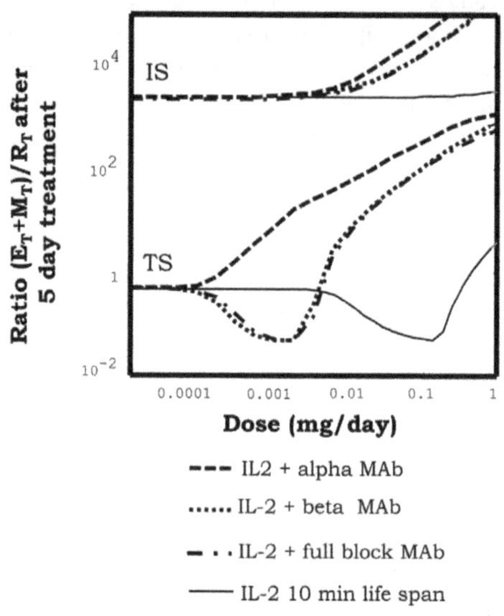

FIGURE 8 | Effect of injections for five days of the indicated doses of immune-complexes of IL2 plus antibodies anti-IL2, on the ratio of helper + memory T cells versus regulatory T cells [ratio (E + M)/R], in a system initialized either in tolerant (TS) or the autoimmune (IS) steady state. Different immune-complexes differ on the class of mAb used to form it (face alpha, face beta or fully blocking mAbs). immune-complexes are always formed with a 1:2 molar ratio of mAbs:IL2 and the dose applied is reported in terms of the mass of IL2 injected. If the simulations start with a system at the TS, immune-complexes formed with face beta or fully blocking mAbs reduce the ratio (E + M)/R for some intermediate dose values and then increases it for higher dose values. This is a pattern of response, qualitatively similar to that obtained with IL2 injection, but significantly displaced to the range of lower doses of IL2. If face alpha mAbs are used to form the complex the pattern of response obtained is qualitatively different. The ratio (E + M)/R always increase (favoring the expansion of E and M cells) and the larger the dose applied the larger the increment. If the simulations start with a system at the IS, all the possible immune-complexes behave qualitatively like the IL2 alone, they promote in dose-dependent way a further expansion of E and R cells, increasing the ratio (E + M)/R.

the therapies based on its basic components, but their comparative efficacy shall depend on the class and the affinity of the mAbs used.

In our simulations, immune-complexes can either reinforce or weaken a preexistent tolerant steady state depending on the class of mAb used on its formulation. **Figure 5**, shows how the injection of immune-complexes significantly changes the number of E, R, and M cells in the system initially set to the tolerant steady state. Immune-complexes formed with beta face or fully blocking mAbs induce a quite significant transient expansion of Regulatory T cells (reinforcing the tolerant state). This transient expansion of the Regulatory T cells is significantly larger than the one induced by an equivalent treatment with IL2 alone and it is maximal for mAbs with some intermediate affinity for the IL2 (27). However, immune-complexes formed with face alpha mAbs have a quite different effect in these simulations (**Figure 8**). They could also expand the R cells, but they expand much more in comparison the M cells in the lymph node. The capacity of this immune complex to expand M cells became larger as their affinity for the IL2 is increased (27). Interestingly for the three classes of immune-complexes a sufficiently high dose of the latter treatment could induce a breakdown of tolerance. But only immune-complexes based on face alpha mAbs perform better in this task than the therapy based on the anti-IL2 mAb or the IL2 alone (**Figure 9**).

When applied to initially autoimmune steady states, all immune-complexes fail to reestablish tolerance steady state. As the injection of IL2 the immune-complexes further reinforce a preexistent autoimmune steady state, expanding the helper and memory T cells (**Figure 8**).

Summarizing the results above shows that immune complex can sometimes synergistically potentiate the effects of IL2 and mAbs. Complexes based on face alpha mAbs do promote immunity primarily by expanding the M cells, and leading ultimately to a quite efficient breakdown of a preexistent tolerant steady state. Complexes based on face beta mAbs, can efficiently reinforce tolerance expanding significantly the R cells preexistent in the tolerant steady state. Face alpha mAbs for immune-complexes are better with the highest possible affinity, but face beta mAbs could be better with some intermediate affinity values.

Qualitatively the effects of immune-complexes can be explained based on two main dynamical properties in the model: (A) In the immune complex the IL2 is protected from degradation. While bind to the mAbs the IL2 has a life span of 3 days (like the mAbs), which is significantly larger than the life span of 10 min reported for free IL2. (B) Immune-complexes block different sites in the surface of IL2 conditioning its preferential interaction with different cell populations, accordingly to their differential expression of the IL2 receptor chains. Face alpha mAbs, form immune-complexes that bind and signal through the beta + gamma pair of IL2 receptors. Thus, since beta chain is over-expressed by the M cells, this complex preferentially redirect the IL2 signal to these cells. Following this analysis one could easily explain why this type of immune complex has a maximal efficiency when the affinity of the face alpha mAbs used is high. With high affinity mAbs, the IL2 is more protected from degradation, and the signaling is maximally

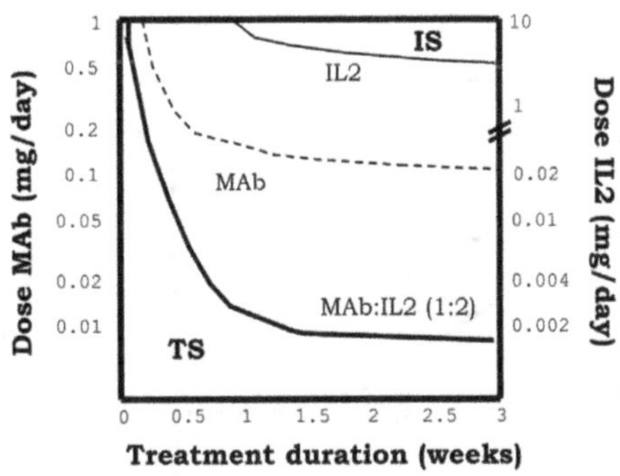

FIGURE 9 | The graph shows the minimal effective dose of mAb (left *y* axis) or IL2 (right *y* axis) versus treatment duration, required to induce the transition to the IS in a system initialized in the TS, for the treatment with immune-complexes formed with face alpha mAbs in the optimal molar proportion 1:2 (mAb:IL2). For direct comparison the equivalent curves obtained for treatments with the same mAbs alone or the IL2 alone are also depicted. It can be seen that the injection of this class of immune complex is more efficient than the injection of the mAb or the IL2 alone to breakdown tolerance in an initial tolerant system, i.e., it requires less dose of either the mAbs or IL2 as compared to the independent treatments.

redirected to the M cells. Face beta mAbs form immune-complexes unable to signal in any class of IL2 receptor. Thus to mediate any biological activity this type of complex has to partially dissociate, working as a controlled source of free IL2. If the affinity of the face beta mAbs in the complex is too high then the IL2 is never released and the immune-complexes have no effect at all. If the affinity of the face beta mAbs is too low, then injecting the complex is like injecting IL2 alone. However, if the affinity of the face beta mAbs in the complex is larger than the affinity of the dimeric IL2 receptor (beta + gamma chain), but lower than the affinity of the trimeric IL2 receptor (alpha + beta + gamma chain), the IL2 in the complex is easily release to provide signal through the high affinity trimeric IL2 receptor, but not through the intermediate affinity dimeric IL2 receptor. In this way the face beta based immune-complexes provided a preferential signaling to the regulatory cells, which overexpress the alpha chain of the IL2 receptor.

Interestingly the model results explain available pre-clinical data on the use of immune-complexes of IL2-anti-IL2 mAbs. Our observations that immune-complexes formed with face alpha or face beta mAbs expand different cell populations when injected *in vivo* into a normal (tolerant) mouse are fully compatible with the results reported in Ref. (18, 20, 39). In these experiments, the S4B6 mAb (a face alpha mAbs) is shown to form immune-complexes that strongly expands $CD8^+CD44^+$ T cells and to a lesser extent the R cells (20). This face alpha immune complex has been also used to increment the immune response induced with a vaccine (17), showing a significantly higher efficiency than IL2 alone. Moreover, the group of Jonathan Sprent have shown that JES6-1 (originally described as a face beta mAbs (20), although it has been recently observed that it also blocks the interaction with CD25, behaving more like a fully blocking mAbs) induce a larger expansion of Tregs ($CD4^+CD25^+Foxp3^+$ T cells) than the injection of IL2 alone in the same experimental setting (20). Remarkably, this latter type of immune complex has been shown to reinforce a preexistent tolerance state, preventing graft rejection or autoimmune disease induction in mice (18). But it showed no effect when applied in a therapeutic setting, this is just after the onset of the autoimmune disease or the initiation of skin graft rejection process (18).

The simulations, however, propose some interesting guidelines to improve the therapeutic effect of immune-complexes. They predict that in the case of complexes using face alpha mAbs, the best strategy is to use mAbs with the higher affinity available. But in the case of immune-complexes formed with face Beta or fully blocking mAbs, the use of intermediate affinity mAbs is recommended. Other important prediction of our model simulations is that treatment with immune-complexes based on face beta or fully blocking mAbs are useful to reinforce a preexistent tolerant state preventing the induction of autoimmunity, but it would be quite inefficient to therapeutically treat an already established autoimmune disorder. For the later task, the best strategy would be to use the anti-IL2 mAbs alone following the strategies described in Section "Simulating the Injections of Different Anti-IL2 mAbs."

Simulating the injection of IL2 mutants

Several mutant variants of IL2 have been designed aiming to improve the therapeutic efficacy of wild-type IL2 in cancer therapy. Most strategies, so far explored, involve the development of IL-2 variants with an either reduced or increased binding affinity for the alpha or the beta chain of the IL2R. In this section three particular classes of mutants are simulated: (a) IL2 Mutant with a reduced conjugation affinity for the alpha chain of the IL-2R as the one described in Ref. (40) (referred here as No-alpha mutants); (b) IL2 Mutant with an increased conjugation affinity for the alpha chain of IL-2R as the one described in Ref. (41) (referred here as Alpha-Plus mutants); (c) IL2 Mutant with an increased affinity for the beta chain of the IL2R as the one described in Ref. (42) (referred here as Beta-Plus mutant). These three classes of IL2 mutants provide a functional IL2 signal to T cells, since they keep binding beta and gamma unit of the IL2 receptor (i.e., they are IL2 agonists). But they might be expected to alter the natural balance in which wild-type IL2 is consumed by different T cell types, resulting on a significantly different overall dynamics.

Figure 10A show the effect of injecting different IL2 variants in a system initially set in the tolerant steady state. As described in Section "Simulating the Injection of IL2," injection of wild-type IL2 transiently reinforce this preexistent tolerant steady state, preferentially expanding the Regulatory T cells in the system. Alpha-Plus IL2 mutants, exhibit a similar response pattern than wtIL2, but with an even more marked preferential expansion of the regulatory T cells. In contrast, No-Alpha and Beta-Plus mutants show a completely different response pattern than wild-type IL2. This class of mutants expand preferentially the helper T cells (E + M), rather than the regulatory T cells at all injection doses. Moreover injections of the three classes of mutants, as for the wild-type IL2, could lead to a breakdown of tolerance in the system when the dose used is significantly increased. However, the minimal dose required for such effect is significantly lower for the No-Alpha mutants and Beta-Plus mutant **Figure 10B**, than for wild-type IL2 and Alpha-Plus mutants.

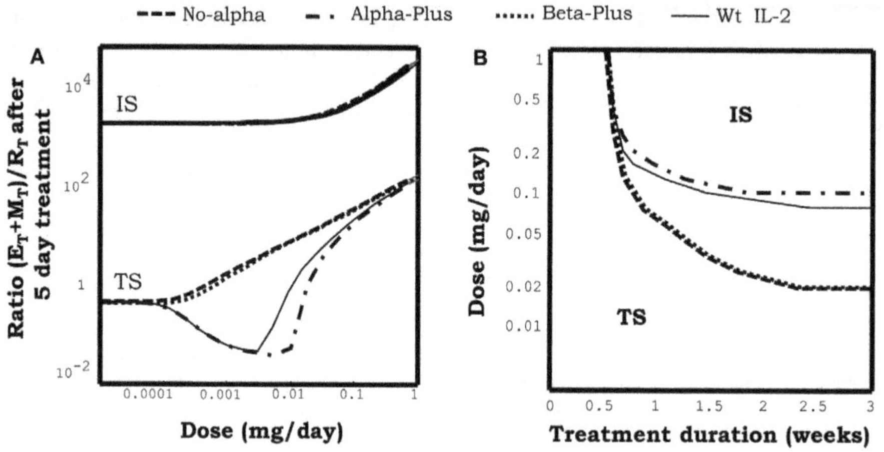

FIGURE 10 | The graph in (A) shows the effect of injections for 5 days at the indicated dose of different mutant variants of IL2 on the ratio of helper + memory T cells versus regulatory T cells [ratio (E + M)/R], in a system initialized either in the tolerant (TS) or the autoimmune (IS) steady state. Mutants differ on their capacity to bind to the different chains of the IL2R. Alpha-plus and Beta-plus mutants have higher binding affinity than wild-type IL2 respectively for the alpha chain ($f_\alpha = 1000$, $f_\beta = 1$) and the beta chain ($f_\alpha = 1$, $f_\beta = 1000$), while No-alpha mutant lack the binding to the alpha chain ($f_\alpha = 0.001$, $f_\beta = 1$). All mutant variants were simulated with a life span of 7 h. If the simulations start with a system at the TS, Alpha-plus mutant reduces the ratio (E + M)/R for some intermediate dose values and then increases it for higher dose values. This is a pattern of response, qualitatively similar to that obtained with IL2 injection, although with a slighter wider range of treatment dose with ratio (E + M)/R reduced from its starting value. If No-alpha or Beta-plus mutants are used the pattern of response obtained is qualitatively different. The ratio (E + M)/R always increase (favoring the expansion of E and M cells) and the larger the dose applied the larger the increment. If the simulations start with a system at the IS, all the mutants variants behave like the wild-type IL2, they promote in dose-dependent way a further expansion of E and R cells, increasing the ratio (E + M)/R. The graph in **(B)** shows the minimal effective dose versus the treatment duration, required to induce the transition to the IS in a system initialized in the TS, for the treatment with different variants of IL2 mutants. It can be seen that the injection of No-alpha and Beta-Plus IL2 mutants is more efficient than the injection of wild-type IL2 alone to breakdown tolerance in an initial tolerant system, i.e., it requires less dose to achieve a similar effect.

Figure 10A also shows the effect of injecting different classes of IL2 mutants in a model system initially set in the autoimmune steady state. In this case the three classes of mutants behave quite similarly to wild-type IL2, i.e., None of them is able to promote a transition to a tolerant steady states, at any dose and treatment duration. Moreover, they reinforce the preexistent autoimmune steady state, further expanding the Helper and Memory T cells.

Overall the result in this section show that No-Alpha and Beta-Plus IL2 mutants behave quite similarly, being significantly better than wild-type IL2 to promote immunity. While Alpha-Plus mutants could be slightly better that wild-type IL2 to reinforce a preexistent tolerant state, expanding more the regulatory T cells. Qualitatively, the latter results could be easily understood in the model, by taking into account the differential expression of the high affinity/trimeric form (alpha + beta + gamma) and intermediate affinities/dimeric form (beta + gamma) of the IL2 receptors on the different T cell populations. Regulatory T cells, relay on the overexpression of the alpha chain of the IL2R, to have the highest expression of the high affinity form of the IL2R. Memory T cells relay in the overexpression of the beta chain of the IL2 R to have the higest expression level of the intermediate affinity form of the IL2R. The No-Alpha and Beta-Plus mutants have a similar impact in the balance of use of IL2 related signal in the model. In both cases the resulting mutants lack the preferential capacity to signal over Regulatory T cells at low concentration, which is characteristic of the wild-type IL2. Furthermore they will preferentially redirect the signal toward the memory T cells, and strongly promote immunity. As the reverse case the Alpha-Plus mutant, reinforce the capacity of the wild-type IL2 to signal preferentially over the Regulatory T cells, resulting on a better tool to reinforce a preexistent tolerance state.

The results obtained above are compatible with existent experimental data. Both No-alpha (40) and Beta-Plus (42) mutants have been shown to induce a more potent anti-tumoral response than wild-type IL2 in several transplantable tumor models in mice. The dynamic effects predicted *in silico* for these types of IL-2 mutants is qualitatively similar to those described in Sections "Simulating the Injection of IL2/mAb Immune-Complexes" for treatments with immune-complexes of IL-2 and anti-IL-2 mAbs, when face alpha mAb are used. Indeed No-Alpha mutants can be easily conceptualized as an extreme case of such immune-complexes if the affinity of the mAbs for the IL2 tends to infinity. From a quantitative point of view, in the model, IL2 mutants can become as efficient as the immune-complexes, only when its life span is set to be greater than 24 h. If the life span of the mutant is taken to be of 7 h (the one used in **Figure 10**), which is the one reported for a wtIL2 fused to a constant region of IgG (43), then one might need around 5–10 time more mutant than wtIL2 in the immune-complex to obtain an equivalent effect. However, since immune-complexes work *in vivo* at very low concentrations of IL2, 1–2 micrograms in mice (20), a quite reasonably small amount of the IL2 mutants would be required to induce a similar effect. Thus, these IL2 mutants can be useful tools to promote immunity, for instance to treat tumors or to enhance the response to cancer vaccines. It is important to note that mutants might have some regulatory/developmental advantages as potential drugs in comparison to the immune-complexes, given the fact that they are single molecules.

The predicted capacity of Alpha-Plus mutants to reinforce preexistent tolerant steady state, expanding the regulatory T cells, has never been evaluated. A mutant variant of IL2 with 1000 times' higher affinity for the IL-2Ra was developed by Rao et al. (41). But only the *in vitro* effect of this mutant on different T cell lines was evaluated. Potentially the Alpha-Plus mutant could be used to treat patients that would receive an organ transplant to reduce the risk of graft rejection. However from a quantitative point of view the mutant efficacy expanding regulatory T cells is predicted only as slightly better than that of wild-type IL2. Moreover, it is quite similar to that obtained with immune-complexes of IL2-anti-IL2 mAbs formed with face beta or fully blocking mAbs (see Simulating the injection of IL2/mAb immune-complexes), when its life span is set to be of around 7 h (the value used in **Figure 10**). This is when its life span is similar to that reported for a wtIL2 fused to a constant region of IgG (43). Therefore this Alpha-plus mutant or just simply the wild-type IL2 fused to Fc of IgG, could be a reasonable drug to prevent allograft rejection. They might have a similar effect to that reported for immune-complexes in mice, but being much simpler drugs to develop. Indeed a version of IL2 fused to Fc portions of immunoglobulin is already available (43).

CONCLUDING REMARKS

Mathematical modeling of the IL2 and T-cell dynamics, considering the dual role of IL2 in its interaction with regulatory and helper CD4$^+$ T cells, is able to explain the complexity observed in the effects of IL2 modulating treatments. In this sense, we show that the model explains a large amount of available clinical and pre-clinical data. Moreover, it predicts optimal strategies for the future application of these treatments:

(A) Mutant variants of IL2, either with reduced affinity for CD25 (the alpha chain of IL2 receptor) or an increased affinity for CD122 (the beta chain of IL2 receptor), and with an increased life span in circulation (for instance fusing them to Fc portion of IgG), are the best strategy to potentiate immunity alone or in combination with vaccines.

(B) Increasing IL2 life span in circulation, either by fusing it with larger proteins or forming complexes with mAbs that block the interaction of IL2 and CD122 (the beta chain of the IL2 receptor), significantly potentiate its capacity to reinforce a preexistent natural tolerance, further expanding the regulatory T cells. This effect might be useful to treat patients that would receive an organ transplant, reducing the risk of graft rejection.

(C) Anti-IL2 antibodies which block the interaction of IL2 with CD122, CD25, or both can be used to treat an ongoing autoimmune disorder, promoting the induction of tolerance. The best schedule for this therapy is to start treatment with a high dose of the mAb (one capable to induce some immune suppression) and then scale the dose down slowly the dose in subsequent applications.

Last, but not least, it is important to highlight that our model has focused on the control that IL2 exerts on T cell cycle progression, impacting both in T cell proliferation and survival. We have neglected some other reported roles of IL2 in T cell differentiation. For instance, IL2 has been reported to increase the suppressive capacity of the Regulatory T cells (12); to condition the differentiation of CD8 T cells into a memory phenotype (44, 45); to induce together with TGFb, the generation of the so called induced Tregs from naïve CD4$^+$ T cells (46). We believe these phenomena, although important in some experimental contexts, are not essential to understands the main phenomenology studies in this paper. In future studies, the current model could be extended to include some or all of the above referred interactions of IL2.

Moreover, severe toxicity, i.e., the appearance of the cytokine storm and the vascular leak syndrome, is perhaps the major limitation known today of the practical application of IL2 modulation treatments in clinics. Our model cannot be used to simulate directly the toxic effects of the different IL2 modulation treatments studied. It could only be used to predict strategies that optimize the expected therapeutic efficacy related to the balance between regulatory and effector CD4$^+$ T cells. However, a recent report by the group of Boyman (47) has shown that vascular leak syndrome, which leads to severe pulmonary edema, is caused by the direct interaction of IL2 with its high affinity receptor expressed in lung epithelial cells. They demonstrated that treatment with immune-complexes of IL2 + S4B6 mAbs (anti-IL2 mAb which interferes the binding of IL2 to the alpha chain of IL2 receptor), prevents vascular leak syndrome while inducing a potent anti-tumor response. Furthermore, in Carmenate el al. (40), treatment with IL2 mutants with a reduced affinity for CD25 (no-alpha mutant) was shown to be less toxic than treatment with wild-type IL2. These experimental observations support the practical feasibility of some of our model predictions.

REFERENCES

1. Kudo-Saito C, Garnett CT, Wansley EK, Schlom J, Hodge JW. Intratumoral delivery of vector mediated IL-2 in combination with vaccine results in enhanced T cell avidity and anti-tumor activity. *Cancer Immunol Immunother* (2007) **56**(12):1897–910. doi:10.1007/s00262-007-0332-1
2. Fishman M, Hunter TB, Soliman H, Thompson P, Dunn M, Smilee R, et al. Phase II trial of B7-1 (CD-86) transduced, cultured autologous tumor cell vaccine plus subcutaneous interleukin-2 for treatment of stage IV renal cell carcinoma. *J Immunother* (2008) **31**(1):72–80. doi:10.1097/CJI.0b013e31815ba792
3. Lin CT, Tsai YC, He L, Yeh CN, Chang TC, Soong YK, et al. DNA vaccines encoding IL-2 linked to HPV-16 E7 antigen generate enhanced E7-specific CTL responses and antitumor activity. *Immunol Lett* (2007) **114**(2):86–93. doi:10.1016/j.imlet.2007.09.008
4. Tarpey I, van Loon AA, de Haas N, Davis PJ, Orbell S, Cavanagh D, et al. A recombinant turkey Herpesvirus expressing chicken interleukin-2 increases the protection provided by in ovo vaccination with infectious bursal disease and infectious bronchitis virus. *Vaccine* (2007) **25**(51):8529–35. doi:10.1016/j.vaccine.2007.10.006
5. Davey RT Jr, Murphy RL, Graziano FM, Boswell SL, Pavia AT, Cancio M, et al. Immunologic and virologic effects of subcutaneous interleukin 2 in combination with antiretroviral therapy: a randomized controlled trial. *JAMA* (2000) **284**(2):183–9. doi:10.1001/jama.284.2.183
6. Kovacs JA, Vogel S, Albert JM, Falloon J, Davey RT Jr, Walker RE, et al. Controlled trial of interleukin-2 infusions in patients infected with the human immunodeficiency virus. *N Engl J Med* (1996) **335**(18):1350–6. doi:10.1056/NEJM199610313351803

7. Sereti I, Martinez-Wilson H, Metcalf JA, Baseler MW, Hallahan CW, Hahn B, et al. Long-term effects of intermittent interleukin 2 therapy in patients with HIV infection: characterization of a novel subset of CD4(+)/CD25(+) T cells. *Blood* (2002) **100**(6):2159–67.
8. Natarajan V, Lempicki RA, Sereti I, Badralmaa Y, Adelsberger JW, Metcalf JA, et al. Increased peripheral expansion of naive CD4+ T cells in vivo after IL-2 treatment of patients with HIV infection. *Proc Natl Acad Sci U S A* (2002) **99**(16):10712–7. doi:10.1073/pnas.162352399
9. Ahmadzadeh M, Rosenberg SA. IL-2 administration increases $CD4^+$ CD25(hi) $Foxp3^+$ regulatory T cells in cancer patients. *Blood* (2006) **107**(6):2409–14. doi:10.1182/blood-2005-06-2399
10. Montero E, Alonso L, Perez R, Lage A. Interleukin-2 mastering regulation in cancer and autoimmunity. *Ann N Y Acad Sci* (2007) **1107**:239–50. doi:10.1196/annals.1381.026
11. Tang Q, Adams JY, Penaranda C, Melli K, Piaggio E, Sgouroudis E, et al. Central role of defective interleukin-2 production in the triggering of islet autoimmune destruction. *Immunity* (2008) **28**(5):687–97. doi:10.1016/j.immuni.2008.03.016
12. Grinberg-Bleyer Y, Baeyens A, You S, Elhage R, Fourcade G, Gregoire S, et al. IL-2 reverses established type 1 diabetes in NOD mice by a local effect on pancreatic regulatory T cells. *J Exp Med* (2010) **207**(9):1871–8. doi:10.1084/jem.20100209
13. Setoguchi R, Hori S, Takahashi T, Sakaguchi S. Homeostatic maintenance of natural Foxp3(+) CD25(+) CD4(+) regulatory T cells by interleukin (IL)-2 and induction of autoimmune disease by IL-2 neutralization. *J Exp Med* (2005) **201**(5):723–35. doi:10.1084/jem.20041982
14. Onizuka S, Tawara I, Shimizu J, Sakaguchi S, Fujita T, Nakayama E. Tumor rejection by in vivo administration of anti-CD25 (interleukin-2 receptor alpha) monoclonal antibody. *Cancer Res* (1999) **59**(13):3128–33.
15. Church AC. Clinical advances in therapies targeting the interleukin-2 receptor. *QJM* (2003) **96**(2):91–102. doi:10.1093/qjmed/hcg014
16. Kamimura D, Sawa Y, Sato M, Agung E, Hirano T, Murakami M. IL-2 in vivo activities and antitumor efficacy enhanced by an anti-IL-2 mAb. *J Immunol* (2006) **177**(1):306–14.
17. Mostbock S, Lutsiak ME, Milenic DE, Baidoo K, Schlom J, Sabzevari H. IL-2/anti-IL-2 antibody complex enhances vaccine-mediated antigen-specific CD8(+) T cell responses and increases the ratio of effector/memory CD8(+) T cells to regulatory T cells. *J Immunol* (2008) **180**(7):5118–29.
18. Webster KE, Walters S, Kohler RE, Mrkvan T, Boyman O, Surh CD, et al. In vivo expansion of Treg cells with IL-2-mAb complexes: induction of resistance to EAE and long-term acceptance of isletallografts without immunosuppression. *J Exp Med* (2009) **206**(4):751–60. doi:10.1084/jem.20082824
19. Boyman O, Surh CD, Sprent J. Potential use of IL-2/anti-IL-2 antibody immune complexes for the treatment of cancer and autoimmune disease. *Expert Opin Biol Ther* (2006) **6**(12):1323–31. doi:10.1517/14712598.6.12.1323
20. Boyman O, Kovar M, Rubinstein MP, Surh CD, Sprent J. Selective stimulation of T cell subsets with antibody-cytokine immune complexes. *Science* (2006) **311**:1924–7. doi:10.1126/science.1122927
21. Smith KA. Interleukin-2: inception, impact, and implications. *Science* (1988) **240**(4856):1169–76. doi:10.1126/science.3131876
22. Almeida AR, Legrand N, Papiernik M, Freitas AA. Homeostasis of peripheral $CD4^+$ T cells: IL-2R alpha and IL-2 shape a population of regulatory cells that controls CD4+ T cell numbers. *J Immunol* (2002) **169**(9):4850–60.
23. Grinberg-Bleyer Y, Saadoun D, Baeyens A, Billiard F, Goldstein JD, Grégoire S, et al. Pathogenic T cells have a paradoxical protective effect in murine autoimmune diabetes by boosting Tregs. *J Clin Invest* (2010) **120**(12):4558–68. doi:10.1172/JCI42945
24. Almeida AR, Zaragoza B, Freitas AA. Indexation as a novel mechanism of lymphocyte homeostasis: the number of CD4+CD25+ regulatory T cells is indexed to the number of IL-2-producing cells. *J Immunol* (2006) **177**(1):192–200.
25. Barthlott T, Moncrieffe H, Veldhoen M, Atkins CJ, Christensen J, O'Garra A, et al. CD25+ CD4+ T cells compete with naive CD4+ T cells for IL-2 and exploit it for the induction of IL-10 production. *Int Immunol* (2005) **17**(3):279–88. doi:10.1093/intimm/dxh207
26. Thornton AM, Shevach EM. CD4+CD25+ immunoregulatory T cells suppress polyclonal T cell activation in vitro by inhibiting interleukin 2 production. *J Exp Med* (1998) **188**(2):287–96. doi:10.1084/jem.188.2.287
27. Garcia-Martinez K, Leon K. Modeling the role of IL-2 in the interplay between CD4+ helper and regulatory T cells: studying the impact of IL2 modulation therapies. *Int Immunol* (2012) **24**(7):427–46. doi:10.1093/intimm/dxr120
28. Garcia-Martinez K, Leon K. Modeling the role of IL-2 in the interplay between CD4+ helper and regulatory T cells: assessing general dynamical properties. *J Theor Biol* (2010) **262**(4):720–32. doi:10.1016/j.jtbi.2009.10.025
29. Smith KA. The structure of IL2 bound to the three chains of the IL2 receptor and how signaling occurs. *Med Immunol* (2006) **5**:3. doi:10.1186/1476-9433-5-3
30. Smith KA. The quantal theory of how the immune system discriminates between "self and non-self." *Med Immunol* (2004) **3**(1):3. doi:10.1186/1476-9433-3-3
31. Kuniyasu Y, Takahashi T, Itoh M, Shimizu J, Toda G, Sakaguchi S. Naturally anergic and suppressive CD25(+)CD4(+) T cells as a functionally and phenotypically distinct immunoregulatory T cell subpopulation. *Int Immunol* (2000) **12**(8):1145–55. doi:10.1093/intimm/12.8.1145
32. Létourneau S, Krieg C, Pantaleo G, Boyman O. IL-2- and CD25-dependent immunoregulatory mechanisms in the homeostasis of T-cell subsets. *J Allergy Clin Immunol* (2009) **123**(4):758–62. doi:10.1016/j.jaci.2009.02.011
33. León K, Peréz R, Lage A, Carneiro J. Modelling T-cell-mediated suppression dependent on interactions in multicellular conjugates. *J Theor Biol* (2000) **207**(2):231–54. doi:10.1006/jtbi.2000.2169
34. Carneiro J, Leon K, Caramalho I, van denDoolC, Gardner R, Oliveira V, et al. When three is not a crowd: a crossregulation model of the dynamics and repertoire selection of regulatory CD4+ T cells. *Immunol Rev* (2007) **216**:48–68.
35. Blattman JN, Grayson JM, Wherry EJ, Kaech SM, Smith KA, Ahmed R. Therapeutic use of IL-2 to enhance antiviral T-cell responses in vivo. *Nat Med* (2003) **9**(5):540–7. doi:10.1038/nm866
36. Cesana GC, DeRaffele G, Cohen S, Moroziewicz D, Mitcham J, Stoutenburg J, et al. Characterization of CD4+CD25+ regulatory T cells in patients treated with high-dose interleukin-2 for metastatic melanoma or renal cell carcinoma. *J Clin Oncol* (2006) **24**(7):1169–77. doi:10.1200/JCO.2005.03.6830
37. Sereti I, Imamichi H, Natarajan V, Imamichi T, Ramchandani MS, Badralmaa Y, et al. In vivo expansion of CD4CD45RO-CD25 T cells expressing foxP3 in IL-2-treated HIV-infected patients. *J Clin Invest* (2005) **115**(7):1839–47. doi:10.1172/JCI24307
38. Rojas G, Pupo A, Leon K, Avellanet J, Carmenate T, Sidhu S. Deciphering the molecular bases of the biological effects of antibodies against Interleukin-2: a versatile platform for fine epitope mapping. *Immunobiology* (2013) **218**(1):105–13. doi:10.1016/j.imbio.2012.02.009
39. Létourneau S, van Leeuwen EM, Krieg C, Martin C, Pantaleo G, Sprent J, et al. IL-2/anti-IL-2 antibody complexes show strong biological activity by avoiding interaction with IL-2 receptor alpha subunit CD25. *Proc Natl Acad Sci U S A* (2010) **107**(5):2171–6. doi:10.1073/pnas.0909384107
40. Carmenate T, Pacios A, Enamorado M, Moreno E, Garcia-Martínez K, Fuente D, et al. Human IL-2 mutein with higher antitumor efficacy than wild type IL-2. *J Immunol* (2013) **190**(12):6230–8. doi:10.4049/jimmunol.1201895
41. Rao BM, Driver I, Lauffenburger DA, Wittrup KD. High-affinity CD25-binding IL-2 mutants potently stimulate persistent T cell growth. *Biochemistry* (2005) **44**(31):10696–701. doi:10.1021/bi050436x
42. Levin AM, Bates DL, Ring AM, Krieg C, Lin JT, Su L, et al. Exploiting a natural conformational switch to engineer an interleukin-2 'superkine.' *Nature* (2012) **484**(7395):529–33. doi:10.1038/nature10975
43. Harvill ET, Fleming JM, Morrison SL. In vivo properties of an IgG3-IL-2 fusion protein. A general strategy for immune potentiation. *J Immunol* (1996) **157**(7):3165–70.
44. Williams MA, Tyznik AJ, Bevan MJ. Interleukin-2 signals during priming are required for secondary expansion of CD8+ memory T cells. *Nature* (2006) **441**(7095):890–3. doi:10.1038/nature04790
45. Kamimura D, Bevan MJ. Naive CD8+ T cells differentiate into protective memory-like cells after IL-2 anti IL-2 complex treatment in vivo. *J Exp Med* (2007) **204**(8):1803–12. doi:10.1084/jem.20070543
46. Zheng SG, Wang J, Wang P, Gray JD, Horwitz DA. IL-2 is essential for TGF-beta to convert naive CD4+CD25− cells to CD25+Foxp3+ regulatory T cells and for expansion of these cells. *J Immunol* (2007) **178**(4):2018–27.
47. Krieg C, Letourneau S, Pantaleo G, Boyman O. Improved IL-2 immunotherapy by selective stimulation of IL-2 receptors on lymphocytes and endothelial cells. *Proc Natl Acad Sci U S A* (2010) **107**:11906. doi:10.1073/pnas.1002569107

48. Wolf M, Schimpl A, Hunig T. Control of T cell hyperactivation in IL-2-deficient mice by CD4(+)CD25(−) and CD4(+)CD25(+) T cells: evidence for two distinct regulatory mechanisms. *Eur J Immunol* (2001) **31**(6):1637–45. doi:10.1002/1521-4141(200106)31:6<1637::AID-IMMU1637>3.0.CO;2-T

49. Malek TR, Porter BO, Codias EK, Scibelli P, Yu A. Normal lymphoid homeostasis and lack of lethal autoimmunity in mice containing mature T cells with severely impaired IL-2 receptors. *J Immunol* (2000) **164**(6):2905–14.

APPENDIX A

DYNAMICS IN THE BLOOD COMPARTMENT

Equations for the dynamics in the blood compartment are the following:

$$\frac{d\mathrm{IL2_S}}{dt} = K_{\mathrm{off}}^{\mathrm{Ab}} \times \mathrm{IL2_S^{Ab}} - K_{\mathrm{on}}^{\mathrm{Ab}} \times \frac{1}{N_\mathrm{A} \times V_\mathrm{S}} \times \mathrm{IL2_S} \times \mathrm{Ab_S} + N_{\mathrm{LN}} \times \left(D_{\mathrm{il}} \frac{\mathrm{IL2}}{\mathrm{fve} \times V_{\mathrm{LN}}} - D_{\mathrm{il}} \frac{\mathrm{IL2_S}}{V_\mathrm{S}} \right) - K_{\mathrm{di}} \times \mathrm{IL2_S} + \Gamma_\mathrm{i} \quad (A1)$$

$$\frac{d\mathrm{IL2m_S}}{dt} = N_{\mathrm{LN}} \times \left(D_{\mathrm{il}} \frac{\mathrm{IL2m}}{\mathrm{fve} \times V_{\mathrm{LN}}} - D_{\mathrm{il}} \frac{\mathrm{IL2m_S}}{V_\mathrm{S}} \right) - K_{\mathrm{di}} \times \mathrm{IL2m_S} + \Gamma_{\mathrm{mi}} \quad (A2)$$

$$\frac{d\mathrm{Ab_S}}{dt} = K_{\mathrm{off}}^{\mathrm{Ab}} \times \mathrm{IL2_S^{Ab}} - K_{\mathrm{on}}^{\mathrm{Ab}} \times \frac{1}{N_\mathrm{A} \times V_\mathrm{S}} \times \mathrm{IL2_S} \times \mathrm{Ab_S} + N_{\mathrm{LN}} \times \left(D_{\mathrm{ab}} \frac{\mathrm{Ab}}{\mathrm{fve} \times V_{\mathrm{LN}}} - D_{\mathrm{ab}} \frac{\mathrm{Ab_S}}{V_\mathrm{S}} \right) - K_{\mathrm{da}} \times \mathrm{Ab_S} + \Gamma_{\mathrm{ab}} \quad (A3)$$

$$\frac{d\mathrm{IL2_S^{Ab}}}{dt} = -K_{\mathrm{off}}^{\mathrm{Ab}} \times \mathrm{IL2_S^{Ab}} + K_{\mathrm{on}}^{\mathrm{Ab}} \times \frac{1}{N_\mathrm{A} \times V_\mathrm{S}} \times \mathrm{IL2_S} \times \mathrm{Ab_S} + N_{\mathrm{LN}} \times \left(D_{\mathrm{ab}} \frac{\mathrm{IL2^{Ab}}}{\mathrm{fve} \times V_{\mathrm{LN}}} - D_{\mathrm{ab}} \frac{\mathrm{IL2_S^{Ab}}}{V_\mathrm{S}} \right) - K_{\mathrm{da}} \times \mathrm{IL2_S^{Ab}} \quad (A4)$$

Equations A1–A3 model the dynamics of IL2 ($\mathrm{IL2_s}$), IL2 mutant variants ($\mathrm{IL2m_s}$), and anti-IL2 antibodies ($\mathrm{Ab_s}$) number respectively, while the dynamics of the number of immune-complexes IL2 + anti-IL2 antibodies ($\mathrm{IL2_s^{Ab}}$) is modeled by Eq. A4. The variables and parameters involved in these equations are defined in **Table 1**.

Equations A1, A3, and A4 consider the increase in the number of IL2 and mAbs in the blood due to the dissociation process of immune-complexes with a constant rate ($K_{\mathrm{off}}^{\mathrm{Ab}}$), which corresponds to a decrease in the amount of these complexes (first term in Eqs A1, A3, and A4). The process of formation of immune-complexes, through the association of IL2 and mAb with a constant rate ($K_{\mathrm{on}}^{\mathrm{Ab}}$), is taken into account in the second term in Eqs A1, A3, and A4. The exchange of molecules between blood and peripheral lymph nodes is modeled as a simple diffusion process that balances the molecule concentrations in both compartments (third term in Eqs A1, A3, and A4; first term in Eq. A2). The number of molecules decays exponentially with a constant rate ($K_{\mathrm{di}}, K_{\mathrm{da}}$), due to renal elimination in kidney (fourth term in Eqs A1, A3, and A4 and second term in Eq. A2). Finally, an external source for IL2, IL2m, and mAbs is considered, which causes an increase in the number of these molecules in the compartment (last term in Eqs A1–A3).

APPENDIX B

DYNAMICS OF T CELLS IN THE LYMPH NODE COMPARTMENT

The dynamics of the number of T cells in the lymph node compartment, following the process described above, are modeled with the following set of equations:

$$\frac{d\,E_\mathrm{N}}{dt} = \Gamma_\mathrm{e} - K_\mathrm{A}^\mathrm{E} \times E_\mathrm{N}^\mathrm{B} \times \left(1 - \frac{R_\mathrm{T}^\mathrm{B}}{s \times A}\right)^{(s-1)} + \alpha_\mathrm{E} \times K_\mathrm{S}^\mathrm{E} \times \left(1 - \frac{(\mathrm{SigE})^\mathrm{h}}{(S_\mathrm{E})^\mathrm{h} + (\mathrm{SigE})^\mathrm{h}}\right) \times E_\mathrm{A} + 2\,K_\mathrm{P}^\mathrm{E} \times E_\mathrm{C} - K_\mathrm{d}^\mathrm{E} \times E_\mathrm{N}^\mathrm{F} \quad (B1)$$

$$\frac{d\,E_\mathrm{A}}{dt} = K_\mathrm{A}^\mathrm{E} \times E_\mathrm{N}^\mathrm{B} \times \left(1 - \frac{R_\mathrm{T}^\mathrm{B}}{s \times A}\right)^{(s-1)} - K_\mathrm{S}^\mathrm{E} \times E_\mathrm{A} \quad (B2)$$

$$\frac{d\,E_\mathrm{C}}{dt} = K_\mathrm{S}^\mathrm{E} \times \left(\frac{(\mathrm{SigE})^\mathrm{h}}{(S_\mathrm{E})^\mathrm{h} + (\mathrm{SigE})^\mathrm{h}}\right) \times E_\mathrm{A} - K_\mathrm{P}^\mathrm{E} \times E_\mathrm{C} \quad (B3)$$

$$\frac{d\,R_\mathrm{N}}{dt} = \Gamma_\mathrm{r} - K_\mathrm{A}^\mathrm{R} \times R_\mathrm{N}^\mathrm{B} + \alpha_\mathrm{R} \times K_\mathrm{S}^\mathrm{R} \times \left(1 - \frac{(\mathrm{SigR})^\mathrm{h}}{(S_\mathrm{R})^\mathrm{h} + (\mathrm{SigR})^\mathrm{h}}\right) \times R_\mathrm{A} + 2\,K_\mathrm{P}^\mathrm{R} \times R_\mathrm{C} - K_\mathrm{d}^\mathrm{R} \times R_\mathrm{N}^\mathrm{F} \quad (B4)$$

$$\frac{d\,R_\mathrm{A}}{dt} = K_\mathrm{A}^\mathrm{R} \times R_\mathrm{N}^\mathrm{B} - K_\mathrm{S}^\mathrm{R} \times R_\mathrm{A} \quad (B5)$$

$$\frac{d\,R_\mathrm{C}}{dt} = K_\mathrm{S}^\mathrm{R} \times \left(\frac{(\mathrm{SigR})^\mathrm{h}}{(S_\mathrm{R})^\mathrm{h} + (\mathrm{SigR})^\mathrm{h}}\right) \times R_\mathrm{A} - K_\mathrm{P}^\mathrm{R} \times R_\mathrm{C} \quad (B6)$$

$$\frac{d\,M_\mathrm{A}}{dt} = -K_\mathrm{S}^\mathrm{M} \times \left(\frac{(\mathrm{SigM})^\mathrm{h}}{(S_\mathrm{M})^\mathrm{h} + (\mathrm{SigM})^\mathrm{h}}\right) \times M_\mathrm{A} + 2 \times K_\mathrm{P}^\mathrm{M} \times M_\mathrm{C} - K_\mathrm{d}^\mathrm{M} \times M_\mathrm{A} \quad (B7)$$

$$\frac{d\,M_\mathrm{C}}{dt} = K_\mathrm{S}^\mathrm{M} \times \left(\frac{(\mathrm{SigM})^\mathrm{h}}{(S_\mathrm{M})^\mathrm{h} + (\mathrm{SigM})^\mathrm{h}}\right) \times M_\mathrm{A} - K_\mathrm{P}^\mathrm{M} \times M_\mathrm{C} \quad (B8)$$

$$\frac{K^\mathrm{E}}{V_{\mathrm{LN}}} = E_\mathrm{l}^\mathrm{B}/(E_\mathrm{l}^\mathrm{F} \times F); \quad \frac{K^\mathrm{R}}{V_{\mathrm{LN}}} = R_\mathrm{l}^\mathrm{B}/(R_\mathrm{l}^\mathrm{F} \times F); \quad \frac{K^\mathrm{M}}{V_{\mathrm{LN}}} = M_\mathrm{l}^\mathrm{B}/(M_\mathrm{l}^\mathrm{F} \times F) \quad (B9)$$

$$F = s \times A - \sum_l E_\mathrm{l}^\mathrm{B} - \sum_l R_\mathrm{l}^\mathrm{B} - \sum_l M_\mathrm{l}^\mathrm{B}; \quad \forall l \in \{\mathrm{N, A, C}\} \quad (B10)$$

The dynamics of the number of Helper and Regulatory CD4$^+$ T cells, on their three different functional states of their life cycle [resting (E_N, R_N), activated (E_A, R_A) and cycling (E_C, R_C) cells], is modeled using Eqs B1–B6, respectively; while the dynamics of the number of Memory CD8$^+$ T cells on its two functional states [activated (M_A) and cycling (M_C) cells] is modeled with Eqs B7 and B8. The process of conjugation of T cells, on their different functional states, with their cognate APCs is modeled assuming quasi-steady state equilibrium, which leads to the equations presented in Eq. B9 [see a more detailed explanation of the derivation of these equations in (28)]. In Eq. B9, the symbolic label l denotes the functional state of the cell ($l = N$: resting, $l = A$: activated, $l = C$: cycling); and the superscript B and F denotes the cells conjugated to APC or free, respectively. The definitions of variables and parameters in Eqs B1–B9 are resumed in **Table 2**.

Equations B1–B6 considered that resting E and R cells are produced by the thymus (first term in Eqs B1 and B4), and they die with a constant rate K_d^E and K_d^R, respectively (last term in Eqs B1 and B4). Resting cells become activated after conjugation with APCs, process which is inhibited in E cells by the presence of co-conjugated R cells in the same APC (second term in Eqs B1 and B4; first term in Eqs B2 and B5). Activated T cells require enough cytokine derived signals to become cycling cells (first term in Eqs B3 and B6). The fraction of activated cells obtaining these signals is computed with a sigmoid function of the mean number of bound cytokines signaling receptors per cell (SigE, SigR). In the absence of these signals, a fraction α of the activated cells revert to the resting state (third term in Eqs B1 and B4) and the remaining fraction $(1-\alpha)$ simply die. The cycling E and R cells divide producing two new resting cells with a constant rate K_p^E and K_p^R, respectively (fourth term in Eqs B1 and B4; second term in Eqs B3 and B6).

The Eqs B7 and B8 describe the dynamics of memory CD8$^+$ T cells. In these equations, is modeled the dynamics of M cells analogous that for E cells. The only difference is that M cells are considered pre-activated cells, which become cycling in response to cytokine signals (first term in Eqs B7 and B8). The cycling M cells divide producing two new activated cells with a constant rate K_p^M (second term in Eqs B7 and B8). The activated cells die with a constant rate K_d^M (last term in Eq. B7).

APPENDIX C

DYNAMICS OF MOLECULES IN THE LYMPH NODE

The equations in the model describing the dynamics of the number of molecules circulating in the Lymph Node (IL2, anti-IL2 antibodies, and immune-complexes) and the number of complexes IL2-IL2R and IL2-mAb-IL2R formed in a single cell membrane are the following:

$$\begin{aligned}\frac{d\mathrm{IL2}}{dt} &= K_{\mathrm{off}}^{\mathrm{Ab}} \times \mathrm{IL2}^{\mathrm{Ab}} - \frac{1}{N_A \times \mathrm{fve} \times V_{\mathrm{LN}}} K_{\mathrm{on}}^{\mathrm{Ab}} \times \mathrm{IL2} \times \mathrm{Ab} \\ &\quad - \left(D_{\mathrm{il}} \frac{\mathrm{IL2}}{\mathrm{fve} \times V_{\mathrm{LN}}} - D_{\mathrm{il}} \frac{\mathrm{IL2_S}}{V_S}\right) + K_{\mathrm{pi}} \times K_A^E \times E_N^B \\ &\quad \times \left(1 - \frac{R_T^B}{s \times A}\right)^{(s-1)} + \sum_j K_{\mathrm{off}}^j \\ &\quad \times \left[\sum_l (C_j^{E_l} \times E_l) + \sum_l (C_j^{R_l} \times R_l) + \sum_l (C_j^{M_l} \times M_l)\right] \\ &\quad - \sum_j \frac{1}{N_A \times \mathrm{fve} \times V_{\mathrm{LN}}} K_{\mathrm{on}}^j \times \mathrm{IL2} \\ &\quad \times \left[\sum_l (P_j^{E_l} \times E_l) + \sum_l (P_j^{R_l} \times R_l) + \sum_l (P_j^{M_l} \times M_l)\right]\end{aligned} \quad \text{(C1)}$$

$$\begin{aligned}\frac{d\mathrm{IL2m}}{dt} &= -\left(D_{\mathrm{il}} \frac{\mathrm{IL2m}}{\mathrm{fve} \times V_{\mathrm{LN}}} - D_{\mathrm{il}} \frac{\mathrm{IL2m_S}}{V_S}\right) + \sum_j K_{\mathrm{off}}^j \\ &\quad \times \left[\sum_l (\mathrm{Cm}_j^{E_l} \times E_l) + \sum_l (\mathrm{Cm}_j^{R_l} \times R_l)\right. \\ &\quad \left. + \sum_l (\mathrm{Cm}_j^{M_l} \times M_l)\right] \\ &\quad - \sum_j f_j \times \frac{1}{N_A \times \mathrm{fve} \times V_{\mathrm{LN}}} K_{\mathrm{on}}^j \times \mathrm{IL2m} \\ &\quad \times \left[\sum_l (P_j^{E_l} \times E_l) + \sum_l (P_j^{R_l} \times R_l) + \sum_l (P_j^{M_l} \times M_l)\right]\end{aligned} \quad \text{(C2)}$$

$$\begin{aligned}\frac{d\mathrm{Ab}}{dt} &= K_{\mathrm{off}}^{\mathrm{Ab}} \times \mathrm{IL2}^{\mathrm{Ab}} - \frac{1}{N_A \times \mathrm{fve} \times V_{\mathrm{LN}}} K_{\mathrm{on}}^{\mathrm{Ab}} \\ &\quad \times \mathrm{IL2} \times \mathrm{Ab} - \left(D_{\mathrm{ab}} \frac{\mathrm{Ab}}{\mathrm{fve} \times V_{\mathrm{LN}}} - D_{\mathrm{ab}} \frac{\mathrm{Ab_S}}{V_S}\right) \\ &\quad + \sum_j (1 - N_j) \times \left[K_{\mathrm{off}}^{\mathrm{Ab}} \times \sum_l (\mathrm{CAb}_j^{E_l} \times E_l\right. \\ &\quad \left. + \mathrm{CAb}_j^{R_l} \times R_l + \mathrm{CAb}_j^{M_l} \times M_l)\right] \\ &\quad - \sum_j (1 - N_j) \times \left[\frac{1}{N_A \times \mathrm{fve} \times V_{\mathrm{LN}}} K_{\mathrm{on}}^{\mathrm{Ab}} \times \mathrm{Ab}\right. \\ &\quad \left. \times \sum_l \left(C_j^{E_l} \times E_l + C_j^{R_l} \times R_l + C_j^{M_l} \times M_l\right)\right]\end{aligned} \quad \text{(C3)}$$

$$\begin{aligned}\frac{d\mathrm{IL2}^{\mathrm{Ab}}}{dt} &= -K_{\mathrm{off}}^{\mathrm{Ab}} \times \mathrm{IL2}^{\mathrm{Ab}} + \frac{1}{N_A \times \mathrm{fve} \times V_{\mathrm{LN}}} K_{\mathrm{on}}^{\mathrm{Ab}} \\ &\quad \times \mathrm{IL2} \times \mathrm{Ab} - \left(D_{\mathrm{ab}} \frac{\mathrm{IL2}^{\mathrm{Ab}}}{\mathrm{fve} \times V_{\mathrm{LN}}} - D_{\mathrm{ab}} \frac{\mathrm{IL2_S^{Ab}}}{V_S}\right)\end{aligned}$$

$$+\sum_j (1-N_j)\times K_{off}^{j}\times\left[\sum_l(\mathrm{CAb}_j^{E_l}\times E_l)+\sum_l(\mathrm{CAb}_j^{R_l}\times R_l)+\sum_l(\mathrm{CAb}_j^{M_l}\times M_l)\right]-\sum_j(1-N_j)\times\frac{1}{N_A\times \mathrm{fve}\times V_{LN}}K_{on}^{j}\times \mathrm{IL2}^{Ab}\times\left[\sum_l(P_j^{E_l}\times E_l)+\sum_l(P_j^{R_l}\times R_l)+\sum_l(P_j^{M_l}\times M_l)\right] \quad (C4)$$

$$\frac{d\mathrm{Cm}_\alpha^{E_l}}{dt}=f_\alpha\times K_{on}^{\alpha}\times\frac{1}{N_A\times \mathrm{fve}\times V_{LN}}\times \mathrm{IL2m}\times P_\alpha^{E_l}-K_{off}^{\alpha}\times \mathrm{Cm}_\alpha^{E_l}-f_\beta\times K_{on}^{\alpha\beta}\times \mathrm{Cm}_\alpha^{E_l}\times P_\beta^{E_l}+K_{off}^{\alpha\beta}\times \mathrm{Tm}^{E_l} \quad (C5)$$

$$\frac{d\mathrm{Cm}_\beta^{E_l}}{dt}=f_\beta\times K_{on}^{\beta}\times\frac{1}{N_A\times \mathrm{fve}\times V_{LN}}\times \mathrm{IL2m}\times P_\beta^{E_l}-K_{off}^{\beta}\times \mathrm{Cm}_\beta^{E_l}-f_\alpha\times K_{on}^{\beta\alpha}\times \mathrm{Cm}_\beta^{E_l}\times P_\alpha^{E_l}+K_{off}^{\beta\alpha}\times \mathrm{Tm}^{E_l}-K_{in}\times \mathrm{Cm}_\beta^{E_l} \quad (C6)$$

$$\frac{d\mathrm{Tm}^{E_l}}{dt}=f_\beta\times K_{on}^{\alpha\beta}\times \mathrm{Cm}_\alpha^{E_l}\times P_\beta^{E_l}-K_{off}^{\alpha\beta}\times \mathrm{Tm}^{E_l}+f_\alpha\times K_{on}^{\beta\alpha}\times \mathrm{Cm}_\beta^{E_l}\times P_\alpha^{E_l}-K_{off}^{\beta\alpha}\times \mathrm{Tm}^{E_l}-K_{in}\times \mathrm{Tm}^{E_l} \quad (C7)$$

$$\frac{dC_\alpha^{E_l}}{dt}=K_{on}^{\alpha}\times\frac{1}{N_A\times \mathrm{fve}\times V_{LN}}\times \mathrm{IL2}\times P_\alpha^{E_l}-K_{off}^{\alpha}\times C_\alpha^{E_l}-K_{on}^{\alpha\beta}\times C_\alpha^{E_l}\times P_\beta^{E_l}+K_{off}^{\alpha\beta}\times T^{E_l}+(1-N_\alpha)\times\left(-\frac{1}{N_A\times \mathrm{fve}\times V_{LN}}K_{on}^{Ab}\times C_\alpha^{E_l}\times \mathrm{Ab}+K_{off}^{Ab}\times \mathrm{CAb}_\alpha^{E_l}\right) \quad (C8)$$

$$\frac{dC_\beta^{E_l}}{dt}=K_{on}^{\beta}\times\frac{1}{N_A\times \mathrm{fve}\times V_{LN}}\times \mathrm{IL2}\times P_\beta^{E_l}-K_{off}^{\beta}\times C_\beta^{E_l}-K_{on}^{\beta\alpha}\times C_\beta^{E_l}\times P_\alpha^{E_l}+K_{off}^{\beta\alpha}\times T^{E_l}+(1-N_\beta)\times\left(-\frac{1}{N_A\times \mathrm{fve}\times V_{LN}}K_{on}^{Ab}\times C_\beta^{E_l}\times \mathrm{Ab}+K_{off}^{Ab}\times \mathrm{CAb}_\beta^{E_l}\right)-K_{in}\times C_\beta^{E_l} \quad (C9)$$

$$\frac{dT^{E_l}}{dt}=K_{on}^{\alpha\beta}\times C_\alpha^{E_l}\times P_\beta^{E_l}-K_{off}^{\alpha\beta}\times T^{E_l}+K_{on}^{\beta\alpha}\times C_\beta^{E_l}\times P_\alpha^{E_l}-K_{off}^{\beta\alpha}\times T^{E_l}-K_{in}\times T^{E_l} \quad (C10)$$

$$\frac{d\mathrm{CAb}_\alpha^{E_l}}{dt}=(1-N_\alpha)\times\left(K_{on}^{\alpha}\times\frac{1}{N_A\times \mathrm{fve}\times V_{LN}}\times \mathrm{IL2}^{Ab}\times P_\alpha^{E_l}-K_{off}^{\alpha}\times \mathrm{CAb}_\alpha^{E_l}\right)+(1-N_\alpha)\times\left(\frac{1}{N_A\times \mathrm{fve}\times V_{LN}}K_{on}^{Ab}\times C_\alpha^{E_l}\times \mathrm{Ab}-K_{off}^{Ab}\times \mathrm{CAb}_\alpha^{E_l}\right) \quad (C11)$$

$$\frac{d\mathrm{CAb}_\beta^{E_l}}{dt}=(1-N_\beta)\times\left(K_{on}^{\beta}\times\frac{1}{N_A\times \mathrm{fve}\times V_{LN}}\times \mathrm{IL2}^{Ab}\times P_\beta^{E_l}-K_{off}^{\beta}\times \mathrm{CAb}_\beta^{E_l}\right)+(1-N_\beta)\times\left(\frac{1}{N_A\times \mathrm{fve}\times V_{LN}}K_{on}^{Ab}\times C_\beta^{E_l}\times \mathrm{Ab}-K_{off}^{Ab}\times \mathrm{CAb}_\beta^{E_l}\right)-K_{in}\times \mathrm{CAb}_\beta^{E_l} \quad (C12)$$

$$P_\alpha^{E_l}=\mathrm{Ra}^{E_l}-C_\alpha^{E_l}-\mathrm{CAb}_\alpha^{E_l}-T^{E_l}-\mathrm{Cm}_\alpha^{E_l}-\mathrm{Tm}^{E_l},$$

$$P_\beta^{E_l}=\mathrm{Rb}^{E_l}-C_\beta^{E_l}-\mathrm{CAb}_\beta^{E_l}-T^{E_l}-\mathrm{Cm}_\beta^{E_l}-\mathrm{Tm}^{E_l} \quad (C13)$$

$$\mathrm{SigE}=C_\beta^{E_A}+T^{E_A}+\mathrm{Cm}_\beta^{E_A}+\mathrm{Tm}^{E_A}+\mathrm{CAb}_\beta^{E_A}+\mathrm{il}\alpha_{E_A},$$

$$\mathrm{SigR}=C_\beta^{R_A}+T^{R_A}+\mathrm{Cm}_\beta^{R_A}+\mathrm{Tm}^{R_A}+\mathrm{CAb}_\beta^{R_A}, \quad (C14)$$

$$\mathrm{SigM}=C_\beta^{M_A}+T^{M_A}+\mathrm{Cm}_\beta^{M_A}+\mathrm{Tm}^{M_A}+\mathrm{CAb}_\beta^{M_A}+\mathrm{il}\alpha_{M_A}$$

The dynamics of the number of IL2 (IL2), IL2 mutants (IL2m), mAbs (Ab), and immune-complexes ($\mathrm{IL2}^{Ab}$) in the lymph node is modeled using Eqs C1 and C4; while the dynamics of the number of IL2-IL2R complexes (C_α^E, C_β^E, T^E); IL2m-IL2R complexes (Cm_α^E, Cm_β^E, Tm^E); and IL2-IL2R-mAbs complexes CAb_α^E, CAb_β^E per cell are modeled following equations (22–24); (19–21); and (25, 26), respectively. Note that, to simplify, we only present here the equations corresponding to the IL2 and IL2m complexes formed at the E cell membrane. Equivalent equations are written for R and M cells. Algebraic relations are provided in Eqs C13 and C14, for the amount of free alpha (P_α^E) and beta chains (P_β^E) of the IL2 receptor per E cell, and the mean number of bound cytokines signaling receptors per activated E (SigE), R (SigR), and M (SigM) cell. Note that, the terms SigE, SigR, and SigM in Eq. C14 are the one used in the equations for the dynamics of T cells, related with the process of cells receiving cytokine derived signals from IL2 or alternative cytokines (see section 1.2). The variables and parameters used in Ref. (15–28) are defined in **Tables 1–3**.

In Eqs C1, C3, and C4, the first and second terms correspond to the processes of dissociation and formation of immune-complexes. Additionally, due to the presence of T cells in the Lymph Node, we consider in these equations the dissociation and association processes of IL2 and IL2-mAb complexes with the alpha or beta IL2R chains in the cell membranes. In this sense, is taken into account the increase in the amount of free IL2, IL2m, and immune-complexes, due to the dissociation process of IL2-IL2R, IL2m-IL2R, and IL2-mAb-IL2R complexes respectively (third terms in Eqs C1 and C4 and second term in Eq. C2). On the other hand, the association of free IL2, IL2m, and immune-complexes to free alpha or beta IL2R chains is considered to increase the amount of IL2-IL2R and IL2-mAb-IL2R complexes (fourth terms in Eqs C1 and C4, third term in Eq. C2). Additionally, is modeled the processes where mAbs can be dissociated from IL2-mAb-IL2R complexes, increasing the number of free mAbs (third terms in Eq. C3); and the process where free mAbs associate to IL2-IL2R complexes in the cell membrane (fourth terms in Eq. C3). The symbolic labels l and j, appearing in the equations (15–18), denote respectively the functional state of the cell ($l = N$: resting, $l = A$: activated, $l = C$: cycling) and the different IL2R chains ($j = \alpha$ alpha chain and $j = \beta$ beta dimer chain). Finally, the production of IL2 endogenous by activated E cells, which can be inhibited during cell activation by the presence of R cells co-conjugated in the same APC, is considered to increase the amount of this cytokine in the Lymph Node (last term in Eq. C1). The properties of different IL2m is controlled in the model by the parameters f_α and f_β which multiply the association of constant of this molecules to the alpha and beta chain of the IL2 receptor.

The formation of high affinity IL2-IL2R and IL2m-IL2R complexes in a cell membrane is modeled as a two-step process, using equations (22–24) and (19–21) respectively. Firstly, free IL2 or IL2m binds to the available free alpha or beta chains of the IL2R, forming the intermediate or low affinity IL2-IL2R complexes respectively (first terms in Eqs C8, C9 and C5, C6), as mentioned above for the dynamics of IL2. By the corresponding dissociation process are recovered free molecules and receptor chains (second term in Eqs C8, C9 and C5, C6). The association process of intermediate or low affinity IL2-IL2R complexes with the remaining IL2 receptor chain, leads to the formation of high affinity IL2-IL2R complexes (third term in Eqs C8, C9 and C5, C6), and first and third terms in Eqs C10 and C7. The dissociation of these complexes is modeled in the fourth term in Eqs C9, C10 and C5, C6 and second and fourth terms in Eqs C10 and C7. The internalization of IL2 and IL2m forming complexes with IL2Rs is modeled considering that it only occurs for signaling IL2-IL2R complexes requiring binding to the beta chain (last term in Eqs C9, C10 and C6, C7).

The formation of IL2-mAb-IL2R complexes in the cell membrane is modeled in Eqs C11 and C12, and in the fifth term in Eqs C8 and C9. In this sense, we consider the association and dissociation processes of free immune-complexes with the alpha or beta IL2R chains (first term in Eqs C11 and C12); and the same processes for free mAbs with IL2-IL2R complexes in the cell membrane (fifth term in Eqs C8 and C9); second term in Eqs C11 and C12). The possibility of formation of intermediate or low affinity IL2-mAb-IL2R complexes depend on the IL2 interface that mAbs recognize (controlled in simulations by the parameter N_j, see **Table 3**). We don't consider the formation of high affinity IL2-mAb-IL2R complexes, due to association of antibodies with the high affinity IL2-IL2R complexes or the association of intermediate or low affinity IL2-mAb-IL2R complexes with the remaining IL2 receptor chain, because we are studying mAbs that bind to the alpha or beta interface of the IL2 which will block the formation of these complexes. Finally, the internalization of IL2 as immune-complexes bound to the beta chains of IL2Rs in the cell membrane is also modeled (last term in Eq. C12).

19

Modulation of antigen-specific T-cells as immune therapy for chronic infectious diseases and cancer

Suling Li [1]***, Alistair L. J. Symonds*** [2]***, Tizong Miao*** [2]***, Ian Sanderson*** [2] ***and Ping Wang*** [2]*******

[1] *Bioscience, Brunel University, London, UK*
[2] *Blizard Institute (BICMS), Barts and the London School of Medicine and Dentistry, London, UK*

Edited by:
Fang-Ping Huang, Imperial College London, UK

Reviewed by:
Jianping Huang, University of Florida, USA
Alex Yee-Chen Huang, Case Western Reserve University School of Medicine, USA

****Correspondence:***
Ping Wang, 4 Newark Street, London E1 2AT, UK
e-mail: p.wang@qmul.ac.uk

T-cell responses are induced by antigen presenting cells (APC) and signals from the microenvironment. Antigen persistence and inflammatory microenvironments in chronic infections and cancer can induce a tolerant state in T-cells resulting in hyporesponsiveness, loss of effector function, and weak biochemical signaling patterns in response to antigen stimulation. Although the mechanisms of T-cell tolerance induced in chronic infection and cancer may differ from those involved in tolerance to self-antigen, the impaired proliferation and production of IL-2 in response to antigen stimulation are hallmarks of all tolerant T cells. In this review, we will summarize the evidence that the immune responses change from non-self to "self"-like in chronic infection and cancer, and will provide an overview of strategies for re-balancing the immune response of antigen-specific T cells in chronic infection and cancer without affecting the homeostasis of the immune system.

Keywords: tolerance induction, antigen-specific T cells, bystander T-cells, nanoAPC, reverse tolerance

INTRODUCTION

T cells are essential for robust adaptive immune responses against pathogen invasion, as well as maintaining immune tolerance to self-antigens. In the tolerant state, T cells generally fail to proliferate and produce IL-2 in response to antigen stimulation (1, 2). Anergy and immune regulation are two interconnected mechanisms that maintain peripheral tolerance to self-antigens *in vivo*. In contrast to the biochemical events induced during effective responses to pathogenic antigens, in anergy the biochemical signaling pathways in T cells are only partially activated. Activation of the calcium/calcineurin/nuclear factor of activated T cells (NFAT) pathway, but not AP1 and NFκB pathways (1–3), in anergic conditions results in the expression of tolerance associated genes such as E3-ligases (1–3). This partial TCR signaling is largely due to the lack of additional signals such as costimulatory signals and activating cytokines such as IL-2, or due to direct regulation by Treg (2). Therefore, altered expression of costimulatory signals and/or activating cytokines, or defective Treg function, results in full activation of TCR signals in response to self-antigens and may induce autoimmune responses. Recent studies have uncovered hyporesponsive phenotypes with partial activation of biochemical events in virus specific T cells in chronic infectious diseases (4, 5) and models mimicking chronic infectious conditions (5, 6). These findings indicate that during chronic infection the T-cells switch from mounting robust non-self responses to a state similar to self-tolerance due to antigen persistence and/or changes in the microenvironment. Similar to the immunological milieu of chronic infection, the tumor microenvironment contains a multitude of suppressive mechanisms that allow tumors to escape immune surveillance (4, 7). Immune hyporesponsive states have been studied in many different models *in vitro* and *in vivo* and have been categorized based on the phenotypes discovered in each tolerant state (8).

This review will briefly summarize the extracellular signals that affect self-tolerance or effector function of antigen-specific T cells. We will describe the application of these signals in therapeutic intervention and focus on the recently developed nano-technologies that can reverse the tolerant state of viral specific T cells by delivering costimulatory or cytokine signals to antigen-specific T cells.

ALTERED T-CELL RESPONSES DURING CHRONIC VIRUS INFECTION AND CANCER

Chronic virus infections are associated with impaired anti-viral immunity, particularly in the infections caused by highly replicative viruses such as HIV, HBV, and HCV. In chronic infection, persistent viral antigen, and often chronic inflammation, renders T-cells dysfunctional. The mechanisms underlying dysfunctional immune responses in patients are largely unknown. Based on experimental systems studied *in vitro* and *in vivo*, different states of T-cell dysfunction have been discovered and are classified as exhaustion, tolerance, anergy, senescence, deletion, induced Treg, and ignorance based on the phenotypes, production of inhibitory cytokines such as IL-10 and TGFβ, impairment of T-cell receptor signaling molecules, and apoptosis of the T-cells in these models (**Figure 1**) (4–6, 8–10). These findings have been extensively reviewed (4–6, 8–10). Despite the differences in dysfunctional T-cells characterized in different model systems, the common feature is proliferative hyporesponsiveness, and impaired production of IL-2 following antigen stimulation *in vivo* or *in vitro* (4–6, 8–10). The chronic LCMV infection model resembles the observations from patients with chronic virus infections more closely than other models in terms of induction of dysfunctional T cells (4, 5). The phenotype of exhaustion of CD8 T cells in the chronic LCMV model is well-characterized, with hierarchical loss of effector cytokine production, including IL-2, TNFα, and IFNγ and

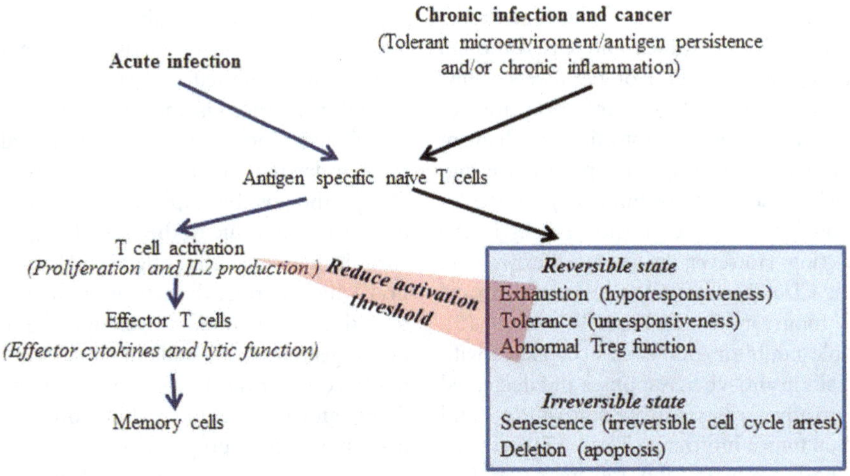

FIGURE 1 | Differential responses of T cells during acute and chronic infection or cancer.

impaired proliferation in response to antigen receptor stimulation *in vitro* (4, 5). In addition to this hyporesponsive phenotype, increased expression of the inhibitory costimulatory molecule PD-1 and production of the repressive cytokine IL-10 are also found in T cells from chronic LCMV infected mice (9, 10). Notably, similar phenotypes have been found in T cells from HIV, HBV, and HCV patients (11–14). Under chronic infectious conditions, viral specific CD8 T cells often lose cytotoxic function (15, 16). At the late stages of exhaustion, viral specific CD8 T cells may be deleted (5, 6). However, in contrast to CD8 T cells, viral specific CD4 T cells can persist under chronic infectious conditions, but in a hyporesponsive state (17). Therefore, there is the potential to restore CD4 responses, which may thereafter help CD8 function. It has been reported that Treg cells are increased or induced in chronic infection (18, 19). The increased Treg cells can reduce chronic inflammation from persistent viral antigen stimulation, but may also contribute to the establishment of immune tolerance toward the virus (18, 19).

Comparable to chronic infection, high levels of tumor antigens and chronic inflammation can establish an immunosuppressive microenvironment. Tumor reactive T cells have been shown to respond to tumor antigens in a similar fashion to viral specific T cells in chronic infection with expression of high levels of inhibitory costimulatory molecules such as PD-1, CTLA-4, and LAG-3 and impaired production of effector cytokines including IFNg, TNFa, and IL-2 (7, 20–22). It has been shown that advanced tumors with high loads of tumor antigens cause functional exhaustion and rapid elimination of tumor reactive T cells (23). However, in contrast to chronic viral infections, tumor antigens are generally poorly antigenic. Therefore, the frequency and avidity of tumor reactive T cells are low.

IMPAIRED TCR SIGNALING DURING CHRONIC VIRUS INFECTION

We have found that antigen persistence can impair TCR signaling resulting in hyporesponsiveness (24). This hyporesponsiveness is gradually induced during antigen persistence with reduction of NFkB and AP1 activation (2, 24). This characteristic phenotype of T-cell tolerance is similar to that observed in chronic HBV infection (25). Down-regulation of TCR proximal signaling molecules has been found in CD8 T cells from chronic HBV patients (25). The impaired TCR signaling in CD8 T cells from chronic HBV patients is partly due to the down-regulation of CD3ζ (25). The reduced expression of CD3ζ is associated with up-regulation of PD-1 and impaired production of IL-2, suggesting that it is part of the mechanism leading to exhaustion (25). Viral protein Nef of HIV and E2 and core protein of HCV directly modulate TCR signaling (26). HIV Nef protein interacts with a number of TCR signaling molecules including Lyn, Hck, and Lck (27). The interaction stimulates the TCR signaling pathways in the absence of antigens leading to maintenance of viral replication (26, 27). The altered TCR signaling induced by Nef negatively affects antigen-mediated TCR signaling (28). Similarly, viral proteins from HCV also modulate TCR signaling (29). E2 protein of HCV binds CD81 and promotes TCR signaling while the core protein inhibits JNK signaling and IL-2 expression (29). However, HCV does not infect T cells. Therefore, the altered TCR responses during chronic HCV infection are largely due to the persistence of viral antigens. Whether the persistent, but abnormal, TCR signaling induced by viral proteins causes the development of T-cell exhaustion is yet to be investigated.

It has been found that the tumor microenvironment impairs the formation of T-cell immunological synapses; supramolecular structures that assemble at the T cell-APC interface (30). Dysregulated synapse formation is associated with impaired activation of Rho-GTPases and can lead to partial activation or anergy of T cells.

INDUCTION OF NEGATIVE COSTIMULATORY MOLECULES

One of the important changes to the phenotype of CD8 T cells in chronic LCMV infection is the increased expression of the negative costimulatory molecules PD-1, 2B4, CTLA-4, and LAG-3 (5). A similar phenotype of increased negative costimulatory molecules has been discovered in CD4 and CD8 T cells from chronic HBV and HIV patients (5, 15, 31–35). The function of these negative costimulatory molecules is important in the maintenance of immune tolerance toward self-antigens. Although the mechanisms underlying the induction of negative costimulatory molecules in T cells during chronic infection are not clear, it may be part of a physiological protection mechanism to reduce immunopathology induced by viral persistence and chronic inflammation. These negative costimulatory molecules are transiently up-regulated in activated effector T cells in the early stages of acute infection. However, the sustained expression of PD-1 on virus-specific CD8 T cells is associated with chronic infection, both in LCMV mouse models and in HBV patients (5). Co-expression of multiple inhibitory molecules correlates with increased functional deficits in anti-virus responses and decreased control of viral loads. Similarly, increased expression of PD-1 and CTLA-4 has been found on tumor infiltrating T cells (TIL), which can be associated with E3-ligase expression and increased Treg cells (7). Thus, the overexpression of inhibitory molecules results in shifting the balance of the immune responses from effective anti-virus or -cancer responses toward tolerance.

ALTERED CYTOKINE PRODUCTION IN T CELLS

One of the most pronounced changes in T cells in chronic infectious conditions is the altered production of cytokines (4–6). In contrast to acute infection, antigen-specific T cells from chronic infectious diseases fail to produce IL-2 and TNFα, but express the regulatory cytokine IL-10 (4–6). We have discovered that antigen-specific CD4 T cells gradually alter their cytokine profile in response to antigen persistence *in vivo* (24). Initial antigen stimulation effectively induces IL-2 production in antigen-specific CD4 T cells *in vivo*, while repeated exposure to the same antigen yields CD4 T cells that produce both IL-2 and IL-10 (24). Antigen persistence can finally switch off the expression of IL-2 in T cells, but these cells still produce high levels of IL-10 (24). This altered cytokine profile is associated with impaired proliferative responses and reduced AP1 and NFκB activation in response to antigen stimulation *in vivo* (24). Impaired production of effector cytokines such as IL-2, TNFα, and IFNγ is also associated with the defective activation of TCR signaling pathways and effector function of viral-specific CD4 and CD8 T cells in chronic HBV, HCV, and HIV infections (5, 6, 25). The up-regulation of inhibitory molecules, especially PD-1, is closely associated with the production of IL-10 and/or TGFβ (5, 6). Thus, virus persistence skews the T-cell response from activation and differentiation into effector cells toward antigen-specific immune tolerance. However, the mechanisms whereby IL-10 and/or TGFβ result in tolerance in chronic infections are still undefined. In the LCMV model, the lack of IL-10 or a defect in IL-10 signaling improves CD8 T-cell responses and drastically enhances the control of the infection (36, 37). TIL also display an altered cytokine profile, which is similar to that seen in chronic infections. High levels of IL-10 producing Treg cells have been found in TILs, which is associated with impaired production of IL-2, TNFa and IFNg (7, 38).

THERAPEUTIC INTERVENTIONS TO REVERSE IMMUNE TOLERANCE IN CHRONIC INFECTION AND CANCER

Therapeutic interventions for chronic viral infection and cancer aim to counter the effects of the immunosuppressive microenvironment and skew responses toward antigenic determinants that are highly immunogenic. Various approaches have been tried to increase antigen presentation quality via immunization with selected antigenic peptides, using methods such as recombinant vaccinia vaccines, DNA vaccines, peptide vaccines, and DC vaccines, to boost the anti-viral and -tumor responses (39). So far these therapeutic vaccines have not been successful. One of the possible explanations is that the hyporesponsiveness of T cells is not due to the lack of antigens, but to aspects of the chronic disease such as antigen persistence and chronic inflammation, which increase the activation threshold of T cells in response to antigen. Therefore, to overcome the high activation threshold of antigen-specific T cells in these conditions, immune therapy has to consider the antagonizing tolerogenic environment. Thus, therapeutic vaccines in combination with targeted immune modulation have been proposed as a more effective strategy to reverse the hyporesponsive state of T cells in chronic infections and cancer. In ovarian cancer, improved anti-tumor immune responses were observed after blockade of PD-1 (40). Similarly, in the LCMV model, immunization with LCMV GP33 encoding vaccinia virus coupled with administration of anti-PD-L1 blocking antibody significantly improved viral-specific CD8 T-cell responses and reduced viral load (41). Moreover, in chronic LCMV, combined therapy with a DNA vaccine and IL-10 neutralizing antibody effectively reversed viral specific CD8 T-cell tolerance (42). Immune tolerance induced by virus persistence is due to a network with multiple suppressive components. Blockade of multiple inhibitory receptors including PD-1, LAG-3, and CTLA-4 or combined blockade of inhibitory receptors and immunosuppressive cytokines achieves greater efficacy than blockade of a single inhibitory molecule in chronic LCMV models (43, 44). Although the increased T-cell function and concomitant decrease in viral load in these interventions are transient, these data support the hypothesis that reversing immune tolerance to the virus or tumor is the key for successful immunotherapy. While blockade of PD-1 and IL-10 resulted in restoration of viral specific CD8 T-cell function in a mouse model (45), the mechanisms underlying this recovery of effector function are still unknown. As many of these interventions do not specifically target the virus- or tumor-specific T cells and these pathways are important for maintenance of peripheral tolerance, it is essential to control the balance between restoration of anti-viral or -tumor responses and prevention of autoimmune diseases (5, 7). The ideal intervention will be to specifically reverse the tolerance of viral or tumor specific T cells, while maintaining the overall self-tolerance of the immune system.

RESTORING NON-SELF-RESPONSES OF VIRAL SPECIFIC T CELLS, WHILE MAINTAINING THE SELF-TOLERANCE OF BYSTANDER T CELLS IN CHRONIC INFECTION

The differential responses of antigen-specific T cells result from biochemical signals induced in T cells following interaction with antigen-MHC complexes, costimulatory molecules, and cytokines. When the mitogenic biochemical signals break the activation threshold, the T cell will enter into the cell cycle and produce growth cytokines such as IL-2 to promote clonal expansion. Due to the persistence of viral antigen, the chronic inflammatory environment and the increased production of inhibitory molecules, the activation threshold of viral specific T cells is increased and the T cells are unable to enter the cell cycle following antigen stimulation (5, 24). However, chronic infection normally does not induce tolerance in T cells responding to antigens other than those derived from the virus itself. Therefore, systemic intervention may reverse the tolerance of viral-specific T cells, but also break the self-tolerance of bystander T cells potentially resulting in autoimmunity (5). Therefore, the ideal strategy is to reverse tolerance via modulations that increase positive and/or dampen negative costimulatory signals thereby breaking the activation threshold and driving clonal expansion of virus responding T cells, but importantly, without affecting bystander T cells. Cytokine modified and viral antigen pulsed DCs have been used to deliver antigen and positive costimulatory signals to viral specific T cells in chronic infection (46–48). However, DCs are unstable and very heterogeneous in terms of population and function. It is therefore difficult to target and deliver additional positive signals to antigen-specific T cells (49). We found that an increase in the amount of antigen presented by activated dendritic cells (DC) cannot reverse tolerance (50, 51). Although exogenous IL-2 can effectively overcome tolerance and restore the full activation of tolerant T cells in response to antigen stimulation in animal models and HBV specific CD8 T cells, systemic administration of high doses of IL-2 not only induces severe side effects, such as cardiovascular, pulmonary, hematological, hepatic, neurological, endocrine, renal, and/or dermatological complications (52), but may also promote Treg function, which can further increase the activation threshold of antigen-specific T cells (53).

In order to use IL-2 and/or anti-PD1 to overcome the hyporesponsiveness of viral specific T cells induced in chronic HBV infection while avoiding the side effects of systemic administration, we have developed a novel therapeutic vaccine (nanoAPC). These nanoAPC are derived from an APC line; the human B cell line 721.221. This cell line is MHC deficient, but expresses high levels of costimulatory molecules (51). The nanoAPC are prepared from the endoplasmic reticulum (ER) membranes of 721.221 cells (51), that are genetically engineered to express ER retained MHC class I alleles and membrane-bound IL-2. Therefore, MHC and IL-2 are synthesized physiologically in 721.221 human B cells and immobilized on ER-membranes (**Figure 2**) (51). After assembly with HBV antigenic peptide *in vitro*, the nanoAPC contain peptide-MHC complexes, costimulatory molecules, and IL-2. Unlike therapeutic DCs, the nanoAPC are homogeneous, stable, and can be stored at −80°C (50, 51). Equipped with defined viral-peptide-MHC complexes, the administered nanoAPC can directly interact with antigen-specific T cells *in vivo* (51). Due to the native structure of their membranes, nanoAPC effectively induce immune synapses and expression of the high affinity IL-2 receptor on T cells (**Figure 2**) (51). The IL-2 delivered by nanoAPC enhanced antigen-specific T-cell responses and effector function, but did not affect bystander T cells or Treg cells. When assembled with a pool of HLA A2 associated HBV peptides and HBV peptides associated with HLA DR and DP, IL-2-nanoAPC induced strong CD4 and CD8 T-cell responses in peripheral lymphocytes from chronic HBV patients (51). We demonstrated that IL-2 on nanoAPC is able to enhance TCR signaling and downregulate PD-1 expression on virus responding CD8 T cells from chronic HBV patients, which could effectively reverse tolerance as demonstrated by induction of IFNγ producing CD8 T cells in lymphocytes from chronic HBV patients (51). In

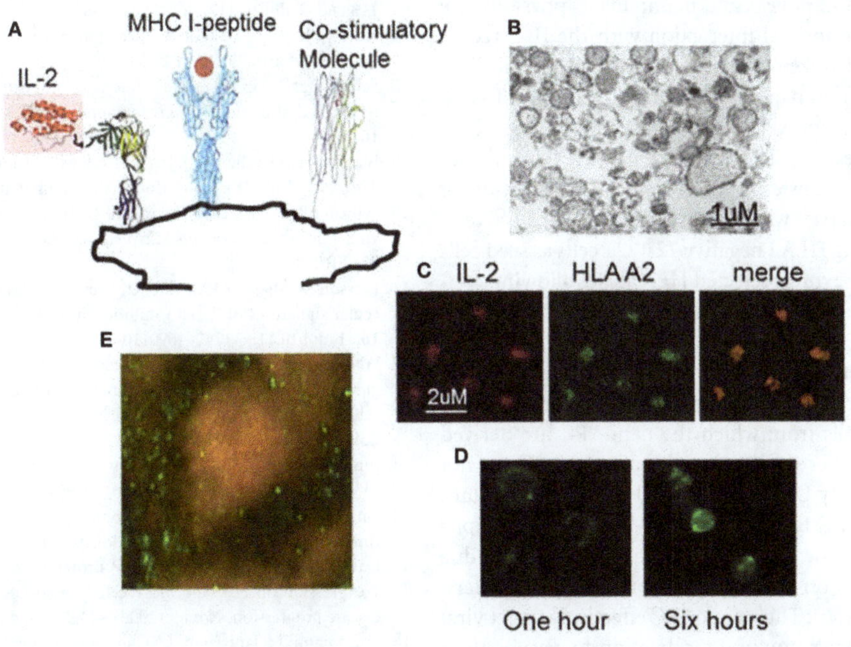

FIGURE 2 | Example of nanoAPC designed to deliver peptide-MHC complexes and IL-2 to their receptors on antigen-specific T lymphocytes. **(A)** Graphical representation of nanoAPC. **(B)** Electron microscopy shows purified nanoAPC from IL-2 engineered 721.221 B cells. **(C)** Confocal microscopy shows nanoAPC stained with anti-IL-2 (red) and anti-HLA A2 (green). **(D)** Confocal microscopy shows interaction of nanoAPC (green) with T lymphocytes after 1 and 6 h *in vitro*. After 6 h, nanoAPCs are internalized into T cells. **(E)** Distribution of nanoAPC (green) prepared from mouse dendritic cells in T lymphocyte areas of mouse lymph node 48 h after i.v. injection. B cells were stained by B220 (orange).

addition to TCR signaling, MAPK activation can result directly from IL-2R signaling (53). It has been found that the activation of MAPK and PI3K through Shc recruited by the IL-2R is independent of STAT5 signaling in effector T cells, which differs from that in Treg cells, and is important for the expansion of activated CD8 T cells (54). We have demonstrated that nanoAPC can induce CD25 expression and immune synapse formation, which not only enables the induction of T-cell activation but also brings engineered bio-adjuvants such as IL-2 stably into signalsomes of effector T cells (51). The increased expression of CD25 on CMV antigen-specific CD8 T cells by IL-2-CMV$_{\text{nlv}}$A2-nanoAPC is consistent with the well-known observation that IL-2 can induce CD25 expression on pre-activated CD8 T cells (51). Thus, together with peptide-MHC complexes and costimulatory molecules, the selective delivery of IL-2 is important in inducing activation of HBV responding T cells in chronic HBV patients. As the overall pharmacological dose remains low, the IL-2-nanoAPC do not activate Treg cells indicating that this approach can be adapted for use with other bio-adjuvants. Our results demonstrate that IL-2-nanoAPC, which deliver both antigen and IL-2 to antigen-responding T cells, can significantly increase functional anti-viral responses, thereby overcoming the immune tolerance induced by persistent viral load.

Nano-particles prepared from synthetic materials or genetically engineered microbes have been used to deliver antigens to DC for induction of anti-viral or -cancer immune responses (55). In contrast to these particles, nanoAPC are prepared from the ER-membranes of bio-engineered APC. Therefore, they are not only more biocompatible than synthetic nano-particles or microbes, but also deliver therapeutic molecules that are physiologically synthesized by APC seed cells. Thus, the IL-2 on IL-2-nanoAPC is more stable than free IL-2 *in vivo*, and maintains its physiological conformation allowing optimal interaction with the IL-2 receptor (data not shown). Unlike other nano-particle based vaccines, we have demonstrated that nanoAPC can directly activate T cells. NanoAPC are derived from APC cells and contain high levels of costimulatory molecules (51). Therefore, the nanoAPC mimic live DC to induce lipid raft clustering on T cells and formation of an immunological synapse, which is essential for T-cell activation. Furthermore, using HLA I negative 721.221 cells as seed cells allows us to specifically express selected HLA alleles allowing construction of HLA allele matched nanoAPC for individual patient populations.

Previously, we observed nanoAPC homing to T-cell areas of peripheral lymphoid organs, largely due to the expression of homing receptors by the cells from which the nanoAPC are derived (50). We have now further demonstrated that nanoAPC are not efficiently endocytosed by DC *in vivo* (50, 51). This is important as it allows the nanoAPC to remain as free-particles in peripheral lymphoid organs. The absence of endocytosis may be due to the lack of molecules on nanoAPC recognized by DC pattern recognition molecules (56). Thus, nanoAPC effectively target viral specific T cells and deliver immune modulation to reverse their tolerant state.

SUMMARY

In chronic infection and cancer, T cells are continuously confronted with moderate to high levels of antigens, which, in combination with the induced immunosuppressive microenvironment resulting from high antigen load and dysregulated immune responses, leads to increased activation thresholds and, subsequently, a reduction in effector function resulting in a tolerant state. This tolerant state can be reversed by positive regulatory molecules such as IL-2, IL-7, and/or blockade of PD-1 and CTLA-4. However, systemic administration of positive regulatory cytokines, or blocking antibodies, may cause autoimmunity. Therefore, one of the major challenges for immunotherapy against chronic infectious diseases and cancer is to reverse the tolerance of antigen-specific T cells, without affecting bystander T cells, thereby maintaining immune homeostasis to self-antigens. The development of delivery vehicles targeting antigen-specific T cells allows the provision of not only antigen but also engineered bio-adjuvant(s), which can restore effector function.

ACKNOWLEDGMENTS

This work was supported by Arthritis Research UK and Medical Research Council UK.

REFERENCES

1. Nurieva RI, Liu X, Dong C. Molecular mechanisms of T-cell tolerance. *Immunol Rev* (2011) **241**:133–44. doi:10.1111/j.1600-065X.2011.01012.x
2. Schwartz RH. T cell anergy. *Annu Rev Immunol* (2003) **21**:305–34. doi:10.1146/annurev.immunol.21.120601.141110
3. Baine I, Abe BT, Macian F. Regulation of T-cell tolerance by calcium/NFAT signaling. *Immunol Rev* (2009) **231**:225–40. doi:10.1111/j.1600-065X.2009.00817.x
4. Kim PS, Ahmed R. Features of responding T cells in cancer and chronic infection. *Curr Opin Immunol* (2010) **22**:223–30. doi:10.1016/j.coi.2010.02.005
5. Frebel H, Richter K, Oxenius A. How chronic viral infections impact on antigen-specific T-cell responses. *Eur J Immunol* (2010) **40**:654–63. doi:10.1002/eji.200940102
6. Colonna M. Viral immunosuppression: disabling the guards. *J Clin Invest* (2004) **113**:660–2. doi:10.1172/JCI200421166
7. Nurieva R, Wang J, Sahoo A. T-cell tolerance in cancer. *Immunotherapy* (2013) **5**:513–31. doi:10.2217/imt.13.33
8. Schietinger A, Greenberg PD. Tolerance and exhaustion: defining mechanisms of T cell dysfunction. *Trends Immunol* (2014) **35**:51–60. doi:10.1016/j.it.2013.10.001
9. Blackburn SD, Wherry EJ. IL-10, T cell exhaustion and viral persistence. *Trends Microbiol* (2007) **15**:143–6. doi:10.1016/j.tim.2007.02.006
10. Wilson EB, Brooks DG. The role of IL-10 in regulating immunity to persistent viral infections. *Curr Top Microbiol Immunol* (2011) **350**:39–65. doi:10.1007/82_2010_96
11. Larsson M, Shankar EM, Che KF, Saeidi A, Ellegård R, Barathan M, et al. Molecular signatures of T-cell inhibition in HIV-1 infection. *Retrovirology* (2013) **10**:31. doi:10.1186/1742-4690-10-31
12. Wedemeyer H, He XS, Nascimbeni M, Davis AR, Greenberg HB, Hoofnagle JH, et al. Impaired effector function of hepatitis C virus-specific CD8+ T cells in chronic hepatitis C virus infection. *J Immunol* (2002) **169**:3447–58. doi:10.4049/jimmunol.169.6.3447
13. Jung MC, Pape GR. Immunology of hepatitis B infection. *Lancet Infect Dis* (2002) **2**:43–50. doi:10.1016/S1473-3099(01)00172-4
14. Guidotti LG, Chisari FV. Immunobiology and pathogenesis of viral hepatitis. *Annu Rev Pathol* (2006) **1**:23–61. doi:10.1146/annurev.pathol.1.110304.100230
15. Day CL, Kaufmann DE, Kiepiela P, Brown JA, Moodley ES, Reddy S, et al. PD-1 expression on HIV-specific T cells is associated with T-cell exhaustion and disease progression. *Nature* (2006) **443**:350–4. doi:10.1038/nature05115
16. Trautmann L, Janbazian L, Chomont N, Said EA, Gimmig S, Bessette B, et al. Upregulation of PD-1 expression on HIV-specific CD8+ T cells leads to reversible immune dysfunction. *Nat Med* (2006) **12**:1198–202.
17. Yi J, Cox M, Zajac A. T cell exhaustion: characteristics, causes and conversion. *Immunology* (2010) **129**:474–81. doi:10.1111/j.1365-2567.2010.03255.x
18. Maizels RM, Smith KA. Regulatory T cells in infection. *Adv Immunol* (2011) **112**:73–136. doi:10.1016/B978-0-12-387827-4.00003-6

19. Belkaid Y, Rouse BT. Natural regulatory T cells in infectious disease. *Nat Immunol* (2005) **6**:353–60. doi:10.1038/ni1181
20. Mumprecht S, Schürch C, Schwaller J, Solenthaler M, Ochsenbein AF. Programmed death 1 signaling on chronic myeloid leukemia-specific T cells results in T-cell exhaustion and disease progression. *Blood* (2009) **114**:1528–36. doi:10.1182/blood-2008-09-179697
21. Matsuzaki J, Gnjatic S, Mhawech-Fauceglia P, Beck A, Miller A, Tsuji T, et al. Tumor-infiltrating NY-ESO-1-specific CD8+ T cells are negatively regulated by LAG-3 and PD-1 in human ovarian cancer. *Proc Natl Acad Sci U S A* (2010) **107**:7875–80. doi:10.1073/pnas.1003345107
22. Kroemer G, Galluzzi L, Kepp O, Zitvogel L. Immunogenic cell death in cancer therapy. *Annu Rev Immunol* (2013) **31**:51–72. doi:10.1146/annurev-immunol-032712-100008
23. Klein L, Trautman L, Psarras S, Schnell S, Siermann A, Liblau R, et al. Visualizing the course of antigen-specific CD8 and CD4 T cell responses to a growing tumor. *Eur J Immunol* (2003) **33**:806–14.
24. Anderson PO, Sundstedt A, Yazici Z, Minaee S, O'Neill EJ, Woolf R, et al. IL-2 overcomes the unresponsiveness but fails to reverse the regulatory function of antigen-induced T regulatory cells. *J Immunol* (2005) **174**:310–9. doi:10.4049/jimmunol.174.8.5133-a
25. Das A, Hoare M, Davies N, Lopes AR, Dunn C, Kennedy PT, et al. Functional skewing of the global CD8 T cell population in chronic hepatitis B virus infection. *J Exp Med* (2008) **205**:2111–24. doi:10.1084/jem.20072076
26. Jerome K. Viral modulation of T cell receptor signalling. *J Virol* (2008) **82**:4194–204. doi:10.1128/JVI.00059-08
27. Abraham L, Fackler OT. HIV-1 Nef: a multifaceted modulator of T cell receptor signaling. *Cell Commun Signal* (2012) **10**:39. doi:10.1186/1478-811X-10-39
28. Baur AS, Sawai ET, Dazin P, Fantl WJ, Cheng-Mayer C, Peterlin BM. HIV-1 Nef leads to inhibition or activation of T cells depending on its intracellular localization. *Immunity* (1994) **1**:373–84. doi:10.1016/1074-7613(94)90068-X
29. Soldaini E, Wack A, D'Oro U, Nuti S, Ulivieri C, Baldari CT, et al. T cell costimulation by the hepatitis C virus envelope protein E2 binding to CD81 is mediated by Lck. *Eur J Immunol* (2003) **33**:455–64.
30. Ramsay AG, Clear AJ, Fatah R, Gribben JG. Multiple inhibitory ligands induce impaired T-cell immunologic synapse function in chronic lymphocytic leukemia that can be blocked with lenalidomide: establishing a reversible immune evasion mechanism in human cancer. *Blood* (2012) **120**:1412–21. doi:10.1182/blood-2012-02-411678
31. Kasprowicz V, Schulze Zur Wiesch J, Kuntzen T, Nolan BE, Longworth S, Berical A, et al. High level of PD-1 expression on hepatitis C virus (HCV)-specific CD8+ and CD4+ T cells during acute HCV infection, irrespective of clinical outcome. *J Virol* (2008) **82**:3154–60. doi:10.1128/JVI.02474-07
32. Waggoner SN, Kumar V. Evolving role of 2B4/CD244 in T and NK cell responses during virus infection. *Front Immunol* (2012) **3**:377. doi:10.3389/fimmu.2012.00377
33. Kaufmann DE, Walker BD. PD-1 and CTLA-4 inhibitory cosignaling pathways in HIV infection and the potential for therapeutic intervention. *J Immunol* (2009) **182**:5891–7. doi:10.4049/jimmunol.0803771
34. Ahmadzadeh M, Johnson LA, Heemskerk B, Wunderlich JR, Dudley ME, White DE, et al. Tumor antigen-specific CD8 T cells infiltrating the tumor express high levels of PD-1 and are functionally impaired. *Blood* (2009) **114**:1537–44. doi:10.1182/blood-2008-12-195792
35. Kroy DC, Ciuffreda D, Cooperrider JH, Tomlinson M, Hauck GD, Aneja J, et al. Liver environment and HCV replication affect human T-cell phenotype and expression of inhibitory receptors. *Gastroenterology* (2014) **146**:550–61. doi:10.1053/j.gastro.2013.10.022
36. Brooks DG, Trifilo MJ, Edelmann KH, Teyton L, McGavern DB, Oldstone MB. Interleukin-10 determines viral clearance or persistence *in vivo*. *Nat Med* (2006) **12**:1301–9. doi:10.1038/nm1492
37. Ejrnaes M, Filippi CM, Martinic MM, Ling EM, Togher LM, Crotty S, et al. Resolution of a chronic viral infection after interleukin-10 receptor blockade. *J Exp Med* (2006) **203**:2461–72. doi:10.1084/jem.20061462
38. Bergmann C, Strauss L, Wang Y, Szczepanski MJ, Lang S, Johnson JT, et al. T regulatory type 1 cells in squamous cell carcinoma of the head and neck: mechanisms of suppression and expansion in advanced disease. *Clin Cancer Res* (2008) **14**:3706–15. doi:10.1158/1078-0432.CCR-07-5126
39. Berzofsky JA, Ahlers JD, Janik J, Morris J, Oh S, Terabe M, et al. Progress on new vaccine strategies against chronic viral infections. *J Clin Invest* (2004) **114**:450–62. doi:10.1172/JCI22674
40. Duraiswamy J, Freeman GJ, Coukos G. Therapeutic PD-1 pathway blockade augments with other modalities of immunotherapy T-cell function to prevent immune decline in ovarian cancer. *Cancer Res* (2013) **73**:6900–12. doi:10.1158/0008-5472.CAN-13-1550
41. Ha SJ, Mueller SN, Wherry EJ, Barber DL, Aubert RD, Sharpe AH, et al. Enhancing therapeutic vaccination by blocking PD-1-mediated inhibitory signals during chronic infection. *J Exp Med* (2008) **205**:543–55. doi:10.1084/jem.20071949
42. Brooks DG, Lee AM, Elsaesser H, McGavern DB, Oldstone MB. IL-10 blockade facilitates DNA vaccine-induced T cell responses and enhances clearance of persistent virus infection. *J Exp Med* (2008) **205**:533–41. doi:10.1084/jem.20071948
43. Vezys V, Penaloza-MacMaster P, Barber DL, Ha SJ, Konieczny B, Freeman GJ, et al. 4-1BB signaling synergizes with programmed death ligand 1 blockade to augment CD8 T cell responses during chronic viral infection. *J Immunol* (2011) **187**:1634–42. doi:10.4049/jimmunol.1100077
44. Brooks DG, Ha SJ, Elsaesser H, Sharpe AH, Freeman GJ, Oldstone MB. IL-10 and PD-L1 operate through distinct pathways to suppress T-cell activity during persistent viral infection. *Proc Natl Acad Sci U S A* (2008) **105**:20428–33. doi:10.1073/pnas.0811139106
45. Barber DL, Wherry EJ, Masopust D, Zhu B, Allison JP, Sharpe AH, et al. Restoring function in exhausted CD8 T cells during chronic viral infection. *Nature* (2006) **439**:682–7. doi:10.1038/nature04444
46. Akbar SM, Horiike N, Onji M. Immune therapy including dendritic cell based therapy in chronic hepatitis B virus infection. *World J Gastroenterol* (2006) **12**:2876–83.
47. Zhou Y, Zhang Y, Yao Z, Moorman JP, Jia Z. Dendritic cell-based immunity and vaccination against hepatitis C virus infection. *Immunology* (2012) **136**:385–96.
48. Lu W, Arraes LC, Ferreira WT, Andrieu JM. Therapeutic dendritic-cell vaccine for chronic HIV-1 infection. *Nat Med* (2004) **10**:1359–65. doi:10.1038/nm1147
49. Steinman RM, Hawiger D, Nussenzweig MC. Tolerogenic dendritic cells. *Annu Rev Immunol* (2003) **21**:685–711. doi:10.1146/annurev.immunol.21.120601.141040
50. Sofra V, Mansour S, Liu M, Gao B, Primpidou E, Wang P, et al. Antigen-loaded ER microsomes from APC induce potent immune responses against viral infection. *Eur J Immunol* (2009) **39**:85–95. doi:10.1002/eji.200838443
51. Liu M, Miao T, Zhu H, Symonds AL, Li L, Schurich A, et al. IL-2-engineered nano-APC effectively activates viral antigen-mediated T cell responses from chronic hepatitis B virus-infected patients. *J Immunol* (2012) **188**:1534–43. doi:10.4049/jimmunol.1102709
52. Mier JW, Aronson FR, Numerof RP, Vachino G, Atkins MB. Toxicity of immunotherapy with interleukin-2 and lymphokine activated killer cells. *Pathol Immunopathol Res* (1988) **7**:459. doi:10.1159/000157075
53. Malek TR, Castro I. Interleukin-2 receptor signaling: at the interface of tolerance and immunity. *Immunity* (2010) **33**:153–65. doi:10.1016/j.immuni.2010.08.004
54. Bensinger SJ, Walsh PT, Zhang J, Carroll M, Parsons R, Rathmell JC, et al. Distinct IL-2 receptor signaling pattern in CD4+CD25+ regulatory T cells. *J Immunol* (2004) **172**:5287–96. doi:10.4049/jimmunol.172.9.5287
55. Nandedkar TD. Nanovaccines: recent developments in vaccination. *J Biosci* (2009) **34**:995–1003. doi:10.1007/s12038-009-0114-3
56. Geijtenbeek TB, van Vliet SJ, Engering BA, Hart A, van Kooyk Y. Self- and nonself-recognition by C-type lectins on dendritic cells. *Annu Rev Immunol* (2004) **22**:33–54. doi:10.1146/annurev.immunol.22.012703.104558

Permissions

All chapters in this book were first published in TICSP, by Frontiers; hereby published with permission under the Creative Commons Attribution License or equivalent. Every chapter published in this book has been scrutinized by our experts. Their significance has been extensively debated. The topics covered herein carry significant findings which will fuel the growth of the discipline. They may even be implemented as practical applications or may be referred to as a beginning point for another development.

The contributors of this book come from diverse backgrounds, making this book a truly international effort. This book will bring forth new frontiers with its revolutionizing research information and detailed analysis of the nascent developments around the world.

We would like to thank all the contributing authors for lending their expertise to make the book truly unique. They have played a crucial role in the development of this book. Without their invaluable contributions this book wouldn't have been possible. They have made vital efforts to compile up to date information on the varied aspects of this subject to make this book a valuable addition to the collection of many professionals and students.

This book was conceptualized with the vision of imparting up-to-date information and advanced data in this field. To ensure the same, a matchless editorial board was set up. Every individual on the board went through rigorous rounds of assessment to prove their worth. After which they invested a large part of their time researching and compiling the most relevant data for our readers.

The editorial board has been involved in producing this book since its inception. They have spent rigorous hours researching and exploring the diverse topics which have resulted in the successful publishing of this book. They have passed on their knowledge of decades through this book. To expedite this challenging task, the publisher supported the team at every step. A small team of assistant editors was also appointed to further simplify the editing procedure and attain best results for the readers.

Apart from the editorial board, the designing team has also invested a significant amount of their time in understanding the subject and creating the most relevant covers. They scrutinized every image to scout for the most suitable representation of the subject and create an appropriate cover for the book.

The publishing team has been an ardent support to the editorial, designing and production team. Their endless efforts to recruit the best for this project, has resulted in the accomplishment of this book. They are a veteran in the field of academics and their pool of knowledge is as vast as their experience in printing. Their expertise and guidance has proved useful at every step. Their uncompromising quality standards have made this book an exceptional effort. Their encouragement from time to time has been an inspiration for everyone.

The publisher and the editorial board hope that this book will prove to be a valuable piece of knowledge for researchers, students, practitioners and scholars across the globe.

List of Contributors

Kathleen M. Kokolus, Haley M. Spangler, Benjamin J. Povinelli, Matthew R. Farren, Kelvin P. Lee and Elizabeth A. Repasky
Department of Immunology, Roswell Park Cancer Institute, Buffalo, NY, USA

Miri Michaeli, Gitit Shahaf, Yishai Pickman, Lena Hazanov and Ramit Mehr
The Mina and Everard Goodman Faculty of Life Sciences, Bar-Ilan University, Ramat Gan, Israel

Iris Barshack
Department of Pathology, Sheba Medical Center, Ramat Gan, Israel
Sackler Faculty of Medicine, Tel Aviv University, Tel Aviv, Israel

Hilla Tabibian-Keissar
The Mina and Everard Goodman Faculty of Life Sciences, Bar-Ilan University, Ramat Gan, Israel
Department of Pathology, Sheba Medical Center, Ramat Gan, Israel

Ginette Schiby and Kinneret Rosenblatt
Department of Pathology, Sheba Medical Center, Ramat Gan, Israel

Deborah K. Dunn-Walters
Division of Immunology, Infection, and Inflammatory Diseases, King's College London School of Medicine, London, UK

Jing Liu
Cancer Research Center, Shantou University Medical College, Shantou, China

Jia-Xin Shen and Jia-Lin Hu
Cancer Research Center, Shantou University Medical College, Shantou, China
Breast Center, Cancer Hospital of Shantou University Medical College, Shantou, China

Wen-He Huang and Guo-Jun Zhang
Breast Center, Cancer Hospital of Shantou University Medical College, Shantou, China

Adrien Six and Wahiba Chaara
UPMC University Paris 06, UMR 7211, Immunology-Immunopathology-Immunotherapy (I3), Paris, France
CNRS, UMR 7211, Immunology-Immunopathology-Immunotherapy (I3), Paris, France
INSERM, UMR_S 959, Immunology-Immunopathology-Immunotherapy (I3), Paris, France
AP-HP, Hôpital Pitié-Salpêtrière, CIC-BTi Biotherapy, Paris, France
AP-HP, Hôpital Pitié-Salpêtrière, Département Hospitalo-Universitaire (DHU), Inflammation-Immunopathology-Biotherapy (i2B), Paris, France

Susana Magadan and Pierre Boudinot
Institut National de la Recherche Agronomique, Unité de Virologie et Immunologie Moléculaires, Jouy-en-Josas, France

Hang-Phuong Pham
UPMC University Paris 06, UMR 7211, Immunology-Immunopathology-Immunotherapy (I3), Paris, France
CNRS, UMR 7211, Immunology-Immunopathology-Immunotherapy (I3), Paris, France

Marie-Paule Lefranc
IMGT®, The International ImMunoGeneTics Information System®, Institut de Génétique Humaine, UPR CNRS 1142, Université Montpellier 2, Montpellier, France

Thierry Mora
Laboratoire de Physique Statistique, UMR8550, CNRS and Ecole Normale Supérieure, Paris, France

Aleksandra M. Walczak
Laboratoire de Physique Théorique, UMR8549, CNRS and Ecole Normale Supérieure, Paris, France

Maria Encarnita Mariotti-Ferrandiz and Véronique Thomas-Vaslin
UPMC University Paris 06, UMR 7211, Immunology-Immunopathology-Immunotherapy (I3), Paris, France
CNRS, UMR 7211, Immunology-Immunopathology-Immunotherapy (I3), Paris, France
INSERM, UMR_S 959, Immunology-Immunopathology-Immunotherapy (I3), Paris, France
AP-HP, Hôpital Pitié-Salpêtrière, Département Hospitalo-Universitaire (DHU), Inflammation-Immunopathology-Biotherapy (i2B), Paris, France

Eva Szymanska Mroczek
Department of Microbiology, University of Alabama at Birmingham, Birmingham, AL, USA

Gregory C. Ippolito
Department of Molecular Biosciences, University of Texas at Austin, Austin, TX, USA

Tobias Rogosch and Michael Zemlin
Laboratory for Neonatology and Pediatric Immunology, Department of Pediatrics, Philipps-University, Marburg, Germany

Kam Hon Hoi
Department of Chemical Engineering, University of Texas at Austin, Austin, TX, USA
Department of Biomedical Engineering, University of Texas at Austin, Austin, TX, USA

Tracy A. Hwangpo, Marsha G. Brand, Yingxin Zhuang and Cun Ren Liu
Department of Medicine, University of Alabama at Birmingham, Birmingham, AL, USA

David A. Schneider
Department of Biochemistry and Molecular Genetics, University of Alabama at Birmingham, Birmingham, AL, USA

Elizabeth E. Brown
Department of Epidemiology, University of Alabama at Birmingham, Birmingham, AL, USA

George Georgiou
Department of Molecular Biosciences, University of Texas at Austin, Austin, TX, USA
Department of Chemical Engineering, University of Texas at Austin, Austin, TX, USA
Department of Biomedical Engineering, University of Texas at Austin, Austin, TX, USA

Harry W. Schroeder Jr.
Department of Microbiology, University of Alabama at Birmingham, Birmingham, AL, USA
Department of Medicine, University of Alabama at Birmingham, Birmingham, AL, USA

Ole Audun Werner Haabeth, Anders Aune Tveita, Marte Fauskanger, Fredrik Schjesvold, Kristina Berg Lorvik, Hilde Omholt and Ludvig A. Munthe
Department of Immunology, Centre for Immune Regulation, Oslo University Hospital, University of Oslo, Oslo, Norway

Peter O. Hofgaard
KG Jebsen Centre for Research on Influenza Vaccines, Institute of Immunology, Oslo University Hospital, University of Oslo, Oslo, Norway

Zlatko Dembic
Faculty of Dentistry, Molecular Genetics Laboratory, Department of Oral Biology, University of Oslo, Oslo, Norway

Alexandre Corthay
Department of Biosciences, University of Oslo, Oslo, Norway
Tumor Immunology Group, Department of Pathology, Oslo University Hospital, University of Oslo, Oslo, Norway

Bjarne Bogen
Department of Immunology, Centre for Immune Regulation, Oslo University Hospital, University of Oslo, Oslo, Norway
KG Jebsen Centre for Research on Influenza Vaccines, Institute of Immunology, Oslo University Hospital, University of Oslo, Oslo, Norway

Chang Gong
Department of Computational Medicine and Bioinformatics, University of Michigan, Ann Arbor, MI, USA

Jennifer J. Linderman
Department of Chemical Engineering, University of Michigan, Ann Arbor, MI, USA

Denise Kirschner
Department of Microbiology and Immunology, University of Michigan Medical School, Ann Arbor, MI, USA

Till S. M. Mathan, Carl G. Figdor and Sonja I. Buschow
Department of Tumor Immunology, Nijmegen Centre for Molecular Life Sciences, Radboud University Nijmegen Medical Centre, Nijmegen, Netherlands

Alexandre Corthay
Tumor Immunology Group, Department of Pathology, Oslo University Hospital Rikshospitalet, Oslo, Norway
Department of Biosciences, University of Oslo, Oslo, Norway
Centre for Immune Regulation, University of Oslo, Oslo, Norway

Joseph Reynolds, Grant Lythe and Carmen Molina-París
Department of Applied Mathematics, School of Mathematics, University of Leeds, Leeds, UK

Mark Coles
Centre for Immunology and Infection, University of York, York, UK

Rebecca R. Laborde, Michael P. Gustafson, Peggy A. Bulur and Allan B. Dietz
Human Cellular Therapy Laboratory, Division of Transfusion Medicine, Department of Laboratory Medicine and Pathology, Mayo Clinic, Rochester, MN, USA

Yi Lin
Division of Hematology, Department of Medicine, Mayo Clinic, Rochester, MN, USA

Veronika I. Zarnitsyna and Rustom Antia
Department of Biology, Emory University, Atlanta, GA, USA

Brian D. Evavold
Department of Microbiology and Immunology, Emory University, Atlanta, GA, USA

Louis N. Schoettle and Joseph N. Blattman
Center for Infectious Diseases and Vaccinology, School of Life Sciences, Arizona State University, Tempe, AZ, USA

John R. Gordon, Yanna Ma, Laura Churchman, Sara A. Gordon and Wojciech Dawicki
Department of Medicine, University of Saskatchewan, Saskatoon, SK, Canada

Gregory W. Schwartz
Systems Immunology Laboratory, School of Biomedical Engineering, Science, and Health Systems, Drexel University, Philadelphia, PA, USA

Uri Hershberg
Systems Immunology Laboratory, School of Biomedical Engineering, Science, and Health Systems, Drexel University, Philadelphia, PA, USA
Department of Microbiology and Immunology, College of Medicine, Drexel University, Philadelphia, PA, USA

Ricardo A. Chaurio, Thomas Harrer, Luis E. Muñoz, Georg Schett and Martin Herrmann
Department of Internal Medicine, Friedrich-Alexander University of Erlangen-Nuremberg, Erlangen, Germany

Christian Maueröder
Department of Internal Medicine, Friedrich-Alexander University of Erlangen-Nuremberg, Erlangen, Germany
Department of Biology, Friedrich-Alexander University of Erlangen-Nuremberg, Erlangen, Germany

Christina Janko
Department of Otorhinolaryngology, Head and Neck Surgery, Section for Experimental Oncology and Nanomedicine (SEON), University Hospital Erlangen, Erlangen, Germany

Barbara G. Fürnrohr
Division of Molecular Immunology, Department of Internal Medicine, Friedrich-Alexander University of Erlangen-Nuremberg, Erlangen, Germany
Division of Biological Chemistry, Medical University Innsbruck, Innsbruck, Austria

Michael Niederweis
Department of Microbiology and Biochemistry, University of Alabama at Birmingham, Birmingham, AL, USA

Rostyslav Bilyy
Institute of Cell Biology, National Academy of Sciences of Ukraine, Lviv, Ukraine

Christian Berens
Department of Biology, Friedrich-Alexander University of Erlangen-Nuremberg, Erlangen, Germany

Paola Carrillo-Bustamante, Can Kesmir and Rob J. de Boer
Theoretical Biology and Bioinformatics, Department of Biology, Utrecht University, Utrecht, Netherlands

Theofilos Poutahidis
Division of Comparative Medicine, Massachusetts Institute of Technology, Cambridge, MA, USA
Laboratory of Pathology, Faculty of Veterinary Medicine, Aristotle University of Thessaloniki, Thessaloniki, Greece

Markus Kleinewietfeld
Departments of Neurology and Immunobiology, Yale School of Medicine, New Haven, CT, USA
Broad Institute, Massachusetts Institute of Technology and Harvard University, Cambridge, MA, USA
Faculty of Medicine, Dresden University of Technology (TUD), Dresden, Germany

Susan E. Erdman
Division of Comparative Medicine, Massachusetts Institute of Technology, Cambridge, MA, USA

Kalet León, Karina García-Martínez and Tania Carmenate
Systems Biology Department, Center of Molecular Immunology, Habana, Cuba

Suling Li
Bioscience, Brunel University, London, UK

Alistair L. J. Symonds, Tizong Miao, Ian Sanderson and Ping Wang
Blizard Institute (BICMS), Barts and the London School of Medicine and Dentistry, London, UK

Index

R

S

T

V

W

www.ingramcontent.com/pod-product-compliance
Lightning Source LLC
LaVergne TN
LVHW060548210926
848485LV00005B/1281